Molecular Pathology of Breast Cancer

Sunil Badve · Yesim Gökmen-Polar
Editors

Molecular Pathology of Breast Cancer

Springer

Editors

Sunil Badve
Department of Pathology and Laboratory Medicine
Indiana University School of Medicine
Indianapolis, IN
USA

Yesim Gökmen-Polar
Department of Pathology and Laboratory Medicine
Indiana University School of Medicine
Indianapolis, IN
USA

ISBN 978-3-319-41759-2 ISBN 978-3-319-41761-5 (eBook)
DOI 10.1007/978-3-319-41761-5

Library of Congress Control Number: 2016950893

Printed on acid-free paper

This Springer imprint is published by Springer Nature
The registered company is Springer International Publishing AG
The registered company address is: Gewerbestrasse 11, 6330 Cham, Switzerland

Preface

Data is not information, information is not knowledge, knowledge is not understanding, understanding is not wisdom

—Clifford Stoll
Lawrence Berkeley National Laboratory, USA

The last few years has seen the deluge of data regarding the alterations in breast cancers. Recent advances in technology also permit analysis of single cells for these alterations. However, clinicians and scientists faced with an onslaught of this data from the scientific and lay press are finding it difficult to distinguish data from information. The major question that arises is—how does it affect the lives of my patients? My research?

Molecular Pathology of Breast Cancer seeks to provide an overview of the recent advances in breast cancer and bring together the techniques, data, and knowledge to provide some understanding and wisdom. We believe that this work will represent a new and important resource for clinicians and scientists, by serving as a "ready reckoner." The chapters, written by experts in the field, provide valuable information to those already involved in and familiar with the complexities of breast cancer. In order to introduce the territory to the novices, the chapters, while being detailed, have been kept short and the discussions brief. The hope is to make the topics "meaningful" but less intimidating for the audience.

It is clear that advances in molecular biology have provided exhaustive data regarding breast cancer. However, it is necessary to separate the wheat from the chaff. We are extremely grateful to the cadre of authors, who have graciously donated their time and energy to make this hard work possible. In a series of chapters within the book, these experts have presented most recent research and highlighted the direction for future research.

Indianapolis, IN, USA

Sunil Badve
Yesim Gökmen-Polar

Contents

Translation of Biomarkers into Clinical Practice

1

Lisa Meier McShane, Tracy G. Lively and Hala R. Makhlouf

Biomarkers have long played a key role in the clinical management of breast cancer. Their use continues to expand beyond the classic biomarkers such as hormone receptors (ER and PR) for guiding use of endocrine therapy and HER2 status for guiding use of HER2-targeting agents. In recognition of the critical role that biomarkers play in drug development and in patient care, the U.S. Food and Drug Administration (FDA) and the U.S. National Institutes of Health (NIH) have recently partnered to develop a standardized glossary of terminology related to biomarkers and clinical outcomes. In that glossary, it is stated that a biomarker is "a defined characteristic that is measured as an indicator of normal biological processes, pathogenic processes, or responses to an exposure or intervention, including therapeutic interventions. Molecular, histologic, radiographic, or physiologic characteristics are types of "biomarkers" (FDA-NIH Biomarker Working Group 2016). Biomarkers can be used individually, or in combination as a "signature", at multiple points along a patient's clinical trajectory to guide clinical care decisions.

The American Society of Clinical Oncology (ASCO) recently issued guidelines for clinical use of biomarkers (beyond T, N and M staging) to aid in decisions on systemic therapy for women with metastatic breast cancer (Van Poznak et al. 2015) and to aid in decisions on adjuvant systemic therapy for women with early-stage invasive breast cancer (Harris et al. 2016). For the metastatic setting, no biomarkers were fully endorsed by the guideline committee except for estrogen receptor (ER), progesterone receptor (PR), and HER2 (Human Epidermal Growth Factor Receptor 2) status in combination with clinical evaluation, patient preferences, and judgment; CEA, CA 15-3, and CA 27.29 were regarded by the committee as appropriate for use adjunctive to decisions regarding therapy but not for use in isolation (Van Poznak et al. 2015). The committee that examined biomarkers for the early-stage invasive breast cancer setting found sufficient evidence to recommend clinical use of OncotypeDX®, EndoPredict®, Prosigna™, Breast Cancer Index℠ and uPA/PAI-1 in specific subgroups of breast cancer, in addition to the well-established estrogen and progesterone receptor (ER/PR) and HER2 biomarkers (Harris et al. 2016). Although the number of biomarkers recommended for clinical use has increased in

L.M. McShane (✉) · T.G. Lively · H.R. Makhlouf
Division of Cancer Treatment and Diagnosis, National Cancer Institute, 9609 Medical Center Drive, Bethesda, MD 20892, USA
e-mail: lisa.mcshane@nih.gov

H.R. Makhlouf
Department of Pathology, Faculty of Medicine, Ain Shams University, 38 Al Abbassia, Greater Cairo, Cairo 11566, Egypt

S. Badve and Y. Gökmen-Polar (eds.), *Molecular Pathology of Breast Cancer*, DOI 10.1007/978-3-319-41761-5_1

the last few years, there is still a large gap between that number and the number of biomarker studies published, perhaps reflecting a lack of appreciation of requirements for translation of a biomarker into clinical practice or other challenges inherent in that process.

There are several challenges in translation of biomarker research results to a clinical test that is useful for making patient treatment decisions. Variation in assay methods used to measure the biomarker (or signature) across potentially many studies comprising the evidence base can make it difficult to interpret the literature and determine the specific assay methods that are optimal. Additionally, pre-analytical factors, which refer to the conditions under which biospecimens are collected, processed or stored prior to analysis, can sometimes have a profound impact on the ability to measure a biomarker reliably or even to measure it at all (Moore et al. 2011). Heterogeneity due to pre-analytic and analytic factors may be further compounded by differences in clinical populations or treatment settings studied. All of the pre-analytical, analytical, and clinical issues must be confronted when developing a biomarker test or evaluating its usefulness for clinical care. Multi-disciplinary expertise is needed to determine which biomarkers are the most informative and reliable for making specific clinical decisions, and to develop the most promising biomarkers into clinical-grade tests.

Biomarker tests need to be rigorously evaluated to establish their readiness for clinical use. Pathologists and clinicians must understand how to appropriately select, apply, and interpret clinical tests, be able to judge if a test has been appropriately validated, and have an appreciation of the potential risks and benefits associated with use of a given test. These requirements apply regardless of whether pathologists or laboratorians develop a version of a biomarker test for use in their laboratory or provide advice concerning use of biomarker tests performed by outside laboratories. Understanding the general process by which biomarker tests are developed and validated is critical in making an informed judgement about the clinical readiness of any particular biomarker-based test.

1.1 From Biomarker to Biomarker Test

Clinical use of a biomarker requires a reliable method to measure it. The constellation of elements that enable measurement comprise the *biomarker test*, which is defined as "an assessment system comprising three essential components: (1) materials for measurement; (2) an assay for obtaining the measurement; and (3) method and/or criteria for interpreting those measurements" (FDA-NIH Biomarker Working Group 2016). For biomarker signatures, the test would also include a procedure for combining measurements of multiple biomarkers, such as output from omics assays which include those based in the disciplines of "genomics, transcriptomics, proteomics, metabolomics, and epigenomics" (Micheel et al. 2012). The result of combining the measurements is typically a risk score developed from a statistical model or a categorization output by an algorithm that classifies each case into one of multiple possible categories based on the pattern detected in the biomarker measurements. Such models or algorithms will be referred to here as *multivariable biomarker predictors* or in the case of high throughput omics technologies, *omics predictors*.

Many biomarkers used in treatment decisions for breast cancer have undergone an evolution in methods for measurement. For example, clinical measurement methods for estrogen receptor (ER) have evolved from ligand binding assays performed on tumor cytosols which produced continuous measurements in units of fmol/mg (typically with ≥ 3 or 20 called positive) to immunohistochemical assays that could be performed on formalin-fixed tumor tissue and which produced semi-quantitative measurements (Hammond et al. 2010). For some biomarkers, acceptable measurement methods have been well established; whereas, for other biomarkers a variety of measurement methods exist, often with little understanding of the degree of concordance that might be expected among results obtained by different methods. The clinical impact of discordance in biomarker measurements due to assay methodology may vary depending on the density of biomarker values in the patient population that are near key clinical decision points and the degree of discordance between assays near those points. Committees convened jointly by the American Society of Clinical Oncology (ASCO) and the College of American Pathologists (CAP) developed best practice guidelines for testing HER2 status (Wolff et al. 2007, 2013) and the hormone receptors ER and PR (Hammond et al. 2010) which specify acceptable pre-analytic and analytic conditions and procedures in order to promote consistency and reliability of testing.

In contrast, there are examples of biomarkers used with some regularity for the care of patients with breast cancer that continue to be measured by a variety of different approaches with insufficient attention paid to the impact of the different measurement methodologies. Stuart-Harris et al. (2008) reviewed literature on the nuclear proliferation marker Ki67 in breast cancer. They reported that among the 43 studies reporting use of an immunohistochemical assay for assessment of Ki67 in early breast cancer, 7 different antibodies for IHC, single or in combination had been used; among those studies, 19 different cutpoints, ranging from 0 to 30 %, had been used for determination of high expression. Further, recent reports by Polley et al. (2013a, b) demonstrated a concerning lack of concordance due to scoring approach alone when eight different laboratories across the world experienced in Ki67 immunohistochemistry evaluated a common set of stained breast cancer tissues represented on a tissue microarray slide. Pathmanathan et al. (2014) demonstrated how varying the Ki67 cutpoint in increments of 5 % could substantially alter the accuracy with which Ki67 assessments could predict survival following breast cancer diagnosis. Together with the lack of concordance found by Polley et al. (2013a, b), this sensitivity of prognostic ability to cutpoints suggests that the clinical value of Ki67 assessments will likely vary across laboratories performing the testing. These examples illustrate the need for greater attention to the specific methods used to measure biomarkers and better understanding of the impact of pre-analytic and analytic heterogeneity on clinical performance of biomarkers.

Details of both pre-analytic conditions and analytical methods should be provided when investigators publish reports of biomarker studies and these should also be provided by laboratories offering biomarker tests. Checklists have been developed to provide guidance on what information is important to report in publications involving use of biospecimens (Moore et al. 2011) and biomarkers used in prognostic (McShane et al. 2005; Altman et al. 2012) and diagnostic (Bossuyt et al. 2003a, b, 2015) studies. Further useful information can be found on the EQUATOR website (EQUATOR Network 2016) which provides a wealth of checklists and guidance for reporting a wide variety of health research studies. Laboratories that offer biomarker tests for clinical use should clearly state any important pre-analytical requirements for biospecimens, provide information about the particular testing procedures they use, and provide clear instructions about how test results should be interpreted. Such details should also be provided in any clinical study protocol that involves investigational use of a biomarker test. These steps would help to make biomarker test development more efficient and ensure that clinical biomarker tests were properly used and their results interpreted appropriately.

1.2 Clinical Uses for Biomarker Tests

Evaluation of clinical performance of a biomarker test must start with a clear statement of the intended use of the test in clinical decision making. Uses most relevant to therapy decisions include forecasting prognosis, therapy selection, or monitoring for disease recurrence or progression; these will be the focus in this chapter. Intended use must also consider the clinical context, including disease stage and treatments received, or other clinical or pathologic factors that define subgroups of patients whose disease is managed differently in routine practice. A major reason for failure of many biomarkers to be translated to a test used in clinical practice is that correlations between biomarker values and outcomes observed in exploratory studies in heterogeneous patient populations often do not translate to information that is meaningful or useful in clinical management.

Prognostic biomarkers are "used to identify likelihood of a clinical event, disease recurrence or progression" (FDA-NIH Biomarker Working Group 2016). Presence of malignant cells in lymph nodes of patients who undergo surgical resection of their tumor predicts higher likelihood of developing recurrent disease. Patients with breast cancer who carry certain germline BRCA1 or BRCA2 mutations are at higher risk of developing a second primary breast cancer or ovarian cancer (Brekelmans et al. 2007; Bergfeldt et al. 2002). In oncology, the term prognosis has generally been used in the clinical context of patients receiving either no therapy (beyond primary surgery) or a uniform standard therapy that all patients are likely to receive. If the term prognosis is used in other settings, for example in the context of a targeted therapy, or in a setting where patients could have received any of several therapies, then there is risk that prognostic and predictive effects (see definition of predictive biomarker below) can become confused. Indeed, potential targets for new therapies are often first discovered as prognostic biomarkers. If a new therapeutic can inhibit a biomarker with negative prognostic effect, that new therapy might improve clinical outcome. This was the situation with HER2 overexpression which was first identified as a negative prognostic factor; HER2-targeted therapies were subsequently developed that substantially improved survival for patients in both the metastatic and adjuvant settings. The importance of distinguishing these terms is discussed further in the section **Evaluation of clinical utility**.

Predictive biomarkers are "used to identify individuals who are more likely than similar patients without the biomarker to experience a favorable or unfavorable effect from a specific intervention or exposure" (FDA-NIH Biomarker Working Group 2016). The term "predictive" has been used somewhat variably in oncology so it is important to be clear about the context. One way in which the term predictive biomarker has been used is in the setting of selecting between two different treatments (one of which could be no further treatment (beyond surgery, possibly with radiation) as in an adjuvant setting for early stage breast cancer), usually with focus on a time-to-event endpoint (e.g., overall survival, recurrence-free survival, disease-free survival, progression-free survival). In this context alternate terms for predictive biomarker are *treatment-effect modifier*, *treatment-guiding* or *treatment-selection biomarker*. The term *treatment-selection biomarker* will be used here; it means that the effect of a particular treatment relative to some other treatment varies depending on the value of the biomarker. The biomarker could predict benefit, lack of benefit, or even harm from a particular treatment. In the simplest setting of a binary biomarker, one could say that a positive biomarker result defines a population that benefits from treatment A relative to B (e.g., longer survival when a patient receives treatment A compared to treatment B) but the biomarker negative group either does equally well under A and B or does better under B than A. A classic example of a treatment-selection predictive biomarker in breast cancer is hormone receptor status to guide use of endocrine therapy. Patients whose tumors are negative for hormone receptors are unlikely to benefit from endocrine therapy (with or without concomitant chemotherapy), whereas the group of patients whose tumors are positive will have an overall reduced rate of recurrence and longer survival if they receive endocrine therapy.

Biomarkers are increasingly used to enrich or select the patient population for clinical trials of targeted anti-cancer agents. This is an approach used for development of new therapeutics, but it has implications for the eventual regulatory approval of the new therapeutic and its approved indications for clinical use. Varied terminology has been used to refer to such biomarkers, including predictive biomarkers, selection biomarkers, or enrichment biomarkers. This type of biomarker will be referred to here as an *enrichment-predictive biomarker*. The key distinction between an enrichment-predictive biomarker and a treatment-selection biomarker is that for an enrichment-predictive biomarker there is no or very little clinical evaluation of the new drug in the "biomarker negative" subgroup. This drug development path might have been chosen because there was little or no biological rationale for why the new drug should work in the biomarker negative group or because in pre-clinical studies drug effects were observed only in models (e.g., cell lines, animal models, xenografts) that were positive for the biomarker. For example, if the drug is a monoclonal antibody one might not expect it to work for patients whose tumors do not express the target antigen. However, such assumptions are sometimes too simplistic and might not account for off-target effects of the drug or might be based on cutpoints for defining positivity that are not optimal. When varied assays are used to assess an enrichment-predictive biomarker it is important to consider whether any particular assay being used identifies a patient population similar to the one identified by the enrichment biomarker actually used in the pivotal clinical trials of the therapeutic agent. Further elaboration with an example is discussed in the section **Evaluation of clinical utility**.

In settings where chemotherapy is given as the first treatment with or without subsequent surgery (e.g., as neoadjuvant therapy or for metastatic disease), biomarkers which can predict tumor response (or possibly prolonged progression-free survival or stable disease) may be of interest. Such biomarkers are often called predictive biomarkers, but they are indicated for a purpose slightly different than the predictive biomarkers just described for therapy selection. They will be denoted *response-predictive biomarkers* here. Rather than comparing between treatments, response predictive biomarkers may be used to indicate likelihood of drug activity—either tumor objective response (complete or partial response) or prolonged stable disease or time to progression. Importantly, drug activity as assessed by tumor response does not necessarily translate to a clinical benefit in terms of prolonged overall or disease-free survival.

Monitoring biomarkers are "measured serially for assessing status of a disease or medical condition or for evidence of exposure to (or effect of) an environmental agent or medical product. Monitoring biomarkers may also be used to indicate toxicity or assess safety, or to provide evidence of exposure, including exposures to medical products" (FDA-NIH Biomarker Working Group 2016). In oncology, blood-based biomarkers and image-based biomarkers are widely used for monitoring patients following initial therapy to detect signs of persistent, recurrent or progressive disease. CT scans to assess tumor burden (which can be considered a "biomarker") are used routinely to monitor for progression in advanced disease. Serum biomarkers such as CEA, CA 15-3, and CA 27.29 have also been widely used for monitoring in metastatic disease (Van Poznak et al. 2015), and more recently circulating tumor cells or cell-free DNA have been investigated for their potential usefulness in monitoring [e.g., circulating tumor cell evaluation in the randomized trial S0500 (NCT00382018; Smerage et al. 2014)].

1.3 Principles in Determination of Fitness of a Biomarker Test for an Intended Clinical Use

Evaluation of the suitability of a biomarker test for a particular clinical use requires a series of studies to address analytical validity, clinical validity, and clinical utility. The nature of these studies will depend on the type of assay methodology used for measurement and the intended use of the biomarker test. Some biomarker tests used in clinical care for breast cancer, for example, CELLSEARCH® Circulating Tumor Cell Kit, Prosigna™, and MammaPrint® have been reviewed and cleared by the FDA (U. S. FDA 2006, 2013, 2015). Others such as standard immunohistochemical tests including ER, PR, and HER2 are performed routinely in essentially all laboratories which analyze breast tumor specimens; they may be performed using a commercial assay kit or using a test developed in the laboratory offering it. Other tests such as OncotypeDX® (Genomic Health 2016) are performed at a central commercial laboratory. Biomarker tests performed in CLIA-certified laboratories may have never been reviewed by the FDA; however, CLIA-certified laboratories are required to validate their assays and perform quality monitoring, and many participate in proficiency testing and education programs such as those offered by the College of American Pathologists (College of American Pathologists 2016). Regardless of the level of FDA or other external review that a biomarker test has undergone, it is important that the appropriate evaluations have been performed by some qualified party to ensure that the test can be used safely and its results can be relied upon to have a particular clinical interpretation.

1.3.1 Analytical validity

Analytical validity refers to "establishing that the performance characteristics of a test, tool, or instrument are acceptable in terms of its sensitivity, specificity, accuracy, precision, and other relevant performance characteristics using a specified technical protocol (which may include specimen collection, handling and storage procedures)" (FDA-NIH Biomarker Working Group 2016). Analytical validity pertains to a test's technical performance but says nothing about its clinical usefulness. Design of analytic validation studies will depend on the specific type of assay under evaluation, but there are several helpful references providing general guidance (Jennings et al. 2009; Linnet and Boyd 2012; Pennello 2013; Becker 2015). A particularly good reference for analytic validation of immunohistochemical assays is CLSI document I/LA28-A2 (CLSI 2010). Some researchers have published analytical validation studies that they conducted and these may also serve as useful guides; examples of published analytical validation studies for tests used for breast cancer include those for CELLSEARCH® (Allard et al. 2004) and several for omics tests including Prosigna™ gene expression ROR score (Nielsen et al. 2014) and the OncotypeDX® Risk Score (Cronin et al. 2007). Publication of skillfully executed analytical validation studies should be encouraged to disseminate best practices.

1.3.2 Clinical validity

Clinical validity refers to "establishing that the test, tool, or instrument acceptably identifies, measures, or predicts the concept of interest where "concept" refers to a "clinical, biological, physical, or functional state, or experience" (FDA-NIH Biomarker Working Group 2016). Clinical validity is established by showing that the biomarker test results are related to the concept of interest in the relevant clinical setting, typically by demonstrating a statistically significant association and quantifying its strength in an appropriately designed study. For example, if a biomarker test is intended to predict disease-free survival, one might demonstrate that patient biomarker values measured at diagnosis are statistically significantly associated with disease-free survival time using Cox proportional hazards regression (Cox 1972) or other type of survival analysis, as appropriate. To demonstrate clinical validity of a biomarker test for monitoring for recurrence following treatment in the adjuvant setting one might, for example, demonstrate that the biomarker value measured at one year after the end of therapy is associated with likelihood of disease recurrence within the following year using an approach such as a landmark analysis (Anderson et al. 1983). For a response-predictive biomarker test that reports a continuous biomarker value, one could show that the biomarker value associates with likelihood of tumor response, for example by showing that the area under the receiver operating characteristic curve is significantly greater than the chance value of 0.5 (Hanley and McNeil 1982; Zou et al. 2007). Although these examples illustrate how associations could be estimated and tested, more is needed to establish that it is beneficial to use a biomarker test to guide clinical care. This concept of benefit from use of a test relates to the notion of clinical utility, which is discussed in depth in the next section.

1.3.3 Clinical Utility

Clinical utility for a biomarker test refers to a conclusion that use of the test "will lead to a net improvement in health outcome or provide useful information about diagnosis, treatment, management, or prevention of a disease. Clinical utility includes the range of possible benefits or risks to individuals and populations" (FDA-NIH Biomarker Working Group 2016). Assessment of clinical utility for a biomarker test is predicated on the test's analytical and clinical validity already having been established.

A laboratory or clinician may wish to evaluate the evidence for clinical utility of a biomarker test that is offered by another laboratory, or they may wish to evaluate clinical utility for a test that they newly developed. A laboratory might also wish to offer its own version of a biomarker test which has already been developed and confirmed to have clinical utility as performed by another laboratory. For the last situation in which a laboratory's intent is to transport the biomarker test to an in-house test, it is important for the laboratory to confirm that the test, as that specific laboratory performs it, delivers results highly concordant with those of the test as it was performed in prior studies that established the test's analytical and clinical validity and confirmed its clinical utility; if test results are not highly concordant, it is incumbent upon the laboratory to demonstrate that the test as performed in-house maintains its clinical performance and utility. For all of these situations a thorough understanding of acceptable approaches for establishing clinical utility is necessary.

The approach to demonstrating clinical utility of a biomarker test will depend on the intended clinical use. The three clinical uses as prognostic, predictive, and monitoring tests are elaborated on here. The first step in evaluation of clinical utility is a clear statement of the intended use; this includes careful definition of the patient population to which the test will be applied and the clinical decision that the test will inform. Too often biomarker studies are carried out using convenience sets of specimens with more attention paid to discovering statistically significant correlations than to what clinical decision the biomarker might help to inform. Such studies of convenience rarely lead to clinically helpful or viable biomarker tests (McShane and Polley 2013; Simon et al. 2009). Investigators aiming to develop biomarker tests for clinical care should focus on the intended clinical use as early as possible in the development process to ensure that the clinical studies forming the evidence base are performed in the relevant patient population and clinical context.

1.4 Evaluation of Clinical Utility

1.4.1 Prognostic Biomarker Utility

To establish that a prognostic biomarker test has clinical utility one should be able to demonstrate that it can identify patients for whom different prognoses, as forecast by the test, would lead to different clinical management decisions and that those decisions lead to a net benefit for the patient. Additionally, the information provided by the test should either add to existing routinely used prognostic indicators or the test should provide information comparable to existing indicators and be more reliable, convenient, or less invasive or expensive.

The 2016 *ASCO Clinical Practice Guideline for Biomarkers to Guide Decisions on Adjuvant Systemic Therapy for Women with Early-Stage Invasive Breast Cancer* cites evidence of clinical utility for prognosis for OncotypeDX®, EndoPredict®, Prosigna™, Breast Cancer Index℠ and uPA/PAI-1 for women with ER/PgR positive/HER2-negative (node-negative) breast cancer (Harris et al. 2016). In the indicated group of patients each of these tests was able to identify a subgroup with sufficiently good outcome in the absence of chemotherapy (e.g., low risk of disease recurrence) that chemotherapy would not be recommended. The ASCO guidelines committee did not find sufficient evidence for clinical utility for prognosis for any biomarkers in node-positive or HER2-positive disease.

Reasons that the ASCO biomarkers guidelines for early stage breast cancer did not recommend all prognostic biomarkers assessed or any prognostic markers outside of the setting of ER/PgR positive/HER2-negative node-negative breast cancer were the lack of sufficient data in the other subgroups or presentation of results only from patient cohorts heterogeneous with respect to standard prognostic variables and or treatments. As an example of why it can be important to study a group of patients who are relatively homogeneous with respect to standard prognostic variables, one can compare the prognostic ability of the

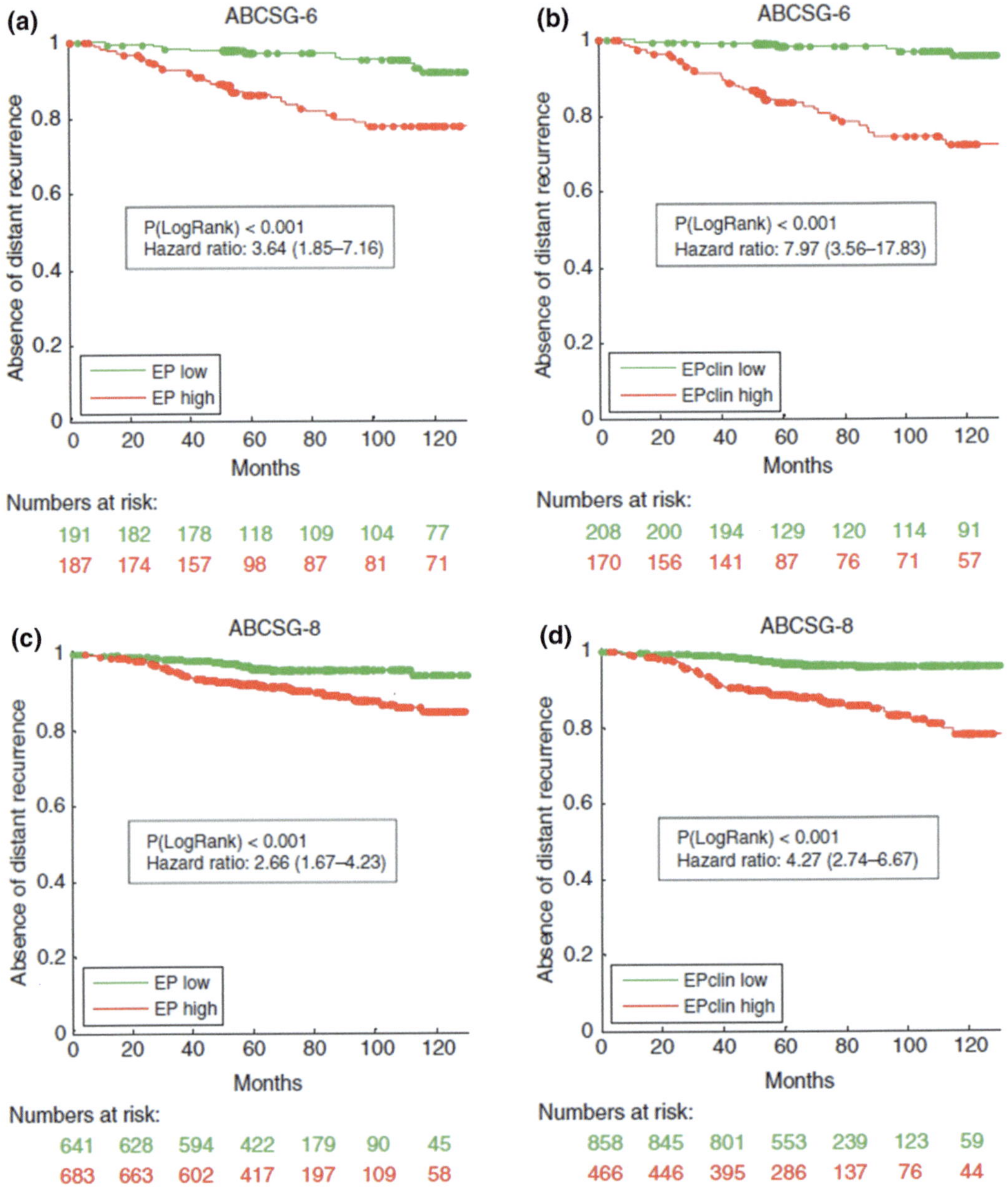

Fig. 1.1 Kaplan-Meier plots of distant recurrence by EP and EPclin risk groups. Distant recurrence according to EP risk groups (**a** and **c**) and EPclin risk groups (**b** and **d**) in patients from the 2 validation cohorts (ABCSG-6 *top*; ABCSG-8 *bottom*). Cutoff points for EP were prespecified at 5 (3.3 for EPclin) in the training set. *Numbers in parentheses* indicate the 95 % CI of the HR (Reprinted from Fig. 2 in Filipits et al. 2011)

dichotomized EndoPredict® EP score within subgroups defined by standard prognostic variables (Filipits et al. 2011). Significant differences in distant recurrence rate between EP low-risk and EP high-risk patients were observed in validation sets from the ABCSG-6 (Fig. 1.1a) and ABCSG-8 (Fig. 1.1c) trials. At 10 years, the distant recurrence rates for patients with EP low and EP high were 8 % (3–13 %) and 22 % (15–29 %) in ABCSG-6 ($P < 0.001$) and 6 % (2–9 %) and 15 % (11–20 %) in ABCSG-8 ($P < 0.001$), respectively. The subgroup defined as low risk by dichotomized EP score in both trials demonstrated 10-year distant recurrence rate less than 10 %. Similar results are shown for the EPclin score which incorporates additional prognostic variables nodal status and tumor size, although the separation between the survival curves appears wider (Figs. 1.1b, d). If the analyses are segregated by nodal status, then in the combined trial cohorts only the low risk group within the node-negative patients, and not the low risk group within the node-positive patients, achieves a distant recurrence rate less than 10 % (Fig. 1.2).

For the MammaPrint® test (Agendia, Inc. Irvine CA), the ASCO guidelines committee could not establish clinical utility due to ambiguity regarding the patient population and treatment setting in which it could be confidently used. The studies of the 70-gene prognosis signature (which was commercially developed into MammaPrint®) included patients with mixed prognostic variables such as positive and negative nodal status and both hormone receptor positive and negative tumors. Patients with hormone receptor positive tumors did not uniformly receive endocrine therapy, and some patients received chemotherapy while others did not (Harris et al. 2016). This heterogeneity among the studied patients made it impossible to determine whether the risk groups identified by the 70-gene prognosis signature were useful independently of standard prognostic variables or were indicating patients most likely to benefit or not from endocrine therapy or from chemotherapy. These examples illustrate that clinical context is critically important for determination of the clinical utility of a prognostic biomarker and studies should be designed with clinical context in mind.

Although it is customary for biomarkers to be categorized into two or more risk groups for clinical decision making, it is important to understand that any type of categorization of a continuous risk score results in a loss of information. For continuous prognostic risk scores it is usually possible to display the risk of the event (e.g., recurrence) at some fixed timepoint as a function of the risk score value, and these risk scores may include standard prognostic variables.

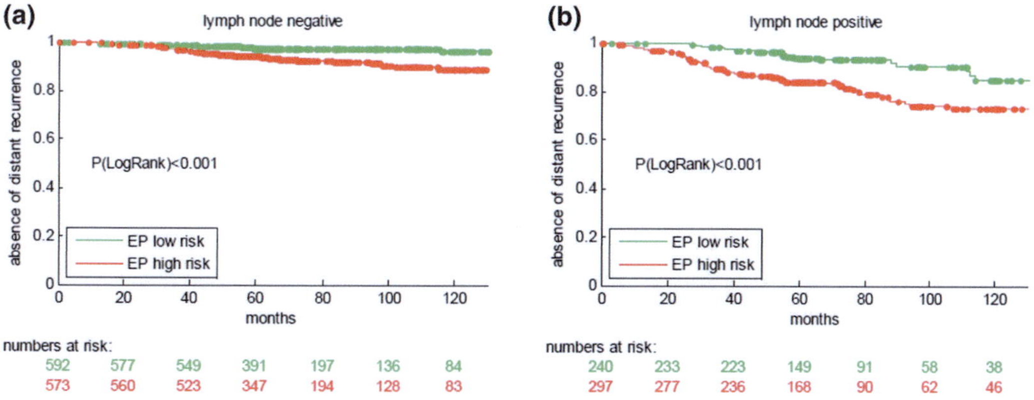

Fig. 1.2 Kaplan-Meier plots of distant recurrence by EP risk groups. Distant recurrence according to EP risk groups separately by nodal status (lymph node negative *left*; lymph node positive *right*) for combined ABCSG-6 and ABCSG-8 validation cohorts. Cutoff points for EP were prespecified at 5 in the training set. Ten-year distant recurrence-free survival is less than 90 % in the low risk lymph node positive group (Extracted from Fig. 9S in Filipits et al. 2011 online supplement)

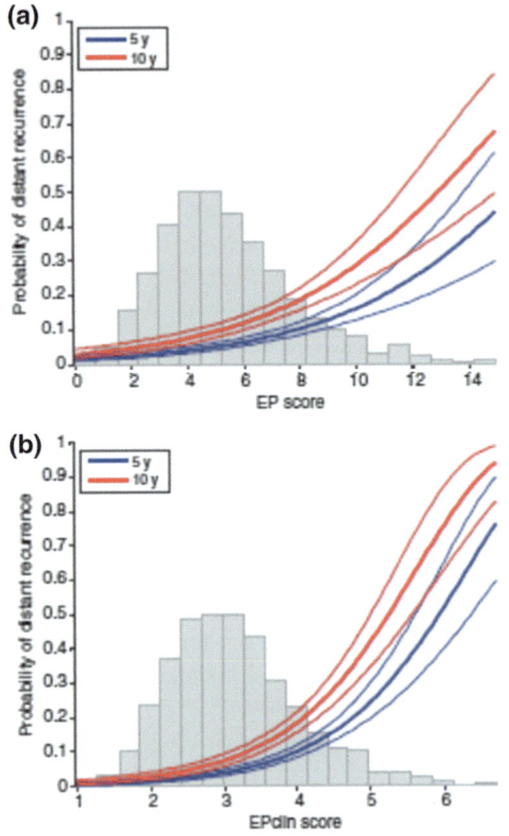

Fig. 1.3 Estimated probability of distant recurrence as continuous functions of the EP risk score (**a**) and the EPclin risk score (**b**). The continuous relation between the respective score and the probability of developing a distant recurrence within the first 5 and 10 years after surgery is described by an independent model for each score generated from all ABCSG-6 and ABCSG-8 data (n = 1702). The thin curves indicate the 95 % CI. The gray histogram in the background shows the distribution of scores for the patients (Reprinted from Fig. 1 in Filipits et al. 2011)

The Kaplan-Meier plots shown in Fig. 1.3a, b depict the prognostic ability of the EP and EPclin continuous scores in the combined ABCSG-6 and ABCSG-8 trial cohorts. These plots allow one to predict distant recurrence risk within 5 years and 10 years as a function of a risk score. The gray-shaded histograms also provide a visualization of the distribution of risk scores in the study population. Variation in absolute risk within each of the low and high risk scores is evident in these figures. This variation is not captured if the risks are reported only in aggregate for each of the low and high risk groups.

1.4.2 Predictive Biomarker Utility

The goal in demonstrating clinical utility for a predictive biomarker is to establish that the biomarker will guide a decision to select a particular treatment over a certain other treatment (the second treatment potentially being no further treatment) and that the selected treatment is associated with benefit for the patient. Criteria for establishing clinical utility vary somewhat for the three types of predictive biomarkers (treatment selection, enrichment-predictive, and response-predictive). Here we highlight some basic design considerations, and references are provided for readers interested in more extensive discussions. An excellent book length treatment of trial designs for predictive medicine is the book edited by Matsui et al. (2015).

1.4.2.1 Considerations for Treatment-Selection or Enrichment-Predictive Biomarker Utility

To establish clinical utility for a treatment-selection or enrichment-predictive biomarker, data from a trial in which there is a randomization between the treatments of interest is generally needed. Either the trial must be conducted prospectively or there must be an adequate number of specimens available from an appropriate completed randomized trial. Note that while it may be tempting to claim that a biomarker is predictive for benefit from a particular therapy when it is associated with more favorable outcome for those patients, such an effect may only be reflecting a prognostic effect that would be present independent of treatment (Polley et al. 2013a, b). Three basic phase III trial designs, or combinations or variations of these designs, are typically used to demonstrate clinical utility for treatment-selection or enrichment-predictive biomarkers: (1) the enrichment design, (2) the stratified design, and (3) the strategy design (Sargent et al. 2005; Freidlin et al. 2010). As will be discussed next, all of these designs require randomization, but they differ in other respects such as patient selection, treatment allocation, and the conclusions they support.

The enrichment design measures the biomarker on each patient at study entry and then randomizes only those patients whose tumors are positive between the experimental therapy (which is hypothesized to be better for patients who are biomarker positive) and some alternative standard therapy; this design can establish definitive evidence for clinical utility of the experimental therapy in the population selected by the enrichment-predictive biomarker if the experimental therapy is demonstrated to be superior to the standard therapy in that group. No information is provided by this design regarding which treatment is better for biomarker-negative patients; it is assumed that existing evidence suggests that biomarker-negative patients are not likely to benefit from the experimental therapy and thus they are not randomized. An enrichment design does not require that the biomarker used for enrichment perfectly identifies the group of patients who benefit from the experimental therapy. The biomarker only needs to be "good enough" so that the treatment effect is sufficiently amplified to be detected statistically in the enriched patient group. Even if imperfect, biomarker enrichment will have implications for the labeling of the new therapy, if the experimental agent is successful in trials leading to approval.

The drug development path for trastuzumab in breast cancer is an example for which the pivotal trials used biomarker enrichment. The metastatic trials enrolled only patients whose tumors were positive by a clinical-trial grade immunohistochemical assay for HER2, and in the adjuvant setting the pivotal trials enrolled patients whose tumors were positive for HER2 by either immunohistochemical (IHC; protein) or in situ hybridization (ISH; gene amplification) assays (Wolff et al. 2007). Due to apparent benefit of trastuzumab in patients whose tumors were negative on central testing but positive on a local assay used for study entry in the pivotal adjuvant studies, a new adjuvant trial, NSABP B-47 (NCT01275677), is underway to determine whether there is benefit of trastuzumab for patients whose tumors are HER2-Low. HER2-Low is defined in the B-47 trial as follows: 1 + by IHC; or 2 + by IHC and ratio of HER2 to chromosome enumeration probe 17 (CEP17) must be <2.0 or, if a ratio-based test was not performed, the HER2 gene copy number must be <4 per nucleus. Patients whose tumors are negative by both IHC and ISH are not eligible for the B-47 trial. This example illustrates the difficulties in the initial identification and subsequent refinement of an enrichment-predictive biomarker.

If it is desired to establish that a biomarker has clinical utility for treatment selection, then the stratified design is the most efficient design to use in most situations. The stratified design randomizes all patients between treatment A (thought to be better for biomarker positive patients) and treatment B (usually some standard therapy used irrespective of biomarker status) with stratification of the randomization by biomarker status to ensure balance of the biomarker values across treatment arms. To show clinical utility of the biomarker for identifying the population of patients who will have an overall better outcome with treatment A compared to treatment B, one must demonstrate that in the biomarker positive subgroup (in the simplest case of a binary biomarker) outcome is superior with treatment A, whereas, in the biomarker negative subgroup treatment B is ether the same or better than A. This design is the most informative in that it clearly distinguishes which treatment has greatest overall benefit in each biomarker subgroup.

A variant of the stratified design is what is sometimes referred to as an *all-comers design*. For this design only the analysis, and not the randomization, is stratified by the biomarker. The biomarker analysis may occur at the same time as the primary trial analysis or many years later using archived specimens. If carried out with appropriate rigor, such retrospective analyses of specimens from all-comers trials (a type of prospective-retrospective study) can provide a high level of evidence for clinical utility (Simon et al. 2009). Risks in using the all-comer design are that the biomarker measurements might not be available on some portion of the patients who are randomized (reducing the statistical power for the analyses) or the group of patients for whom biomarker measurements are available are

Table 1.1 Comparison of biomarker-driven clinical trial designs

Feature	Biomarker-stratified design	Enrichment design	Biomarker-strategy design, with biomarker assessment in the control arm	Biomarker-strategy design, without biomarker assessment in the control arm
Questions design can answer	What is the best treatment in each biomarker-defined subgroup? What is the best treatment in the overall study population? Is the biomarker-directed treatment strategy better than the control in the overall study population? (indirect assessment) Is the biomarker prognostic? Predictive?	What is the best treatment in the biomarker-positive patients?	Is the biomarker-directed treatment strategy better than the control treatment in the overall study population? (direct assessment) What is the best treatment in the biomarker-positive subgroup? Is the biomarker prognostic?	Is the biomarker-directed treatment strategy better than the control treatment in the overall study population? (direct assessment) What is the best treatment in the biomarker-positive subgroup? (indirect assessment) Is the biomarker prognostic? (indirect assessment)
Questions design cannot answer		What is the best treatment in the biomarker-negative subgroup? Is the biomarker prognostic? Predictive?	What is the best treatment in the biomarker-negative subgroup? Is the biomarker predictive?	What is the best treatment in the biomarker-negative subgroup? Is the biomarker predictive?
Advantages	Provides efficient assessment of relative treatment efficacy in each biomarker-defined subgroup and in the whole group	If the assumption that the biomarker reliably identifies the group likely to benefit from the experimental therapy is true, then the design provides an efficient test of efficacy of the experimental treatment in that subgroup, particularly if the biomarker positivity rate is low	Can be used for evaluation of complex biomarker-guided treatment strategies with a large number of treatment options or biomarker categories	Biomarker assessment is limited to the biomarker-directed arm (resource consideration) No issues associated with withholding the biomarker status from the control-arm patients Compliance not influenced by patient knowledge of the biomarker status in the control arm Can be used for evaluation of complex biomarker-guided treatment strategies with a large number of treatment options or biomarker categories
Disadvantages	The design is not feasible for evaluation of biomarker strategies with a large number of treatment options	If the experimental therapy is beneficial in a subgroup but the biomarker does not correctly identify this subgroup, a promising therapy may be missed A positive trial does not prove the utility of the biomarker because the relative treatment efficacy may be the same in the unevaluated biomarker-negative patients	A positive trial does not prove the utility of the biomarker because the experimental treatment may be better than the control treatment for all patients regardless of biomarker status Inefficiency	A positive trial does not prove the utility of the biomarker because the experimental treatment may be better than the control treatment for all patients regardless of biomarker status Inefficiency

Reprinted from Table 1 in Freidlin et al. (2010)

non-representative of the full patient group in such a way that the relationship between biomarker and treatment effect is distorted. In many situations these potential biases will not be a major problem, particularly if specimen collection is mandatory for trial eligibility.

The strategy design is another design which is sometimes used to establish that a biomarker has clinical utility for treatment selection, but it has some limitations. This design can be viewed as a test of the combination of the biomarker test and associated treatment assignment algorithm; patients are randomized to have biomarker testing or not. Patients randomized to the arm with biomarker testing receive the treatment designated by a pre-defined algorithm based on biomarker value (e.g., experimental targeted therapy for biomarker-positive patients and standard therapy for biomarker-negative patients in the simplest case of a binary biomarker). Patients assigned to the no-testing arm receive a standard treatment. Use of the strategy design is usually discouraged because it is statistically inefficient (because biomarker-negative patients receive the same treatment on both arms) and does not allow for separation of biomarker and treatment effects; however, it may be the only viable option in situations where a biomarker takes many possible values or the treatment assignment algorithm is complex.

Summaries of biomarker-driven clinical trial designs and questions they are able to address are given by Table 4.1 in Micheel et al. (2012). Freidlin et al. (2010) discuss advantages and disadvantages for these designs (Table 1.1) and interim monitoring considerations as well as providing many examples of actual trials that used these designs or hybrids of them (Freidlin et al. 2010). Additionally, care must be taken in the statistical design of the stratified (or all comers) design to consider sequence of testing within biomarker subgroups and appropriate type I error control (Freidlin and Korn 2014). Further statistical details are beyond the scope of this discussion.

1.4.2.2 Considerations for Response-Predictive Biomarker Utility

Evaluation of clinical utility for a response-predictive biomarker requires consideration of both long and short term endpoints due to the uncertainties in the association between a near term response endpoint and a long term event-free survival (EFS) endpoint which may include overall survival as well as recurrence, progression, or other events. In a neoadjuvant setting, the ability to achieve a tumor response might offer the advantage of allowing change in surgical management from mastectomy to lumpectomy, resulting in less morbidity and a more favorable cosmetic outcome for a patient. However, it must also be considered whether the reduced surgery could lead to less favorable long term event free survival (EFS) or whether a delay in surgery due to administration of pre-operative therapy could have a detrimental effect on long term EFS, especially if the pre-operative therapy is at best modestly effective. In an advanced disease setting where surgery is not an option and where it is believed that a therapeutic agent will have long term EFS benefit only if it demonstrates activity in the form of tumor shrinkage, a biomarker would have clinical utility as a response-predictive biomarker if it can be established to reliably predict when a tumor will not respond. The clinical utility of such a biomarker would lie in its ability to identify futile treatments, sparing the patient toxicity and potentially allowing selection of an effective treatment more quickly.

To demonstrate clinical utility of a response-predictive biomarker in either the neoadjuvant or metastatic setting, generally a randomized trial would be needed comparing use of the biomarker to not using it; or, in rare instances it might be possible to rely on extensive historical data to establish that acting on the response-predictive biomarker leads to a net benefit to patients through some combination of positive effects on short and long term endpoints. Another challenge is that a biomarker could predict response for two different treatments but provide no information about which treatment would lead to better survival; higher response rate does not necessarily translate to better survival outcome. For example, meta-analyses of neoadjuvant clinical trials in breast cancer that collected both pathologic complete response and event-free survival outcomes were unable to demonstrate that a certain magnitude of difference in pathologic complete response rates reliably translates to a particular magnitude of difference in event-free survival (Cortazar et al. 2014; Berruti et al. 2014; Korn et al. 2016). All of these examples highlight the need for clinical evaluation of

Table 1.2 Comparison of clinical trial phases I–IV of therapeutic trials and tumor biomarker-monitoring trials

Phases of clinical trials, clinical validity				
Type of trial	Phase I	Phase II	Phase III	Phase IV
Therapeutic oncology trial	Explores toxicity and optimal dosage and/or schedule of a new therapy or a new use of an old therapy	Estimates whether the new therapy shows evidence of antineoplastic activity. Usually conducted for a specific disease condition	Compares, through randomization, the new therapy that showed promising results in phase II trials with the current standard of care	Evaluates the benefits, side effects, risks, and optimal use of the therapy over an extended period through long-term surveillance of patients
Tumor biomarker-monitoring trial	Explores the kinetics of the biomarker and the correlation between a change in tumor burden and a change in serial biomarker concentrations	Estimates the monitoring performance of serial biomarker measurements to identify, exclude, and predict a change in tumor burden	Compares, through randomization, whether early biomarker-guided intervention produces a clinical change that improves patient outcomes	Evaluates the change in long-term outcome in terms of overall survival and adverse effects after the biomarker-guided intervention has been introduced into routine use

Reprinted from Table 1 in Söletormos et al. (2013)

response-predictive biomarkers to consider the impact of their use on both short and long term endpoints.

1.4.3 Monitoring Biomarker Utility

Biomarkers are frequently used to monitor disease status during therapy for signs of treatment response, toxicity, resistance or disease progression, or after therapy to detect signs of recurrence or progression. In order to establish clinical utility of such biomarkers it must be shown that clinically significant changes can be detected above the background noise and that detecting those signals leads to a benefit that can be realized by changing therapeutic management. Demonstration of an association between a monitoring biomarker and a clinical outcome may be sufficient to establish clinical validity but it is insufficient to establish clinical utility. Generally it must be shown that the monitoring biomarker test can detect the change in disease status with sufficient lead time before the appearance of clinical signs and that with that lead time there are clinical decisions or actions which can be taken to improve outcome for the patient. Examples of clinical management changes when biomarker monitoring occurs during therapy include a switch to a new therapeutic agent or to a different treatment modality, a change in dose or schedule of the current therapeutic agent, or possibly terminating treatment completely. After completion of therapy, biomarker monitoring may be used to detect recurrent or progressive disease to allow for decisions regarding resumption of therapy. Monitoring biomarkers could also be used to guide decisions regarding initiation of therapy in an active monitoring situation for some in situ breast cancers. Demonstration of clinical utility for a monitoring biomarker typically requires a randomized trial in which patient clinical outcomes resulting from a strategy which acts on the biomarker is compared to that from a strategy independent of the biomarker. The *European Group on Tumor Markers* outlined a process for the rigorous evaluation of tumor biomarker-monitoring trials (Söletormos et al. 2013) as summarized in Table 1.2.

The S0500 trial is an example of a biomarker-monitoring trial in which the role of circulating tumors cells (CTCs) in managing chemotherapy for women receiving first line chemotherapy for metastatic breast cancer (newly metastatic disease or progressive metastatic disease while on hormonal therapy) was assessed (Smerage et al. 2014). Patients were first grouped according to CTC level at baseline. Arm A comprised those patients who did not have increased CTCs at baseline and who were recommended to remain on initial therapy until progression. Those patients who initially had increased CTCs but experienced a decrease in CTCs after 21 days of therapy were recommended to remain on initial therapy (arm B). Patients with persistently increased CTCs after 21 days of therapy were randomly assigned to continue initial therapy (arm C1) or change to an alternative chemotherapy (arm C2). This trial design permitted several questions to be addressed about the role of CTCs in the monitoring setting. A comparison of arm A to arms B + C1 addresses the prognostic ability of baseline CTCs in the context of unchanging standard therapy. A comparison of arms C1 and C2 addresses whether patients with persistently elevated CTCs after 21 days of therapy benefit from a change in chemotherapy; this treatment comparison constitutes an enrichment trial (enrichment for patients with persistently elevated CTCs after 21 days of therapy) embedded in the larger trial. The S0500 study confirmed that baseline CTCs were prognostic but was unable to demonstrate that a switch of cytotoxic chemotherapy was beneficial for those patients with persistently elevated CTCs. A question that is not addressed is whether patients who did not have elevated CTCs at day 21 would have benefitted from a change in chemotherapy. Nonetheless, it is unlikely that there would be interest in addressing that question given the null trial results for those patients with persistently elevated CTCs.

1.5 Regulatory Considerations

In the United States, CLIA regulations require that laboratories performing biomarker tests and returning the results to a patient or the patient's physician must follow good laboratory practices (CMS 2016), but there are not specific CLIA requirements for clinical validation or documentation of comparability of test results between different laboratories. The FDA has longstanding regulatory processes for approval or clearance of biomarker tests which are marketed as devices, but there has been confusion regarding what types of tests meet the definition of a laboratory developed test (LDT) not requiring FDA review, versus fall under the regulatory system for medical devices. Consequently there is the potential for gaps in the evidence supporting biomarker tests offered by some laboratories, particularly if those laboratories do not participate in other quality assurance programs such as those offered through the College of American Pathologists (College of American Pathologists 2016).

Historically FDA has defined an LDT as "an IVD [in vitro diagnostic] that is intended for clinical use and designed, manufactured and used within a single laboratory" (U.S. FDA 2014b). This definition would not cover, for example, a laboratory test developed by a commercial or health system central laboratory and offered through multiple laboratories within its network; such tests are technically subject to FDA review because, strictly speaking, they are not LDTs although rarely have they been reviewed by FDA. FDA's recent draft guidance on a proposed new regulatory approach for LDTs signals its intent to consider increased regulation of both IVDs meeting the traditional LDT definition as well as an expanded definition that would include IVDs that are offered by a CLIA-certified laboratory as an "LDT" (and have not undergone any FDA review for clearance or approval) even though they might not meet the strict historical definition of an LDT (U.S. FDA 2014b).

CLIA requirements, which apply any time a test result is retuned to a patient or the patient's physician, must be adhered to regardless of whether the biomarker test is being performed for investigational purposes in the context of a clinical trial or is being used for routine clinical care. Researchers conducting clinical trials in which biomarker tests will be used must also be aware that such use might require an Investigational Device Exemption (IDE) (U.S. FDA 2014a). Applications for IDEs undergo review for evaluation of the potential risks associated with use of the test weighed against possible benefits with particular emphasis on analytical performance of the biomarker tests.

It is important for laboratories and clinical investigators to remain current in their understanding of, and compliance with, regulatory requirements. A large percentage of biomarker tests currently in use for guiding clinical care decisions have received little external review. Whether through increased regulatory oversight, or wider adoption of best practices for development and evaluation of biomarker tests, it is critical to ensure the safety and efficacy of biomarker tests used in clinical decision making.

1.6 Discussion

Biomarker-based tests are increasingly being used in oncology and are integral to the implementation of precision medicine. Best practices for the development and evaluation of these tests need to be followed, just as rigorous processes are required for the development of new therapeutics. Of paramount importance to this evaluation process is careful consideration of intended use, which includes the clinical setting, patient and specimen characteristics, and the decisions that are to be informed by use of the biomarker test. The goal of this chapter was to outline the principles of analytical and clinical validation and considerations for assessment of clinical utility to promote enhanced understanding of the translational process and wider adoption of best practices. Adherence to these best practices will increase the chances that biomarker tests will perform reliably on real-world clinical materials and that the results can be relied upon to have particular clinical interpretations leading to clinical decisions that benefit patients.

References

Allard WJ, Matera J, Miller MC et al (2004) Tumor cells circulate in the peripheral blood of all major carcinomas but not in healthy subjects or patients with nonmalignant diseases. Clin Cancer Res 10:6897–6904

Altman DG, McShane LM, Sauerbrei W et al (2012) Reporting recommendations for tumor marker prognostic studies (REMARK): explanation and elaboration. BMC Med 10:51. http://www.biomedcentral.com/1741-7015/10/51

Anderson JR, Cain KC, Gelber RD (1983) Analysis of survival by tumor response. J Clin Oncol 1(11):710–719

Becker R Jr (2015) Analytical validation of in vitro diagnostic tests. In: Matsui S, Buyse M, Simon R (eds) Design and analysis of clinical trials for predictive medicine. Chapman and Hall/CRC, Boca Raton, pp 33–49

Bergfeldt K, Rydh B, Granath F et al (2002) Risk of ovarian cancer in breast-cancer patients with a family history of breast or ovarian cancer: a population-based cohort study. Lancet 360:891–894

Berruti A, Amoroso V, Gallo F et al (2014) Pathologic complete response as a potential surrogate for the clinical outcome in patients with breast cancer after neoadjuvant therapy: a meta-regression of 29 randomized prospective studies. J Clin Oncol 32:3883–3891

Bossuyt PM, Reitsma JB, Bruns DE et al (2003a) Towards complete and accurate reporting of studies of diagnostic accuracy: the STARD initiative. Standards for reporting of diagnostic accuracy. Clin Chem 49(1):1–6

Bossuyt PM, Reitsma JB, Bruns DE et al (2003b) The STARD statement for reporting studies of diagnostic accuracy: explanation and elaboration. Clin Chem 49(1):7–18

Bossuyt PM, Reitsma JB, Bruns DE et al (2015) An updated list of essential items for reporting diagnostic accuracy studies. Clin Chem 61(12):1446–1452. doi:10.1373/clinchem.2015.246280

Brekelmans CTM, Tilanus-Linthorst MMA, Seynaeve C et al (2007) Tumour characteristics, survival and prognostic factors of hereditary breast cancer from BRCA2-, BRCA1- and non-BRCA1/2 families as compared to sporadic breast cancer cases. Eur J Cancer 43:867–876

Centers for Medicare & Medicaid Services (CMS) (2016) Clinical laboratory improvement amendments (CLIA).

http://www.cms.gov/CLIA/05_CLIA_Brochures.asp. Accessed 29 Feb 2016

Clinical Laboratory Standards Institute (CLSI) (2010) I/LA28-A2: quality assurance for design control and implementation of immunohistochemistry assays, approved guideline, 2nd edn. Clinical Laboratory Standards Institute, Wayne, PA

College of American Pathologists (2016) 2016 surveys and anatomic pathology education programs. http://www.cap.org/ShowProperty?nodePath=/UCMCon/Contribution%20Folders/WebContent/pdf/2016-surveys-catalog.pdf. Accessed 29 Feb 2016

Cortazar P, Zhang L, Untch M (2014) Pathological complete response and long-term clinical benefit in breast cancer: the CTNeoBC pooled analysis. Lancet 384:164–172

Cox DR (1972) Regression models and life-tables. J R Stat Soc B 34(2):187–220

Cronin M, Sangli C, Liu M-L et al (2007) Analytical validation of the Oncotype DX genomic diagnostic test for recurrence prognosis and therapeutic response prediction in node-negative, estrogen receptor–positive breast cancer. Clin Chem 53(6):1084–1091

EQUATOR Network (2016) Enhancing the quality and transparency of health research. http://www.equator-network.org/reporting-guidelines/. Accessed 29 Feb 2016

FDA-NIH Biomarker Working Group (2016) Glossary. In: BEST (Biomarkers, EndpointS, and other Tools) resource. U.S. Food and Drug Administration (FDA) and National Institutes of Health (NIH). Available via Internet. http://www.ncbi.nlm.nih.gov/books/NBK338448/. Accessed 29 Feb 2016

Filipits M, Rudas M, Jakesz R et al (2011) A new molecular predictor of distant recurrence in ER-positive HER2-negative breast cancer adds independent information to conventional clinical risk factors. Clin Cancer Res 17:6012–6020

Freidlin B, Korn EL (2014) Biomarker enrichment strategies: matching trial design to biomarker credentials. Nat Rev Clin Oncol 11:81–90

Freidlin B, McShane LM, Korn EL (2010) Randomized clinical trials with biomarkers: design issues. J Natl Cancer Inst 102(3):152–160

Genomic Health (2016) Oncotype DX breast cancer assay. http://www.oncotypedx.com/. Accessed 29 Feb 2016

Hammond MEH, Allred DC, Dowsett M et al (2010) American Society of Clinical Oncology/College of American Pathologists guideline recommendations for immunohistochemical testing of estrogen/progesterone receptors in breast cancer. J Clin Oncol 28(16):2784–2795

Hanley JA, McNeil BJ (1982) The meaning and use of the area under a receiver operating characteristic (ROC) curve. Radiology 143:29–36

Harris LN, Ismaila N, McShane LM et al (2016) Use of biomarkers to guide decisions on adjuvant systemic therapy for women with early-stage invasive breast cancer: American Society of Clinical Oncology clinical practice guideline. J Clin Oncol 34 (10):1134–1150

Jennings L, Van Deerlin VM, Gulley ML et al (2009) Recommended principles and practices for validating clinical molecular pathology tests. Arch Pathol Lab Med 133:743–755

Korn EL, Sachs MC, McShane LM (2016) Statistical controversies in clinical research: assessing pathologic complete response as a trial-level surrogate end point for early-stage breast cancer. Ann Oncol 27:10–15

Linnet K, Boyd JC (2012) Selection and analytical evaluation of methods with statistical techniques. In: Burtis CA, Ashwood ER, Bruns DE (eds) Tietz textbook of clinical chemistry and molecular diagnostics, 5th edn. Elsevier Saunders, St Louis, pp 7–47

Matsui S, Buyse M, Simon R (eds) (2015) Design and analysis of clinical trials for predictive medicine. Chapman and Hall/CRC, Boca Raton

McShane LM, Polley M-YC (2013) Development of omics-based clinical tests: the challenge of achieving statistical robustness and clinical utility. Clin Trials 10:653–665

McShane LM, Altman DG, Sauerbrei W et al (2005) Reporting recommendations for tumor marker prognostic studies (REMARK). J Natl Cancer Inst 97 (16):1180–1184

Micheel CM, Nass S, Omenn GS (eds) (2012) Evolution of translational omics: lessons learned and the path forward. The National Academies Press, Institute of Medicine, Washington DC

Moore HM, Kelly AB, Jewell SD et al (2011) Biospecimen reporting for improved study quality (BRISQ). Cancer Cytopathol 119:92–101

Nielsen T, Wallden B, Schaper C et al (2014) Analytical validation of the PAM50-based Prosigna Breast Cancer Prognostic Gene Signature Assay and nCounter Analysis System using formalin-fixed paraffin-embedded breast tumor specimens. BMC Cancer 14:177

Pathmanathan N, Balleine RL, Jayasinghe UW et al (2014) The prognostic value of Ki67 in systemically untreated patients with node-negative breast cancer. J Clin Pathol 67:222–228. doi:10.1136/jclinpath-2013-201793

Pennello GA (2013) Analytical and clinical evaluation of biomarkers assays: when are biomarkers ready for prime time? Clin Trials 10:666–676

Polley M-YC, Freidlin B, Korn EL et al (2013a) Statistical and practical considerations for clinical evaluation of predictive biomarkers. J Natl Cancer Inst 105(22):1677–1683

Polley M-YC, Leung SCY, McShane LM et al (2013b) An international Ki67 reproducibility study. J Natl Cancer Inst 105(24):1897–1906

Sargent DJ, Conley BA, Allegra C et al (2005) Clinical trial designs for predictive marker validation in cancer treatment trials. J Clin Oncol 23:2020–2027

Simon RM, Paik S, Hayes DF (2009) Use of archived specimens in evaluation of prognostic and predictive biomarkers. J Natl Cancer Inst 101:1446–1452

Smerage JB, Barlow WE, Hortobagyi GN et al (2014) Circulating tumor cells and response to chemotherapy in metastatic breast cancer: SWOG S0500. J Clin Oncol 32:3483–3489

Söletormos G, Duffy MJ, Hayes DF et al (2013) Design of tumor biomarker-monitoring trials: a proposal by the European group on tumor markers. Clin Chem 59 (1):52–59

Stuart-Harris R, Caldas C, Pinder SE et al (2008) Proliferation markers and survival in early breast cancer: a systematic review and meta-analysis of 85 studies in 32,825 patients. Breast 17:323–334

U.S. Food and Drug Administration (FDA) (2006) 510(k) Summary for CELLSEARCH® circulating tumor cell kit. http://www.accessdata.fda.gov/cdrh_docs/pdf6/k062013.pdf. Accessed 29 Feb 2016

U.S. Food and Drug Administration (FDA) (2013) 510(k) Summary for Prosigna™ breast cancer prognostic gene signature assay. http://www.accessdata.fda.gov/cdrh_docs/pdf13/k130010.pdf. Accessed 29 Feb 2016

U.S. Food and Drug Administration (FDA) (2014a) FDA decisions for investigational device exemption clinical investigations: guidance for sponsors, clinical investigators, institutional review boards, and Food and Drug Administration staff. U.S. Department of Health and Human Services, Food and Drug Administration, Rockville MD. Available via Internet. http://www.fda.gov/downloads/medicaldevices/deviceregulationandguidance/guidancedocuments/ucm279107.pdf. Accessed 29 Feb 2016

U.S. Food and Drug Administration (FDA) (2014b) Framework for regulatory oversight of laboratory developed tests (LDTs): draft guidance for industry, Food and Drug Administration staff, and clinical laboratories. U.S. Department of Health and Human Services, Food and Drug Administration, Rockville MD. Available via Internet. http://www.fda.gov/downloads/medicaldevices/deviceregulationandguidance/guidancedocuments/ucm416685.pdf. Accessed 29 Feb 2016

U.S. Food and Drug Administration (FDA) (2015) MammaPrint® FFPE 510(k) substantial equivalence determination decision memorandum: assay and instrument combination template. http://www.accessdata.fda.gov/cdrh_docs/reviews/k141142.pdf. Accessed 29 Feb 2016

Van Poznak C, Somerfield MR, Bast RC et al (2015) Use of biomarkers to guide decisions on systemic therapy for women with metastatic breast cancer: American Society of Clinical Oncology clinical practice guideline. J Clin Oncol 33(24):2695–2704

Wolff AC, Hammond ME, Schwartz JN et al (2007) American Society of Clinical Oncology/College of American Pathologists guideline recommendations for Human Epidermal Growth Factor Receptor 2 testing in breast cancer. J Clin Oncol 25(1):118–145

Wolff AC, Hammond ME, Hicks DG et al (2013) Recommendations for Human Epidermal Growth Factor Receptor 2 testing in breast cancer: American Society of Clinical Oncology/College of American Pathologists clinical practice guideline update. J Clin Oncol 31(31):3997–4013

Zou KH, O'Malley AJ, Mauri L (2007) Receiver-operating characteristic analysis for evaluating diagnostic tests and predictive models. Circulation 115:654–657

2 Preanalytic Variables, Tissue Quality and Clinical Samples from Breast Cancer Patients: Implications for Treatment Planning, Drug Discovery and Translational Research

David G. Hicks

Abstract

There are an increasing number of cancer therapies that target specific molecular pathways that drive disease progression in a number of solid tumors requiring companion diagnostic assays. The testing for these tumors usually involves analyzing the tumor on a molecular level for the presence or absence of certain cancer gene signatures or biomarkers. In order for the correct treatment regimen to be determined, the test results need to be an accurate picture of what the patient's tumor is in vivo. With the increase of this type of molecular testing on solid tumors, there has developed an urgent need to preserve the integrity of these molecular markers in the tissues being tested. A long delay between removal of the tissue from the patient and preservation of the tissue can result in degradation or alterations in the molecular integrity of the tissue, confounding analysis. This chapter will review the data about these important preanalytic variables; discuss the need for standardized tissue handling procedures, and offer solutions.

Keywords

Pre-analytical variables · Tissue fixation · Processing

2.1 Introduction

The introduction of targeted cancer therapies into routine clinical practice, in which new treatment regimens are selected based on companion diagnostic testing of tumor tissues, is rapidly ushering in a new era of individualized 'precision' cancer care (Hicks 2012). The analysis of human tissue with high throughput molecular technologies has been used to help define new prognostic and predictive biomarkers and gene

D.G. Hicks (✉)
Surgical Pathology Unit, Department of Pathology and Laboratory Medicine, University of Rochester Medical Center, Rochester, NY, USA
e-mail: David_Hicks@URMC.Rochester.edu

S. Badve and Y. Gökmen-Polar (eds.), *Molecular Pathology of Breast Cancer*, DOI 10.1007/978-3-319-41761-5_2

signatures that have been shown to outperform the standard clinical/pathologic variables used in current clinical practice (Van de Vijver et al. 2002). These discoveries are rapidly being translated into new treatment paradigms, and going forward we will see cancer diagnoses and treatments which include companion diagnostic molecular testing performed to guide the selection of the most appropriate therapies for individual patients, on a case by case basis (Hicks et al. 2008). For hematologic malignancies and certain solid tumors such as breast, lung, gastric and colon cancer, this new era has already arrived (Romond et al. 2005; Hicks and Whitney-Miller 2013). These advancements in diagnosis and management are being driven by rapid technologic advances in our ability to profile routine clinical samples on a molecular level, as well as by ever present and increasing economic pressures. Rising health care costs, along with the increasing number of new and costly targeted cancer drugs, necessitates the development and adoption of new diagnostic strategies and the implementation of new standards that will enable more effective patient selection, therapeutic decisions and treatment options that improve patient outcomes (Parkinson et al. 2014; Barron et al. 2009). As the molecular analysis of diagnostic human tissue samples enters into clinical practice, the accuracy, reliability and relevance of this approach need to be critically evaluated. These important issues apply equally to the discovery of new targeted cancer drugs and to the development of companion diagnostic molecular tests that will help identify the most suitable patients and guide the use of new targeted agents.

The procedures for collecting and preserving diagnostic clinical samples in current medical practice are for the most part decades old and involve the use of 10 % neutral buffered formalin as a fixative to stabilize and preserve tissue for morphologic evaluation. This preservation of human tissue for the morphologic analysis of routinely prepared hematoxylin and eosin stained sections has historically been the gold standard for diagnosis in anatomic pathology. The methods of tissue handling, fixation, processing and sectioning were developed to ensure adequate tissue preservation and acceptable morphology, and it is important to emphasize that accurate morphologic assessment will continue to be relevant as an important part of the diagnostic evaluation in this new era of individualized or 'precision' cancer care (Hicks and McMahon 2010).

These standard practices, however, have paid little attention to the suitability of these tissues for further molecular analysis (Hicks and Boyce 2012). Increasingly the evaluation of diagnostic tissue samples demands further information beyond pure morphology, including an assessment of tumor biology and the level of expression of important target molecules within the diseased tissues. Significant variability in tissue handling and fixation in clinical laboratories has the potential to adversely affect the quality of these clinical samples for both diagnostic evaluation and translational research. This is particularly true in breast cancer, where the evaluation of molecular pathways involving the estrogen receptor (ER), progesterone receptor (PR) and the tyrosine kinase human epidermal growth factor receptor-2 (HER2) is now a part of the standard initial work up for all newly diagnosed breast cancer patients and is important for clinical decisions concerning the selection of the most appropriate adjuvant treatment regimen. These critically important biomarkers help to identify subsets of patients who are appropriate candidates for treatments that target these specific molecular drivers of disease progression (Yaziji et al. 2008; Hicks and Kulkarni 2008a, b). The tissue sample now needs to be considered an analyte, and specification of tissue quality becomes an important aspect of any validated molecular assay performed on these samples (Hewitt et al. 2008). However, the accurate, reliable and reproducible assessment of these biomarkers in clinical specimens represents a significant challenge for surgical pathology laboratories.

2.2 Pre-analytical Variables

The emerging field of biospecimen science has recognized the significant impact of tissue handling and other preanalytical variables on the expression of biomarkers and the suitability of biospecimens for molecular analysis (Moore et al. 2011; Betsou et al. 2009; De Cecco et al. 2009). Preanalytical procedures affecting tissue quality are not generally standardized and have historically been poorly controlled. In addition to prolonged ischemia, many other preanalytic variables have been identified; including the type of fixative used, the size of the tissue, time of fixation, temperature during fixation and processing as well as the type of tissue processing. The ligation of the blood supply to a living tissue being resected during a surgical procedure will induce hypoxia and metabolic stress, resulting in progressive changes in the levels of gene expression along with the degradation of macromolecules that are of potential clinical interest (Liu et al. 2013). The time interval between arterial ligation and tissue removal from the patient has been termed the 'warm ischemic time' and can vary considerably depending on the experience of the surgeon and the complexity of the surgical procedure (Liu et al. 2013). The 'cold ischemic time' is the interval from removal of the sample from the surgical field until incision of the tissue in the laboratory and placement into a suitable fixative. While the 'warm ischemic time' is difficult to control because it is dependent on the surgeon and the surgical procedure, the 'cold ischemic time' is dependent only on the proximity of the operating rooms to the laboratory and having procedures in place to quickly transport the tissue to the laboratory so that it can be prepared for tissue fixation (Hicks et al. 2011). Differing intervals of cold ischemic time due to variable tissue handling remains an important technical hurdle for the study of molecular targets in clinical samples. The current reality is that specimen handling can be quite diverse across different institutions and most routine clinical practices and lacks strict standardization or well-defined standard operating procedures (Hicks and Boyce 2012). Furthermore, in many places both the time interval and the degree of variability are virtually unknown. With this in mind, recent national guidelines have recommended both prompt gross examination and the establishment of minimal and maximal fixation times for breast samples in an attempt to reduce the reported variability that exists in breast tumor predictive assays such as HER2 (Wolff et al. 2007). New ER, PR and HER2 testing guidelines from the ASCO/CAP task force have taken this one step further and now require that breast biopsies and excised breast tissue samples be assessed grossly as rapidly as possible, sectioned and placed in formalin, ideally within 1 h from excision and removal from the patient, and that these times be recorded for each specimen (Hammond et al. 2010; Wolff et al. 2014). While the authors of the guidelines attempted to have each of the recommendations supported by scientific evidence, quantitative data are sparse for many preanalytic variables, including the effects of cold ischemic times. Subsequently, the new guidelines have prompted a re-evaluation of protocols and procedures involving tissue handling for breast specimen and more globally for all surgically removed tissues in a number of institutions. With the rising importance of being able to obtain molecular and genetic information from clinical samples, both surgeons and pathologists will need to be more cognizant of these changes and reevaluate the traditional ways in which tissue samples coming from the operating rooms have been handled as they are transported to the pathology laboratory (Balch 2011). In light of these national guidelines, we have assessed the degree of variability in tissue handing from the operating rooms in our institution and, on the basis of our findings, took steps to try to standardize this potentially important preanalytic variable for all tissue samples that are handled and processed in the surgical pathology unit at our medical center.

2.2.1 The Rapid Tissue Acquisition Program

To address the problem of variable tissue handling in our medical center, we have implemented a new standard operating procedure that we call the "rapid tissue acquisition program" (RTAP), in which pathology has assumed the responsibility for the collection and transport of tissue samples coming from the operating room to the pathology laboratory (Hicks and Boyce 2012; Hicks and Kulkarni 2008a; Hicks 2014). Technical personnel from pathology are stationed in the operating room area during regular hours, equipped with cell phones. These 'pathology-runners' are notified when a specimen has been removed from a patient and are responsible for pickup and rapid transport of the resected tissue to the laboratory. The 'runner' verifies that the specimen is properly labeled, that clinical history is provided and that the collection time, laboratory receipt time and fixation start time are all recorded and tracked for each specimen. Since implementation of this new system, we have seen significant improvement in the median time to fixation and the total number of specimens incised and placed into formalin within one hour from surgical removal from the patient.

2.2.2 How Important Is Standardizing Tissue Handling?

With the implementation of a rapid tissue acquisition program, we have shown that the proactive, rapid retrieval and delivery of tissue specimens from the operating room to the surgical pathology laboratory is possible and can significantly reduce the time interval from collection to the start of fixation for tissue samples removed during surgery (Hicks and Boyce 2012; Hicks and Kulkarni 2008a; Hicks 2014). But the question remains, how important is this for patient care, translational research and potential molecular analysis?

The increasing utilization of molecular analysis and biomarkers in clinical practice as well as in translational research has begun to raise awareness of issues surrounding tissue quality and has led to an increasing emphasis on optimal sample preparation for molecular interrogation (Sherman et al. 2010). The ligation of the blood supply to living tissues being excised during surgery will lead to hypoxia, ischemia and the progressive degradation of macromolecules that are of potential clinical interest. Studies have shown that the level of expression of gene transcripts and proteins can change significantly during this ischemic interval (Hewitt et al. 2008; Liu et al. 2013; Dash et al. 2002; Miyatake et al. 2004). These changes include degradation of RNA, increased levels of expression of hypoxia-induced factor, as well as markers of post-translational modification as a consequence of ischemia and delayed time to formalin fixation (Neumeister et al. 2012). The degradation and/or changes in expression of different target molecules with increasing ischemia will almost certainly confound research studies that are performed on clinical samples with variable or unknown tissue handling (van Maldegem et al. 2008). Additionally, for solid tumors such as breast cancer in which current targeted therapies represent a potential treatment option, the potential impact of the quality of the tissue for diagnostic evaluation remains unclear, and there are few studies available dealing with the impact of tissue handling on the accuracy of breast predictive factor assays (Khoury et al. 2009). Pinhel et al. (2010) have shown that while ER, PR and Ki67 immunohistochemical expression levels were similar between needle core biopsies (which are typically placed into fixative immediately after removal) and breast cancer excisions. However, the immunohistochemical reactivity for phospho-Akt and phospho-Erk1/2 was markedly reduced in the latter specimen type from the same patient. These differences are most likely attributable to variations in tissue handling of excisional samples. Vassilakopoulou et al. (2015) have evaluated the change in antigenicity of a series of phosphoproteins in paraffin-embedded samples for breast tumors as a function of time to formalin fixation. The analysis was performed using the AQUA technology for quantitative immunofluorescence, and showed that the majority of epitopes tested revealed changes in expression with increasing cold ischemic times. Some phosphorylated proteins, such as phosphor-HSP27 and phosphor-S6 RP, which are involved in posttranslational modification and stress response pathways, showed an increase in expression or phosphorylation levels. Other phosphor-epitopes, like phosphor-AKT, phosphor-ERK1/2, phosphor-Tyrosine, and phosphor-MET, were found to be quite labile with loss of antigenicity within 1–2 h of cold ischemic time. This data strongly suggests that there is an important dephosphorylation of proteins in surgical specimens as a result of endogenous tumor phosphatase activity related to delayed fixation, and that the subsequent results of these assay might not be reflective of the in vivo status of the tumor (Vassilakopoulou et al. 2015; Espina et al. 2008). Given that protein kinases are targets for a significant number of new drugs under development for oncology, potentially important pharmacodynamic end points may be deleteriously affected by tissue handling practices that are routine but suboptimal. These differences will have major implications for future translational research, drug development, companion diagnostics test development, as well as clinical management, and must be taken into consideration in the design of ongoing clinical trials of new therapeutic agents, which have a linked companion diagnostic and a correlative science component.

Neumeister et al. (2012) have studied changes in antigenicity as a function of cold ischemic time in a series of 93 breast cancers with known time to fixation using the AQUA method of quantitative immunofluorescence. They found no evidence of loss of antigenicity with time-to-fixation in a 4 h time window. However, with a bootstrapping analysis, they observed a trend toward loss for ER and PR, a statistically significant loss of antigenicity for phosphorylated tyrosine ($P = 0.0048$), and trends toward loss for other proteins. They reported evidence of significantly increased antigenicity in acetylated lysine, AKAP13, and HIF1A, which are proteins known to be expressed in conditions of hypoxia. The loss of antigenicity for phosphorylated tyrosine, and increase in expression of AKAP13 and HIF1A, were confirmed in another cohort of biopsies compared with resection specimens from the same patients. These authors concluded that there is a need for further studies that extend the time range and normalize for intratumoral heterogeneity that can provide more comprehensive information on preanalytic variation due to cold ischemic time and its potential impact on protein biomarker analysis. Neumeister et al. (2014) have also used the AQUA technology to attempt the construction of a tissue quality index (TQI) that could serve as an intrinsic control that would allow a global assessment of protein status based on quantitative measurement of a small number of selected, informative epitopes based on observed changes as a function of delayed time to formalin fixation. Using the quantitative expression levels of three epitopes on separate cohorts of training and validation specimens, these investigators were able to show an association of negative TQI values (an indicator for loss of tissue quality) with increasing cold ischemic times. The authors conclude that although this work is preliminary and requires further optimization and validation, it represents a proof of concept for the potential to provide a surrogate for monitoring tissue quality that could help to inform companion diagnostic testing for clinical trial enrollment or clinical decision making.

2.3 Pre-analytical Variable and Breast Cancer Diagnosis

Accurate and reliable assessment of estrogen and progesterone receptors is important in adjuvant treatment planning for breast cancer patients (Yaziji et al. 2008; Hammond et al. 2010; Goldstein 2010). ER and PR are thermolabile proteins whose levels of expression have been shown to be altered by prolonged cold ischemic times (Nkoy et al. 2010; Yildiz-Aktas et al. 2012). Recent studies have suggested that delays from tissue collection to the initiation of formalin fixation may adversely affect ER and PR assessment (Khoury et al. 2009; Nkoy et al. 2010) as well as HER2 analysis (Khoury et al. 2009). In a study reported by Yildiz-Aktas et al. (2012), breast resection specimens were subjected to variable cold ischemic times within the refrigerator and at room temperature. These samples were processed and stained for ER, PR and HER2 and the results compared with the prior needle core biopsies from the same patient, which would have had a negligible cold ischemic time period before fixation. Significant reduction in IHC staining for hormone receptors and HER2 were not detected until 4 h for refrigerated samples and after 2 h for non-refrigerated samples. The authors concluded that the ASCO/CAP guideline of a cold ischemic time period of <1 h is a prudent guideline to follow and that refrigeration of specimens that may encounter delays until the start of fixation may be warranted. In a similar study, Khoury et al. (2009), showed that the staining for ER and PR were negatively impacted between 1 and 2 h and that fluorescence in situ hybridization for HER2 started to be significantly compromised after 2 h. The negative effect of delay to fixation for ER and PR were also seen when different antibody clones for these proteins were investigated (Qiu et al. 2010).

The results of these studies suggest that variable tissue handling leading to excessive cold ischemic times for excised breast tumor specimens could potentially result in patients being falsely classified as receptor negative. The consequence of invalid breast cancer testing for these important therapeutic targets has the potential to change the type of adjuvant therapeutic regimen offered, which in turn could adversely affect patient outcome. New ER, PR and HER2 testing guidelines from the ASCO/CAP task force now require that breast biopsies and excised breast tissue samples be incised and placed into formalin within 1 h from excision (Wolff et al. 2007, 2014; Hammond et al. 2010). Accomplishing this goal will require that collection times and the fixation start times are recorded and tracked so that the cold ischemic time for each clinical sample can be calculated and monitored. Our experience after implementing the 'rapid tissue acquisition program' at our institution suggests that the one-hour window proposed by the ASCO/CAP task force is challenging and will require an emphasis on standardization of tissue handling as well as a commitment of resources and personnel, along with close collaboration with surgeons and operating room staff to accomplish this goal (Kulkarni and Hicks 2008).

2.3.1 Conclusions

There is a growing need for high quality human biospecimens for translational research as well as in clinical care. Advancements in our ability to profile human tissues on a molecular level has led to a better understanding of tumor biology, which in turn has led to new therapeutic targets and novel treatment approaches. This movement toward "precision medicine" and individualizing treatment to address disease biology will be heavily dependent on high quality tissue samples removed for diagnosis and molecular analysis. Efforts to minimize and document the cold ischemic time will be important as we move forward with clinical/translational research and will allow investigators to determine which genes and proteins are potentially valid and reliable as biomarkers for clinical decision-making (Hewitt et al. 2008). A greater emphasis needs to be placed on developing standardized methods of tissue procurement for diagnosis and molecular testing that are evidence-based, and this issue must be addressed by future biospecimen research. Defining the preanalytical requirements for the molecular analysis of clinical samples will be critical for moving next generation molecular testing from the research laboratories into clinical practice, and will help achieve the goals and potential of 'precision' cancer care. Such studies will in all likelihood lead to evidence-based guidelines for best practices in surgical pathology with regards to tissue handling and molecular testing. Taking ownership of specimen acquisition and transport on the part of our laboratory has led to improved standardization in tissue handling in our institution. Ensuring proper tissue handling of clinical samples is the joint responsibility of pathologists, surgeons, radiologists, and their respective staff (Kulkarni and Hicks 2008) and will require good communication, collaboration and partnership to help ensure the best possible clinical care. The standardization of tissue handling will, in all likelihood, lead to improvements in the overall quality of patient specimens, which will benefit both clinical and research efforts.

Acknowledgments The author would like to thank Ms. Mary Jackson for her assistance in manuscript preparation. The author would also like to thank and acknowledge the work of Emma Tillett, Kristin McCarthy, Robyn Sage, Laurie Baxter, and Michelle Fuller from the department of Pathology as well as the operating room staff for their help and support for improving the quality of human tissue samples collected in our institution.

References

Balch CM (2011) Reexamining our routines of handing surgical tissue in the operating room. J Natl Cancer Inst Monogr 2011(42):39–40

Barron JJ, Cziraky MJ, Weisman T, Hicks DG (2009) HER2 testing and subsequent trastuzumab treatment for breast cancer in a managed care environment. Oncologist 14:760–768

Betsou F, Barnes R, Burke T et al (2009) International Society for Biological and Environmental Repositories (ISBER) Working Group on Biospecimen Science. Human biospecimen research: experimental protocol and quality control tools. Cancer Epidemiol Biomarkers Prev 18:1017–1025

Dash A, Maine IP, Varambally S et al (2002) Changes in differential gene expression because of warm ischemia time of radical prostatectomy specimens. Am J Pathol 161:1743–1748

De Cecco L, Musella V, Veneroni S et al (2009) Impact of biospecimens handling on biomarker research in breast cancer. BMC Cancer 9:409

Espina V, Edmiston KH, Heiby M et al (2008) A portrait of tissue phosphoprotein stability in the clinical tissue procurement process. Mol Cell Proteomics 7:1998–2018

Goldstein NS (2010) Standardized predictive receptor immunohistochemical assays: the view forward from our past. Am J Clin Pathol 133:681–683

Hammond ME, Hayes DF, Dowsett M et al (2010) American Society of Clinical Oncology/College of American Pathologists guideline recommendations for immunohistochemical testing of estrogen and progesterone receptors in breast cancer. J Clin Oncol 28:2784–2795

Hewitt SM, Lewis FA, Cao Y et al (2008) Tissue handling and specimen preparation in surgical pathology: issues concerning the recovery of nucleic acids from formalin-fixed, paraffin-embedded tissue. Arch Pathol Lab Med 132:1929–1935

Hicks DG (2012) Targeted therapies in breast cancer: tailoring treatment to the molecular drivers of disease progression. MLO Med Lab Obs 44:38–39

Hicks DG (2014) Standardization of tissue handling from the OR to the laboratory. AORN J 99:810–813

Hicks DG, Boyce BF (2012) The challenge and importance of standardizing preanalytical variables in surgical pathology specimens for clinical care and translational research. Biotech Histochem 87:14–17

Hicks DG, Kulkarni S (2008a) Trastuzumab as adjuvant therapy for early breast cancer: the importance of accurate human epidermal growth factor receptor 2 testing. Arch Pathol Lab Med 132:1008–1015

Hicks DG, Kulkarni S (2008b) HER2 + breast cancer: review of biologic relevance and optimal use of diagnostic tools. Am J Clin Pathol 129:263–273

Hicks DG, McMahon L (2010) The pros and cons of automation for immunohistochemistry from the prospective of the pathology laboratory. In: Shi S, Taylor C (eds) Immunohistochemistry & Antigen Retrieval Technique Based Research & Diagnostics. John Wiley & Sons, Inc., Hoboken, NJ, pp 151–163

Hicks D, Whitney-Miller C (2013) The evolving role of HER2 evaluation for diagnosis and clinical decision making for breast and gastric adenocarcinoma. Biotech Histochem 88:121–131

Hicks DG, Kulkarni S, Hammond ME (2008) The role of the indispensable surgical pathologist in treatment planning for breast cancer. Arch Pathol Lab Med 132:1226–1227

Hicks DG, Kushner L, McCarthy K (2011) Breast cancer predictive factor testing: the challenges and importance of standardizing tissue handling. J Natl Cancer Inst Monogr 2011:43–45

Khoury T, Sait S, Hwang H et al (2009) Delay to formalin fixation effect on breast biomarkers. Mod Pathol 22:1457–1467

Kulkarni S, Hicks DG (2008) HER2-positive early breast cancer and trastuzumab: a surgeon's perspective. Ann Surg Oncol 15:1677–1688

Liu NW, Sanford T, Srinivasan R et al (2013) Impact of ischemia and procurement conditions on gene expression in renal cell carcinoma. Clin Cancer Res 19:42–49

Miyatake Y, Ikeda H, Michimata R et al (2004) Differential modulation of gene expression among rat tissues with warm ischemia. Exp Mol Pathol 77:222–230

Moore HM, Compton CC, Alper J, Vaught JB (2011) International approaches to advancing biospecimen science. Cancer Epidemiol Biomarkers Prev 20:729–732

Neumeister VM, Anagnostou V, Siddiqui S et al (2012) Quantitative assessment of effect of preanalytic cold ischemic time on protein expression in breast cancer tissues. J Natl Cancer Inst 104:1815–1824

Neumeister VM, Parisi F, England AM et al (2014) A tissue quality index: an intrinsic control for measurement of effects of preanalytical variables on FFPE tissue. Lab Invest 94:467–474

Nkoy FL, Hammond ME, Rees W et al (2010) Variable specimen handling affects hormone receptor test results in women with breast cancer: a large multihospital retrospective study. Arch Pathol Lab Med 134:606–612

Parkinson B, Pearson SA, Viney R (2014) Economic evaluations of trastuzumab in HER2-positive metastatic breast cancer: a systematic review and critique. Eur J Health Econ 15:93–112

Pinhel IF, MacNeill FA, Hills MJ (2010) Extreme loss of immunoreactive p-Akt and p-Erk1/2 during routine fixation of primary breast cancer. Breast Cancer Res 12:R76

Qiu J, Kulkarni S, Chandrasekhar R et al (2010) Effect of delayed formalin fixation on estrogen and progesterone receptors in breast cancer: a study of three different clones. Am J Clin Pathol 134:813–819

Romond EH, Perez EA, Bryant J et al (2005) Trastuzumab plus adjuvant chemotherapy for operable HER2-positive breast cancer. N Engl J Med 353:1673–1684

Sherman ME, Howatt W, Blows FM et al (2010) Molecular pathology in epidemiologic studies: a primer on key considerations. Cancer Epidemiol Biomarkers Prev 19:966–972

Van de Vijver MJ, He YD, van't Veer LJ et al (2002) A gene-expression signature as a predictor of survival in breast cancer. N Engl J Med 347:1999–2009

van Maldegem F, de Wit M, Morsink F et al (2008) Effects of processing delay, formalin fixation, and immunohistochemistry on RNA Recovery From Formalin-fixed Paraffin-embedded Tissue Sections. Diagn Mol Pathol 17:51–58

Vassilakopoulou M, Parisi F, Siddiqui S et al (2015) Preanalytical variables and phosphoepitope expression in FFPE tissue: quantitative epitope assessment after variable cold ischemic time. Lab Invest 95(3):334–341

Wolff AC, Hammond ME, Hicks DG, et al, American Society of Clinical Oncology; College of American Pathologists (2014) Recommendations for human epidermal growth factor receptor 2 testing in breast cancer: American Society of Clinical Oncology/College of American Pathologists clinical practice guideline update. Arch Pathol Lab Med 138(2):241–256

Wolff AC, Hammond ME, Schwartz JN et al, American Society of Clinical Oncology/College of American Pathologists (2007) American Society of Clinical Oncology/College of American Pathologists guideline recommendations for human epidermal growth factor receptor 2 testing in breast cancer. Arch Pathol Lab Med 131:18–43

Yaziji H, Taylor CR, Goldstein NS et al (2008) Consensus recommendations on estrogen receptor testing in breast cancer by immunohistochemistry. Appl Immunohistochem Mol Morphol 16:513–520

Yildiz-Aktas IZ, Dabbs DJ, Bhargava R (2012) The effect of cold ischemic time on the immunohistochemical evaluation of estrogen receptor, progesterone receptor, and HER2 expression in invasive breast carcinoma. Mod Pathol 25:1098–1105

3 Impact of Analytical Variables in Breast Cancer Biomarker Analysis

Anthony Warford and Bharat Jasani

Abstract

Assessment of biomarkers for tissues is a demanding science. Scientific rigor in the analytical methodology is the key to obtaining standardized and consistent results. In this chapter, we focus on the analytical variables, both assay variables and reporting variables, in biomarker analysis. Each and every step in the assay process needs to be carefully monitored, optimized and standardized. Using immunohistochemistry and in situ methods as a background, we describe in detail the parameters required for staining. Assessment of the staining requires the evaluation of not only the tumor staining but also presence of staining in the internal controls such as normal breast epithelium. Strict laboratory quality control using both internal and external quality assessment metrices is necessary. Adoption of national and international guidelines such as ASCO-CAP guidelines, when available, is necessary to provide high degree of confidence required for biomarker analysis that is critical in this era of precision medicine.

Keywords

Analytical variable · Immunohistochemistry · In situ hybridization · Quality control · Quality assurance

3.1 Introduction

Precision medicine is the current buzz phrase that captures the concept of treating a patient in accordance with a more accurately defined understanding of their condition. In the context of oncology this means prescribing the right drug regime on the basis of a diagnosis that involves an accurate morphological and molecular understanding of an individual's cancer. This paradigm has been

A. Warford (✉)
University of Westminster, 115 New Cavendish Street, London W1W 6UW, UK
e-mail: A.Warford@westminster.ac.uk

B. Jasani
Department of Pathology, Targos Molecular Pathology GmbH, D-34119 Kassel, Germany

S. Badve and Y. Gökmen-Polar (eds.), *Molecular Pathology of Breast Cancer*, DOI 10.1007/978-3-319-41761-5_3

spearheaded by breast cancer and currently involves the combination of clinical presentation with morphological typing and molecular analysis for hormone receptor status and the human epithelial growth factor 2 (HER2). Demonstration of positive estrogen and/or progesterone receptor status is an indicator that the cancer should respond to the anti-estrogen drug tamoxifen (Jordan 2006) and/or endogenous estrogen depleting aromatase inhibitors (Geisler 2008). While HER2 protein over expression and/or HER2 gene copy number increase is a predictive indicator that the breast cancer should be treated with HER2 targeted drug regimens of which there are now several variants available that include; Trastuzumab (Herceptin), Pertuzumab (Perjeta), Ado-trastuzumab emtansine (Kadcyla) and Lapatinib (Tykerb). The absence of hormone receptors and HER2 overexpression/ amplification, termed triple negative breast cancer, will indicate alternative treatment regimes. Accordingly, getting the right morphological diagnosis together with an accurate molecular characterisation of a breast cancer sample is of critical importance. Its relevance to the patient is obvious in providing a treatment regime that is most likely to challenge tumor growth. Its importance to the clinical team is to provide the most appropriate and efficacious treatment regime.

The association between hormonal status and breast cancer can be traced back to the work of Charles Beatson at the end of the nineteenth century (see Stockwell 1983; Love and Philips 2002, for reviews). It was not until the emergence of drugs to target hormone receptor positive tumors that the necessity to segregate lesions for potential treatment became necessary. Initially a ligand binding assay, that required the use of freshly frozen unfixed homogenized tissue, was used to assess hormone receptor status (Hähnel and Twaddle 1973; Leclercq et al. 1973). This was subsequently replaced by the current immunohistochemical (IHC) method using sections of formalin fixed paraffin embedded tissue sections (FFPE) (Barnes et al. 1996; Harvey et al. 1999).

The association between gene amplification and the overexpression of HER2 and poor prognosis for invasive breast cancer was elucidated during the 1980s and 1990s (as reviewd by Bazell 1998). In the same time frame the anti HER2 monoclonal antibody Trastuzumab (Herceptin) was shown to be beneficial in extending HER2 positive patients survival in cases of invasive metastatic cancer. This led, in September 1998, to the approval of the monoclonal antibody based drug for use with patients with HER2 positive metastatic breast cancer and the simultaneous introduction of the FDA approved HercepTest for the IHC evaluation of HER2 expression in FFPE sections. Subsequent investigations and clinical trials have demonstrated that HER2 targeted therapy is of value to all patients with invasive breast cancer regardless of the stage with surface membrane over expression of the growth factor receptor (Figueroa-Magalhães et al. 2014).

The purpose of this chapter is to survey and comment on the analytical variables that influence the reliability and accuracy of results for the assessment of hormone receptor status and HER2 expression within the routine diagnostic cellular pathology department. These considerations are presented within context of international guidelines that define boundaries for preanalytical, analytical and postanalytical aspects of the laboratory procedures (Hammond et al. 2010; Rakha et al. 2015; Wolff et al. 2014; summarized in Tables 3.1 and 3.2). Adherence to these is an enforceable requirement and ensures that the clinical oncologist is provided with an accurate molecular assessment of a breast cancer sample leading to the prescribing of the correct treatment regime for the patient in their care.

In the context of the diagnostic and molecular characterisation of breast cancer for hormone receptor status and HER2 expression core biopsy or resection tissue are recommended (Rakha et al. 2015) as providing representative samples for cellular pathology analysis. Accordingly the preparation of cell samples for cytological analysis is not considered.

Table 3.1 Summary of US and UK analytical guidelines for HER2 assessment

Step		American Society of Clinical Oncology/College of American Pathologists Clinical Practice Guideline Update Recommendations for Human Epidermal Growth Factor Receptor 2 Testing in Breast Cancer 2014	National Coordinating Committee for Breast Pathology Updated UK Recommendations for HER2 assessment in breast cancer 2015
Preanalytical	Tissue		Core biopsy recommended. Incisional or excisional sample if former not available
	Cold ischaemic time	≤ 1 h	As ASCO/CAP guidelines
	Fixation type/time	Buffered formalin/6–72 h	As ASCO/CAP guidelines
	Section preparation	Stain within six weeks of cutting	Dry sections at 60 °C for 1 h or 37 °C overnight and stain within 1–2 days
Analytical	Controls		Tissue or cell line derived positive controls of positive, equivocal and negative HER2 preparations
	Assay	Preferentially, FDA approved	Must be validated. Dual HER2/C17 ISH recommended over single HER2 probe ISH. Commercial reagents/assays recommended
Postanalytical	Positive	Intense complete membrane staining of >10 % of tumor cells by IHC (3+) *or* average HER2 gene copy number ≥ 6 by ISH using single probe *or*, using dual probes, HER2/CEP17 ratio is ≥ 2.0 with an average HER2 copy number ≥ 4.0 signals per cell	As ASCO/CAP guidelines
	Negative	Weak or negative staining of <10 % of tumor cells by IHC *or* average HER2 gene copy number <4 by ISH using single probe *or*, using dual probes, HER2/CEP17 ratio is <2.0 with an average HER2 copy number <4.0 signals per cell	As ASCO/CAP guidelines
	Scoring	For ISH survey slide then count copy number in 20 nonoverlapping tumor cell nuclei	As ASCO/CAP guidelines, plus up to 60 cells in cases with tumor heterogeneity
Quality	Internal	Includes use of standard operating procedures, equipment maintenance, qualified and trained staff	
	External	Mandatory with a minimum of two testing events per year	Mandatory
	Laboratory	At least one external inspection every two years	

Table 3.2 Summary of US analytical guidelines for hormone receptor status assessment

Step		American Society of Clinical Oncology/College of American Pathologists Guideline Recommendations for Immunohistochemical Testing of Estrogen and Progesterone Receptors in Breast Cancer 2010
Preanalytical	Tissue	Representative large and, preferably, multiple core biopsies
	Cold ischaemic time	≤ 1 h
	Fixation type/time	Buffered formalin/6–72 h
Analytical	Reagents	Antibodies with well-established specificity and sensitivity that have been clinically validated and demonstrating good correlation with patient outcomes in published reports *or* Laboratory sourced antibodies with 90 % concordance with ER/PR positive and 95 % concordance with ER/PR negative cases as established with an antibody from the former category
	Controls	Positive, with moderate expression of receptor, and negative in all runs Internal positive control within test sample is presence of normal epithelial cells
	Slides	Stain within six weeks of cutting
Postanalytical	Positive	≥ 1 % of tumor cell nuclei are immunoreactive
	Negative	Tumors that are negative, but do not contain normal breast epithelium should be reported as uninterpretable
	Scoring	H score, Allred score or Quick score, with or without image analysis
Quality	Internal	Includes use of standard operating procedures, equipment maintenance, qualified and trained staff
	External	Mandatory with a minimum of two testing events per year
	Laboratory	At least one external inspection every two years

3.2 Preanalytical Stage

This stage covers the ischaemic phase up to the completion of the tissue fixation step and subsequent processing and paraffin wax embedding.

3.2.1 Ischaemic Phase

Ischaemic change begins as soon as the blood supply is severed during a surgical procedure. Warm ischaemia defines the phase when the sample is still within the body and cold ischaemia the phase after its removal from the patient before the commencement of fixation. As a general rule the longer the time of either or both of these phases the more prone the sample is likely to morphological and/or molecular degradation. Different components of cells and tissues are more susceptible to ischaemic change, with phosphorylated proteins being amongst the fastest to be degraded (Baker et al. 2005), protein and mRNA intermediate (Atkin et al. 2006) and DNA often the most resilient, as judged by its analysis for forensic analysis. For hormone receptor and HER2 assessment the recommended cold ischaemia time should be less than 1 h (Tables 3.1 and 3.2).

3.2.2 Tissue Fixation

Fixation of the tissue is aimed at the permanent preservation of cell and tissue architecture and, ideally, the retention of molecular constituents in a form that allows their subsequent microscopic visualisation. For histological examination buffered formalin solutions are commonly used for this purpose. This fixative initially hydroxymethylates basic amino acid groups of proteins and can also react in an additive fashion with nucleic acid bases when they are not involved in base pairing. The subsequent formation of methylene bridges between hydroxymethylated proteins and formaldehyde modified proteins and nucleic acids results in a cross linked meshwork that stabilizes the morphology of the sample by either directly fixing tissue components or entrapping them in this framework. Under fixation will result in the poor conservation of morphology and loss of soluble molecular components. Over fixation can degrade nucleic acids and render demonstration of proteins by analytical methods such as IHC difficult as epitopes are not fully accessible in the tightly cross linked meshwork of the sample.

Core biopsies, that are typically no more than 2 mm in diameter, can be immersed in buffered formalin directly and the fixative will penetrate these quickly. Core biopsy samples are recommended for evaluation of hormone receptor and HER2 status (Tables 3.1 and 3.2; Uy et al. 2010). To ensure the even and adequate fixation of excisional/incisional samples 'bread loafing' of the tissue is recommended when slices should not be more than 2–3 mm thick to ensure adequate fixation. After an initial fixation period representative blocks of tumor tissue, other regions of interest and lymph nodes can be taken forward for paraffin processing. The exact location of these blocks must be recorded so as to relate them to the initial sample. This is often done by reference to ink markings made when the tissue was surgically removed or when first received in the laboratory.

The guidelines for hormone receptor and HER2 assessment (Tables 3.1 and 3.2) recommend minimum fixation of 6 h and maximum of 72 h in buffered formalin before paraffin processing. Fixation time for core biopsies does not need to exceed 24 h, but excisional/incisional samples may require longer fixation. It should be noted that fixation in Bouin fluid, a solution containing formalin, picric acid and acetic acid, is not recommended (Rakha et al. 2015). This fixative does not penetrate tissue of any substantial volume well and it rapidly degrades DNA making it unsuitable for in situ hybridisation (ISH) based analysis (Apple et al. 2011; Moatamed et al. 2011).

3.2.3 Processing and Embedding

Before the analytical phase can commence the fixed samples are processed to replace the water in the tissue with paraffin wax to provide support for the cutting of sections for staining. As water and wax are immiscible processing involves the removal of water using ascending grades of alcohol that is then replaced by a solvent such as xylene, which is finally replaced by infiltration with paraffin wax. The whole procedure is automated. For core biopsy samples rapid processing schedules that employ heat and vacuum replacement of the reagents are suitable. However, with excisional/incisional tissue the larger tissue blocks often require a longer schedule to ensure that all solutions are adequately replaced. Failure to attend to the differing optimum time requirements during paraffin processing and attending to the quality control of the solvents used for the tissue dehydration steps can result in compromised morphology and variable IHC and ISH results.

The final step in FFPE process is to surround the processed tissue with paraffin wax contained within a mould in the embedding step to provide external support for sectioning. To avoid sample loss during sectioning care must be taken during this step to ensure that the samples are embedded on the same plane. This is particularly important when core samples are being embedded as, due to their small diameter, precious tissue could otherwise be lost during sectioning.

3.2.4 Achieving Optimal Conditions

The guidelines for optimal handling of the tissue at the preanalytical stage for hormone receptor and HER2 assessment are based on accumulated experience and data available at their time of writing (Dabbs and Bhargava 2011). While this is very important, due to the implications of diagnosis, they have also made it very difficult to assemble sufficient residual surgical tissue to assess whether the current recommendations for controlling preanalytical variables are robust and reliable. Furthermore, as highlighted in the literature review conducted by Kalkman et al. (2014), the majority of these investigations have used high scoring cases as the controls that makes the application of these results uncertain for intermediate to borderline cases. The investigations and results for some of these studies are summarized in Table 3.3 for HER2 and hormone receptors in Table 3.4. Taken together the results indicate that further and more exhaustive studies are required before the guidelines as presently stipulated for pre analytical tissue handling can be safely altered to allow clinically critical assessments and decisions to be made.

3.3 Analytical Stage

This covers sectioning and staining to allow microscopic visualisation of tissue architecture and molecular components.

3.3.1 Sectioning and Storage

Serial sections cut at a uniform thickness set between 2 and 4 μm should be mounted on adhesive coated slides to prevent detachment during staining. There is no general consensus on the temperature for drying sections onto slides, storage conditions thereafter or interval between cutting and IHC or ISH staining. For the demonstration of HER2 the latest UK guidelines recommend drying sections at 60 °C for 1 h or 37 °C overnight and staining within 1–2 days (Rakha et al. 2015) while the ASCO/CAP guidelines state that staining should be undertaken within six weeks of cutting (Wolff et al. 2014). A sensible approach is to standardize cutting, drying conditions and time interval to staining as this will eliminate these steps as a potential source of variability.

3.3.2 Staining

3.3.2.1 Morphological Analysis

For morphological diagnosis sections are first stained with the haematoxylin and eosin (H&E). DNA is stained blue with haematoxylin and cytoplasmic and connective tissue components

Table 3.3 Summary of studies investigating the effect of preanalytical variables on HER2

Investigation	Results	Reference
10 cases used. Fixation delayed by 0, 10, 30 min, 1, 2, 4, and 8 h at ambient temperature and overnight at 4 °C. Fixation time in buffered formalin was not identical in for all samples	Delayed fixation had no effect on the IHC 3+ case. Results for other cases graded as IHC 2 or 1+ were technically unsuitable for analysis. Fixation delay introduced variability in ISH results affecting HER2 probe staining more than the C17 control probe Recommended not to delay fixation beyond 1 h	Khoury et al. (2009)
10 IHC 3+ cases with fixation time in buffered formalin from 3 to 120 h	No difference in HER2 IHC staining	Ibarra and Rogers (2010)
One IHC 3+ sample, ischaemic time of 96 h and multiple fixation types used thereafter	Ischaemic time did not affect IHC or ISH. Buffered formalin, to 168 h fixation, best fixative. Bouin fixation acceptable for IHC but not for ISH. Other fixatives not as good as buffered formalin	Moatamed et al. (2011)
84 cases. Cold ischaemic time; <1 h (45 cases), 1–2 h (27 cases), 2–3 h (6 cases), and >3 h (6 cases). Fixation was in buffered formalin	Ischaemic time of up to 3 h had no effect on IHC or ISH results	Portier et al. (2013)

Table 3.4 Summary of studies investigating the effect of preanalytical variables on hormone receptor status

Investigation	Results	Reference
10 cases used. Fixation delayed by 0, 10, 30 min, 1, 2, 4, and 8 h at ambient temperature and overnight at 4 °C. Fixation time in buffered formalin was not identical in for all samples	Quick score declined at 2 h delayed fixation for ER and 1 h delayed fixation for PR. Lowest scores were after 8 h delayed fixation for ER and overnight for PR. The differences were not statistically significant. Recommended not to delay fixation beyond 1 h	Khoury et al. (2009)
10 cases, high ER expressing 'core' tissue used, 1 to 10 h fixation time in buffered formalin	1–9 h fixation and rapid processing did not affect ER IHC	Ibarra et al. (2010)
One high expressing ER/PR case used. Fixation delayed for 96 h at 4 °C. Several fixatives used for between 1 and 168 h	No effect on ER/PR IHC after storage before fixation. No difference in IHC after fixation although Bouin results were variable	Apple et al. (2011)

Key: *ER* estrogen receptor, *PR* progesterone receptor

various hues of red with eosin. Attention to the quality and consistency of the H&E preparation is paramount as the primary diagnosis is derived from it. Diagnosis of invasive cancer will lead to HER2 and hormone receptor status determination, but for ductal carcinoma in situ these are not required as they will, at present, have no bearing on subsequent targeted therapeutic options.

3.3.2.2 Immunohistochemistry and In Situ Hybridisation

IHC is used for the demonstration of HER2 and estrogen/progesterone hormone receptor protein expression. The method harnesses the specificity of antibodies to recognize and bind to epitopes that should only be present on the protein to be demonstrated. ISH can be used as either a primary or secondary tool, in the instance of borderline IHC results, for assessing HER2 gene copy number status. ISH shares many procedural steps with IHC, but employs nucleic acid probes that attach to target genes by complementary base pairing to allow their demonstration. It is essential that antibodies, nucleic acid probes and their associated assays are validated for specificity, sensitivity and reproducibility before they are used for any diagnostic purpose and this is especially important in the context assessments that will guide therapy (Howat et al. 2014; Taylor 2014; Smith and Womack 2014). In a complimentary paper to that of the ASCO/CAP hormone receptor guidelines Fitzgibbons et al. (2010) describes procedures for hormone receptor antibody and assay validation. The need for this is also emphasized in the guidelines for HER2 and hormone receptor status determination; see Tables 3.1 and 3.2.

In practice the use of regulatory authority approved commercial kits (http://www.fda.gov/medicaldevices/productsandmedicalprocedures/invitrodiagnostics/ucm301431.htm) for IHC and ISH combined with their use on automated staining platforms is recommended. The combination should provide consistency of staining, providing preanalytical variables are controlled. When laboratory reagents are used instead of approved commercial offerings then concordance must be demonstrated against previously validated reagents/kits (Fitzgibbons et al. 2010; Hammond et al. 2010). When manual staining is used then this should be rigorously standardized and undertaken with a full understanding of the influence each procedural step on the potential staining result. In particular of duration of formalin fixation time on optimal antigen retrieval (unmasking) for IHC or exposure of DNA from surrounding fixed proteins for ISH techniques must be considered very carefully (Warford et al. 2014; Warford 2016).

For the demonstration of gene copy change for HER2, fluorescent ISH (FISH) methods were initially described (Wang et al. 2000) and are still most frequently used. With the fluorescent end point it is necessary to read the slides using a microscope fitted with epi-fluorescent illumination and appropriate excitation and emission filter sets for demonstration of HER2 target, and optionally, centromeric control gene sequences present on the same chromosome 17, within intact interphase nuclei counterstained with DAPI. Selection of appropriate tumor areas for scoring and the process of scoring itself can be challenging when viewing 'bright dots' within nuclei without the morphological signposts afforded by the bright field microscopy being available for reference (Fig. 3.1). In response to these challenges several ISH assays with chromogenic end points have been described and some of these have now received regulatory approval for assessment of HER2 gene copy number change (Gruver et al. 2010; Kosa et al. 2013; Mollerup et al. 2012; Penault-Llorca et al. 2009). It is likely that these bright field ISH assays will replace FISH for the assessment of HER2 gene copy change.

Algorithms for assessment of HER2 status usually place IHC ahead of ISH. This has been based on assay cost, turnaround times and ease of interpretation. When unequivocal IHC positive staining is observed there is no need to confirm this using ISH. However when borderline results are recorded then reflex ISH is undertaken. With the advent of bright field ISH this algorithm may change to use of this assay alone.

3.3.3 Internal Quality Control

Regardless of the type of assay, controls must be incorporated with every running of patient samples. Controls are of two types; positive controls that harbor the target that the assay is to

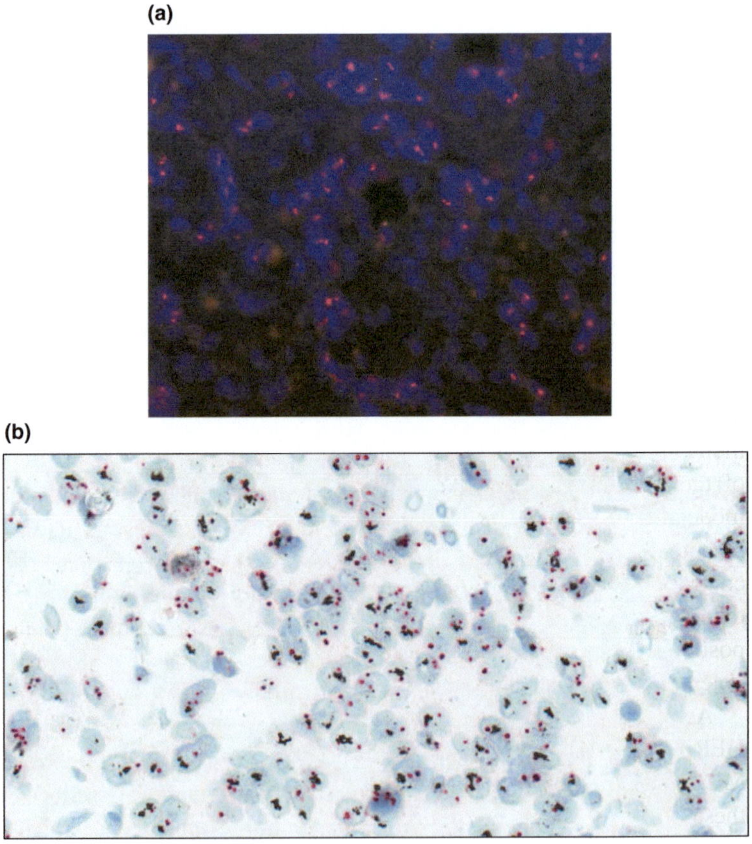

Fig. 3.1 Examples of HER2 gene amplification using dual probe in situ hybridisation.
a Fluorescent in situ hybridisation. HER2 *red*; CEP17, *green*. ×63 magnification.
b Chromogenic in situ hybridisation. HER2 black, CEP17, *red*. ×40 magnification. Images courtesy of G Baenfer, Targos GMBH

demonstrate and negative controls that are used to assess for any nonspecific reaction that may be associated with the assay. For HER2 and hormone receptor IHC it is recommended that several positive controls are included that demonstrate a range of protein expression levels. The inclusion of residual sections of patient samples is one way of fulfilling this requirement, but for HER2 IHC a much better solution is to stain FFPE preparations of cultured cells that express different levels of the receptor as these provide a consistent and replenishable source of positive control material (Rhodes et al. 2002a, b, Jasani et al. 2010). As described in these papers FFPE cell blocks were produced from SKOV-3, MDAMB-453, BT-20, and MCF-7 cell lines that are, respectively, IHC HER2 3+, 2+, 1+, and negative. The same cell blocks were also shown to be suitable for demonstration of FISH copy number change and are therefore suitable for use when this assay is run.

By embedding the cell block pellets together as composites, sections can be cut and placed on the same microscope slides onto which the patient's section is also placed. This on slide positive control confirms reagents have reacted with each individual test slide and therefore increases the level of quality control over the separate inclusion of sections of positive material as extra slides in a run.

The positive control for ER/PR hormone receptor status is often 'on slide', but relies on the demonstration of normal strong expression of the receptors in normal ductal elements (Hammond et al. 2010). In the absence of the presence of these an external positive control slide with moderate expression levels of the hormone receptors should be included. By using a positive control with moderate expression levels weaker than the expected intensity and distribution of positive cells provides for early warning of potential assay under performance.

As described above negative controls for HER2 IHC and ISH can be provided by using MCF7 cell block preparations. While staining of these would signal an alert about the possible presence of nonspecific staining, the test tissue sections need to be carefully assessed as this could be due to intrinsic factors such as necrosis or sub-optimal tissue preparation and/or an overall assay related issue. When unexpected nonspecific staining is present over several different patients test slides then this is more likely to indicate assay related nonspecific staining.

3.4 Postanalytical Stage

This encompasses microscopic assessment, reporting and quality assurance.

3.4.1 Assessment

Clear and detailed guidelines are provided for these largely the Pathologist led activities (Hammond et al. 2010; Rakha et al. 2015; Wolff et al. 2014) and the cut offs for determining HER2 gene expression and hormone receptor status as positive or negative are summarized in Tables 3.1 and 3.2. It is important to note that the possibility of tumor heterogeneity, challenging morphological presentations and the interpretation based on sections of core biopsy samples that may contain only a few invasive cancer cells can all complicate assessment. Furthermore the potential impact of preanalytical and analytical steps on the validity of assessment must also be considered (Lee et al. 2013). For this reason the Pathologist should be presented with a full audit trail of these steps.

Before any assessment of patient sections is made the Pathologist will need to review the controls that are included with these and to either accept or reject them. Interpretation, for example, of a section for estrogen or progesterone status where the staining of normal ductal elements is lacking must lead to reflex testing to exclude technical issues and if the situation persists then the case should be reported as uninterpretable (Hammond et al. 2010). Similarly, as previously discussed, there is a need to consider the reasons for any unexpected staining.

IHC is often used as the primary analytical method to assess HER2 status. Examples of HER2 IHC staining from IHC 1+ to 3+ positive are provided in Fig. 3.2. It should be noted that only cell membrane staining is relevant for interpretation. In cases where the 10 % or more of the tumor cells show strong and complete cell membrane staining for HER2 it is reported as IHC 3+ and positive for the receptor. In situations where there is a complete absence of HER2 staining or weak and incomplete membrane staining of less than 10 % of the tumor cells then the case is reported as HER2 receptor negative. However in cases where there is moderate cell membrane staining in 10 % or more tumor cells then further assessment by ISH for gene copy number is required (Wolff et al. 2014; Rakha et al. 2015).

For ISH assessment great care must be taken to identify the interphase nuclei to be counted. This can be particularly challenging when FISH techniques are used (see Fig. 3.1). Only nonoverlapping and well preserved tumor cell nuclei should be assessed, and a minimum of 20 of these need to be present. In situations where a dual probe ISH technique has been employed then a case where the HER2/CEP17 ratio is ≥ 2.0 with an average HER2 copy number ≥ 4.0 signals per cell should be reported as positive. When using only the HER2 probe the average copy number over the cells counted must be ≥ 6 for positive receptor status to be reported. Cases are negative for HER2 when the average HER2/CEP17 ratio is <2.0 with an average HER2 copy number <4.0 signals per cells or, when using only the HER2 probe alone, the average copy number is <4 copies per cell. In equivocal cases then the signals in up to a further 40 nuclei, preferably from three distinct tumor regions, should be counted and the same assessment criteria applied, but beyond this no further assessment of a case is recommended (Wolff et al. 2014; Rakha et al. 2015).

For the assessment of hormone receptor status the cellular compartmentalisation of staining must first be considered. Only nuclear staining is valid and if staining of other cellular compartments is observed this must be discounted and a decision taken as to whether the preparation is technically acceptable for assessment. If assessment can proceed then calculation of the percentage and intensity of nuclear staining of the invasive carcinoma component of the sample is required. In accordance with the CAP/ASCO guidelines (Hammond et al. 2010) for either estrogen or progesterone receptor staining a minimum of ≥ 1 % of the tumor population must be stained to qualify as hormone receptor positive and suitable for consideration for targeted therapy. The 'Ontario' guidelines (Nofech-Mozes et al. 2012) refine this by suggesting that a score of between 1 and 10 % should lead to careful clinical consideration of the benefit of hormone directed therapy while a score of ≥ 10 % would normally qualify a patient as suitable for targeted intervention.

To establish the percentage of stained nuclei a semi-quantitative scoring method should be used. Three scoring methods are commonly employed for this purpose: H score (McCarty et al. 1986), Allred score (Allred et al. 1998), and 'quickscore' (Detre et al. 1995). The mathematical basis for these semi-quantitative scoring methods is provided in Box 1. It is important that when employing any of these that all invasive carcinoma areas present on the stained section/s are included to produce the score. In Figs. 3.3 and 3.4 examples of estrogen and progesterone staining are shown. If taken as representative of distribution of staining across a whole diagnostic section then the staining for estrogen receptor in Fig. 3.3a, b and that for progesterone in Fig. 3.4a would be unequivocally positive. While the staining for progesterone receptor as illustrated in Fig. 3.4b is heterogeneous, a positive hormone receptor status would result from the application of any of the scoring systems. However, in Fig. 3.3c only weak staining for estrogen receptor is present and the number of these cells would be below 1 % cut off and therefore it would be categorized as hormone receptor negative.

3.4.2 Reporting

Guidance for the reporting of HER2 and hormone receptor staining is provided in the recommendations of Hammond et al. (2010), Rakha et al. (2015) and Wolff et al. (2014). To aid clinical decisions reports should include

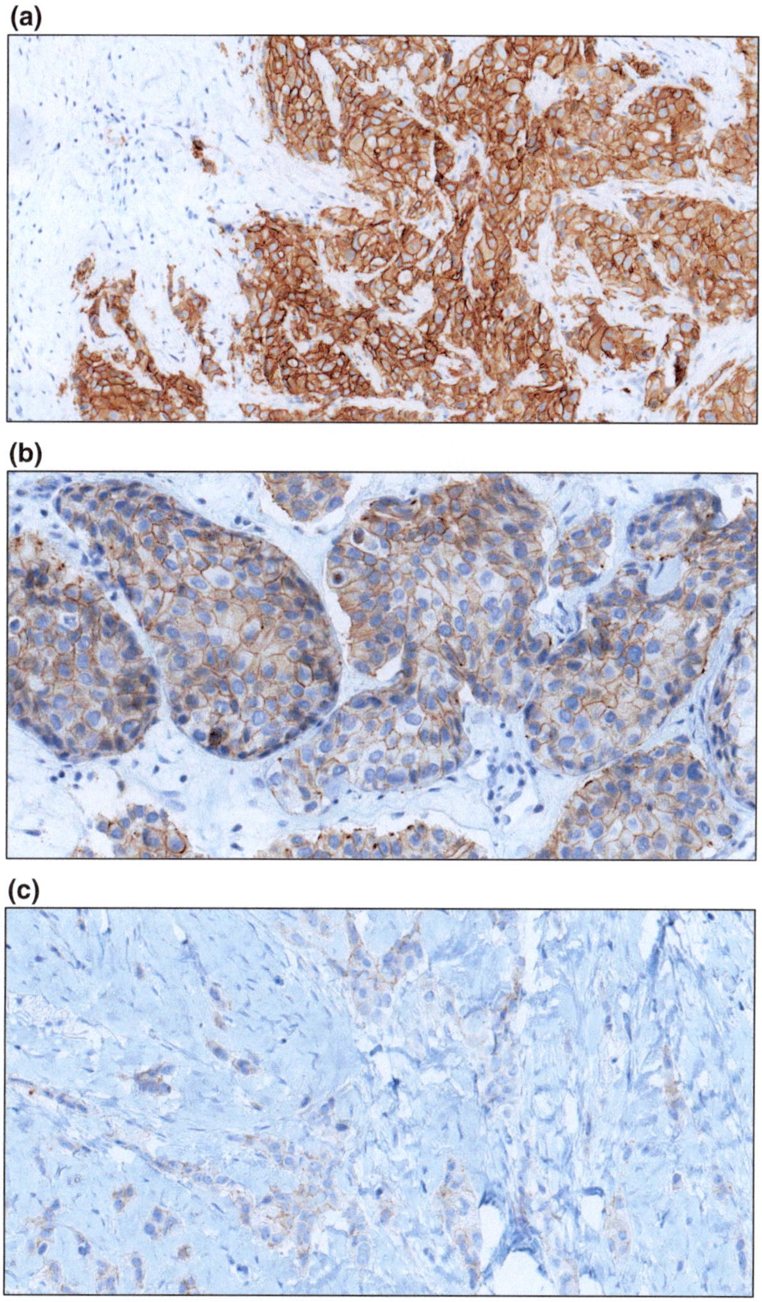

Fig. 3.2 Examples of immunohistochemical demonstration of HER2 protein expression in invasive breast cancer. **a** HER2 3+ (×10 magnification); **b** HER2 2 +; **c** HER2 1+ (× 20 magnification). Images courtesy of G Baenfer, Targos GMBH

preanalytical, analytical information as well as the morphological diagnosis, HER2 and hormone receptor status and scores when positive staining has been recorded. The adoption of a standard template for reporting is also emphasized in the 'Ontario' guidelines for hormone receptor assessment (Nofech-Mozes et al. 2012) and this should provide the clinical oncologist with consistent information on which he/she can make a decision on treatment.

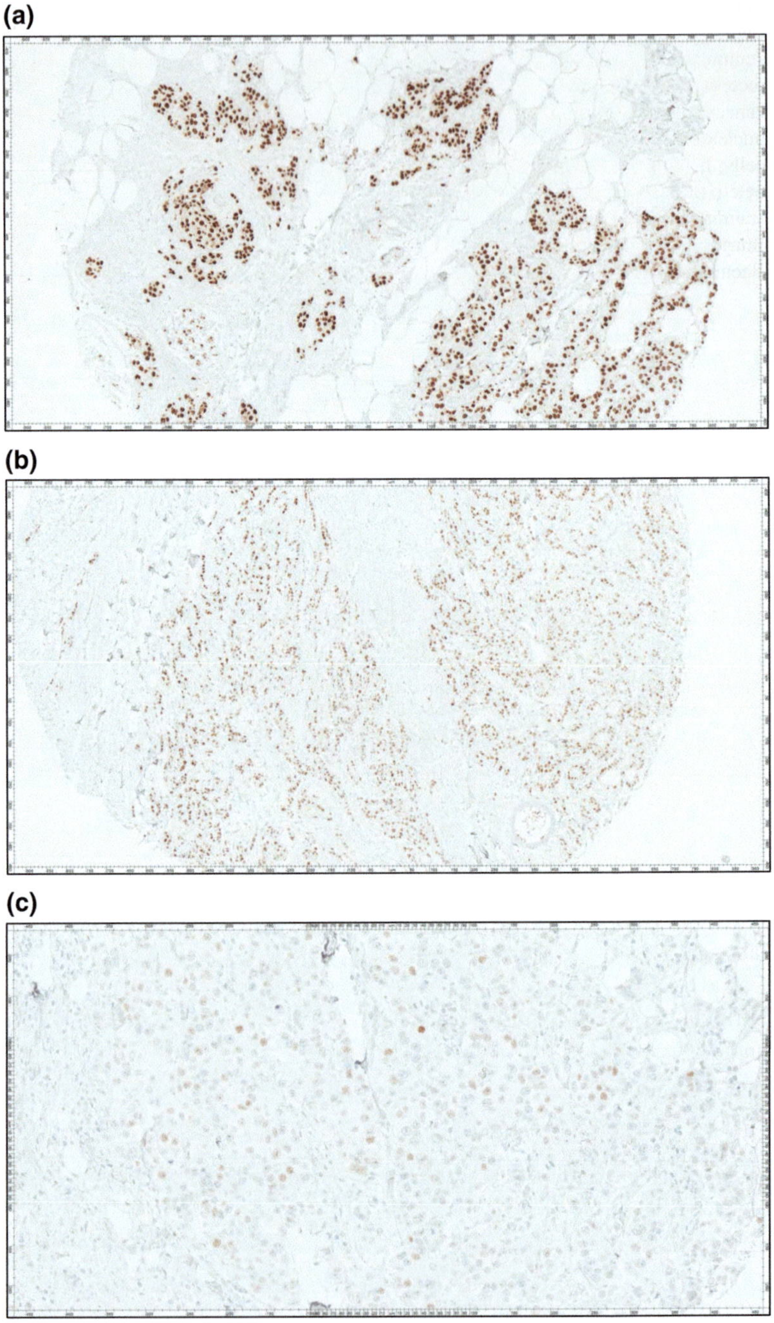

Fig. 3.3 Examples of immunohistochemical staining for estrogen receptor in invasive breast cancer. **a** Strong uniform nuclear staining. **b** Medium uniform nuclear staining. **C** Weak nuclear staining of occasional cells within the tumour. Images courtesy of G Baenfer, Targos GMBH

3.4.3 Quality Assurance

Quality assurance (QA) includes quality control (see analytical step), but as a component of a larger system of checks and balances that confirm that a testing laboratory is operating in a manner confirming it is able to provide results that are consistent and reliable. The necessity for external verification of the meeting of QA standards was emphasized by the discovery of a 39.1 % false negative rate for hormone receptor staining recorded in centralized testing

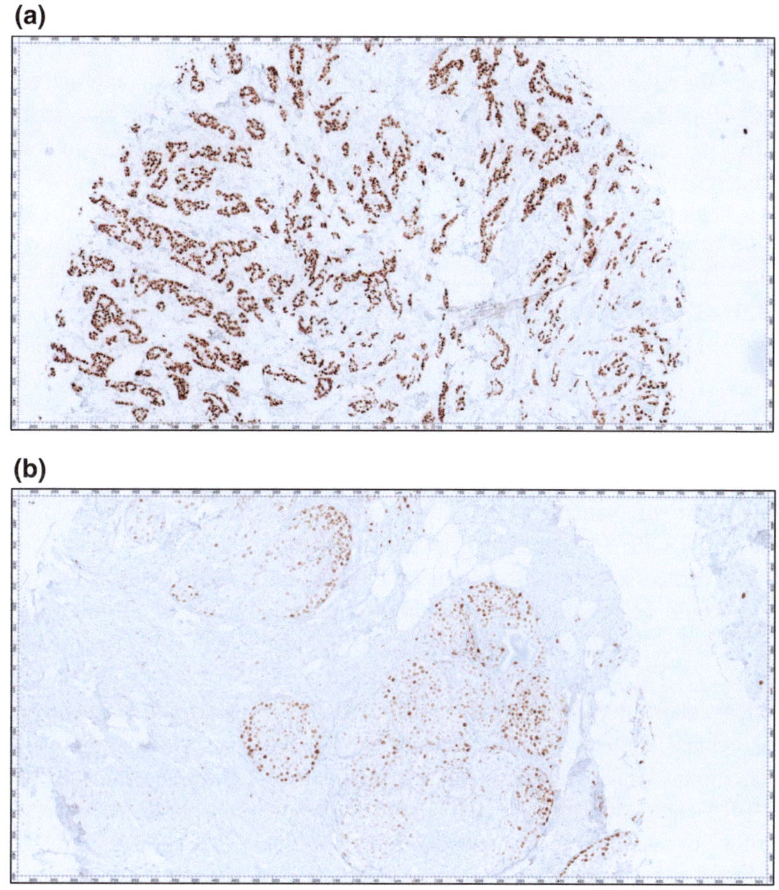

Fig. 3.4 Examples of immunohistochemical staining for progesterone receptor in invasive breast cancer. **a** Strong uniform nuclear staining of tumour cells; **b** strong heterogeneous nuclear staining of tumor cells. Images courtesy of G Baenfer, Targos GMBH

laboratories in Newfoundland and Labrador in Canada over the period of 1997–2005. This was attributed to preanalytical, analytical and post-analytical issues that were compounded by the presence of general laboratory deficiencies (Gregory and Parfrey 2010).

As highlighted by Hammond et al. (2010) and Wolff et al. (2014) QA must include accreditation of the laboratory as a whole; i.e., facilities; staff training, equipment validation and the use of up-to-date standard operating procedures, together with participation of the testing laboratory in external quality assessment schemes. The latter is also emphasized as an essential requirement for undertaking HER2 status testing in the UK guidelines (Rakha et al. 2015). Indeed, when it is considered that laboratories offering this service in the UK must be accredited to ISO 15189 (www.iso.org/iso/catalogue_detail?csnumber=56115) then the wider context of QA is implicitly included in these guidelines.

External QA, as exemplified by the UK NEQAS, Nordic QA and equivalent US/Canadian schemes for HER2 and hormone receptor ICC (UK; http://www.ukneqasiccish.org/ Nordic; http://www.nordiqc.org/ US; http://www.cap.org/) involve the regular circulation of slides for staining in participating laboratories. These are then returned and reviewed by an expert panel of assessors and given a rating. Individual feedback is then provided to the participating laboratory together with summary information on the QA run that includes valuable information on the overall performance of all participating laboratories. This information covers such items as the type of pretreatments used, antibody clones and use of automated platforms. With this information, a participating laboratory may consider the need to revise current testing protocols. If a laboratory fails to attain the pass score for a run then steps must be taken to rectify this situation and, in the case of a repeated failure, the laboratory can be prevented from undertaking further testing until remedial action has been taken and shown to be successful.

3.5 Conclusions and Future Directions

Precision medicine for breast cancer is here and here to stay. For hormone receptor status a debate continues as to whether this is important for the treatment of patients with ductal carcinoma in situ (DCIS) (Allred 2010). In terms of laboratory processes, the assessment of DCIS samples could be accommodated without alteration of existing guidelines. Intriguingly Borgquist et al. (2015) have recently demonstrated in a large cohort study that HER2 positive DCIS is associated with lower rate of recurrent invasive carcinoma. Thus, the potential of assessment of HER2 expression as a positive prognostic indicator in cases of DCIS may become a future laboratory protocol.

It is becoming apparent that at the molecular level breast cancer is complex (Blows et al. 2010; Simpson et al. 2005) and it is possible that in the future therapeutic decisions could be made on the basis of nucleic acid based molecular profiling and/or IHC/ISH for new prognostic and predictive biomarkers (Patani et al. 2013). Prototypically this has been shown by the commercially available RNA expression based Oncotype DX (http://www.oncotypedx.com/) and MammaPrint (http://www.agendia.com/) panels that include assessment of HER2 and hormone receptor gene expression together with the expression of many other genes. In a comparative study of hormone receptor expression using Oncotype DX and IHC receptor status the latter was shown to be more sensitive (Kraus et al. 2012). The same was apparently also found to be true for the estimation of the HER2 status (Dabbs et al. 2011). Importantly, additional factors that include the speed of test turnaround, its lower cost and the presence of morphology when using IHC also favor the use of this assay in a routine setting.

As an alternative to homogenate molecular assays, the assessment of mRNA expression by ISH has been demonstrated for HER2 using the extremely sensitive branched DNA methodology (Wang et al. 2013). If, as suggested by the authors, this technology is effective in clarifying HER2 expression in equivocal cases then its speed and presence of morphology could make it a worthwhile adjunct to current laboratory assessment using IHC.

If new biomarkers and alternative readout technologies are to be introduced then one further hurdle has to be overcome. This relates to the demonstration of benefit in large clinical cohorts (Lee et al. 2013; Nofech-Mozes et al. 2012) that is used as a safeguard for the reliability of current procedures. What the alternative route or routes are to refining existing procedures and validating new molecular panels for use in precision medicine is not readily apparent. One suggestion could be to adopt 90 % agreement for positive results and 95 % agreement for negative results in the same way as recommended for the validation of 'in house antibody testing' an alternative to use of a regulatory approved antibody clone for hormone receptor staining (Fitzgibbons et al. 2010).

If this validation criterion were adopted then a move away from semi-quantitative scoring to the application of quantitative and automated image analysis might be more readily accepted. At present the application of this technology hangs in the balance, due to 'insufficient evidence for … routine use' being available (Rakha et al. 2015). Algorithms have been described for HER2 and hormone receptor IHC image analysis (Chung et al. 2007; Skaland et al. 2008). For the development of algorithms for HER2 ISH, where only well preserved and nonoverlapping nuclei can be counted and the presentation of signal can be complex, more work may be required. However, it is likely that image analysis will replace the use of manual semi-quantitative assessment in the short to medium term.

The introduction of laboratory methods to assess HER2 expression and hormone receptor status in breast cancer has pioneered the involvement of the cellular pathology in precision medicine. It is probable that as underlying molecular basis of the disease is better understood and more closely coupled to specific treatment, this could lead to the introduction of tests for new molecular targets. These developments would directly benefit the patient by providing more precise and reliable information regarding the diagnosis, prognosis and treatment responsiveness or resistance of the breast cancer to therapy.

Box 1 Semiquantitative Scoring Methods for Immunohistochemical Assessment of Staining

H score: This is based on the counting of nuclear staining intensities in a population of 100 tumour cells. For weak staining each cell is counted as 1, for moderate staining 2 and for strong staining 3. Once this has been completed a cumulative score, between 1 and 300 is produced. For example, if in a population of 100 cells, 20 stained at weak intensity the sum is 20, if an additional 20 cells are stained at moderate intensity the sum is 40 (20×2) and if 10 cells are stained at strong intensity the sum is 30 (10×3). In this example the final H score is 90.

Allred score: This is based on the estimation of the percentage of stained tumor cells across the whole of the preparation under microscopic examination. The percentage of cells that are stained is estimated as either 1 = <1 %; 2 = 5–10 %; 3 = 11–33 %; 4 = 34–66 %; 5 = $\geq$67 % and average intensity as either 1 for weak, 2 for moderate or 3 for strong staining across the tumor. The score is arrived at by adding the percentage score and intensity score together giving a final score between 0 and 8.

Quickscore: This is similar to the Allred scoring system, but the final score is a multiplication of the percentage and intensity of staining. The percentage of cells that are stained is estimated as either 1 = 0–4 %; 2 = 5–19 %; 3 = 20–39 %; 4 = 40–59 %; 5 = 60–79 %; 6 = 80–100 % and intensity as either 1 for weak, 2 for moderate or 3 for strong staining across the tumor. The score is arrived at by multiplying the percentage score and intensity score together giving a final score between 0 and 18.

References

Allred DC, Harvey JM, Berardo M, Clark GM (1998) Prognostic and predictive factors in breast cancer by immunohistochemical analysis. Mod Pathol 11:155–168

Allred DC (2010) Issues and updates: evaluating estrogen receptor-a, progesterone receptor, and HER2 in breast cancer. Mod Pathol 23:S52–S59

Apple S, Pucci R, Lowe AC, Shintaku I, Shapourifar-Tehrani S, Moatamed N (2011) The effect of delay in fixation, different fixatives, and duration of fixation in estrogen and progesterone receptor results in breast carcinoma. Am J Clin Pathol 135:592–598

Atkin G, Daley FM, Bourne S, Glynne-Jones R, Northover J, Wilson GD (2006) The effect of surgically induced ischaemia on gene expression in a colorectal cancer xenograft model. Br J Cancer. 94:121–127

Baker AF, Dragovich T, Ihle NT, Williams R, Fenoglio-Preiser C, Powis G (2005) Stability of phosphoprotein as a biological marker of tumor signaling. Clin Cancer Res 11:4338–4340

Barnes DM, Harris WH, Smith P, Millis RR, Rubens RD (1996) Immunohistochemical determination of estrogen receptor: comparison of different methods of assessment of staining and correlation with clinical outcome of breast cancer patients. Br J Cancer 74:1445–1451

Bazell R (1998) HER-2: the making of herceptin, a revolutionary treatment for breast cancer. Random House, USA

Blows FM, Driver KE, Schmidt MK et al (2010) Subtyping of breast cancer by immunohistochemistry to investigate a relationship between subtype and short and long term survival: a collaborative analysis of data for 10,159 cases from 12 studies. PLoS Med 7: e1000279

Borgquist S, Zhou W, Jirström K et al (2015) The prognostic role of HER2 expression in ductal breast carcinoma in situ (DCIS); a population-based cohort study. BMC Cancer 15:468

Chung GG, Zerkowski MP, Ghosh S, Camp RL, Rimm DL (2007) Quantitative analysis of estrogen receptor heterogeneity in breast cancer. Lab Invest 87:662–669
Dabbs DJ, Bhargava R (2011) Fixation time does not affect the expression of estrogen receptor. Am J Clin Pathol 135:171–172; author reply 172
Dabbs DJ, Klein ME, Mohsin SK, Tubbs RR, Shuai Y, Bhargava R (2011) High false-negative rate of HER2 quantitative reverse transcription polymerase chain reaction of the Oncotype DX test: an independent quality assurance study. J Clin Oncol 29:4279–4285
Detre S, Saccani Jotti G, Dowsett M (1995) A "quick-score" method for immunohistochemical semiquantitation: validation for estrogen receptor in breast carcinomas. J Clin Pathol 48:876–878
Figueroa-Magalhães MC, Jelovac D, Connolly RM, Wolff AC (2014) Treatment of HER2-positive breast cancer. Breast 23:128–136
Fitzgibbons PL, Murphy DA, Hammond ME, Allred DC, Valenstein PN (2010) Recommendations for validating estrogen and progesterone receptor immunohistochemistry assays. Arch Pathol Lab Med 134:930–935
Geisler J (2008) Aromatase inhibitors: from bench to bedside and back. Breast Cancer 15:17–26
Gregory DM, Parfrey PS (2010) The breast cancer hormone receptor retesting controversy in Newfoundland and Labrador, Canada: lessons for the health system. Healthc Manage Forum 23:114–118
Gruver AM, Peerwani Z, Tubbs RR (2010) Out of the darkness and into the light: bright field in situ hybridisation for delineation of ERBB2 (HER2) status in breast carcinoma. J Clin Pathol 63:210–219
Hähnel R, Twaddle E (1973) Estimation of the association constant of the estrogen-receptor complex in human breast cancer. Cancer Res 33:559–566
Hammond ME, Hayes DF, Dowsett M et al (2010) American Society of Clinical Oncology/College of American Pathologists guideline recommendations for immunohistochemical testing of estrogen and progesterone receptors in breast cancer (unabridged version). Arch Pathol Lab Med 134:48–72
Harvey JM, Clark GM, Osborne CK, Allred DC (1999) Estrogen receptor status by immunohistochemistry is superior to the ligand-binding assay for predicting response to adjuvant endocrine therapy in breast cancer. J Clin Oncol 17:1474–1481
Howat WJ, Lewis A, Jones P et al (2014) Antibody validation of immunohistochemistry for biomarker discovery: recommendations of a consortium of academic and pharmaceutical based histopathology researchers. Methods 70:34–38
Ibarra JA, Rogers LW (2010) Fixation time does not affect expression of HER2/neu a pilot study. Am J Clin Pathol 134:594–596
Ibarra JA, Rogers LW, Kyshtoobayeva A, Bloom K (2010) Fixation time does not affect the expression of estrogen receptor. Am J Clin Pathol 133:747–755
Jasani B, Reid V, Tristram C et al (2010) Standard reference material: cell lines development and use of reference cell lines as standards for external quality assurance of HER2 IHC and ISH Testing. In: Taylor C, Shi S (eds) Antigen retrieval immunohistochemistry based research and diagnostics, 1st edn. Hobeken, NJ, Wiley-Blackwell, pp 101–122
Jordan VC (2006) Tamoxifen (ICI46,474) as a targeted therapy to treat and prevent breast cancer. Br J Pharmacol 147(Suppl 1):S269–S276
Kalkman S, Barentsz MW, van Diest PJ (2014) The effects of under 6 hours of formalin fixation on hormone receptor and HER2 expression in invasive breast cancer: a systematic review. Am J Clin Pathol 142:16–22
Khoury T, Sait S, Hwang H et al (2009) Delay to formalin fixation effect on breast biomarkers. Mod Pathol 22:1457–1467
Kosa C, Kardos L, Kovacs J, Szollosi Z (2013) Comparison of dual-color dual-hapten brightfield in situ hybridization (DDISH) and fluorescence in situ hybridization in breast cancer HER2 assessment. Pathol Res Pract 209:147–150
Kraus JA, Dabbs DJ, Beriwal S, Bhargava R (2012) Semi-quantitative immunohistochemical assay versus oncotype DXs qRT-PCR assay for estrogen and progesterone receptors: an independent quality assurance study. Mod Pathol 25:869–876
Leclercq G, Heuson JC, Schoenfeld R, Mattheiem WH, Tagnon HJ (1973) Estrogen receptors in human breast cancer. Eur J Cancer 9:665–673
Lee M, Lee CS, Tan PH (2013) Hormone receptor expression in breast cancer: postanalytical issues. J Clin Pathol 66:478–484
Love RR, Philips J (2002) Oophorectomy for breast cancer: history revisited. J Natl Cancer Inst 94:1433–1434
McCarty KS Jr, Szabo E, Flowers JL et al (1986) Use of a monoclonal anti-estrogen receptor antibody in the immunohistochemical evaluation of human tumors. Cancer Res 46(Suppl):4244s–4248s
Moatamed NA, Nanjangud G, Pucci R et al (2011) Effect of ischemic time, fixation time, and fixative type on HER2/neu immunohistochemical and fluorescence In situ hybridization results in breast cancer. Am J Clin Pathol 136:754–761
Mollerup J, Henriksen U, Müller S, Schønau A (2012) Dual color chromogenic in situ hybridization for determination of HER2 status in breast cancer: a large comparative study to current state of the art fluorescence in situ hybridization. BMC Clin Pathol 14(12):3
Nofech-Mozes S, Vella ET, Dhesy-Thind S, Hanna WM (2012) Cancer care Ontario guideline recommendations for hormone receptor testing in breast cancer. Clin Oncol 24:684–696
Patani N, Martin L-A, Dowsett M (2013) Biomarkers for the clinical management of breast cancer: international perspective. Int J Cancer 133:1–13

Penault-Llorca F, Bilous M, Dowsett M et al (2009) Emerging technologies for assessing HER2 amplification. Am J Clin Pathol 132:539–548

Portier BP, Wang Z, Downs-Kelly E et al (2013) Delay to formalin fixation 'cold ischemia time': effect on ERBB2 detection by in-situ hybridization and immunohistochemistry. Mod Pathol 26:1–9

Rakha EA, Pinder SE, Bartlett JM et al (2015) Updated UK Recommendations for HER2 assessment in breast cancer. J Clin Pathol 68:93–99

Rhodes A, Jasani B, Couturier J et al (2002a) A formalin-fixed, paraffin-processed cell line standard for quality control of immunohistochemical assay of HER-2/neu expression in breast cancer. Am J Clin Pathol 117:81–89

Rhodes A, Jasani B, Anderson E, Dodson AR, Balaton AJ (2002b) Evaluation of HER-2/neu immunohistochemical assay sensitivity and scoring on formalin-fixed and paraffin-processed cell lines and breast tumors: a comparative study involving results from laboratories in 21 countries. Am J Clin Pathol 118:408–417

Simpson PT, Reis-Filho JS, Gale T, Lakhani SR (2005) Molecular evolution of breast cancer. J Pathol. 205:248–254

Skaland I, Øvestad I, Janssen EA et al (2008) Comparing subjective and digital image analysis HER2/neu expression scores with conventional and modified FISH scores in breast cancer. J Clin Pathol 61:68–71

Smith NR, Womack C (2014) A matrix approach to guide IHC-based tissue biomarker development in oncology drug discovery. J Pathol. 232:190–198

Stockwell S (1983) Classics in oncology. George Thomas Beatson, M.D. (1848-1933). CA Cancer J Clin 33:105–121

Taylor CR (2014) Predictive biomarkers and companion diagnostics. The future of immunohistochemistry: "in situ proteomics," or just a "stain"? Appl Immunohistochem Mol Morphol 22:555–561

Uy GB, Laudico AV, Carnate JM Jr et al (2010) Breast cancer hormone receptor assay results of core needle biopsy and modified radical mastectomy specimens from the same patients. Clin Breast Cancer 10:154–159

Wang S, Saboorian MH, Frenkel E, Hynan L, Gokaslan ST, Ashfaq R (2000) Laboratory assessment of the status of Her-2/neu protein and oncogene in breast cancer specimens: comparison of immunohistochemistry assay with fluorescence in situ hybridisation assays. J Clin Pathol 53:374–381

Wang Z, Portier BP, Gruver AM et al (2013) Automated quantitative RNA in situ hybridization for resolution of equivocal and heterogeneous ERBB2 (HER2) status in invasive breast carcinoma. J Mol Diagn. 15:210–219

Warford A, Akbar H, Riberio D (2014) Antigen retrieval, blocking, detection and visualisation systems in immunohistochemistry: a review and practical evaluation of tyramide and rolling circle amplification systems. Methods 70:28–33

Warford A. (2016) In situ hybridisation: technologies and their application to understanding disease. Prog Histochem Cytochem 50:37–48

Wolff AC, Hammond ME, Hicks DG et al (2014) Recommendations for human epidermal growth factor receptor 2 testing in breast cancer: American Society of Clinical Oncology/College of American Pathologists clinical practice guideline update. Arch Pathol Lab Med 138:241–256

4 Hormone Receptors in Breast Cancer

K.P.M. Suijkerbuijk, E. van der Wall and P.J. van Diest

Abstract

Steroid hormone receptors are critical for the growth and development of breast tissue as well as of breast cancer. The importance of the role estrogens in breast cancer has been delineated for more than 100 years. The analysis of its expression has been used not only to classify breast cancers but also for treating patients. The expression of ER and PR in tumors is associated with better prognosis and sensitivity to endocrine therapy. In this chapter we discuss the role of these receptors in addition to androgen receptor (AR) in breast cancer. A brief overview of the structure and function of these receptors and methods to detect their presence in breast cancer is presented. This includes criteria for scoring positivity and national and international guidelines associated with the scoring. Lastly, data regarding the use of expression of AR as therapeutic target, particularly in triple negative cancers, is presented.

Keywords

Estrogen · Progesterone and androgen receptors · Scoring · ASCO-CAP · Endocrine therapy

4.1 Introduction

In 1896, Beatson reported unexpected tumor responses in women with locally advanced breast cancer that underwent oophorectomy (Beatson 1896). Subsequent studies using other forms of endocrine therapy confirmed this finding and demonstrated the tremendous value of this treatment modality for the majority of breast cancer patients with hormone receptor–positive disease. The introduction of endocrine therapy, which should probably be regarded as the oldest

K.P.M. Suijkerbuijk · E. van der Wall · P.J. van Diest
Departments of Medical Oncology and Pathology, University Medical Center Utrecht, Utrecht, The Netherlands

P.J. van Diest (✉)
Department of Pathology, University Medical Center Utrecht, PO Box 85500, 3508 GA Utrecht, The Netherlands
e-mail: p.j.vandiest@umcutrecht.nl

S. Badve and Y. Gökmen-Polar (eds.), *Molecular Pathology of Breast Cancer*, DOI 10.1007/978-3-319-41761-5_4

form of targeted therapy, has tremendously changed the prognosis of breast cancer patients. Largely depending on the clinical situation (premenopausal or postmenopausal; adjuvant or palliative setting), different forms of endocrine therapy are nowadays used, either in combination or monotherapy:

- Surgical ablation of estrogen-producing organs or medical ablation of the pituitary gland
- Selective estrogen receptor modulators (e.g.,. tamoxifen) or downregulators (e.g., fulvestrant)
- Aromatase inhibitors, nonsteroidal: e.g., anastrozole and letrozole; steroidal: e.g., exemestane
- Progestins, e.g., megesterolacetate

Endocrine therapy is now the most widely applied form of systemic therapy for hormone-sensitive breast cancer and one of the cornerstones of breast cancer treatment in this category. With the increasing knowledge on molecular biology of the disease grew the perception that the therapy needed its target in the tumor, which initiated research into the assessment of hormone receptors in breast cancer tissue. For women with estrogen receptor (ER) positive breast cancer, 5 years tamoxifen treatment has convincingly shown to reduce breast cancer mortality with more than 30 % (Early Breast Cancer Trialists' Collaborative 2005) with an additional benefit only recently shown in high-risk women if its use is extended to 10 years (Davies et al. 2013; Gray 2013). The importance of hormone receptor assessment has initially however been disputed (Barnes et al. 1989), and methods have evolved over the last decades.

4.2 Hormone Receptor Assessment-A Historical View

Methods to measure ER content were introduced in the late 1970s (Dowsett 2006; Jensen 1981). This was especially instigated by the fact that early endocrine treatment was mainly surgical (oophorectomy, adrenalectomy, hypophysectomy) or used native hormones (estrogens and androgens) with significant side effects. Identifying patients with hormone receptor negative tumors thereby bearing a low rate of response would prevent ineffective treatments such as surgery or the administration of pure hormones.

With the development of new drugs like tamoxifen and aromatase inhibitors, which are relatively nontoxic, estrogens and androgens and major ablative surgery fell largely into disuse, and the need for testing hormone receptors shifted from negative to positive predictive value.

From the 1970s to the early 1990s, assays were based on ligand-binding involving incubation with radioactively labeled estradiol of centrifuged cytosol of a homogenized fresh-frozen piece of tumor. Receptor-bound estradiol was usually separated from the unbound fraction with a suspension of dextran-coated charcoal (DCC) that adsorbed the unbound estradiol (Dowsett 2006; Feherty et al. 1971). DCC based methods had the major disadvantage of blindly using a piece of tumor that had unknown tumor content, and frozen material was clearly not always available (King et al. 1985). Further, DCC measured both ERα and ERß (see below). When monoclonal antibodies to ER and the progesterone receptor (PR) became available, the enzyme immunoassay (EIA) was developed as a more precise and less labor-intensive alternative to the DCC (Dowsett 2006), which was specific for ERα. These antibodies also allowed immunohistochemical (IHC) assays on frozen tissue sections, allowing for assessment of tumor content (Andersen et al. 1986), and shifting hormone receptor assessment from clinical chemistry to pathology. ER IHC has been shown to be more accurate in predicting response to endocrine therapy than the ligand-binding assays (Harvey et al. 1999). The breakthrough came with the development of monoclonal antibodies that worked well on paraffin sections after antigen retrieval and allowed ER and PR assessment on regular diagnostic paraffin material. This has now been the standard for many years, with antibodies and staining protocols of ever increasing quality.

Interestingly, there was initially considerable skepticism as to the value of hormone receptor assessment. A historical "Point of view" by several renowned experts in the Lancet concluded that "Appropriate decisions about the management of early and advanced breast cancer can be made without knowledge of the receptor status of the primary tumor. There is no essential role for steroid receptor measurements in the routine management of breast cancer … receptor measurements are not justified in the routine evaluation of patients with breast cancer" (Barnes et al. 1989).

Clearly, we now think differently, and ER and PR testing have an essential and established role in predicting the likelihood of breast cancer patients responding to endocrine therapy, and are recognized prognostic factors. In the following, we will discuss several issue of hormone receptor assessment in breast cancer, with focus on predictive rather than prognostic value.

4.3 General Principles of Hormone Receptor Testing and Standardization of Methodology

It has been estimated that about 20 % of ER and PR testing worldwide is inaccurate (Hammond et al. 2010), although there is a clear issue of a lacking gold standard. Often, "inaccurate" is defined as deviant from the value obtained in a (sometimes self-acclaimed) reference lab. Clinical response to hormonal therapy would be a better gold standard, but this is in practice difficult to realize. False positivity and false negativity can be due to preanalytic, analytic and postanalytic variables, or a combination of those, that need to be standardized for reliable hormone receptor assessment. The following recommendations have been made by the American Society of Clinical Oncology (ASCO) and College of American Pathologists CAP (Hammond et al. 2010).

Reports on hormone receptor status should at least include the percentage of tumor cells with positively staining nuclei, the intensity of the staining relative to the positive control and interpretation of the assay (either positive, negative, or uninterpretable). In order to minimize the influence of cold ischemic time on the assay, efforts should be made to keep the time from biopsy or excision to fixation as short as possible, but no longer than one hour, in the meanwhile keeping specimens cooled. The ASCO/CAP guideline advices fixation in 10 % neutral buffered formaldehyde for 6–72 h for both core needle biopsies (CNB) and resections. However, same day diagnosis has become a trend necessitating much shorter fixation (Barentsz et al. 2014). Fortunately, brief fixation (up to 45 min) does not seem to influence analysis of hormone receptor expression in CNB when compared to conventionally fixed resection specimens of the same tumor (Kalkman et al. 2014).

Although a gold standard is not available, assays are strongly advised to be tested against a clinically validated assay requiring 90 % concordance for ER/PR positivity and 95 % concordance for ER/PR negativity. The use of an internal control (normal epithelial cells) and external positive, negative and variable level positive controls is essential. Obviously, doubt about any of the controls precludes reporting of the results and necessitates repeating of the assay. Participation in regular external Quality Assessment programs (like UK-NEQAS and NordiQC) and quality accreditation of the laboratory are important for safeguarding the validity of the assays.

Scoring of nuclear positivity of hormone receptors is generally done subjectively by eyeballing of a pathologist. A study in nonpalpable breast tumors showed a high interobserver agreement for hormone receptor status when assessed by a routine and expert pathologist. In this study ER and PR discordance was found in only 1 and 2 % of cases, respectively (Postma et al. 2013). Similar concordance rates of 1 and 6 %, respectively, were found in a recent study (Dekker et al. 2015). Indeed, the vast majority of cases are clearly positive or completely negative, inherently leading to high concordance percentages. Problems, however, may arise in cases around the decision threshold. Other studies indeed showed larger differences with interobserver discrepancies in 3–5 % for ER and 12–18 % to for PR (Bueno-de-Mesquita et al. 2010; Viale et al. 2007) when comparing local and central review. Nevertheless, visual scoring is inevitably liable to observer variation, which is relevant in cases close to the threshold. Image analysis may help here, as discussed below.

Generally, hormone receptor score is expressed as a percentage of positive nuclei, irrespective of the intensity of staining (Hammond et al. 2010). Alternatively, scoring systems incorporating both percentage and intensity of staining have been promoted like the Allred score and the H score (Hammond et al. 2010). The Allred score sums up an estimated proportion score on a scale of 0–5 with an intensity score of 0–3, resulting in a dynamic range from 0 to 8. The H score provides an overall score from 0 to 300 based on the sum of ordinal weighted percentiles of cells stained weak, moderate, and strong. These scoring systems do not seem to have clear advantages over the mere percentage of positivity (Hammond et al. 2010).

Although hormone receptor assessment of a full section through the equator of the tumor in the resection specimen probably provides the best overview of staining and its heterogeneity, assessment of CNB is required when neoadjuvant or heat ablation therapy will be applied. For ER status, high concordance rates ranging from 95 to 98 % have been reported when comparing assessment in CNB and excision specimens. Concordance rates for PR are significantly lower and in the range of 85–90 % (Arnedos et al. 2009; Burge et al. 2006; Motamedolshariati et al. 2014; Tamaki et al. 2010).

In case of multiple synchronous tumors, the ASCO/CAP guidelines advise to test at least on one of the tumors, preferably the largest (Hammond et al. 2010). However, multiple primary tumors by definition differ in their genetic makeup and thereby potentially in their receptor status. Since it is unpredictable which tumor may metastasize, we prefer to test all primary tumors irrespective of size, where any hormone receptor positivity sets the indication for adjuvant hormonal therapy.

4.4 The Estrogen Receptor

4.4.1 Variants

There are two major variants of the estrogen receptor (ER), ERα and ERß. Most knowledge has been obtained on ERα. ERα is encoded by the *ESR1* gene located on the long arm of chromosome 6, while ERß is encoded by *ESR2* on chromosome 14. Although encoded by separate genes, there is a high degree of homology between ERα and ERß. ERα and ERß both consist of six domains. The A/B region located at the N-terminus of the protein plays a crucial role in ligand-independent transactivation through the AF1 domain. The C-domain encompasses the DNA Binding Domain. The hinge region in the D-domain connects the C- and E-domain. The E-domain functions as the ligand binding cavity and a binding site for coactivators and corepressors. The C-terminal F-domain has a function in ligand binding and transactivation. Upon activation by a ligand such as estrogen, the ER subunits dimerize and can function as a transcription factor, translocate into the nucleus and bind to estrogen responsive elements (EREs) in the promoters of genes. Thereby, ER can directly regulate transcription of that gene. Besides the canonical mechanism shared with other steroid hormones, E2 also modulates gene expression by a second indirect mechanism that involves the interaction of ER with other transcription factors such as the activator protein-1, nuclear factor-κB and stimulating protein-1 by stabilizing DNA protein complexes and/or recruiting coactivators and a variety of signal transduction pathways such as ERK/MAPK, p38/MAPK, PI3K/AKT, PLC/PKC (Marino et al. 2006). Lastly, the function of ER is controlled by a number of genes that are referred to as co-activators, co-repressors (Shibata et al. 1997) and pioneer factors (Nakshatri and Badve 2007; Jozwik and Carroll 2012) (Fig. 4.1).

Numerous ERα and ERβ splice variants have been identified (Wimberly et al. 2014; Taylor et al. 2010), but their clinical significance has not been fully elucidated.

4.4.2 Definition of Positivity

There is no worldwide consensus on the percentage of nuclei that need to show expression for a tumor to be called hormone receptor positive. The ASCO/CAP guidelines prescribe a 1 % threshold (Hammond et al. 2010), while many European countries use a 10 % threshold. Solid

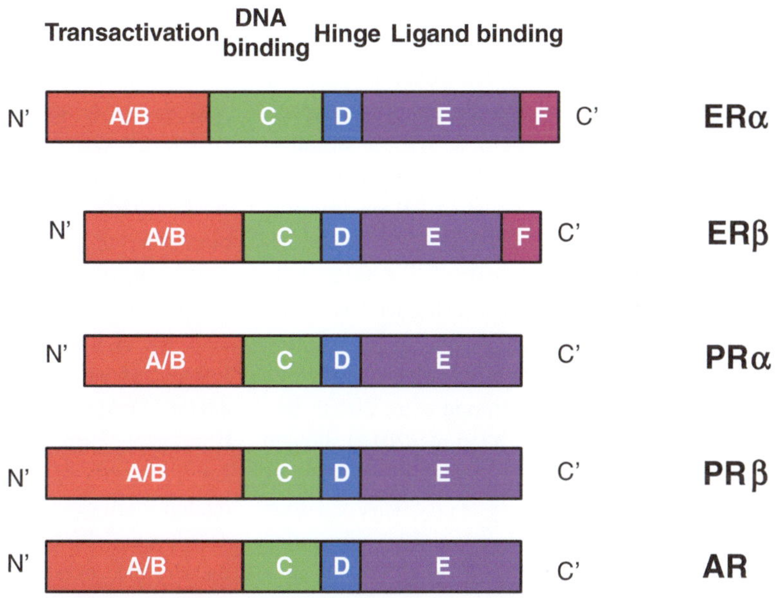

Fig. 4.1 Gene structures of ERalpha, ERbeta, PRalpha, PRbeta, and AR. All genes have a homologous structure with a transactivation domain, a DNA binding domain, a hinge region, and a ligand binding domain

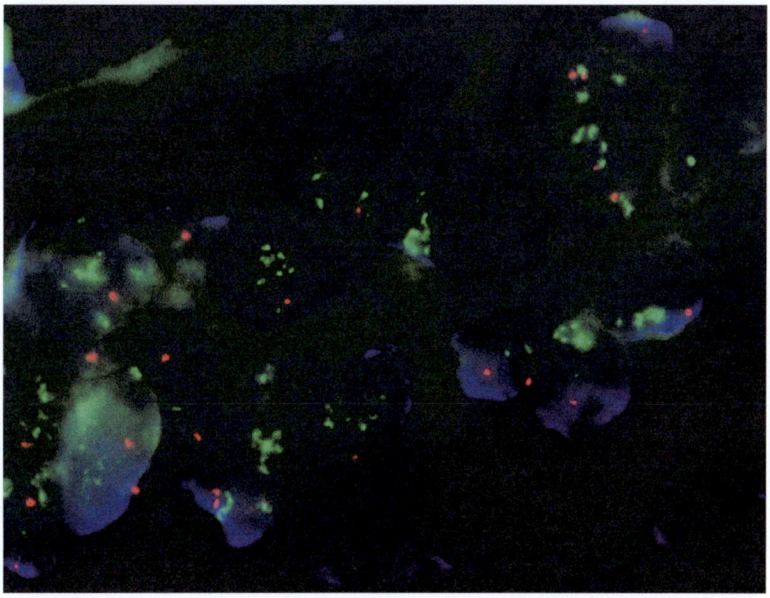

Fig. 4.2 ERalpha amplification of an invasive breast cancer. The ERalpha probe shows multiple copies in *green*, while the control probe shows 1–2 copies per nucleus in *red*

evidence on response rates on endocrine therapy for women with breast tumors showing 1–10 % ER positivity is largely lacking. Using a 1 % threshold, approximately 70 % of primary breast cancer are ER positive (Harvey et al. 1999). Tumors with no more than 1 % positively staining tumor cells show significant response to endocrine therapy (Hammond et al. 2010). Also taking into account the relatively favorable response toxicity profile of these drugs, this has led to the ASCO/CAP recommendation to consider endocrine therapy in patients whose breast tumors exhibit at least 1 % ER positive cells. The question here is whether poor fixation of specimens has played a role here, and 10 % would in fact be a better threshold for well-fixed specimens. Nevertheless, the level of ER positivity is an important predictor of response to endocrine therapy as well as a prognosticator. Patients with higher ER levels experience a higher likelihood of response to endocrine therapy, longer duration of response and consequently longer disease free and overall survival (Hammond et al. 2010). In a large retrospective study, Yi et al. (2014) showed that patients with tumors displaying 1–9 % ER positivity had significantly worse survival than patients with ER ≥10 % positivity, suggesting that tumors with 1–9 % ER positivity behave more like ER negative tumors. Nevertheless, based on expression and survival data a proportion of the 1–9 % ER positive breast cancer patients is thought to benefit from endocrine therapy (Iwamoto et al. 2012). Therefore, treating physicians are advised to weigh toxicity and expected benefit of endocrine therapy, especially in patients with 1–10 % ER positivity and discuss this with their patients. A large meta-analysis confirmed the absence clinical benefit from endocrine therapy for women with ER-negative breast tumors (Early Breast Cancer Trialists' Collaborative 2005). For tumors with less than 100 % positivity, negative nuclei are usually dispersed between the positive ones. However, tumors with completely negative areas do occur, probably reflecting ER negative subclones. The clinical significance of ER negative clones is largely unknown, although tumors with lower percentages of positive nuclei are more prone to receptor negative distant metastases (unpublished results). Obviously, negative (central) zones due to fixation artefacts must be excluded here.

4.4.3 Detection Methods

There are several antibodies on the market that have been clinically validated to assess expression of ERα by IHC. The ASCO/CAP guidelines mention the 6F11, SP1 and 1D5 antibodies. According to NordiQC, the latter has less affinity (http://www.nordiqc.org/Epitopes/ER/er.htm).

The presence of elastosis has been shown to be closely related to ERα positivity (Muresan et al. 1986), and is thereby a morphological biomarker of ERα positivity, useful for quality control, next to the normal mammary epithelium that should shows scattered positivity. The vast majority of lobular, mucinous, papillary, cribriform, tubular, ductulolobular and low grade ductal breast carcinomas are ERα positive. Contrarily, ERα positivity is found in only a small minority of metaplastic, medullary, *BRCA1* related, high grade ductal and salivary gland type carcinomas (Li et al. 2005). Histologic type is thereby also useful for ERα quality control.

ERα can also be determined on the mRNA level by individual assays or as part of a multigene expression assay with greater dynamic range (Hammond et al. 2010). The 21-gene *Oncotype* Dx assay includes ERα. However, comparison between ERα mRNA and protein expression and mRNA by PCR showed a discordance rate of 9 % (Hammond et al. 2010). So far, one study showed the clinical benefit of the individual measures of ERα mRNA from the 21-gene signature. However, the added clinical value over ERα IHC is not yet clear (Dowsett et al. 2015). The latter also holds true for TargetPrint, an expression array test for ERα, that does correlate well with ERα IHC (Roepman et al. 2009). mRNA tests are therefore not yet recommended over IHC, until it is more clear how IHC+/PCR− and IHC−/PCR+ cases behave clinically.

The impact of ERα amplification (Fig. 4.2) in breast cancer has been described for the first time by Holst et al. (2012) who claimed 36 % of breast cancers to be ERα amplified by FISH, with excellent prognosis and response to endocrine therapy. Further studies have either confirmed (Holst et al. 2012) or challenged (Thomas and Gustafsson 2011) that *ESR1* is frequently (low level) gained in breast cancer, related to different copy number enumeration methods and scoring criteria. Likely, the fact that hybridization of the FISH probe to *ESR1* premessenger RNA can result in aggregates of FISH signals which may be misinterpreted as amplification (Ooi et al. 2012). However, RNase treatment can impair FISH analysis by its DNA binding properties. A study comparing FISH with and without RNase treatment showed that 94.6 % of tumors with increased ESR1 gene copy numbers before RNase treatment retained increased ESR1 status after RNase treatment, and RNase eliminated eye catching fuzzy ESR1 clusters of ESR1 signals that made interpretation easier. There was frequent intratumor heterogeneity, so the influence of interobserver and intraobserver differences on ESR1 amplification assessment may be much greater than removal of premessenger RNA (Moelans et al. 2013).

ERß is widely expressed in normal breast as well as in breast tumors. While endocrine therapies mainly seem to target ERα, the clinical significance of ERß is less well known. In ERα negative, but not in ERα positive disease, ERß expression has been suggested to predict response to Tamoxifen (Gruvberger-Saal et al. 2007). ERß has not yet made it to routine assessment in breast cancer.

4.4.4 ER Mutations and Promoter Methylation

Mutations in the coding region of ER are very uncommon in primary tumors and do not account for many ER negative tumors (Roodi et al. 1995). Recently, data have linked the occurrence of *ESR1* mutations in breast cancer metastases to endocrine resistance in these tumors (Jeselsohn et al. 2015; Merenbakh-Lamin et al. 2013). These ESR1 mutations are found in the ligand-binding domain of *ESR1* and lead to a conformation change which mimics activated ligand-bound receptor and can therefore induce ligand-independent ER activity, resulting in tumor growth despite endocrine therapy. Breast tumors of women naïve for endocrine therapy do seem not harbor these mutations. These mutations may perhaps even be monitored in the blood (Sefrioui et al. 2015).

ER promoter methylation has been suggested as a mechanism of loss of ER expression. Methylation of the ER promoter is found in a proportion of the ER negative tumors (Lapidus et al. 1996) and in ER negative cells lines. The use of demethylating agents was shown to reactivate ER expression (Ferguson et al. 1995), which reveals a potential new strategy to overcome endocrine resistance in breast cancer patients. Besides from genetic and epigenetic alterations, posttranslational modifications play an important part in the complex process of ER inactivation in breast cancer (Barone et al. 2010).

4.5 The Progesterone Receptor

4.5.1 Variants

There are 2 variants of the PR, PRα and PRß, that are widely studied. Most knowledge has been obtained on PRα. Both PRα and PRß are encoded by the *PGR* gene located on chromosome 11. Similar to the ER, the PR has a regulatory domain located on the N-terminus, a DNA binding domain, a hinge region and a ligand binding domain at the C-terminus. Unlike PRα, PRß has an extra N-terminal domain called the B-upstream segment (BUS) containing a third transcription activation function (TAF3). TAF3 enables binding of other coactivators that efficiently bind with PRß, but not with PRα. This explains the distinct transactivation properties of PRα and PRß for different genes and in different cells.

Upon binding by progesterone, the PR dimerizes, can bind progesterone responsive elements (PRE) in the promoters of other genes and induce transcription of these genes.

4.5.2 Added Value to ERα

Although most current guidelines recommend PR measurement in all breast cancer patients, its clinical significance is still under debate. Studies questioning the additive value of PR testing over ERα testing for predicting response to endocrine therapy have shown conflicting results. Retrospective data from two large databases suggest that breast cancer patients that are ERα and PR positive benefit more from adjuvant endocrine therapy than ERα positive/PR negative patients (Bardou et al. 2003). On the other hand, a meta-analysis by the Early Breast Cancer Trialists' Collaborative Group (2005) showed that PR status does not add to ERα status in predicting response to Tamoxifen. Even more discussion remains for the ERα negative/PR positive subtype, hampered by the small subset of patients with this phenotype.

4.5.3 Definition of Positivity

Immunohistochemical PR expression ≥1 % is considered positive according to the ASCO/CAP guidelines, but most European countries apply a 10 % threshold for positivity, where similar issues apply as brought forward for ER above. There is even less evidence on the clinical significance of PR expression between 1 and 10 % than for ERα.

4.5.4 Detection Methods

Several antibodies are on the market that have been clinically validated. The ASCO/CAP guidelines mention clones 1294 and 312 (Hammond et al. 2010). According to NordiQC, clones 16, PgR 636 and rmAb clone 1E2 are recommended (http://www.nordiqc.org/Run-42-B18-H6/Assessment/Run_B18_PR.pdf).

Most of lobular, mucinous, papillary and tubular breast carcinomas are PR positive. Comedo and inflammatory tumors are found to be PR positive in only half of cases, while only the minority of medullary tumors of the breast display PR positivity (Li et al. 2005). Histologic type is thereby useful for PR quality control. An association between the presence of elastosis and PR positivity has been found (Muresan et al. 1986), so elastosis is also for PR a morphological biomarker useful for quality control.

As for ERα, for tumors with less than 100 % positivity, negative nuclei are usually dispersed between the positive ones. However, tumors with fully negative areas do occur, probably reflecting PR negative clones. The clinical significance of such PR negative clones is largely unknown, although tumors with lower percentages of positive nuclei are more prone to receptor negative distant metastases (unpublished results). Again, negative (central) zones due to fixation artefacts must be excluded here.

PRα can also be determined on the mRNA level by individual assays or as part of a multigene expression assay (Hammond et al. 2010). The 21-gene OncotypeDx assay includes PR. However, comparison between PR mRNA and protein expression and mRNA by PCR showed a discordance rate of 12 % (Hammond et al. 2010) and there is no evidence on the individual measures of PR mRNA from the 21-gene signature with clinical outcome. The latter also holds for TargetPrint, an expression array test for PR, that does correlate well with PR IHC (Roepman et al. 2009). mRNA test are therefore not recommended over IHC, as for ERα.

4.6 The Androgen Receptor

The androgen receptor (AR) is encoded by the AR gene, located on the X chromosome. AR can be activated by its ligands testosterone and dihydrotestosterone. Apart from its well-known role in developing and maintaining the male phenotype, AR also plays an important role in female fertility (Walters et al. 2010).

Like ER, ARs most well-known function is that of a transcription factor by binding Androgen Responsive Elements (ARE) in promoter regions of other genes. Insulin-like growth factor I receptor (IGF-1R) is one of its target genes. AR can also indirectly activate or inhibit other genes by recruiting other DNA-binding proteins. Lastly, AR has been shown to regulate signal transduction by interacting with signal transduction proteins in the cytoplasm of cells (Heinlein and Chang 2002).

Similarly to ER, AR is composed of 6 functional domains: the A/B regulatory domain at the N-terminus, the C-domain encompassing the DNA Binding Domain that is important for binding AREs, the hinge region in the D-domain, the E-domain important for ligand-binding and the F- C-terminal domain.

Splice variants of the AR have been identified in breast cancer (Hu et al. 2014). Recently, the presence of AR splice variant 7 (AR-V7), a variant lacking the binding domain, has been shown to be related to endocrine resistance in prostate cancer patients (Antonarakis et al. 2014).

In a large cohort of breast cancer patients, considering an AR percentage ≥1 % to be positive, 77 % of tumors showed AR expression (Collins et al. 2011). AR expression is seen across histological subtypes. Increased incidence of AR positivity is found in lobular carcinomas (96 %), mucinous carcinomas (81 %) and tubular carcinomas (Collins et al. 2011). Also apocrine cancers usually express AR. The ratio of nuclear AR to ER has been suggested to be a predictor of response to tamoxifen treatment: patients with a ratio ≥2 had an over 4 times increased risk for failure on tamoxifen (Cochrane et al. 2014). Furthermore, preclinical data suggest antitumor effect of enzalutamide, a potent antiandrogen, in AR positive breast cancer (Cochrane et al. 2014). Clinical studies investigating the clinical value of enzalutamide in this subgroup are currently ongoing, and are especially of interest in a subset of triple negative breast cancer (Lehmann et al. 2011).

4.7 Intrinsic Subtype and Hormone Receptor Expression

Hormone receptor expression clearly relates to the "intrinsic" or "molecular" subtypes primarily defined by gene expression studies. "Luminal" cancers have properties of glandular cells driven by high expression of ER (and to a lesser extent PR), "HER2" driven cancers have amplification and overexpression of HER2 but lack ER/PR expression, and "basal" cancers that lack ER/PR and HER2 ("triple negative") (Sorlie et al. 2001). This underlines the importance of steroid receptor expression in molecularly classifying breast cancers.

AR does not seem to play a major role in this intrinsic subtyping. Besides from frequent expression in luminal A and B and HER2 subtypes, AR expression was found in one third of basal-like breast tumors. AR expression is very frequently found in HER2 positive apocrine cancers (Safarpour et al. 2014).

4.8 Image Analysis

Currently, the common method of scoring IHC stained slides is by visual examination under a microscope by the pathologist. This procedure is prone to variability among pathologists, even when strict guidelines are followed. The ASCO/CAP recommendations for testing of the ER and PR receptor status include encouragement of the use of quantitative image analysis techniques with the goal of improving the consistency of the interpretation (Hammond et al. 2010; Veta et al. 2014), which is especially important for cases close to the threshold. Such image analysis algorithms have been available for decades, but their use has only recently been increasing since it has become possible to digitally scan full IHC stained slides and process them by commercially available image analysis algorithms such as ImageScope (Leica, Vista, CA, USA), TissueStudio (Definiens, Munich, Germany) and Tissuemorph (Visiopharm, Hoersholm, Denmark). A publicly available web application for ER/PR quantification is described in (Tuominen et al. 2010). In various recent studies, automatic scoring has shown high agreement with experts and other methods (Bolton et al. 2010; Lloyd et al. 2010).

4.9 Testing of Breast Cancer Recurrences

Receptor conversion, the phenomenon that describes hormone receptor expression changes from primary tumor to metastasis, is frequently observed in breast cancer (Hoefnagel et al. 2010). ERα and PRα conversion rates of 15 and 33 %, respectively, have been described. Although the change from receptor positivity to negativity is most often observed, conversion from hormone receptor negative to positive breast cancer is still seen in 8 % of cases. Because of the large clinical implications, all breast cancer local and distant recurrences are therefore advised to be retested for ERα and PRα expression (Hammond et al. 2010). The conversion from ER-positive or PgR-positive primary breast carcinoma to a negative distant metastasis is associated with a worse prognosis (Hoefnagel et al. 2012). Receptor conversion should be suspected at the moment of a breast tumor recurrence after adjuvant therapy and at progression of metastatic disease undergoing systemic treatment. Moreover, the phenomenon has been reported to occur during neoadjuvant chemotherapy (Montagna et al. 2015), which certainly is of relevance for endocrine treatment after surgery. No studies have yet investigated receptor conversion for AR.

4.10 Hormone Receptors in Ductal Carcinoma In Situ

Pure and true ductal carcinoma in situ (DCIS) can by definition not metastasize, but microinvasion may be missed, leading to regional and distant metastases in a very small percentage of "DCIS" patients. Thereby, prognosis of DCIS is very good (see Chap. 18 for details). However, the frequency of local recurrence after excision is higher, for which usually adjuvant radiotherapy is indicated and administered.

ERα and PRα are positive in the majority of DCIS, even in high grade lesions. In a recent large study, ERα was positive in 76 % of DCIS patients. Patients with ERα-positive DCIS treated with tamoxifen showed significant decreases in subsequent breast cancer at 10 years versus placebo treated patients, while no significant benefit was observed in ERα-negative DCIS. PRα and either receptor were positive in 66 and 79 % of patients, respectively, and in general, neither was more predictive than ERα alone (Allred et al. 2012). These results await further confirmation. For lobular carcinoma in situ that is also generally ER/PR positive, no such clinical data are available.

4.11 Hormone Receptors in Male Breast Cancer

The vast majority of male breast cancer (MBC) are ERα and/or PR positive. In our own studies, 95 % of MBC were ERα positive and 68 % PR positive (Kornegoor et al. 2012). Indeed, MBC patients benefit from adjuvant hormonal therapy (Giordano et al. 2005). However, many male patients discontinue endocrine treatment due to side effects (Anelli et al. 1994). Aromatase inhibition seems to result in a reduction of the estrogen levels (Doyen et al. 2010) and may play a role in the treatment of MBC.

Interestingly, and in contrast with female breast cancer, elastosis in MBC is rare despite the frequent expression of ER and PR (unpublished results), and is thereby not an ER/PR biomarker in MBC.

4.12 Conclusion

Immunohistochemical ER and PR testing of primary tumors as well as recurrences is of key importance for treatment decisions in men and women with breast cancer. Preliminary data indicate that also DCIS testing may set the indication for adjuvant tamoxifen. Therefore, ensuring the validity of the assays used by standardization and regular quality assessment is critical. Further developments are expected from hormone receptor analysis on the mRNA level. AR positivity is observed in a substantial proportion of breast tumors and is increasingly recognized as a potential therapeutic target, especially for women with ER and PR negative disease.

References

Allred DC, Anderson SJ, Paik S, Wickerham DL, Nagtegaal ID, Swain SM, Mamounas EP, Julian TB, Geyer CE Jr, Costantino JP, Land SR, Wolmark N (2012) Adjuvant tamoxifen reduces subsequent breast cancer in women with estrogen receptor-positive ductal carcinoma in situ: a study based on NSABP protocol B-24. J Clin Oncol 30(12):1268–1273. doi:10.1200/JCO.2010.34.0141

Andersen J, Orntoft T, Poulsen HS (1986) Semiquantitative oestrogen receptor assay in formalin-fixed paraffin sections of human breast cancer tissue using monoclonal antibodies. Br J Cancer 53(5):691–694

Anelli TF, Anelli A, Tran KN, Lebwohl DE, Borgen PI (1994) Tamoxifen administration is associated with a high rate of treatment-limiting symptoms in male breast cancer patients. Cancer 74(1):74–77

Antonarakis ES, Lu C, Wang H, Luber B, Nakazawa M, Roeser JC, Chen Y, Mohammad TA, Chen Y, Fedor HL, Lotan TL, Zheng Q, De Marzo AM, Isaacs JT, Isaacs WB, Nadal R, Paller CJ, Denmeade SR, Carducci MA, Eisenberger MA, Luo J (2014) AR-V7 and resistance to enzalutamide and abiraterone in prostate cancer. N Engl J Med 371 (11):1028–1038. doi:10.1056/NEJMoa1315815

Arnedos M, Nerurkar A, Osin P, A'Hern R, Smith IE, Dowsett M (2009) Discordance between core needle biopsy (CNB) and excisional biopsy (EB) for estrogen receptor (ER), progesterone receptor (PgR) and HER2 status in early breast cancer (EBC). Ann Oncol 20 (12):1948–1952. doi:10.1093/annonc/mdp234

Bardou VJ, Arpino G, Elledge RM, Osborne CK, Clark GM (2003) Progesterone receptor status significantly improves outcome prediction over estrogen receptor status alone for adjuvant endocrine therapy in two large breast cancer databases. J Clin Oncol 21 (10):1973–1979. doi:10.1200/JCO.2003.09.099

Barentsz MW, Wessels H, van Diest PJ, Pijnappel RM, van der Pol CC, Witkamp AJ, van den Bosch MA, Verkooijen HM (2014) Same-day diagnosis based on histology for women suspected of breast cancer: high diagnostic accuracy and favorable impact on the patient. PLoS ONE 9(7):e103105. doi:10.1371/journal.pone.0103105

Barnes DM, Fentiman IS, Millis RR, Rubens RD (1989) Who needs steroid receptor assays? Lancet 1 (8647):1126–1127

Barone I, Brusco L, Fuqua SA (2010) Estrogen receptor mutations and changes in downstream gene expression and signaling. Clin Cancer Res 16(10):2702–2708. doi:10.1158/1078-0432.CCR-09-1753

Beatson GW (1896) On the treatment of inoperable cases of carcinoma of the mamma: suggestions for a new method of treatment with illustrative cases. Lancet 148:104–107

Bolton KL, Garcia-Closas M, Pfeiffer RM, Duggan MA, Howat WJ, Hewitt SM, Yang XR, Cornelison R, Anzick SL, Meltzer P, Davis S, Lenz P, Figueroa JD, Pharoah PD, Sherman ME (2010) Assessment of automated image analysis of breast cancer tissue microarrays for epidemiologic studies. Cancer Epidemiol Biomarkers Prev 19(4):992–999. doi:10.1158/1055-9965.EPI-09-1023

Bueno-de-Mesquita JM, Nuyten DS, Wesseling J, van Tinteren H, Linn SC, van de Vijver MJ (2010) The impact of inter-observer variation in pathological assessment of node-negative breast cancer on clinical risk assessment and patient selection for adjuvant systemic treatment. Ann Oncol 21(1):40–47. doi:10.1093/annonc/mdp273

Burge CN, Chang HR, Apple SK (2006) Do the histologic features and results of breast cancer biomarker studies differ between core biopsy and surgical excision specimens? Breast 15(2):167–172. doi:10.1016/j.breast.2005.06.004

Cochrane DR, Bernales S, Jacobsen BM, Cittelly DM, Howe EN, D'Amato NC, Spoelstra NS, Edgerton SM, Jean A, Guerrero J, Gomez F, Medicherla S, Alfaro IE, McCullagh E, Jedlicka P, Torkko KC, Thor AD, Elias AD, Protter AA, Richer JK (2014) Role of the androgen receptor in breast cancer and preclinical analysis of enzalutamide. Breast Cancer Res 16(1):R7. doi:10.1186/bcr3599

Collins LC, Cole KS, Marotti JD, Hu R, Schnitt SJ, Tamimi RM (2011) Androgen receptor expression in breast cancer in relation to molecular phenotype: results from the Nurses' Health Study. Mod Pathol 24 (7):924–931. doi:10.1038/modpathol.2011.54

Davies C, Pan H, Godwin J, Gray R, Arriagada R, Raina V, Abraham M, Medeiros Alencar VH, Badran A, Bonfill X, Bradbury J, Clarke M, Collins R, Davis SR, Delmestri A, Forbes JF, Haddad P, Hou MF, Inbar M, Khaled H, Kielanowska J, Kwan WH, Mathew BS, Mittra I, Muller B, Nicolucci A, Peralta O, Pernas F, Petruzelka L, Pienkowski T, Radhika R, Rajan B, Rubach MT, Tort S, Urrutia G, Valentini M, Wang Y, Peto R, Adjuvant Tamoxifen: Longer Against Shorter Collaborative G (2013) Long-term effects of continuing adjuvant tamoxifen to 10 years versus stopping at 5 years after diagnosis of oestrogen receptor-positive breast cancer: ATLAS, a randomised trial. Lancet 381 (9869):805–816. doi:10.1016/S0140-6736(12)61963-1

Dekker TJ, ter Borg S, Hooijer GK, Meijer SL, Wesseling J, Boers JE, Schuuring E, Bart J, van Gorp J, Bult P, Riemersma SA, van Deurzen CH, Sleddens HF, Mesker WE, Kroep JR, Smit VT, van de Vijver MJ (2015) Quality assessment of estrogen receptor and progesterone receptor testing in breast cancer using a tissue microarray-based approach.

Breast Cancer Res Treat 152(2):247–252. doi:10.1007/s10549-015-3444-x

Dowsett M (2006) Estrogen receptor: methodology matters. J Clin Oncol 24(36):5626–5628. doi:10.1200/JCO.2006.08.3485

Dowsett M, Sestak I, Buus R, Lopez-Knowles E, Mallon E, Howell A, Forbes JF, Buzdar A, Cuzick J (2015) Estrogen receptor expression in 21-gene recurrence score predicts increased late recurrence for estrogen-positive/HER2-negative breast cancer. Clin Cancer Res 21(12):2763–2770. doi:10.1158/1078-0432.CCR-14-2842

Doyen J, Italiano A, Largillier R, Ferrero JM, Fontana X, Thyss A (2010) Aromatase inhibition in male breast cancer patients: biological and clinical implications. Ann Oncol 21(6):1243–1245. doi:10.1093/annonc/mdp450

Early Breast Cancer Trialists' Collaborative G (2005) Effects of chemotherapy and hormonal therapy for early breast cancer on recurrence and 15-year survival: an overview of the randomised trials. Lancet 365 (9472):1687–1717. doi:10.1016/S0140-6736(05)66544-0

Feherty P, Farrer-Brown G, Kellie AE (1971) Oestradiol receptors in carcinoma and benign disease of the breast: an in vitro assay. Br J Cancer 25(4):697–710

Ferguson AT, Lapidus RG, Baylin SB, Davidson NE (1995) Demethylation of the estrogen receptor gene in estrogen receptor-negative breast cancer cells can reactivate estrogen receptor gene expression. Cancer Res 55(11):2279–2283

Giordano SH, Perkins GH, Broglio K, Garcia SG, Middleton LP, Buzdar AU, Hortobagyi GN (2005) Adjuvant systemic therapy for male breast carcinoma. Cancer 104(11):2359–2364. doi:10.1002/cncr.21526

Gray RG (2013) aTTom: Long-term effects of continuing adjuvant tamoxifen to 10 years versus stopping at 5 years in 6,953 women with early breast cancer. In: Abstract ASCO annual meeting 2013. J Clin Oncol (suppl; abstr 5)

Gruvberger-Saal SK, Bendahl PO, Saal LH, Laakso M, Hegardt C, Eden P, Peterson C, Malmstrom P, Isola J, Borg A, Ferno M (2007) Estrogen receptor beta expression is associated with tamoxifen response in ERalpha-negative breast carcinoma. Clin Cancer Res 13(7):1987–1994. doi:10.1158/1078-0432.CCR-06-1823

Hammond ME, Hayes DF, Dowsett M, Allred DC, Hagerty KL, Badve S, Fitzgibbons PL, Francis G, Goldstein NS, Hayes M, Hicks DG, Lester S, Love R, Mangu PB, McShane L, Miller K, Osborne CK, Paik S, Perlmutter J, Rhodes A, Sasano H, Schwartz JN, Sweep FC, Taube S, Torlakovic EE, Valenstein P, Viale G, Visscher D, Wheeler T, Williams RB, Wittliff JL, Wolff AC (2010) American Society of Clinical Oncology/College Of American Pathologists guideline recommendations for immunohistochemical testing of estrogen and progesterone receptors in breast cancer. J Clin Oncol 28(16):2784–2795. doi:10.1200/JCO.2009.25.6529

Harvey JM, Clark GM, Osborne CK, Allred DC (1999) Estrogen receptor status by immunohistochemistry is superior to the ligand-binding assay for predicting response to adjuvant endocrine therapy in breast cancer. J Clin Oncol 17(5):1474–1481

Heinlein CA, Chang C (2002) The roles of androgen receptors and androgen-binding proteins in nongenomic androgen actions. Mol Endocrinol 16 (10):2181–2187. doi:10.1210/me.2002-0070

Hoefnagel LD, van de Vijver MJ, van Slooten HJ, Wesseling P, Wesseling J, Westenend PJ, Bart J, Seldenrijk CA, Nagtegaal ID, Oudejans J, van der Valk P, van der Groep P, de Vries EG, van der Wall E, van Diest PJ (2010) Receptor conversion in distant breast cancer metastases. Breast Cancer Res 12(5):R75. doi:10.1186/bcr2645

Hoefnagel LD, Moelans CB, Meijer SL, van Slooten HJ, Wesseling P, Wesseling J, Westenend PJ, Bart J, Seldenrijk CA, Nagtegaal ID, Oudejans J, van der Valk P, van Gils CH, van der Wall E, van Diest PJ (2012) Prognostic value of estrogen receptor alpha and progesterone receptor conversion in distant breast cancer metastases. Cancer 118(20):4929–4935. doi:10.1002/cncr.27518

Holst F, Moelans CB, Filipits M, Singer CF, Simon R, van Diest PJ (2012) On the evidence for ESR1 amplification in breast cancer. Nat Rev Cancer 12 (2):149. doi:10.1038/nrc3093-c3

Hu DG, Hickey TE, Irvine C, Wijayakumara DD, Lu L, Tilley WD, Selth LA, Mackenzie PI (2014) Identification of androgen receptor splice variant transcripts in breast cancer cell lines and human tissues. Horm Cancer 5(2):61–71. doi:10.1007/s12672-014-0171-4

Iwamoto T, Booser D, Valero V, Murray JL, Koenig K, Esteva FJ, Ueno NT, Zhang J, Shi W, Qi Y, Matsuoka J, Yang EJ, Hortobagyi GN, Hatzis C, Symmans WF, Pusztai L (2012) Estrogen receptor (ER) mRNA and ER-related gene expression in breast cancers that are 1 % to 10 % ER-positive by immunohistochemistry. J Clin Oncol 30(7):729–734. doi:10.1200/JCO.2011.36.2574

Jensen EV (1981) Hormone dependency of breast cancer. Cancer 47(10):2319–2326

Jeselsohn R, Buchwalter G, De Angelis C, Brown M, Schiff R (2015) ESR1 mutations-a mechanism for acquired endocrine resistance in breast cancer. Nat Rev Clin Oncol 12(10):573–583. doi:10.1038/nrclinonc.2015.117

Jozwik KM, Carroll JS (2012) Pioneer factors in hormone-dependent cancers. Nat Rev Cancer 12 (6):381–385. doi:10.1038/nrc3263

Kalkman S, Barentsz MW, Witkamp AJ, van der Wall E, Verkooijen HM, van Diest PJ (2014) Brief fixation does not affect assessment of hormone receptor expression in invasive breast carcinoma biopsies: paving the road for same-day tissue diagnostics. Am J Surg Pathol 38(8):1071–1078. doi:10.1097/PAS.0000000000000207

King WJ, DeSombre ER, Jensen EV, Greene GL (1985) Comparison of immunocytochemical and

steroid-binding assays for estrogen receptor in human breast tumors. Cancer Res 45(1):293–304
Kornegoor R, Verschuur-Maes AH, Buerger H, Hogenes MC, de Bruin PC, Oudejans JJ, van der Groep P, Hinrichs B, van Diest PJ (2012) Molecular subtyping of male breast cancer by immunohistochemistry. Mod Pathol 25(3):398–404. doi:10.1038/modpathol.2011.174
Lapidus RG, Ferguson AT, Ottaviano YL, Parl FF, Smith HS, Weitzman SA, Baylin SB, Issa JP, Davidson NE (1996) Methylation of estrogen and progesterone receptor gene 5′ CpG islands correlates with lack of estrogen and progesterone receptor gene expression in breast tumors. Clin Cancer Res 2 (5):805–810
Lehmann BD, Bauer JA, Chen X, Sanders ME, Chakravarthy AB, Shyr Y, Pietenpol JA (2011) Identification of human triple-negative breast cancer subtypes and preclinical models for selection of targeted therapies. J Clin Invest 121(7):2750–2767. doi:10.1172/JCI45014
Li CI, Uribe DJ, Daling JR (2005) Clinical characteristics of different histologic types of breast cancer. Br J Cancer 93(9):1046–1052. doi:10.1038/sj.bjc.6602787
Lloyd MC, Allam-Nandyala P, Purohit CN, Burke N, Coppola D, Bui MM (2010) Using image analysis as a tool for assessment of prognostic and predictive biomarkers for breast cancer: how reliable is it? J Pathol Inform 1:29. doi:10.4103/2153-3539.74186
Marino M, Galluzzo P, Ascenzi P (2006) Estrogen signaling multiple pathways to impact gene transcription. Curr Genomics 7(8):497–508
Merenbakh-Lamin K, Ben-Baruch N, Yeheskel A, Dvir A, Soussan-Gutman L, Jeselsohn R, Yelensky R, Brown M, Miller VA, Sarid D, Rizel S, Klein B, Rubinek T, Wolf I (2013) D538G mutation in estrogen receptor-alpha: a novel mechanism for acquired endocrine resistance in breast cancer. Cancer Res 73(23):6856–6864. doi:10.1158/0008-5472.CAN-13-1197
Moelans CB, Holst F, Hellwinkel O, Simon R, van Diest PJ (2013) ESR1 amplification in breast cancer by optimized RNase FISH: frequent but low-level and heterogeneous. PLoS ONE 8(12):e84189. doi:10.1371/journal.pone.0084189
Montagna E, Bagnardi V, Viale G, Rotmensz N, Sporchia A, Cancello G, Balduzzi A, Galimberti V, Veronesi P, Luini A, Mastropasqua MG, Casadio C, Sangalli C, Goldhirsch A, Colleoni M (2015) Changes in PgR and Ki-67 in residual tumour and outcome of breast cancer patients treated with neoadjuvant chemotherapy. Ann Oncol 26(2):307–313. doi:10.1093/annonc/mdu528
Motamedolshariati M, Memar B, Aliakbaian M, Shakeri MT, Samadi M, Jangjoo A (2014) Accuracy of prognostic and predictive markers in core needle breast biopsies compared with excisional specimens. Breast Care (Basel) 9(2):107–110. doi:10.1159/000360787
Muresan Z, Dutu R, Voiculetz N (1986) Relationships of steroid hormone receptors, age and histological characteristics in human breast cancer. Neoplasma 33(3):371–377
Nakshatri H, Badve S (2007) FOXA1 as a therapeutic target for breast cancer. Expert Opin Ther Targets 11 (4):507–514. doi:10.1517/14728222.11.4.507
Ooi A, Inokuchi M, Harada S, Inazawa J, Tajiri R, Kitamura SS, Ikeda H, Kawashima H, Dobashi Y (2012) Gene amplification of ESR1 in breast cancers–fact or fiction? A fluorescence in situ hybridization and multiplex ligation-dependent probe amplification study. J Pathol 227(1):8–16. doi:10.1002/path.3974
Postma EL, Verkooijen HM, van Diest PJ, Willems SM, van den Bosch MA, van Hillegersberg R (2013) Discrepancy between routine and expert pathologists' assessment of non-palpable breast cancer and its impact on locoregional and systemic treatment. Eur J Pharmacol 717(1–3):31–35. doi:10.1016/j.ejphar.2012.12.033
Roepman P, Horlings HM, Krijgsman O, Kok M, Bueno-de-Mesquita JM, Bender R, Linn SC, Glas AM, van de Vijver MJ (2009) Microarray-based determination of estrogen receptor, progesterone receptor, and HER2 receptor status in breast cancer. Clin Cancer Res 15(22):7003–7011. doi:10.1158/1078-0432.CCR-09-0449
Roodi N, Bailey LR, Kao WY, Verrier CS, Yee CJ, Dupont WD, Parl FF (1995) Estrogen receptor gene analysis in estrogen receptor-positive and receptor-negative primary breast cancer. J Natl Cancer Inst 87(6):446–451
Safarpour D, Pakneshan S, Tavassoli FA (2014) Androgen receptor (AR) expression in 400 breast carcinomas: is routine AR assessment justified? Am J Cancer Res 4(4):353–368
Sefrioui D, Perdrix A, Sarafan-Vasseur N, Dolfus C, Dujon A, Picquenot JM, Delacour J, Cornic M, Bohers E, Leheurteur M, Rigal O, Tennevet I, Thery JC, Alexandru C, Guillemet C, Moldovan C, Veyret C, Frebourg T, Di Fiore F, Clatot F (2015) Short report: monitoring ESR1 mutations by circulating tumor DNA in aromatase inhibitor resistant metastatic breast cancer. Int J Cancer 137(10):2513–2519. doi:10.1002/ijc.29612
Shibata H, Spencer TE, Onate SA, Jenster G, Tsai SY, Tsai MJ, O'Malley BW (1997) Role of co-activators and co-repressors in the mechanism of steroid/thyroid receptor action. Recent Prog Horm Res 52:141–164; discussion 164–145
Sorlie T, Perou CM, Tibshirani R, Aas T, Geisler S, Johnsen H, Hastie T, Eisen MB, van de Rijn M, Jeffrey SS, Thorsen T, Quist H, Matese JC, Brown PO, Botstein D, Lonning PE, Borresen-Dale AL (2001) Gene expression patterns of breast carcinomas distinguish tumor subclasses with clinical implications. Proc Natl Acad Sci U S A 98 (19):10869–10874. doi:10.1073/pnas.191367098
Tamaki K, Sasano H, Ishida T, Miyashita M, Takeda M, Amari M, Tamaki N, Ohuchi N (2010) Comparison of core needle biopsy (CNB) and surgical specimens for accurate preoperative evaluation of ER, PgR and HER2

status of breast cancer patients. Cancer Sci 101(9):2074–2079. doi:10.1111/j.1349-7006.2010.01630.x

Taylor SE, Martin-Hirsch PL, Martin FL (2010) Oestrogen receptor splice variants in the pathogenesis of disease. Cancer Lett 288(2):133–148. doi:10.1016/j.canlet.2009.06.017

Thomas C, Gustafsson J-Å (2011) Not enough evidence to include ESR1 amplification. Nat Rev Cancer 11 (11):823

Tuominen VJ, Ruotoistenmaki S, Viitanen A, Jumppanen M, Isola J (2010) ImmunoRatio: a publicly available web application for quantitative image analysis of estrogen receptor (ER), progesterone receptor (PR), and Ki-67. Breast Cancer Res 12(4): R56. doi:10.1186/bcr2615

Veta M, Pluim JP, van Diest PJ, Viergever MA (2014) Breast cancer histopathology image analysis: a review. IEEE Trans Biomed Eng 61(5):1400–1411. doi:10.1109/TBME.2014.2303852

Viale G, Regan MM, Maiorano E, Mastropasqua MG, Dell'Orto P, Rasmussen BB, Raffoul J, Neven P, Orosz Z, Braye S, Ohlschlegel C, Thurlimann B, Gelber RD, Castiglione-Gertsch M, Price KN, Goldhirsch A, Gusterson BA, Coates AS (2007) Prognostic and predictive value of centrally reviewed expression of estrogen and progesterone receptors in a randomized trial comparing letrozole and tamoxifen adjuvant therapy for postmenopausal early breast cancer: BIG 1-98. J Clin Oncol 25(25):3846–3852. doi:10.1200/JCO.2007.11.9453

Walters KA, Simanainen U, Handelsman DJ (2010) Molecular insights into androgen actions in male and female reproductive function from androgen receptor knockout models. Hum Reprod Update 16(5):543–558. doi:10.1093/humupd/dmq003

Wimberly H, Han G, Pinnaduwage D, Murphy LC, Yang XR, Andrulis IL, Sherman M, Figueroa J, Rimm DL (2014) ERbeta splice variant expression in four large cohorts of human breast cancer patient tumors. Breast Cancer Res Treat 146(3):657–667. doi:10.1007/s10549-014-3050-3

Yi M, Huo L, Koenig KB, Mittendorf EA, Meric-Bernstam F, Kuerer HM, Bedrosian I, Buzdar AU, Symmans WF, Crow JR, Bender M, Shah RR, Hortobagyi GN, Hunt KK (2014) Which threshold for ER positivity? A retrospective study based on 9639 patients. Ann Oncol 25(5):1004–1011. doi:10.1093/annonc/mdu053

Human Epidermal Growth Factor Receptor 2 (HER2): Translating the Lab to the Clinic

5

Cesar Santa-Maria, Sarika Jain and William J. Gradishar

Abstract

The overexpression/amplification of HER2 has been classically associated with poor outcomes in breast cancer. However, with the advent of targeted therapies this may no longer be the case. A number of agents that are directed at the HER2 molecule or downstream of it have now become available. Evidence from clinical trials seems to suggest that these agents are potent. More importantly, they exert an additive/synergistic effect resulting in improved patient outcomes. In this chapter, we review the available evidence for the use of these agents in metastatic and early breast cancer. We also briefly discuss the mechanisms that have been implicated in the development of resistance to anti-HER2 therapies.

Keywords

HER2 · Neoadjuvant · Metastatic · Trastuzumab · Pertuzumab · T-DM1

5.1 Introduction

The subset of breast cancer that is characterized as HER2-positive has been the focus of intense laboratory and clinical investigation for the last 2 decades. As a result of these efforts a greater understanding of the complex biology of HER2 disease has translated into several HER2-directed therapies that have dramatically improved the prognosis of patients with both early-stage and advanced stage disease. Additionally, insights into the mechanisms that explain resistance to HER2-directed therapies are now being defined and clinical trials are being conducted to evaluated strategies to overcome resistance.

5.2 HER2 Testing

Identifying patients who are most likely to benefit from a particular treatment strategy, and by extension, identifying those individuals who will

C. Santa-Maria · S. Jain · W.J. Gradishar (✉)
Division of Hematology/Oncology, Department of Medicine, Robert H. Lurie Comprehensive Cancer Center, Northwestern University Feinberg School of Medicine, Chicago, USA
e-mail: w-gradishar@northwestern.edu

W.J. Gradishar
676, North St. Clair, #850, Chicago, IL 60611, USA

S. Badve and Y. Gökmen-Polar (eds.), *Molecular Pathology of Breast Cancer*, DOI 10.1007/978-3-319-41761-5_5

not benefit from a particular therapy, is the cornerstone of precision medicine. Since HER2 status is a predictive factor in breast cancer, HER2 testing is a critical initial step in the pathologic evaluation of breast cancer. In 2007, an expert panel of the American Society of Clinical Oncology (ASCO) and the College of American Physicians (CAP) developed guidelines on the optimal algorithm and interpretation of HER2 testing (Wolff et al. 2007), which were further refined in the current 2013 guidelines (Wolff et al. 2013). It is recommended that HER2 status be determined in all patients with newly diagnosed, recurrent, and metastatic breast cancer. HER2-positive status is determined when there is evidence of protein overexpression (immunohistochemistry [IHC]) 3+ based on circumferential membrane staining that is complete and intense or gene amplification (in situ hybridization [ISH]) based on counting at least 20 cells within the area. IHC is the most commonly used assay as it is easy to perform with relatively low cost. Its scoring is highly applicable to negative cases (0 or 1+) or positive (3+), however equivocal cases (2+) must be evaluated by other methods, such as fluorescence ISH (FISH) analysis (Wolff et al. 2013). The advantage of FISH testing is the quantitative interpretation of results, which increases the concordance rates among observers compared to IHC (Fig. 5.1).

Per the ASCO-CAP 2013 recommendations, if HER2 test results are equivocal, a reflex test is recommended on the same specimen using an alternative test or a new specimen using the same or an alternative test (Wolff et al. 2013). Equivocal findings include IHC 2+ or ISH-equivocal based on single-probe ISH average HER2 copy number 4.0 to <6.0 signals/cell or dual-probe HER2/CEP17 ratio <2.0 with an average HER2 copy number 4.0 to <6.0 signals/cell. Repeat testing should also be considered if histo-pathologic features suggest HER2 discordance, such as HER2 positivity in a grade 1 carcinoma that is hormone receptor-positive or of a favorable histology, or in cases of HER2 negativity in a grade 3 tumor. In particular, the 2013 guidelines included changes to the interpretation of HER2 FISH results (Wolff et al. 2013). A retrospective review of 904 invasive breast cancer cases evaluated the impact of these updated guidelines on HER2 FISH interpretation and found 9.4 % of cases were re-classified (7.3 % went from HER2 negative to equivocal, 1.7 % to HER2 positive and four cases from HER2 equivocal to negative) (Bethune et al. 2015). The increase in uncertain cases will likely augment laboratory resource utilization, cost, and may impact patient care.

Though FISH testing remains the gold standard technique to identify HER2 status in ambiguous cases of breast cancer, it is an expensive and time-consuming test requiring very specific training and is not universally available. Therefore, alternative diagnostic strategies have been evaluated including standard bright-field techniques such as chromogenic in situ hybridization (CISH) and silver-enhanced in situ hybridization (SISH) as well as quantitative real-time polymerase chain reaction (qPCR) (Francis et al. 2009; Tanner et al. 2000; Vanden Bempt et al. 2005). Unlike FISH, CISH combines features of immunohistochemical analysis and in situ hybridization, allowing pathologists to analyze gene amplification simultaneously with detailed tissue morphology. CISH signals do not diminish over time providing useful archival tissue and are associated with less cost. SISH is a technique that offers the advantage of a bright-field FISH test coupled with automation for HER2 amplification, thereby reducing the risk of error. Methods based on PCR have successfully evaluated mRNAs expressed in mixed cell populations, especially those expressed in low copy numbers in a small number of cells or in small quantity of tissue. However, a major drawback to PCR techniques include the high false-negative rate due to the dilution of tumor mRNA by the presence of surrounding non-tumor tissue. Laser microdissection of the tumor may circumvent these issues, but is not practical in routine practice. One study prospectively compared the performance level of CISH, SISH, and qPCR with IHC and FISH for evaluation of HER2 amplification status in 840 breast cancer core biopsies (Jacquemier et al. 2013).

Primary or Metastatic Tumor

Immunohistochemistry (IHC)		In Situ Hybridization (FISH/CISH)
0		
1+	Anti-HER2 therapy NOT Indicated	Negative
2+	Reflux testing	Equivocal
3+	Anti-HER2 therapy Indicated	**Positive**

Fig. 5.1 Algorithm for HER2 assessment in breast cancer

The concordance between IHC and FISH based on HER2/CEN17 ratio and HER2 copy number was 96 and 95 %, respectively. Similarly, the concordance of CISH, SISH, and qPCR with FISH was excellent (range, 95–97 %, based on HER2/CEN17 ratio). While these other strategies are promising, there is insufficient evidence to support its use in unselected patients.

5.3 Approach to Metastatic HER2-Positive Breast Cancer

The development of therapy directed against the human epidermal growth factor receptor 2-neu (HER2) demonstrates the power of how translational science and clinical collaboration can change the lives of patients. The discovery of HER2 in the 1980s led to the development of trastuzumab, a monoclonal antibody against HER2; and eventually to Food and Drug Administration (FDA) approval in 1998 (Coussens et al. 1985; Brenner and Adams 1999). The addition of trastuzumab has been shown to improve survival in patients with HER2-positive metastatic breast cancer (Slamon et al. 2001). Data also exists suggesting that the continuation of trastuzumab after progression on trastuzumab and chemotherapy is beneficial (von Minckwitz et al. 2009). Although continuation of trastuzumab beyond disease progression has not been demonstrated to improve overall survival (OS) prospectively (only nonsignificant improvement in OS, from 20 to 26 months), it does not add significant toxicity, is commonly used and considered a standard of care (Bethune et al. 2015; von Minckwitz et al. 2009).

The CLEOPATRA study compared front line docetaxel and trastuzumab (TH) with or without pertuzumab (THP), a monoclonal antibody against HER2 and human epidermal growth factor receptor 3 (HER3), and changed the treatment paradigm for front line therapy of HER2-positive metastatic breast cancer (Baselga et al. 2012b).

Median progression free survival (PFS) was modestly improved from 12.4 to 18.5 months (hazard ratio [HR] 0.62, 95 % confidence interval [CI] 0.51–0.75, $p < 0.001$), however, an updated analysis demonstrated an unprecedented improvement in OS from 40.8 to 56.5 months (HR 0.68, 95 % CI 0.56–0.84, $p < 0.001$) (Swain et al. 2015). THP is considered standard of care front line therapy for patients with HER-positive metastatic breast cancer based on these data, but many questions remain. Other than HER2 status, there remains no other biomarker that has been proven to identify those patients more likely to benefit from pertuzumab. It remains unknown if there is a benefit to continuing pertuzumab after disease progression, as it appears to be beneficial with trastuzumab. While the development of pertuzumab is an important cornerstone for patients with HER2-positive breast cancer, patients ultimately progress, and additional therapies are needed.

Lapatinib, a tyrosine kinase inhibitor (TKI) reversibly binding and inhibiting the intracellular domain of HER2, was the first second-line anti-HER2 agent approved. A phase 3 study comparing lapatinib and capecitabine to capecitabine alone demonstrated an improvement in time to progression (HR 0.49, 95 % CI 0.34–0.71, $p < 0.001$) and but not OS (HR 0.92; 95 % CI 0.58–1.46, $p = 0.72$) (Geyer et al. 2006). The combination of lapatinib with trastuzumab has been found to improve PFS (8–11 weeks; HR 0.74, 95 % CI 0.58–0.94) and OS (10 to 14 months; HR 0.74, 95 % CI 0.57–0.97) compared to lapatinib alone after progression on one or more trastuzumab-based regimens, and may represent a chemotherapy-free option for select patients with metastatic, HER2-positive breast cancer (Blackwell et al. 2012).

A conceptually simple method of overcoming trastuzumab resistance has been the development of antibody-drug conjugates. This strategy attaches a highly toxic chemotherapeutic to a targeted monoclonal antibody via a linker molecule. This allows for a targeted payload of highly toxic chemotherapy to a cancer cell, which through endocytosis is incorporated into the cancer cell where the linker molecule is degraded and the chemotherapeutic agent becomes active. Trastuzumab emtansine (TDM-1) is an antibody-drug conjugate that has shown significant efficacy in patients with advanced HER2-positive breast cancer. In the EMILIA study TDM-1 was compared to the combination of lapatinib and capecitabine in patients progressing on trastuzumab-based therapy and found to improve PFS (HR 0.65, 95 % CI 0.55–0.77, $p < 0.001$) and OS (HR 0.68, 95 % CI 0.55–0.85, $p < 0.001$) (Verma et al. 2012). These data provide strong support for the use of TDM-1 in the second-line setting and is now considered a standard of care. The TH3RESA study compared TDM-1 to the physicians' choice of treatment in patients progressing on trastuzumab-based therapy and lapatinib-based therapy. In this later line setting TDM-1 had superior PFS (HR 0.53, 95 % CI 0.42–0.66, $p < 0.0001$) and a trend favoring OS (HR 0.55, 95 % CI 0.37–0.83, $p = 0.0034$, stopping boundary not crossed). The recently reported MARIANNE study compared TDM-1, with or without pertuzumab, versus trastuzumab with a taxane, finding that the TDM-1 containing arms were non-inferior, but not superior, to trastuzumab with a taxane (Ellis et al. 2015). These results are difficult to apply to current practice as THP is a standard of care, front-line therapy, but suggests that in patients not able to tolerate chemotherapy, TDM-1 may be a reasonable front-line approach for select patients.

The success of anti-HER2 therapies in the metastatic setting has provided rationale for their investigation in the early stage setting, where they have already changed the treatment paradigm, and increased rates of cure. Additionally, other HER2-directed therapies continue to be developed, as well as novel therapeutics that can be combined with available agents to overcome resistance that develops.

5.4 Approach to Early HER2-Positive Breast Cancer

The incorporation of systemic therapies for early breast cancer has vastly improved outcomes, particularly in HER2-positive breast cancer with the advent of targeted therapies. Early studies determined that whether systemic therapy was given after surgery (adjuvant) or before (neoadjuvant), outcomes were the same in terms of disease-free survival (DFS) and OS (Mauri et al. 2005). Selecting appropriate patients for either adjuvant versus neoadjuvant therapy is dependent on several variables, and requires a multidisciplinary approach including medical, surgical and radiation oncologists, pathologists, and radiologists. Specific indications for administration of neoadjuvant therapy include patients who have inoperable locally advanced breast cancer, those who desire breast conservation surgery (BCS) and are not eligible at diagnosis, and patients with inflammatory breast cancer (King and Morrow 2015). The neoadjuvant setting is furthermore a powerful research tool where anti-tumor effects can be assessed by pathological response, and tissue-based biomarkers can be easily assessed. Pathologic complete response (pCR) after neoadjuvant therapy can predict in individual patients DFS, and has been used as a surrogate for survival in many studies. The longstanding debate focuses on whether pCR can predict the outcome of similar treatment administered postoperatively (adjuvant) in much larger clinical trials (Prowell and Pazdur 2012). If concordant, the implications would be the ability to identify effective therapies in a far shorter time frame, less expense and fewer required patients (Prowell and Pazdur 2012).

Based on success in the metastatic setting, studies investigating trastuzumab in early breast cancer were performed. The landmark study performed by the Breast Cancer International Research Group (BCIRG) demonstrated that the addition of trastuzumab to chemotherapy improved disease free survival (DFS) and OS (Slamon et al. 2011). In this study, the two regimens that were investigated were trastuzumab in combination with docetaxel and carboplatin (TCH), as well as in combination with paclitaxel after standard doxorubicin and cyclophosphamide (AC/TH). Both TCH and AC/TH were superior to chemotherapy without trastuzumab, but there were no differences in survival endpoints between the two trastuzumab-containing regimens, albeit AC/TH did demonstrate a non-significant trend towards superiority. The AC/TH arm, however, had an increased incidence of cardiomyopathy and secondary leukemias compared to the TCH arm (Slamon et al. 2011).

The optimal duration of trastuzumab has also been studied, where a total of one year found to be most effective and safe. The Herceptin Adjuvant (HERA) trial investigated 24 versus 12 months of adjuvant trastuzumab, finding that 24 months was not more effective than 12 months of treatment, but rather increased cardiac toxicity (7.2 % decrease in left ventricular ejection fraction in 24 month group, compared to 4.1 % in 12 month group, $p < 0.0001$) (Goldhirsch et al. 2013). Conversely, the Protocol of Herceptin Adjuvant with Reduced Exposure (PHARE) study, compared 6 versus 12 months of adjuvant trastuzumab, and found that 6 months was not non-inferior to 12 months of treatment, thus failing to meet its primary endpoint (Pivot et al. 2013).

Data from the neoadjuvant setting also supports the benefit of adding trastuzumab to chemotherapy in patients with early breast cancer. The addition of trastuzumab to chemotherapy has been demonstrated to increase pCR rates from 20 to 43 % (relative risk [RR] for pCR 2.07, 95 % CI 1.41–3.03, $p = 0.0002$), and decreased relapse rate from 20 to 12 % (RR for relapse 0.67, 95 % CI 0.48–0.94) (Petrelli et al. 2011). Survival data from the Neoadjuvant Herceptin (NOAH) study presented at the 2013 Annual American Society of Clinical Oncology (ASCO) meeting also demonstrated that event-free survival (EFS) and OS were improved in those taking trastuzumab (HR 0.64, $p = 0.016$ and HR 0.66, $p = 0.055$, respectively) (Gianni et al. 2013, 2015). This is the only neoadjuvant study to demonstrate a statistically significant correlation of improved pCR rates with improved survival endpoints.

Lapatinib has also been studied in several neoadjuvant trials, where its addition to trastuzumab-based therapy has been found to improve pCR rates by 4–21 % (Bonnefoi et al. 2015; Robidoux et al. 2013; Carey et al. 2013; de

Azambuja et al. 2014). The Neoadjuvant Lapatinib and/or Trastuzumab Treatment Optimization (NeoALTTO) study demonstrated the most significant improvement in pCR rates; where the addition of lapatinib to trastuzumab-based therapy improved pCR rates from 30 to 51 % (de Azambuja et al. 2014). The NeoALTTO study did not demonstrate improved event-free survival (EFS, HR 0.78, 95 % CI 0.47–1.28, $p = 0.33$) or OS (HR 0.62, 95 % CI 0.30–1.25, $p = 0.19$), albeit it was not powered to detect small differences in survival outcomes. The larger and confirmatory Adjuvant Lapatinib and/or Trastuzumab Treatment Optimization (ALTTO) study was powered to detect survival differences, however, did not demonstrate improved EFS with the addition of lapatinib (HR 0.84, CI 0.70–1.02, $p = 0.048$, $p \leq 0.025$ needed for statistical significance) (Piccart-Gebhart et al. 2014). While the discordant relationship between pCR and survival endpoints may be in part explained by the fact the anthracycline-based portion of therapy in NeoALTTO was given after surgery and therefore did not impact pCR rates, these data do not support the use of lapatinib in early HER2-positive breast cancer. These data inform future study design in terms of drug development, suggesting that all planned systemic therapy should be given before surgery when interpreting pCR rates.

The novel TKI, neratinib, which irreversibly inhibits HER2, is being developed as an improvement on first generation TKIs. Neratinib was studied in the I-SPY 2 trial where it demonstrated overall pCR rates of 32 % (95 % CI 28–36 %), laying the foundation for a larger registration trial (Park et al. 2014). Neratinib has also been studied adjuvantly after the completion of one year of trastuzumab. In a phase 3 study presented at the ASCO 2015 meeting, treatment with 12 months of neratinib after one year of trastuzumab resulted in lower invasive DFS at 2 years (93.9 % for neratinib arm compared to 91.6 % in placebo, HR 0.67, CI 0.50–0.91, $p = 0.0009$). This modest improvement in 2-year invasive DFS was at the cost of increased toxicity, most notably 40 % grade 3 diarrhea (Chan et al. 2015). These data must be interpreted with caution as the trial underwent significant change over the accrual period and equally important, the role and contribution of adjuvant pertuzumab in combination with trastuzumab is being evaluated in the yet to be reported Adjuvant Pertuzumab and Herceptin in Initial Therapy of Breast Cancer (APHINITY) trial.

Drug development of pertuzumab in early breast cancer took a similar approach as with lapatinib, with neoadjuvant studies performed to assess pCR rates. The addition of pertuzumab to trastuzumab and docetaxel improved pCR rates from 29 to 45.8 % in the Neoadjuvant Study of Pertuzumab and Herceptin in an Early Regimen Evaluation (NeoSPHERE) study, however, in a recent update DFS was not significantly improved (HR 0.60, 95 % CI 0.28–1.27) (Gianni et al. 2012, 2013, 2015). As with the NeoALTTO study, this is study was not powered to detect smaller improvements in survival, and the anthracycline portion of the treatment was not administered until after surgery, and thus does not directly affect pCR rates. The Trastuzumab Plus Pertuzumab in Neoadjuvant HER2 Positive Breast Cancer (TRYPHAENA) study provided more promising data by demonstrating an unprecedented pCR rate of 66.2 % when using the regimen of docetaxel, carboplatin, trastuzumab, and pertuzumab (TCHP) in patients with early HER2-positive breast cancer (Schneeweiss et al. 2013). While these results are very promising, one key limitation in their interpretation is the fact there was no non-pertuzumab control arm. Nevertheless, based on these promising results the FDA granted approval for the use of pertuzumab in the neoadjuvant setting, and the National Comprehensive Cancer Network (NCCN) has made provisional statements to consider its use both in the neoadjuvant and adjuvant settings (Bethune et al. 2015). The eagerly awaited adjuvant APHINITY study, which will investigate the addition of pertuzumab to AC/TH and TCH, will confirm if the addition of pertuzumab truly does improve survival outcomes in patients with early, HER2-positive breast cancer.

Most studies in early HER2-positive breast cancer tend to be in larger and/or axillary node-positive tumors, and while significant improvements in response rates and survival have been made, these regimens include a significant amount of chemotherapy that tends to add toxicity. Such aggressive therapy may not be needed in patients who have smaller axillary node-negative, HER2-positive tumors. Stage I breast cancers generally have good outcomes irrespective of subtype without chemotherapy, however, HER2-positive tumors tend to have an inferior outcomes compared to HER2-negative tumors (Vaz-Luis et al. 2014; Chavez-MacGregor and Gonzalez-Angulo 2009; Gonzalez-Angulo et al. 2009; Curigliano et al. 2009; Fehrenbacher et al. 2014). A large meta-analysis including five of the six adjuvant trastuzumab trials evaluated the addition of trastuzumab in tumors less than 2 cm, and found that the addition of trastuzumab improved DFS and OS, irrespective of hormone receptor status, although in those with one or no positive lymph nodes, particularly in hormone receptor positive tumors, only DFS, and not OS, were was improved (O'Sullivan et al. 2015). These data suggest that patients with one positive axillary node, or negative axillary lymph nodes, particularly in those who are hormone receptor positive, less aggressive treatment regimens may be considered. Indeed, a recent single arm study with paclitaxel and trastuzumab was conducted on patients with HER2-positive tumors less than 3 cm with negative lymph nodes, and found that three-year rates of survival free from invasive disease were 98.7 % (95 %, CI 97.6–99.8). This regimen was well tolerated with only 3.2 % (95 %, CI 1.7–5.4) of patients developing grade 3 neuropathy, and 0.5 % (95 %, CI 0.1–1.8) developing symptomatic heart failure (Tolaney et al. 2015). These early data demonstrate that patients treated with this less aggressive regimen do very well, and provide rationale for future studies.

In summary, anti-HER2 therapy has changed the landscape of treatment for patients with early HER2-positive breast cancer. Thoughtful study design and accurate interpretation of results are key in developing better treatments, balancing efficacy with toxicity.

5.5 Mechanisms of Resistance to HER2-Directed Therapy

An important area of investigation is identifying factors that may predict response or resistance to HER2-directed therapy. As outlined above, initial testing of a tumor sample will identify whether a patient is HER2 positive and therefore a candidate for HER2-directed therapy. In spite of the results from these testing methods, there are patients with HER2-positive tumors who will not respond to HER2-directed therapy and others where disease progression occurs after initially responding to a HER2-directed therapy. Patients with HER2-positive disease exhibit both intrinsic and acquired resistance to trastuzumab (Wong et al. 2014). Intrinsic resistance is observed in ~20 % of patients with early stage breast cancer and ~70 % of patients with MBC treated with trastuzumab monotherapy; acquired resistance affects as many has 50 % of women treated with trastuzumab, and leads to disease progression on therapy (Wong et al. 2014).

Several mechanisms have been explored that may help to predict the likelihood of resistance including hyperactivation of the phosphoinositide 3-kinase (PI3K) pathway by activating mutations, phosphatase and tensin homolog (PTEN) loss, the presence of the truncated form of the extracellular domain of HER2 (p95), dimerization of HER2/IGF-IR (insulin-like growth factor-1 receptor) heterodimerization and Src activation. To date, none of the suggested markers has been validated in prospective clinical trials, but the preoperative setting has proved to be a valuable "laboratory" in which to obtain sequential tumor samples for molecular interrogation.

Multiple clinical trials exploring preoperative HER2-directed therapy (either one agent or a combination of two anti-HER2 agents, with or without chemotherapy) have been consistent in demonstrating that tumors coexpressing HER2 and ER are less likely to attain a pCR compared to tumors treated identically that are molecularly HER2 positive and ER negative. The implication of this discordance in pCR may reflect crosstalk between ER and HER2 pathways resulting in an attenuated response to HER2-directed therapy in ER-positive tumors. Blocking ER with an endocrine agent may be important to optimize the anti-tumor effect of HER2-directed therapy in this setting. Several trials have investigated this approach including combining anastrozole with trastuzumab and letrozole with lapatinib (Johnston et al. 2009; Kaufman et al. 2009). For select patients this type of approach, thereby avoiding chemotherapy, can be considered.

The presence of PI3KCA (catalytic subunit A) mutations in HER2-positive/ER-positive disease have been associated with lower rates of pCR in the neoadjuvant setting compared to tumors lacking a PI3KCA mutations (Loibl et al. 2014; Pernas Simon 2014). However, this finding has not been shown in HER2-positive, ER-negative tumors. A truncated carboxy terminal of the extracellular domain of HER2 (p95) has been associated with resistance to trastuzumab, but not lapatinib (Esteva et al. 2010). Other investigators have not uniformly corroborated these results. Finally, higher levels of circulating HER2 have been associated with a higher pCR rate in patients receiving HER2-directed therapy. At present, none of these molecular markers have been validated for routine clinical use.

There is great interest in immunologic approaches to fighting cancer particularly leveraging host immunity. In particular, the presence of tumor infiltrating lymphocytes (TILs) in tumor tissue has been shown to have prognostic significance in certain subtypes of breast cancer (Ocana et al. 2015). TILs can be further subdivided into intratumoral TILs and stromal TILs. In both triple-negative breast cancer (TNBC) and HER2-positive breast cancer, increasing number of TILs are associated with a reduction in risk of death in adjuvant therapy trials (Tung and Winer 2015; Loi et al. 2014; Adams et al. 2014). Dieci et al. (2015) reported on 816 patients from the Gustave Roussy in France who participated in randomized trials comparing adjuvant anthracyclines versus no chemotherapy. Tumor samples were evaluated using previously validated cut-off for high- and low-TIL number. Patients with high-grade tumors and ER-negative were most likely to be categorized as high TIL. Overall survival (OS) was evaluated according to level of TILs present. The prognostic significance of continuous TIL was limited to patients with TNBC and HER2-positive disease. Ten-year OS in the HER2-positive group was 78 and 57 %, respectively, for the high and low TIL group (Dieci et al. 2015). Although patients did not receive HER2-directed therapy in these trials, the results raise the possibility that other factors may influence the benefit derived from these therapies.

In the Neo ALTTO trial (Neoadjuvant Lapatinib and/or Trastuzumab Treatment Optimization) patients with HER2-positive tumors received preoperative lapatinib, trastuzumab, or the combination of both, followed by weekly paclitaxel ×12, followed by FEC ×3 (Baselga et al. 2012a). A total of 387 tumor samples (out of 455) were used for the analysis of tumors for presence of TILs (Salgado et al. 2015). The median level of TILs was 12.5 % and was higher in ER-negative tumors compared to ER-positive tumors. For the pCR endpoint, levels of TILs greater than 5 % were associated with higher pCR rates independent of treatment group. With a median followup time of 3.7 years, every 1 % increase in TILs was associated with a 3 % decrease in rate of a disease-related event (EFS) regardless of anti-HER2 therapy received (Salgado et al. 2015). There was no association between PI3KCA status of the tumor and different TIL levels at diagnosis (Salgado et al. 2015; Loibl 2015). Recently, Perez et al. (2014) presented data from the Alliance N9831 study in which patients received standard anthracyclines/taxane adjuvant therapy with, or without, adjuvant trastuzumab. Interestingly, patients with lymphocyte-predominant breast cancer (LPBC) had a better survival receiving chemotherapy alone. In contrast, patients with LPBC did not benefit from adjuvant trastuzumab therapy (Perez et al. 2014). Although these data are intriguing, a true understanding of the contribution of TILs requires more study and at present TILs should be viewed as potentially offering prognostic information but they should not be utilized to predict who would benefit from HER2-directed therapy.

It is worth noting that because of their differing mechanisms of action, lapatinib does not have complete cross-resistance with trastuzumab and/or pertuzumab—although there are other resistance mechanisms that can affect lapatinib or other TKI treatments (Oakman et al. 2010). In cell lines, PTEN loss or PIK3CA mutations, were not correlated with response to lapatinib (O'Brien et al. 2010). In contrast, and contrary to these findings, others have shown that transfection of constitutively active AKT reduces sensitivity to lapatinib (Hutchinson 2010; Lee et al. 2013). PTEN loss and activating mutations in PIK3CA can confer resistance to lapatinib. ERα-mediated overexpression of the receptor tyrosine kinase AXL confers resistance to lapatinib (Liu et al. 2009). Activation of the mTORC1 pathway in cell lines, even in the absence of alterations of PI3K/AKT, has been shown to lead to lapatinib resistance (Jegg et al. 2012).

These potential mechanisms of resistance have led to clinical trial designs that partner HER2-directed therapy with a variety of agents targeting specific signaling pathways (i.e., PI3K, mTOR, AKT, etc.) in an effort to prevent, delay or overcome resistance to available HER2 agents. Molecular interrogation of the tumor (repeat biopsy) at the time of disease progression may be required in order to identify the most rationale treatment combinations to optimize the likelihood of treatment benefit in individual patients.

5.6 Conclusions

In summary, significant advances have been made in the treatment of HER2 positive breast cancer. These have resulted in dramatic improvement in patient outcomes. However,

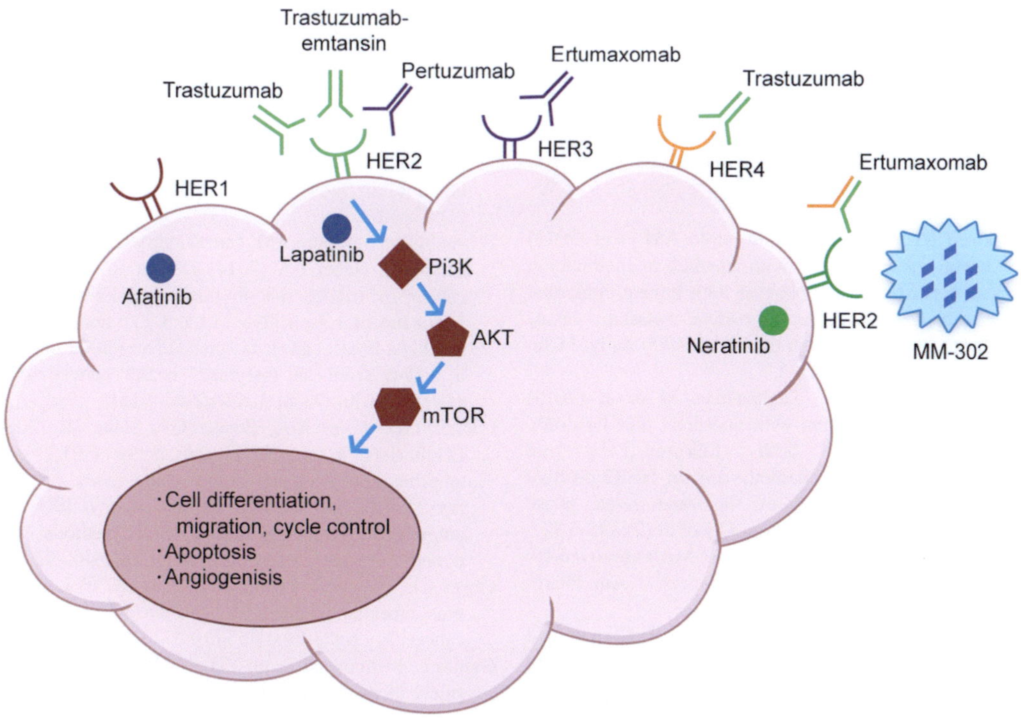

Fig. 5.2 Schematic representation of the agents available for the treatment of HER2-positive breast cancer

approximately 20 % of patients have innate resistance to these therapies. The knowledge regarding the pathways of resistance is still evolving. The role of immune mechanisms and tumor infiltrating lymphocytes in HER2 positive breast cancer is becoming clearer. Better methods for identifying which patients are likely to respond to one or more targeted agents are needed to stratify the patients for combinatorial therapies (Fig. 5.2).

References

Adams S, Gray RJ, Demaria S et al (2014) Prognostic value of tumor-infiltrating lymphocytes in triple-negative breast cancers from two phase III randomized adjuvant breast cancer trials: ECOG 2197 and ECOG 1199. J Clin Oncol 32(27):2959–2966

Baselga J, Bradbury I, Eidtmann H et al (2012a) Lapatinib with trastuzumab for HER2-positive early breast cancer (NeoALTTO): a randomised, open-label, multicentre, phase 3 trial. Lancet 379(9816):633–640

Baselga J, Cortes J, Kim SB et al (2012b) Pertuzumab plus trastuzumab plus docetaxel for metastatic breast cancer. N Engl J Med 366(2):109–119

Bethune GC, Veldhuijzen van Zanten D, MacIntosh RF et al (2015) Impact of the 2013 American Society of Clinical Oncology/College of American Pathologists guideline recommendations for human epidermal growth factor receptor 2 (HER2) testing of invasive breast carcinoma: a focus on tumours assessed as 'equivocal' for HER2 gene amplification by fluorescence in-situ hybridization. Histopathology 67:880–887

Blackwell KL, Burstein HJ, Storniolo AM et al (2012) Overall survival benefit with lapatinib in combination with trastuzumab for patients with human epidermal growth factor receptor 2-positive metastatic breast cancer: final results from the EGF104900 study. J Clin Oncol 30(21):2585–2592

Bonnefoi H, Jacot W, Saghatchian M et al (2015) Neoadjuvant treatment with docetaxel plus lapatinib, trastuzumab, or both followed by an anthracycline-based chemotherapy in HER2-positive breast cancer: results of the randomised phase II EORTC 10054 study. Ann Oncol 26(2):325–332

Brenner TL, Adams VR (1999) First MAb approved for treatment of metastatic breast cancer. J Am Pharm Assoc (Wash) 39(2):236–238

Carey LA, Berry DA, Ollila D et al (2013) Clinical and translational results of CALGB 40601: a neoadjuvant phase III trial of weekly paclitaxel and trastuzumab with or without lapatinib for HER2-positive breast cancer. J Clin Oncol 31(suppl 15; abstr 500)

Chan A, Delaloge S, Holmes FA et al (2015) Neratinib after adjuvant chemotherapy and trastuzumab in HER2-positive early breast cancer: primary analysis at 2 years of a phase 3, randomized, placebo-controlled trial (ExteNET). J Clin Oncol 33 (suppl; abstr 2508)

Chavez-MacGregor M, Gonzalez-Angulo AM (2009) HER2-neu positivity in patients with small and node-negative breast cancer (pT1a, b, N0, M0): a high risk group? Clin Adv Hematol Oncol 7(9):591–598

Coussens L, Yang-Feng TL, Liao YC et al (1985) Tyrosine kinase receptor with extensive homology to EGF receptor shares chromosomal location with neu oncogene. Science 230(4730):1132–1139

Curigliano G, Viale G, Bagnardi V et al (2009) Clinical relevance of HER2 overexpression/amplification in patients with small tumor size and node-negative breast cancer. J Clin Oncol 27(34):5693–5699

de Azambuja E, Holmes AP, Piccart-Gebhart M et al (2014) Lapatinib with trastuzumab for HER2-positive early breast cancer (NeoALTTO): survival outcomes of a randomised, open-label, multicentre, phase 3 trial and their association with pathological complete response. Lancet Oncol 15(10):1137–1146

Dieci MV, Mathieu MC, Guarneri V et al (2015) Prognostic and predictive value of tumor-infiltrating lymphocytes in two phase III randomized adjuvant breast cancer trials. Ann Oncol 26(8):1698–1704

Ellis PA, Barrios CH, Eiermann W et al (2015) Phase III, randomized study of trastuzumab emtansine (T-DM1) ± pertuzumab (P) vs trastuzumab + taxane (HT) for first-line treatment of HER2-positive MBC: primary results from the MARIANNE study. J Clin Oncol 33:507

Esteva FJ, Yu D, Hung MC, Hortobagyi GN (2010) Molecular predictors of response to trastuzumab and lapatinib in breast cancer. Nat Rev Clin Oncol 7 (2):98–107

Fehrenbacher L, Capra AM, Quesenberry CP Jr, Fulton R, Shiraz P, Habel LA (2014) Distant invasive breast cancer recurrence risk in human epidermal growth factor receptor 2-positive T1a and T1b node-negative localized breast cancer diagnosed from 2000 to 2006: a cohort from an integrated health care delivery system. J Clin Oncol 32(20):2151–2158

Francis GD, Jones MA, Beadle GF, Stein SR (2009) Bright-field in situ hybridization for HER2 gene amplification in breast cancer using tissue microarrays: correlation between chromogenic (CISH) and automated silver-enhanced (SISH) methods with patient outcome. Diagn Mol Pathol 18(2):88–95

Geyer CE, Forster J, Lindquist D et al (2006) Lapatinib plus capecitabine for HER2-positive advanced breast cancer. N Engl J Med 355(26):2733–2743

Gianni L, Pienkowski T, Im YH et al (2012) Efficacy and safety of neoadjuvant pertuzumab and trastuzumab in women with locally advanced, inflammatory, or early HER2-positive breast cancer (NeoSphere): a randomised multicentre, open-label, phase 2 trial. Lancet Oncol 13(1):25–32

Gianni L, Eiermann W, Semiglazov V et al (2013) Follow-up results of NOAH, a randomized phase III trial evaluating neoadjuvant chemotherapy with trastuzumab (CT + H) followed by adjuvant H versus CT alone, in patients with HER2-positive locally advanced breast cancer. J Clin Oncol 31(s):503 (abstract)

Gianni L, Pienkowski T, Im YH et al (2015) Five-year analysis of the phase II NeoSphere trial evaluating four cycles of neoadjuvant docetaxel (D) and/or trastuzumab (T) and/or pertuzumab (P). J Clin Oncol 33:(suppl; abstr 505)

Goldhirsch A, Gelber RD, Piccart-Gebhart MJ et al (2013) 2 years versus 1 year of adjuvant trastuzumab for HER2-positive breast cancer (HERA): an open-label, randomised controlled trial. Lancet 382 (9897):1021–1028

Gonzalez-Angulo AM, Litton JK, Broglio KR et al (2009) High risk of recurrence for patients with breast cancer who have human epidermal growth factor receptor 2-positive, node-negative tumors 1 cm or smaller. J Clin Oncol 27(34):5700–5706

Hutchinson L (2010) Targeted therapies: activated PI3K/AKT confers resistance to trastuzumab but not lapatinib. Nat Rev Clin Oncol 7(8):424

Jacquemier J, Spyratos F, Esterni B et al (2013) SISH/CISH or qPCR as alternative techniques to FISH for determination of HER2 amplification status on breast tumors core needle biopsies: a multicenter experience based on 840 cases. BMC Cancer 13:351

Jegg AM, Ward TM, Iorns E et al (2012) PI3K independent activation of mTORC1 as a target in lapatinib-resistant ERBB2+ breast cancer cells. Breast Cancer Res Treat 136(3):683–692

Johnston S, Pippen J Jr, Pivot X et al (2009) Lapatinib combined with letrozole versus letrozole and placebo as first-line therapy for postmenopausal hormone receptor-positive metastatic breast cancer. J Clin Oncol 27(33):5538–5546

Kaufman B, Mackey JR, Clemens MR et al (2009) Trastuzumab plus anastrozole versus anastrozole alone for the treatment of postmenopausal women with human epidermal growth factor receptor 2-positive, hormone receptor-positive metastatic breast cancer: results from the randomized phase III TAnDEM study. J Clin Oncol 27(33):5529–5537

King TA, Morrow M (2015) Surgical issues in patients with breast cancer receiving neoadjuvant chemotherapy. Nat Rev Clin Oncol 12:335–343

Lee YY, Kim HP, Kang MJ et al (2013) Phosphoproteomic analysis identifies activated MET-axis PI3K/AKT and MAPK/ERK in lapatinib-resistant cancer cell line. Exp Mol Med 45:e64

Liu L, Greger J, Shi H et al (2009) Novel mechanism of lapatinib resistance in HER2-positive breast tumor cells: activation of AXL. Cancer Res 69(17):6871–6878

Loi S, Michiels S, Salgado R et al (2014) Tumor infiltrating lymphocytes are prognostic in triple negative breast cancer and predictive for trastuzumab benefit in early breast cancer: results from the FinHER trial. Ann Oncol 25(8):1544–1550

Loibl S (2015) The dual role of tumor-infiltrating lymphocytes in human epidermal growth factor receptor 2-positive primary breast cancer: two sides of the same coin? JAMA Oncol 1(4):455–456

Loibl S, von Minckwitz G, Schneeweiss A et al (2014) PIK3CA mutations are associated with lower rates of pathologic complete response to anti-human epidermal growth factor receptor 2 (her2) therapy in primary HER2-overexpressing breast cancer. J Clin Oncol 32 (29):3212–3220

Mauri D, Pavlidis N, Ioannidis JP (2005) Neoadjuvant versus adjuvant systemic treatment in breast cancer: a meta-analysis. J Natl Cancer Inst 97(3):188–194

Oakman C, Pestrin M, Zafarana E, Cantisani E, Di Leo A (2010) Role of lapatinib in the first-line treatment of patients with metastatic breast cancer. Cancer Manag Res 2:13–25

O'Brien NA, Browne BC, Chow L et al (2010) Activated phosphoinositide 3-kinase/AKT signaling confers resistance to trastuzumab but not lapatinib. Mol Cancer Ther 9(6):1489–1502

Ocana A, Diez-Gonzalez L, Adrover E, Fernandez-Aramburo A, Pandiella A, Amir E (2015) Tumor-infiltrating lymphocytes in breast cancer: ready for prime time? J Clin Oncol 33(11):1298–1299

O'Sullivan CC, Bradbury I, Campbell C et al (2015) Efficacy of adjuvant trastuzumab for patients with human epidermal growth factor receptor 2-positive early breast cancer and tumors ≤2 cm: a meta-analysis of the randomized trastuzumab trials. J Clin Oncol 33 (24):2600–2608

Park JW, Liu MC, Yee D et al (2014) Neratinib plus standard neoadjuvant therapy for high-risk breast cancer: Efficacy results from the I-SPY 2 TRIAL. In: AACR 2014 annual meeting. Abstract # CT227

Perez EA, Ballman KV, Anderson SK et al (2014) Stromal tumor-infiltratinglymphocytes (S-TILs): in the Alliance N9831 trial S-TILS are associated with chemotherapy benefit but not associated with trastuzumab benefit. Breast Cancer Res Treat, Abs S01-06

Pernas Simon S (2014) Neoadjuvant therapy of early stage human epidermal growth factor receptor 2 positive breast cancer: latest evidence and clinical implications. Ther Ad Med Oncol 6:210–221

Petrelli F, Borgonovo K, Cabiddu M, Ghilardi M, Barni S (2011) Neoadjuvant chemotherapy and concomitant trastuzumab in breast cancer: a pooled analysis of two randomized trials. Anticancer Drugs 22(2):128–135

Piccart-Gebhart MJ, Holmes AP, Baselga J et al (2014) First results from the phase III ALTTO trial (BIG 2-06; NCCTG [Alliance] N063D) comparing one year of anti-HER2 therapy with lapatinib alone (L), trastuzumab alone (T), their sequence (T → L), or their combination (T + L) in the adjuvant treatment of

HER2-positive early breast cancer (EBC). J Clin Oncol 32:35s(suppl; abstr LBA)

Pivot X, Romieu G, Debled M et al (2013) 6 months versus 12 months of adjuvant trastuzumab for patients with HER2-positive early breast cancer (PHARE): a randomised phase 3 trial. Lancet Oncol 14(8):741–748

Prowell TM, Pazdur R (2012) Pathological complete response and accelerated drug approval in early breast cancer. N Engl J Med 366(26):2438–2441

Robidoux A, Tang G, Rastogi P et al (2013) Lapatinib as a component of neoadjuvant therapy for HER2-positive operable breast cancer (NSABP protocol B-41): an open-label, randomised phase 3 trial. Lancet Oncol 14(12):1183–1192

Salgado R, Denkert C, Campbell C et al (2015) Tumor-infiltrating lymphocytes and associations with pathological complete response and event-free survival in HER2-positive early-stage breast cancer treated with lapatinib and trastuzumab: a secondary analysis of the NeoALTTO trial. JAMA Oncol 1 (4):448–454

Schneeweiss A, Chia S, Hickish T et al (2013) Pertuzumab plus trastuzumab in combination with standard neoadjuvant anthracycline-containing and anthracycline-free chemotherapy regimens in patients with HER2-positive early breast cancer: a randomized phase II cardiac safety study (TRYPHAENA). Ann Oncol 24(9):2278–2284

Slamon DJ, Leyland-Jones B, Shak S et al (2001) Use of chemotherapy plus a monoclonal antibody against HER2 for metastatic breast cancer that overexpresses HER2. N Engl J Med 344(11):783–792

Slamon D, Eiermann W, Robert N et al (2011) Adjuvant trastuzumab in HER2-positive breast cancer. N Engl J Med 365(14):1273–1283

Swain SM, Baselga J, Kim SB et al (2015) Pertuzumab, trastuzumab, and docetaxel in HER2-positive metastatic breast cancer. N Engl J Med 372(8):724–734

Tanner M, Gancberg D, Di Leo A et al (2000) Chromogenic in situ hybridization: a practical alternative for fluorescence in situ hybridization to detect HER-2/neu oncogene amplification in archival breast cancer samples. Am J Pathol 157(5):1467–1472

Tolaney SM, Barry WT, Dang CT et al (2015) Adjuvant paclitaxel and trastuzumab for node-negative, HER2-positive breast cancer. N Engl J Med 372 (2):134–141

Tung NM, Winer EP (2015) Tumor-infiltrating lymphocytes and response to platinum in triple-negative breast cancer. J Clin Oncol 33(9):969–971

Vanden Bempt I, Vanhentenrijk V, Drijkoningen M, Wlodarska I, Vandenberghe P, De Wolf-Peeters C (2005) Real-time reverse transcription-PCR and fluorescence in-situ hybridization are complementary to understand the mechanisms involved in HER-2/neu overexpression in human breast carcinomas. Histopathology 46(4):431–441

Vaz-Luis I, Ottesen RA, Hughes ME et al (2014) Outcomes by tumor subtype and treatment pattern in women with small, node-negative breast cancer: a multi-institutional study. J Clin Oncol 32(20):2142–2150

Verma S, Miles D, Gianni L et al (2012) Trastuzumab emtansine for HER2-positive advanced breast cancer. N Engl J Med 367(19):1783–1791

von Minckwitz G, du Bois A, Schmidt M et al (2009) Trastuzumab beyond progression in human epidermal growth factor receptor 2-positive advanced breast cancer: a german breast group 26/breast international group 03-05 study. J Clin Oncol 27(12):1999–2006

Wolff AC, Hammond ME, Schwartz JN et al (2007) American Society of Clinical Oncology/College of American Pathologists guideline recommendations for human epidermal growth factor receptor 2 testing in breast cancer. Arch Pathol Lab Med 131(1):18–43

Wolff AC, Hammond ME, Hicks DG et al (2013) Recommendations for human epidermal growth factor receptor 2 testing in breast cancer: American Society of Clinical Oncology/College of American Pathologists clinical practice guideline update. J Clin Oncol 31(31):3997–4013

Wong HH, Collins J, McAdam K, Wilson C (2014) Trastuzumab beyond progression in advanced breast cancer: national guidance versus oncologist's decision. Oncology 86(1):22–23

Triple-Negative Breast Cancer

6

Melinda L. Telli

Abstract

Breast cancer is a heterogeneous disease consisting of distinct biological subtypes and triple-negative breast cancers (TNBC) are those that lack expression of the breast cancer prognostic markers ER, PR and HER2. TNBC often follows an aggressive disease course with poorer disease-specific survival compared to other breast cancer subtypes. Recent increased understanding of the molecular mechanisms responsible for the initiation and propagation of this breast cancer subtype has been gained through gene expression profiling, the study of cancer genetics and the study of host antitumor immunity. A subset of TNBCs express the androgen receptor (AR) and trials are underway to assess the efficacy of androgen receptor antagonists in this subgroup. In addition to germline BRCA1 and BRCA2 mutation status, biomarkers of genomic instability have been developed that detect genomic "scarring" caused by accumulated DNA damage. Therapeutic strategies are currently being investigated to assess whether these germline and genetic biomarkers can identify groups of patients with TNBC with underlying DNA repair deficiency more likely to benefit from DNA repair defect targeted therapies. A role of host antitumor immunity has also been implicated in TNBC and studies are underway to assess immune checkpoint blockade and other immunotherapeutic strategies in these patients. While we currently lack targeted therapeutic strategies for patients with TNBC, the discovery of novel biomarkers and the development of selective therapies targeting these biomarkers offer tremendous promise for the future.

M.L. Telli (✉)
Division of Oncology, Department of Medicine, Stanford University School of Medicine, 875 Blake Wilbur Drive, CC 2241, Stanford, CA 94305-5826, USA
e-mail: mtelli@stanford.edu

S. Badve and Y. Gökmen-Polar (eds.), *Molecular Pathology of Breast Cancer*, DOI 10.1007/978-3-319-41761-5_6

Keywords
Breast cancer subtypes • Basal-like breast cancer • BRCA1 mutation • BRCA2 mutation • Homologous recombination deficiency (HRD) • Tumor-infiltrating lymphocytes • Immune response

6.1 Introduction

Breast cancer is a heterogeneous disease comprised of distinct biological subtypes that carry both prognostic and therapeutic implications. The triple-negative breast cancer (TNBC) subtype accounts for approximately 15 % of all breast cancers, and is defined pathologically by the absence of expression of the estrogen receptor (ER) and progesterone receptor (PR) and lack of overexpression or amplification of the HER2/neu oncogene (Nielsen et al. 2004; Carey et al. 2006; Telli et al. 2011). The disease course for patients diagnosed with TNBC often follows a more aggressive course, with higher rates of early recurrence, visceral and central nervous system metastases and poorer disease-specific survival, compared to hormone receptor-positive breast cancer (Dent et al. 2009; Foulkes et al. 2010). The frequency of TNBC varies by race and ethnicity, with higher rates observed among African American and Hispanic women (Bauer et al. 2007; Carey et al. 2006; Lund et al. 2009). Therapeutics targeting ER, PR and HER2 have no role in the treatment of this disease and, therefore, the standard treatment approach for women with early-stage TNBC remains anthracycline- and taxane-based combination chemotherapy. At present, there are no approved targeted therapeutics for patients with TNBC either in the early-stage or advanced disease setting. Survival after relapse remains poor, with a median survival of just over 1 year. A tremendous amount of effort is currently being directed toward advancing novel targeted therapeutic strategies for patients with TNBC. These strategies have been borne out of an increasing knowledge of the critical molecular mechanisms involved in the initiation and propagation of this breast cancer subtype and will be reviewed in this chapter.

6.2 Insights from Gene Expression Profiling

In a landmark study published in 2000, gene expression profiling of primary breast tumors first described the "intrinsic" breast cancer molecular subtypes, including basal-like, HER2-enriched, luminal A, luminal B and normal-like subtypes (Perou et al. 2000). Over time it has been appreciated that the majority of TNBCs cluster within the basal-like subgroup by gene expression, a molecular subtype characterized by low expression of hormone receptor and HER2-related genes and high expression of proliferation genes characteristic of the basal epithelial cell layer (Sorlie et al. 2001, 2003). Despite this association, substantial molecular heterogeneity in TNBC defined by immunophenotyping exists. In a recent pooled analysis of patient derived samples from three phase III clinical trials in patients with early-stage breast cancer, among HER2-negative tumors with ER and PR staining <1 % (n = 283), 73 % were basal-like, 17 % HER2 enriched, 7.6 % luminal and 2.5 % normal-like using the PAM50 algorithm (Cheang et al. 2015; Parker et al. 2009) (Fig. 6.1). Currently in the clinic, the therapeutic significance of basal-like versus non-basal-like TNBC has yet to be clarified and much of the correlation has been to prognosis, rather than prediction. PAM50 subtype was assessed in a subgroup of 210 of 376 patients enrolled in the phase III Triple Negative Trial (TNT) that evaluated 6 cycles of first line carboplatin versus docetaxel in patients with metastatic TNBC (Tutt et al. 2014). In this subgroup, 83 % of patients were identified as having basal-like breast cancer. There was no significant difference in efficacy between carboplatin versus docetaxel among those patients classified as having basal-like breast cancer, but in the small subset of patients with non-basal-like breast cancer, docetaxel was associated with a significantly higher objective response rate. This apparent improved sensitivity of docetaxel over carboplatin in non-basal-like TNBCs is intriguing, but requires further investigation.

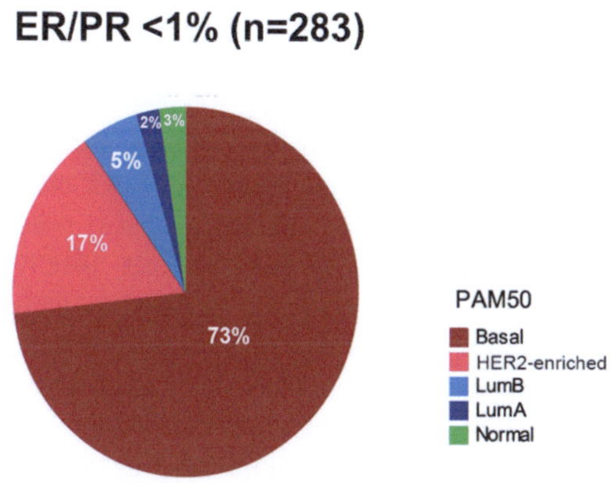

Fig. 6.1 Intrinsic subtype distribution by PAM50 among 283 patients with triple-negative breast cancer. Cheang, M.—Need permission to print (Presented at the 2012 ASCO Annual Meeting)

More recent work in this area has focused on further dissecting the molecular heterogeneity of TNBC using gene expression profiling with the goal of identifying TNBC subtypes with therapeutic implications. A team from Vanderbilt University pooled gene expression data from 21 breast cancer data sets and selected for TNBC by filtering for ER, PR and HER2 by mRNA expression identifying 587 cases (Lehmann et al. 2011). Using hierarchical clustering within this group, six stable TNBC subtypes were identified, including two basal-like (BL-1 and BL-2), an immunomodulatory (IM), a mesenchymal (M), a mesenchymal stem-like (MSL), and luminal androgen receptor (LAR) subtype (Fig. 6.2). Preclinical studies were then performed in breast cancer cell lines representative of these subtypes with the finding of enhanced cisplatin sensitivity, for example, in the BL subtypes, and enhanced sensitivity to antiandrogens among the LAR

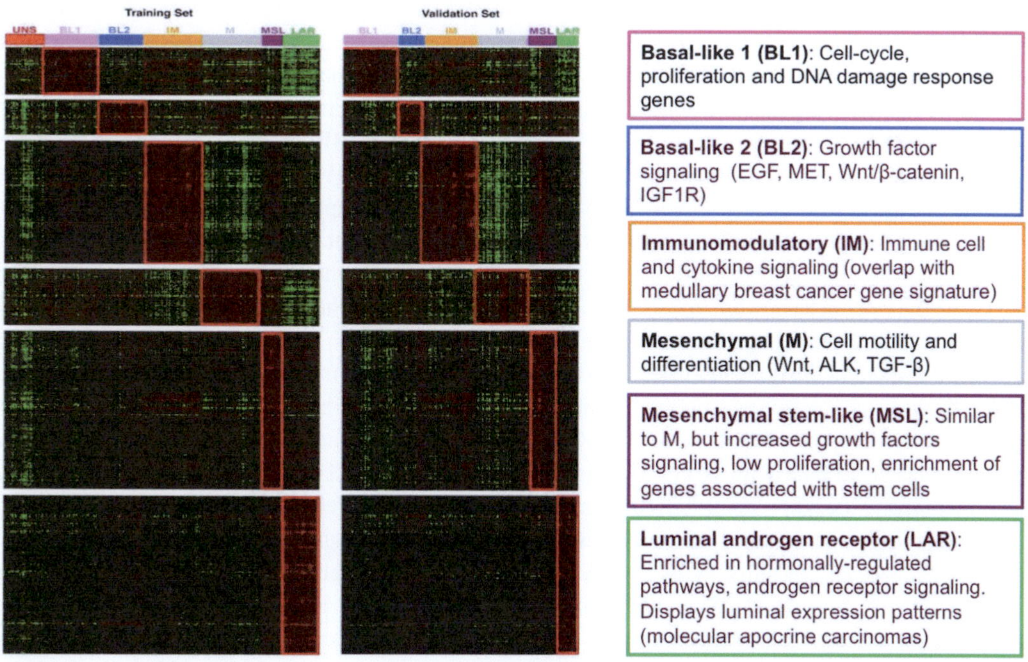

Fig. 6.2 Six stable TNBC subtypes identified from hierarchical clustering of 587 breast tumors filtered by ER, PR and HER2 expression. Adapted from Lehmann BD, et al. Journal of Clinical Investigation, 2011

subtype tumors. The clinical promise of this type of strategy was highlighted by two recent reports evaluating the antiandrogens bicalutamide and enzalutamide in patients with advanced ER-negative breast cancer whose tumors express the androgen receptor. In the first phase II study exploring the efficacy of bicalutamide, of 424 patients with ER-negative (≤10 %) and PR-negative (≤10 %) breast cancer, 12 % expressed AR at a level of >10 % nuclear staining (Gucalp et al. 2013). Of 26 evaluable patients treated with continuous daily dosing with bicalutamide 150 mg orally daily, a clinical benefit rate at 24 weeks of 19 % was observed, however objective tumor responses were not observed. In the second study in patients with advanced TNBC, among patients with AR staining in ≥10 % of tumor nuclei who received enzalutamide 160 mg orally daily, 6/75 patients (8 %) achieved an objective response to therapy and the clinical benefit rate at 16 weeks was 35 % (Traina et al. 2015). Though the objective response rate is low, this is significant as this type of therapy offers an endocrine alternative to chemotherapy in advanced TNBC patients where no such alternative currently exists. Additional clinical trials are now ongoing to further interrogate therapeutic strategies within the distinct Vanderbilt TNBC subtypes.

6.3 Insights from Cancer Genetics

Though the characterization of TNBC using messenger RNA gene expression profiling has provided important insights into the biology of this disease, an evolving understanding of genetic alterations associated with TNBC has been associated to date with more obvious clinical therapeutic insights. In 1994, the original report defining the sequence of the breast and ovarian cancer susceptibility gene BRCA1 was published (Miki et al. 1994). Since that time, the implications of the breast cancer susceptibility genes BRCA1 and BRCA2 in the clinic have continued to evolve. Interestingly, it has long been observed that the breast cancers developing in women with a germline BRCA1 mutation are overwhelmingly triple negative. In addition, in a recently reported prospective study of 211 patients with unselected TNBC, the frequency of deleterious BRCA1 or BRCA2 mutations was high at 15.4 % (Sharma et al. 2014). Pooled data suggest that the lifetime risk of breast cancer approximates 57 % in BRCA1 mutation carriers and 49 % in BRCA2 mutation carriers (Chen and Parmigiani 2007). Similarly, lifetime risks of ovarian cancer are also elevated in BRCA1 mutation carriers (~40 %) and BRCA2 mutation carriers (~18 %). Based on this elevated and quantifiable risks, BRCA1 and BRCA2 mutation screening began to be used to guide screening, medical and surgical risk reducing recommendations for carriers (Daly et al. 2016).

Of great interest has been recent research focused on the use of germline BRCA1 and BRCA2 mutation status as a biomarker for treatment selection. The concept of using this germline information to guide treatment for carriers affected by breast cancer is based on the notion that these defining genetic events carry with them biologic information that can be exploited to therapeutic advantage. Given the known role of BRCA1 and BRCA2 in homologous recombination (HR) DNA repair, therapeutic strategies targeting this DNA repair deficiency in BRCA mutation carriers have now been assessed in multiple studies with proof-of-concept clearly demonstrated. Treatment with platinum chemotherapy, a class of cytotoxic chemotherapy that is directly DNA damaging through the formation of platinum-DNA adducts with subsequent formation of toxic intrastrand and interstrand crosslinks, has been associated with high level activity in both early and advanced BRCA1 and BRCA2 mutation-associated breast cancer (Tutt et al. 2014; Byrski et al. 2009, 2012). Furthermore, robust single agent anticancer activity with poly (ADP-ribose) polymerase (PARP) inhibitors has been observed in BRCA1 and BRCA2 mutation carriers with heavily pretreated advanced breast cancer of various subtypes (Tutt et al. 2010). Poly (ADP-ribose) polymerase-1 (PARP1) is a nuclear enzyme crucial for recruitment of a cell's base excision repair machinery to sites of DNA damage. In 2005, a pair of pivotal papers suggested a novel application of PARP inhibitors in the treatment of cancers demonstrating that the use of inhibitors of PARP in cells deficient in BRCA1 and BRCA2 function resulted in selective cytotoxicity, compared to cells wild type or heterozygous for BRCA1 or BRCA2 (Farmer et al. 2005; Bryant et al. 2005). This concept of 'chemical synthetic lethality' of PARP inhibitors in the treatment of BRCA1 and BRCA2-associated cancer led to rapid clinical investigation in this area. Based on encouraging early studies, multiple phase III studies are currently evaluating the efficacy of PARP inhibitor alone or in combination with cytotoxic chemotherapy in BRCA1 and BRCA2 mutation carriers.

In addition to BRCA1 and BRCA2, many other genes implicated in hereditary breast cancer syndromes have a role in homologous recombination DNA repair and include genes such as PALB2, ATM, BARD1, BRIP1, RAD50, RAD51C, RAD51D, ATR, and the Fanconi anemia complementation group of genes, among others (Couch et al. 2015; Castera et al. 2014). In an important study that assessed over 1800 patients with unselected TNBC, deleterious mutations in 15 non-BRCA1/2 predisposition genes were detected in 3.7 % of patients, with the majority observed in genes involved in homologous recombination, including PALB2 (1.2 %) and BARD1, RAD51D, RAD51C, and BRIP1 (0.3–0.5 %) (Couch et al. 2015). As with BRCA1 and BRCA2, mutations in these genes linked to regulation of the DNA double strand break repair pathway are hypothesized to have similar chemosensitivity to DNA-damaging therapies, such as PARP inhibitors, and clinical trials are currently underway to assess this hypothesis (McCabe et al. 2006).

These insights from germline genetics led to subsequent hypotheses that sporadic triple-negative or basal-like breast tumors may possess similar DNA repair defects and demonstrate similar chemosensitivity as BRCA1 mutation-associated breast tumors. It has been shown that basal-like breast cancer cell lines, like BRCA1-deficient cancer cell lines, demonstrate increased sensitivity to PARP inhibition and platinum (Hastak et al. 2010) and are deficient in base excision repair (Alli et al. 2009). In recent years, investigations focusing on the role of underlying DNA repair deficiency in TNBC and how this may be exploited with DNA damaging chemotherapeutics and novel DNA repair defect targeted agents, such as PARP inhibitors, have been conducted. While the role of PARP inhibition in sporadic TNBC remains unclear, a growing body of clinical data suggests that platinum chemotherapeutic agents may have a role in the standard treatment of both early-stage and advanced TNBC. In the neoadjuvant setting, randomized phase II trials have demonstrated an increase in the rate of pathological complete response (pCR) when platinum is added to a standard anthracycline and taxane-based regimen (Sikov et al. 2015; von Minckwitz et al. 2014). Studies examining the longterm outcomes associated with platinum therapy in early-stage TNBC are currently underway.

Given the heterogeneity in TNBC, a major goal has been to develop methods to identify sporadic TNBC patients most likely to benefit from DNA repair defect treatment strategies. With this goal in mind, many groups have developed measures of genomic instability with potential to serve as biomarkers of response to DNA damaging therapeutics (Abkevich et al. 2012; Birkbak et al. 2012; Popova et al. 2012; Vollebergh et al. 2011). As described above, beyond BRCA1 and BRCA2, there are many additional HR-related genes that may be altered by mutation, rearrangement, DNA methylation or mRNA expression that are hypothesized to result in impairment of the HR pathway. To identify this biology, the Homologous Recombination Deficiency (HRD) assay (Myriad Genetics) has been developed using an indirect approach to allow for the detection of HRD regardless of its etiology or mechanism as measured by levels of genomic instability. The assay is compatible with formalin-fixed paraffin-embedded (FFPE) tumor tissue and BRCA1 and BRCA2 tumor sequence data is simultaneously generated. Early in assay development, genomic regions of loss of heterozygosity (LOH) of intermediate length (>15 Mb and < one chromosome) were shown to

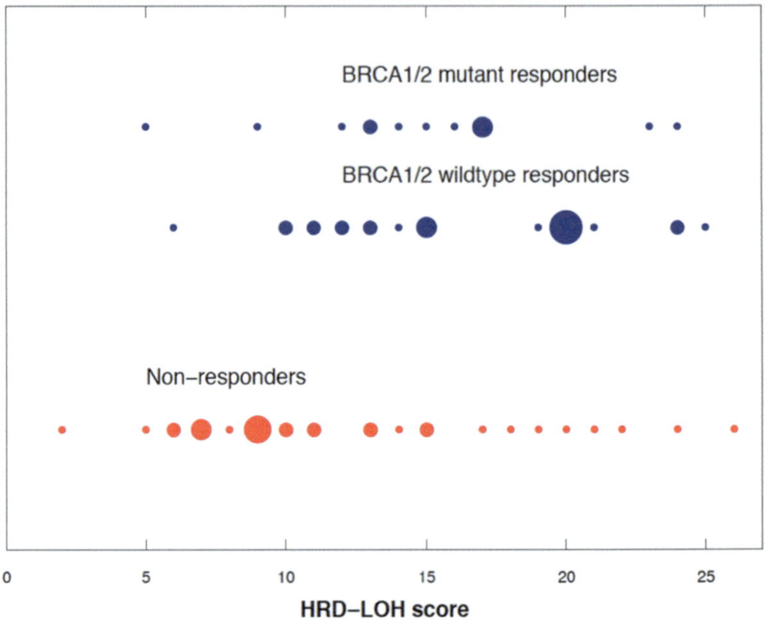

Fig. 6.3 Homologous recombination loss of heterozygosity (HRD-LOH) score association with response to neoadjuvant platinum-based therapy in PRECOG 0105. Telli ML, JCO 2015—Need permission to reprint

be highly associated with HR deficiency and the HRD-LOH score was derived as a count of LOH regions of this length across the tumor genome (Abkevich et al. 2012). Assessment of the HRD-LOH assay score in a phase II neoadjuvant trial of platinum-based therapy showed that responders had significantly higher mean HRD scores compared to nonresponders and that this was true for both BRCA1/2 wild type and mutant responders (Fig. 6.3) (Telli et al. 2015). Recently, the HRD assay has been further optimized and currently incorporates additional measures of genomic instability, including telomeric allelic imbalance (TAI; the number of regions with allelic imbalance that extend to the subtelomere, but do not cross the centromere) and large-scale state transitions (LST; the number of chromosomal breaks between adjacent genomic regions longer than 10 Mb after filtering out regions shorter than 3 Mb) (Timms et al. 2014; Popova et al. 2012; Birkbak et al. 2012). The HRD score is currently calculated by adding the LOH, TAI and LST scores and is reported as a continuous score from 0–100. An HRD score of <41 is defined as HR proficient and HRD score of ≥42 as HR deficient. Assessment of this biomarker in additional neoadjuvant clinical trial cohorts has shown significant correlation with favorable response to platinum-based therapy (Kaklamani et al. 2015). These data strongly suggest that tumor measures of genomic instability may be important biomarkers in the identification of germline BRCA1 and BRCA2 wild type patients who may benefit from DNA repair defect-targeted treatment strategies. Additional prospective validation of this novel genomic instability biomarker is currently underway.

6.4 Role of Host Antitumor Immunity in TNBC

Increasing data has documented the important role of host antitumor immunity in the prognosis and treatment of TNBC (Loi et al. 2013, 2014; Adams et al. 2014; Denkert et al. 2010, 2015; West et al. 2011; Issa-Nummer et al. 2013; Vinayak et al. 2014a). In a study of 1334 breast cancer patients with long-term followup, it was demonstrated that the presence of $CD8^+$ TILs in the tumor microenvironment was strongly associated with improved patient survival (Mahmoud et al. 2011). In this study, the total number of $CD8^+$ cells was positively correlated with tumor grade and inversely correlated with age at diagnosis, ER expression and PR expression. Two recent studies analyzing tumor samples from three large adjuvant chemotherapy breast cancer clinical trials demonstrated a positive correlation between tumor-infiltrating lymphocytes (TILs) and clinical outcomes among patients with TNBC. Among 481 evaluable TNBC tumors from patients enrolled on two Eastern Cooperative Oncology Group studies, stromal TILs were seen in 80 % and intratumoral TILs in 15 % (Fig. 6.4) (Adams et al. 2014). Lymphocyte-predominant breast cancer (LPBC) was defined as that involving ≥50 % lymphocytic infiltration of either tumor stroma or cell nests, and was seen in 4.4 % of cases. With over 10 years of median followup, higher stromal TIL scores were associated with improved disease-free and overall survival and this was independently prognostic in a multivariable analysis. A "dose response" was noted; for every 10 % increase in stromal TILs, a 14 % reduction of risk of recurrence or death ($p = 0.02$), an 18 % reduction of risk of distant recurrence ($p = 0.04$), and 19 % reduction of risk of death ($p = 0.01$) were observed. In the second study, among 256 ER-negative and HER2-negative patients, LPBC was seen in 10.6 % (Loi et al. 2013). In this study the degree of lymphocytic infiltration was also prognostic; for every 10 % increment in stromal and intratumoral lymphocytic infiltration, there was a 15 and 17 % reduction of risk for recurrence or death and 17 and 27 % reduction of risk for death, respectively.

In addition to the role of TILs in prognosis, there is evidence from neoadjuvant studies that the presence of TILs is predictive of chemotherapy response. In two German Breast Group (GBG) neoadjuvant trials, the percentage of intratumoral lymphocytes was a significant independent predictor for pathologic complete response (pCR) (Denkert et al. 2010). Pathologic complete response (pCR) rate were 40 % in

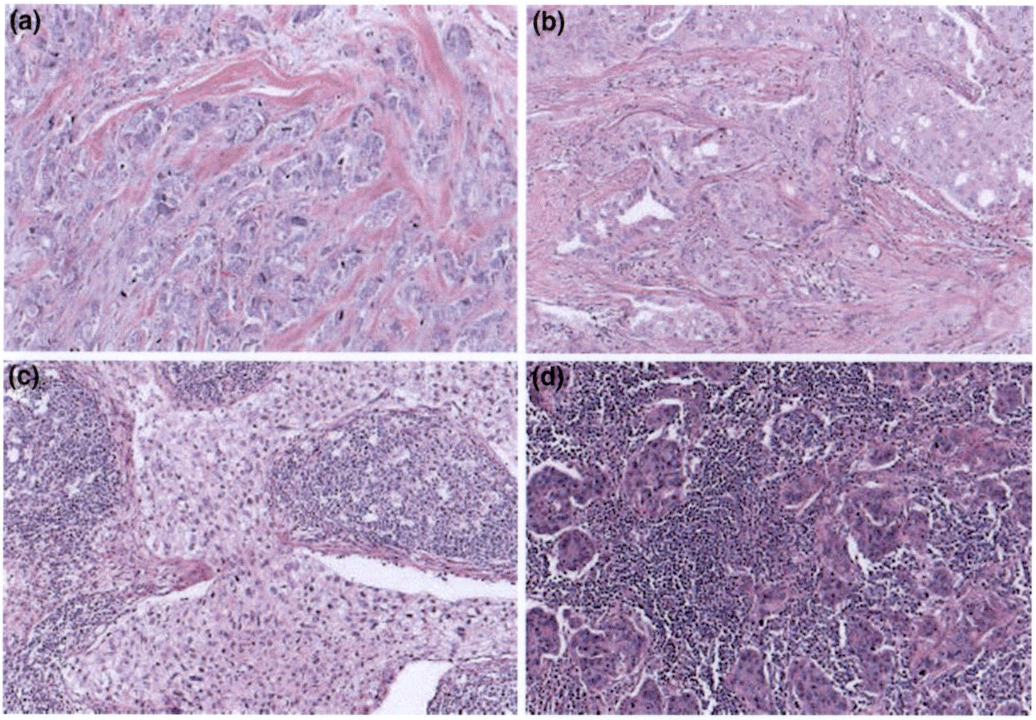

Fig. 6.4 Varying levels of stromal tumor-infiltrating lymphocytes by H&E in triple-negative breast cancer. **a** 0 %, **b** 20 %, **c** Formation of germinal follicles, **b** 80 % (10× magnification). Adams S, et al. JCO 2014

LPBC, while the pCR rates were 7 % in tumors lacking infiltrating lymphocytes. More recent data from the GBG suggests a significant interaction with TILs and carboplatin therapy specifically in patients treated with standard chemotherapy with or without carboplatin (Denkert et al. 2015). In the PrECOG 0105, the percentage of TILs was significantly associated with pathologic complete response to neoadjuvant platinum-based therapy in triple-negative and BRCA1/2 mutation-associated breast cancer (Vinayak et al. 2014a). In this study, TILs as assessed by a pathologist also associated with the immunomodulatory (IM) subtype of TNBC according to the mRNA expression-based Vanderbilt TNBC subtype classification. Using CIBERSORT, a novel method for characterizing cell composition of complex tissues from their gene expression profile, both activated $CD4^+$ memory T cells and $CD8^+$ T cells were associated with pathologic response to neoadjuvant therapy in PrECOG 0105 (Newman et al. 2015) (Fig. 6.1). Intriguingly, while germline BRCA1/2 mutation status was not significantly associated with TILs or immune score in this study, a measure of genomic instability was significantly associated with the CIBERSORT immune score (Vinayak et al. 2014b). These data suggest a potential intimate interplay between genomic instability and immune infiltration, potentially shaping adaptive antitumor immune responses, and thereby affecting neoadjuvant response in TNBC.

In summary, assessment of the preexisting host antitumor immune response in TNBC appears to have both prognostic and predictive value. Attempts to capitalize on this immune response via treatment with immunotherapy are currently underway. Recent proof-of-concept has been demonstrated in advanced TNBC with inhibitors of the PD-1 and PD-L1 checkpoints (Nanda et al. 2014; Emens et al. 2014). Despite an increasing appreciation of the antitumor immune response in TNBC, the immunological determinants of these antitumor immune responses remain poorly understood. A possible major determinant of TNBC immunogenicity may be the presence of neoantigens or mutated tumor antigens. Work in this promising area is currently ongoing and insights gained will be critically important to shape future immune targeted strategies for patients with TNBC.

6.5 Conclusions

While targeted therapies for patients with early and advanced stage TNBC are currently lacking, recent biologic insights into this aggressive breast cancer subtype are beginning to reveal potential therapeutic strategies that are currently being tested in the clinic. Expression profiling has highlighted the heterogeneity of this disease and revealed distinct TNBC subsets with potential therapeutic significance. In addition to germline BRCA1 and BRCA2 mutation status, biomarkers of genomic instability have been developed that detect genomic "scarring" caused by accumulated DNA damage. Therapeutic strategies are currently being investigated to assess whether these germline and genetic biomarkers can identify groups of patients with TNBC with underlying DNA repair deficiency more likely to benefit from DNA repair defect targeted therapies such as platinum and PARP inhibitors. Finally, a role of host antitumor immunity has also been implicated in TNBC and studies are underway to assess immunotherapeutic strategies in these patients. The discovery of clinical biomarkers will enable the development of selective therapies for subgroups of patients with TNBC and has great potential to make clinical impact for patients with this difficult-to-treat disease.

References

Abkevich V, Timms KM, Hennessy BT et al (2012) Patterns of genomic loss of heterozygosity predict homologous recombination repair defects in epithelial ovarian cancer. Br J Cancer 107(10):1776–1782

Adams S, Gray RJ, Demaria S et al (2014) Prognostic value of tumor-infiltrating lymphocytes in triple-negative breast cancers from two phase III randomized adjuvant breast cancer trials: ECOG 2197 and ECOG 1199. J Clin Oncol 32(27):2959–2966

Alli E, Sharma VB, Sunderesakumar P, Ford JM (2009) Defective repair of oxidative dna damage in triple-negative breast cancer confers sensitivity to inhibition of poly(ADP-ribose) polymerase. Cancer Res 69(8): 3589–3596

Bauer KR, Brown M, Cress RD, Parise CA, Caggiano V (2007) Descriptive analysis of estrogen receptor (ER)-negative, progesterone receptor (PR)-negative, and HER2-negative invasive breast cancer, the so-called triple-negative phenotype: a population-based study from the California Cancer Registry. Cancer 109(9):1721–1728

Birkbak NJ, Wang ZC, Kim JY et al (2012) Telomeric allelic imbalance indicates defective DNA repair and sensitivity to DNA-damaging agents. Cancer Discov 2 (4):366–375

Bryant HE, Schultz N, Thomas HD et al (2005) Specific killing of BRCA2-deficient tumours with inhibitors of poly(ADP-ribose) polymerase. Nature 434(7035): 913–917

Byrski T, Huzarski T, Dent R et al (2009) Response to neoadjuvant therapy with cisplatin in BRCA1-positive breast cancer patients. Breast Cancer Res Treat 115 (2):359–363

Byrski T, Dent R, Blecharz P et al (2012) Results of a phase II open-label, non-randomized trial of cisplatin chemotherapy in patients with BRCA1-positive metastatic breast cancer. Breast Cancer Res 14(4):R110

Carey LA, Perou CM, Livasy CA et al (2006) Race, breast cancer subtypes, and survival in the Carolina breast cancer study. JAMA 295(21):2492–2502

Castera L, Krieger S, Rousselin A et al (2014) Next-generation sequencing for the diagnosis of hereditary breast and ovarian cancer using genomic capture targeting multiple candidate genes. Eur J Hum Genet 22(11):1305–1313

Cheang MC, Martin M, Nielsen TO et al (2015) Defining breast cancer intrinsic subtypes by quantitative receptor expression. Oncologist 20(5):474–482

Chen S, Parmigiani G (2007) Meta-analysis of BRCA1 and BRCA2 penetrance. J Clin Oncol 25(11): 1329–1333

Couch FJ, Hart SN, Sharma P et al (2015) Inherited mutations in 17 breast cancer susceptibility genes among a large triple-negative breast cancer cohort unselected for family history of breast cancer. J Clin Oncol 33(4):304–311

Daly MB, Pilarski R, Axilbund JE et al (2016) Genetic/familial high-risk assessment: breast and ovarian, version 2.2015. J Natl Compr Canc Netw 14(2):153–162

Denkert C, Loibl S, Noske A et al (2010) Tumor-associated lymphocytes as an independent predictor of response to neoadjuvant chemotherapy in breast cancer. J Clin Oncol 28(1):105–113

Denkert C, von Minckwitz G, Brase JC et al (2015) Tumor-infiltrating lymphocytes and response to neoadjuvant chemotherapy with or without carboplatin in human epidermal growth factor receptor 2-positive and triple-negative primary breast cancers. J Clin Oncol 33(9):983–991

Dent R, Hanna WM, Trudeau M, Rawlinson E, Sun P, Narod SA (2009) Pattern of metastatic spread in triple-negative breast cancer. Breast Cancer Res Treat 115(2):423–428

Emens LA, Braiteh FS, Cassier P et al (2014) Inhibition of PD-L1 by MPDL3280A leads to clinical activity in patients with metastatic triple-negative breast cancer. San Antonio breast cancer symposium, 10 Dec 2014, Abstract PD1-6

Farmer H, McCabe N, Lord CJ et al (2005) Targeting the DNA repair defect in BRCA mutant cells as a therapeutic strategy. Nature 434(7035):917–921

Foulkes WD, Smith IE, Reis-Filho JS (2010) Triple-negative breast cancer. N Engl J Med 363(20): 1938–1948

Gucalp A, Tolaney S, Isakoff SJ et al (2013) Phase II trial of bicalutamide in patients with androgen receptor-positive, estrogen receptor-negative metastatic breast cancer. Clin Cancer Res 19(19):5505–5512

Hastak K, Alli E, Ford JM (2010) Synergistic chemosensitivity of triple-negative breast cancer cell lines to poly(ADP-Ribose) polymerase inhibition, gemcitabine, and cisplatin. Cancer Res 70(20):7970–7980

Issa-Nummer Y, Darb-Esfahani S, Loibl S et al (2013) Prospective validation of immunological infiltrate for prediction of response to neoadjuvant chemotherapy in HER2-negative breast cancer–a substudy of the neoadjuvant GeparQuinto trial. PLoS ONE 8(12): e79775

Kaklamani VG, Jeruss JS, Hughes E et al (2015) Phase II neoadjuvant clinical trial of carboplatin and eribulin in women with triple negative early-stage breast cancer (NCT01372579). Breast Cancer Res Treat 151(3): 629–638

Lehmann BD, Bauer JA, Chen X et al (2011) Identification of human triple-negative breast cancer subtypes and preclinical models for selection of targeted therapies. J Clin Invest 121(7):2750–2767

Loi S, Sirtaine N, Piette F et al (2013) Prognostic and predictive value of tumor-infiltrating lymphocytes in a phase III randomized adjuvant breast cancer trial in node-positive breast cancer comparing the addition of docetaxel to doxorubicin with doxorubicin-based chemotherapy: BIG 02-98. J Clin Oncol 31(7):860–867

Loi S, Michiels S, Salgado R et al (2014) Tumor infiltrating lymphocytes are prognostic in triple negative breast cancer and predictive for trastuzumab benefit in early breast cancer: results from the FinHER trial. Ann Oncol 25(8):1544–1550

Lund MJ, Trivers KF, Porter PL et al (2009) Race and triple negative threats to breast cancer survival: a population-based study in Atlanta, GA. Breast Cancer Res Treat 113(2):357–370

Mahmoud SM, Paish EC, Powe DG et al (2011) Tumor-infiltrating CD8+ lymphocytes predict clinical outcome in breast cancer. J Clin Oncol 29(15):1949–1955

McCabe N, Turner NC, Lord CJ et al (2006) Deficiency in the repair of DNA damage by homologous recombination and sensitivity to poly(ADP-ribose) polymerase inhibition. Cancer Res 66(16):8109–8115

Miki Y, Swensen J, Shattuck-Eidens D et al (1994) A strong candidate for the breast and ovarian cancer susceptibility gene BRCA1. Science 266(5182):66–71

Nanda R, Chow LQ, Dees EC et al (2014) A phase Ib study of pembrolizumab (MK-3475) in patients with advanced triple-negative breast cancer. In: San Antonio breast cancer symposium, 10 Dec 2014, Abstract S1-09

Newman AM, Liu CL, Green MR et al (2015) Robust enumeration of cell subsets from tissue expression profiles. Nat Methods 12(5):453–457

Nielsen TO, Hsu FD, Jensen K et al (2004) Immunohistochemical and clinical characterization of the basal-like subtype of invasive breast carcinoma. Clin Cancer Res 10(16):5367–5374

Parker JS, Mullins M, Cheang MC et al (2009) Supervised risk predictor of breast cancer based on intrinsic subtypes. J Clin Oncol 27(8):1160–1167

Perou CM, Sorlie T, Eisen MB et al (2000) Molecular portraits of human breast tumours. Nature 406 (6797):747–752

Popova T, Manie E, Rieunier G et al (2012) Ploidy and large-scale genomic instability consistently identify basal-like breast carcinomas with BRCA1/2 inactivation. Cancer Res 72(21):5454–5462

Sharma P, Klemp JR, Kimler BF et al (2014) Germline BRCA mutation evaluation in a prospective triple-negative breast cancer registry: implications for hereditary breast and/or ovarian cancer syndrome testing. Breast Cancer Res Treat 145(3):707–714

Sikov WM, Berry DA, Perou CM et al (2015) Impact of the addition of carboplatin and/or bevacizumab to neoadjuvant once-per-week paclitaxel followed by dose-dense doxorubicin and cyclophosphamide on pathologic complete response rates in stage II to III triple-negative breast cancer: CALGB 40603 (Alliance). J Clin Oncol 33(1):13–21

Sorlie T, Perou CM, Tibshirani R et al (2001) Gene expression patterns of breast carcinomas distinguish tumor subclasses with clinical implications. Proc Natl Acad Sci U S A 98(19):10869–10874

Sorlie T, Tibshirani R, Parker J et al (2003) Repeated observation of breast tumor subtypes in independent gene expression data sets. Proc Natl Acad Sci U S A 100(14):8418–8423

Telli ML, Chang ET, Kurian AW et al (2011) Asian ethnicity and breast cancer subtypes: a study from the California cancer registry. Breast Cancer Res Treat 127(2):471–478

Telli ML, Jensen KC, Vinayak S et al (2015) Phase II study of gemcitabine, carboplatin, and iniparib as neoadjuvant therapy for triple-negative and BRCA1/2 mutation-associated breast cancer with assessment of a tumor-based measure of genomic instability: PrECOG 0105. J Clin Oncol 33(17):1895–1901

Timms KM, Abkevich V, Hughes E et al (2014) Association of BRCA1/2 defects with genomic scores predictive of DNA damage repair deficiency among breast cancer subtypes. Breast Cancer Res 16(6):475

Traina TA, Miller K, Yardley DA et al (2015) Results from a phase 2 study of enzalutamide (ENZA), an androgen receptor (AR) inhibitor, in advanced AR+ triple-negative breast cancer (TNBC). J Clin Oncol 33:(suppl; abstr 1003)

Tutt A, Robson M, Garber JE et al (2010) Oral poly (ADP-ribose) polymerase inhibitor olaparib in patients with BRCA1 or BRCA2 mutations and advanced breast cancer: a proof-of-concept trial. Lancet 376 (9737):235–244

Tutt A, Ellis P, Kilburn L et al (2014) The TNT trial: a randomized phase III trial of carboplatin (C) compared with docetaxel (D) for patients with metastatic or recurrent locally advanced triple negative or BRCA1/2 breast cancer (CRUK/07/012) In: San Antonio breast cancer symposium, San Antonio, Texas, Abstract S3-01

Vinayak S, Gray RJ, Adams S et al (2014a) Association of increased tumor-infiltrating lymphocytes (TILs) with immunomodulatory (IM) triple-negative breast cancer (TNBC) subtype and response to neoadjuvant platinum-based therapy in PrECOG0105. In: American Society of clinical oncology annual meeting, Chicago, IL, 3 June 2014, Abstract 1000

Vinayak S, Newman A, Adams S et al (2014b) Deconvoluting immune cell populations using 'in silico flow cytometry' with CIBERSORT: association with neoadjuvant therapy response and genomic instability in TNBC. In: San Antonio breast cancer symposium, San Antonio, Texas, Abstract P5-04-03

Vollebergh MA, Lips EH, Nederlof PM et al (2011) An aCGH classifier derived from BRCA1-mutated breast cancer and benefit of high-dose platinum-based chemotherapy in HER2-negative breast cancer patients. Ann Oncol 22(7):1561–1570

von Minckwitz G, Schneeweiss A, Loibl S et al (2014) Neoadjuvant carboplatin in patients with triple-negative and HER2-positive early breast cancer (GeparSixto; GBG 66): a randomised phase 2 trial. Lancet Oncol 15:747–756

West NR, Milne K, Truong PT, Macpherson N, Nelson BH, Watson PH (2011) Tumor-infiltrating lymphocytes predict response to anthracycline-based chemotherapy in estrogen receptor-negative breast cancer. Breast Cancer Res 13(6):R126

Proliferation Markers in Breast Cancer

7

Frederique Penault-Llorca and Nina Radosevic-Robin

Abstract

Breast cancer proliferation can be measured by several approaches (mitotic count, S-phase fraction assessment, evaluation of cell cycle-related protein expression, molecular tests). It is used to predict outcome, by discriminating luminal A from luminal B breast cancer, and consequently to guide the choice of chemotherapy in hormone receptor-positive, HER2-negative breast cancer. Proliferation reflects tumor aggressiveness and gives valuable information for the identification of patients at risk of early relapses and thus potentially candidates for chemotherapy. Dynamic evaluation of proliferation allows identification of the patients resistant to neoadjuvant endocrine treatment and, at a lesser degree, to neoadjuvant chemotherapy. Evaluation of proliferation does not bring any added value to the management of HER2-positive, triple negative or metastatic breast cancer.

Keywords

Breast · Cancer · Proliferation · S-phase · Immunohistochemistry · Gene expression · Prognosis

7.1 Introduction

Uncontrolled proliferation is one of the hallmarks of cancer as proposed by Hanahan and Weinberg (2011), so numerous studies have been published about proliferation activity of breast cancer (BC). Before the era of gene expression profiling, proliferation was evaluated by counting mitoses, by flow cytometry to determine the S-phase fraction or by immunohistochemistry (IHC) to assess the expression of proliferating cell nuclear antigen (PCNA), Ki67 or the related proteins.

F. Penault-Llorca (✉) · N. Radosevic-Robin
Department of Pathology, Jean Perrin Comprehensive Cancer Centre, 63011 58 rue Montalembert, Clermont-Ferrand, France
e-mail: frederique.penault-llorca@clermont.unicancer.fr

F. Penault-Llorca · N. Radosevic-Robin
ERTICa Research Group, University of Auvergne (EA4677), 63011 58 rue Montalembert, Clermont-Ferrand, France

S. Badve and Y. Gökmen-Polar (eds.), *Molecular Pathology of Breast Cancer*, DOI 10.1007/978-3-319-41761-5_7

Breast cancer is a heterogeneous disease involving at least four relevant molecular subgroups (two oestrogen receptor (ER)-positive: luminal A and B, and two ER-negative: HER2-enriched and basal-like) (Lakhani et al. 2012; Perou et al. 2000). Those molecular subgroups, known also as breast cancer intrinsic subtypes, are defined by gene expression profiles. They harbour distinct clinical features including prognosis and metastatic behaviour. Luminal breast cancers can be further divided into luminal A and luminal B subtypes, mainly upon the expression level of proliferation genes, such as *MKI67*, *AURKA*, *TOP2A*. Luminal B cancers have higher proliferation rates and poorer prognosis than luminal A cancers. This is the reason why expression of Ki67 (Gerdes et al. 1983) has been used to distinguish immunohistochemically defined luminal A from luminal B breast cancers in the 2013 and 2015 Saint Gallen consensus conference (Goldhirsch et al. 2013; Coates et al. 2015).

In the molecular biology era, the key biological drivers in nine published prognostic signatures were genes involved in proliferation, in addition to ER-signalling and HER2 activation pathways (Wirapati et al. 2008). Recent works from the Perou group, based on the existing 52 gene expression signatures, identified key drivers of proliferation in luminal breast cancers (*FGD5, METTL6, CPT1A, DTX3, MRPS23, EIF2S2, EIF6* and *SLC2A10*) which are uniquely amplified in patients with highly proliferative luminal breast tumours, and could be putative therapeutic targets (Gatza et al. 2014).

Proliferation assessment (IHC-based or not) in breast cancer is used to estimate prognosis by discriminating luminal A from luminal B subtype and consequently to guide the choice of chemotherapy in hormone receptor-positive, HER2-negative breast cancer. Proliferation reflects tumour aggressiveness and gives information for the identification of patients at risk of early relapses.

Proliferation evaluation does not bring any added value to the management of HER2-positive, triple negative, or metastatic disease (Aleskandarany et al. 2012; Van Poznak et al. 2015).

Therefore the degree of tumour cell proliferation is of paramount importance in ER-positive, HER2-negative breast cancers. This chapter is aimed to describe various tools for assessment of proliferation in breast cancer, with a special focus on Ki67 and the commercially available molecular signatures.

7.2 Mitotic Index/SBR Grade

Mitotic count or mitotic index is one of the three features evaluated in the Elston and Ellis modification of Scarff, Bloom and Richardson histologic grading (Rakha et al. 2008). The mitotic count score criteria vary depending on the field diameter of the microscope used by the pathologist (score 1: ≤ 3 mitoses/mm^2, score 2:4–7 mitoses/mm^2, score 3: ≥ 8 mitoses/mm)^2. The pathologist counts mitotic figures within 10 consecutive high-power fields (HPF, usually defined as the combination of 10× eyepiece and 40× objective). When using a HPF of 0.50 mm diameter, the criteria are as follows: (i) score 1: ≤ 7 mitoses per 10 HPF, (ii) score 2:8–14 mitoses per 10 HPF, (iii) score 3: ≥ 15 mitoses per 10 HPF. This is the oldest method to evaluate tumour proliferation. It has been proven to be prognostic of breast cancer-related death (reviewed in Beresford et al. 2006). Nevertheless, it is a subject of considerable variations depending on the thickness of the tissue section, fields chosen (mitotic counts are usually highest at the periphery of a tumour), type of microscope used, delay in fixation time, and observer's experience in the identification of mitotic figures (hyperchromatic, karyorrhexic, or apoptotic nuclei should not be considered as mitotic figures). Furthermore, the duration of the mitotic phase is variable, consequently mitotic count is not always strictly correlated to the proliferation rate in a linear fashion.

7.3 S-Phase Fraction and the Related Tools

The S-phase fraction ("the S-phase") corresponds to the measurement of the fraction of tumour cells engaged in DNA synthesis.

- **Tritiated thymidine** (3HTdR) **labelling index** (LI) was the first method used to evaluate the S-phase fraction. This method measured the incorporation of 3HTdR (a DNA precursor) into the dividing cells. The method required the use of fresh material and was time-consuming as autoradiography was performed on slides, usually several weeks after 3HTdR incorporation. The LI corresponds to the fraction of tumour cells (percentage) labelled by black nuclear dots. If 3HTdR incorporation was performed with cells in suspension, consequently, the isotopic emission is measured by a scintillation beta-counter. The 3HTdR LI tends to be much higher than the mitotic count because the cells stay longer in the S-phase than in the M-phase. The 3HTdR is extremely accurate, reproducible, however it not suitable for a routine use (requirement of fresh tissue, use of radioactive material, long assay duration).
- **5-bromodeoxyuridine (BrdU)** incorporation and its immunohistochemical detection was developed as specific assay for detection of DNA replication, avoiding the use of radiography and radioactive products (Gratzner 1982). BrdU assay showed comparable results to the 3HTdR assay. However, fresh and thin viable tissue is required and endogenous thymidylate activity has to be blocked.
- **Flow cytometry** is a technique that consists of measurement of various parameters while a suspension of cells flows through a beam of light past stationary detectors. The instrument focuses hydrodynamically a cell suspension in a sample chamber and passes single cells through a light source, usually a laser. The light scattered at various angles by the cells is registered by detectors and converted to electronic signals, which are then digitized, stored, and analysed by the computer to produce a histogram. This technique allows the analysis of 5000–10,000 cells per second. Flow cytometry can be used to analyse DNA content (DNA ploidy). Depending on their DNA content, neoplasms are divided into diploid and aneuploid. Diploid tumours have a major population with the normal diploid DNA value. Aneuploid tumours are those having a major cell population with a DNA content other than diploid. The **DNA index (DI)** is the ratio of the DNA content of the aneuploid peak to the DNA content of the diploid peak. The hyperdiploid fraction is the percentage of cells above the upper boundary of the diploid population and constitutes a measure of the S-phase or proliferative fraction of a cell population (S-phase fraction or SPF). Flow cytometry measurements of SPF have been shown to correlate with mitotic counts, histological grades and 3HTdR LI. The prognostic value of S-phase measurement has been shown in various retrospective studies (reviewed in Beresford et al. 2006). The flow cytometry method has two major limitations: (i) the fact that the stromal cells are also present in the population of cells being evaluated, thus the results do not solely reflect the malignant component; (ii) the requirement of fresh tissue, not suitable for a large spread of the technique.

7.4 Nuclear Antigens

Immunohistochemical (IHC) detection of nuclear antigens closely related to proliferation offers a unique opportunity to democratize the evaluation of tumour proliferation on formalin-fixed, paraffin-embedded (FFPE) tissue sections or on cytology specimens. Ki67 IHC assay is the most popular among those techniques and will be addressed at the end of this paragraph.

- **Phosphorylated histone H3** (PhH3) is expressed in the cells in mitotic phase. PhH3 is a nuclear core histone protein that is a component of chromatin. Its phosphorylation at Serine 10 and Serine 28 is implicated in chromosome condensation and cell cycle progression during mitosis and meiosis (Lee et al. 2014). Thus number of cells expressing PhH3 should theoretically correlate with mitotic count. Therefore PhH3 has emerged as a potential IHC marker of mitotic activity and consequently of proliferation. Several reports showing positive correlation between mitotic and PhH3 counts have been published (Beresford et al. 2006). Due to lack of correlation between PhH3 and other markers of proliferation, PhH3 is currently considered more as an aid to the assessment of mitotic count than as a true proliferation marker (Dessauvagie et al. 2015).

- **Proliferating cell nuclear antigen** (PCNA) is an auxiliary protein of DNA polymerase delta. It seems to be essential for DNA synthesis and is expressed in high concentrations during the cell cycle. PCNA is also involved in DNA repair processes. PCNA correlates poorly with the Ki67 labelling index and mitotic count so is of more limited use in assessing proliferation and has become a dead letter (Leonardi et al. 1992).
- **Mitosin**, a nuclear phosphoprotein expressed in the late G1, S, G2, and M phases of the cell cycle but not in G0 has been evaluated as a substitute to S-phase (Clark et al. 1997). Good correlation was observed with the S-phase fraction, without a correlation with overall survival (Clark et al. 1997). This marker is no longer used in breast cancer. Recent publications have evaluated its accuracy as a prognosis marker in astrocytoma (Varughese et al. 2016).
- **Cyclins and cyclin-dependent kinases**: Progression through the cell cycle is dependent on the interactions between cyclins and cyclin-dependent kinases (CDKs). Cyclins are proteins which expression varies during different phases of the cell cycle. Cyclin D1 is expressed during G1 phase, cyclin E during G1 and early S phase, cyclin A during S and G2 phase and cyclin B during late G2 phase. They are, therefore, useful markers of the proportion of cells in a given phase of the cell cycle at any time. High expression of either cyclin A or cyclin E is associated with poor prognosis in breast cancer (Kuhling et al. 2003). Amplifications of the cyclin D1 gene (*CCND1*), found in 40 % of luminal breast cancers, and of the CDK4 gene (*CDK4*) are linked to hormone receptor-positivity and there is some evidence of a relationship between high levels of expression/amplification and poor prognosis (Roy et al. 2010). Correlations between expression of various cyclins and Ki67-based measurements of proliferation have been demonstrated in breast cancer (Beresford et al. 2006).
- **Inhibitors of the CDKs** can also be studied using immunohistochemical techniques: p16INK4a, p21 and p27 bind to and inhibit the activity of cyclin-CDK2 or -CDK4 complexes. Thus they control the cell cycle progression at G1. Low nuclear p27 levels and sequestration of p27 in the cytoplasm are associated with high proliferative activity and have been shown to relate to a high tumour grade and poor prognosis (Catzavelos et al. 1997; Tsuchiya et al. 1999).

In the light of new drugs targeting CDK4/6 such as palbociclib (Roberts et al. 2012), several markers appeared to be potential candidates for response predictors, including retinoblastoma (Rb) protein loss or phosphorylation, inactivation of CDK4/6 inhibitors and amplification of genes for cyclins or CDKs. Inactivation of *RB1* appears to predict resistance to CDK4 and CDK6 inhibitors, but two of the most promising biomarkers, loss of *CDKN2A* (coding for p16INK4a) and gains of *CCND1* (coding for cyclin D1), failed to predict a benefit for palbociclib in ER-positive breast cancer in the PALOMA 1 trial (Finn et al. 2015). More studies are needed to evaluate putative biomarkers to better select patient eligible for CDK4/6 inhibitors (Carey and Perou 2015).

- **Argyrophilic nucleolar organiser regions** (AgNORs) are composed of non-histone proteins associated with loops of DNA transcribing to ribosomal RNA (Pich et al. 2000). The number and size of AgNORs can be assessed by a silver-based staining of the tumour tissue. AgNORs are being aggregated and segregated during the cell cycle. Immediately after mitosis the NORs are dispersed through the nucleus and the nucleolus is not readily apparent. AgNOR staining reveals a large number of dots. The AgNOR count should be higher in cells in late G2 or early G1 when the NORs are segregated and they are more easily discernible. The major caveat with AgNOR assessment is that their number can also be elevated in benign proliferations so an elevated AgNOR count is not per se diagnostic of malignancy. The use of image analysis has improved the specificity of the AgNOR assay (Beresford et al. 2006). It seems that, although the number of AgNORs per cell is not discriminatory enough on its own to determine malignancy, the addition of size or area measurements using image analysis gives improved diagnostic and prognostic specificity in breast cancer (Winzer et al. 2013). Some authors have suggested to use AgNOR staining as an alternative measure of tumour proliferation (Raymond and Leong 1989; Canepa et al. 1990). Nevertheless, the AgNOR assay requires use of image analysis, so is introduced only in some laboratories, for research purposes.

- **Topoisomerase II (topoII)** is a nuclear enzyme which breaks and joins DNA strands. The isoform topoIIα is a marker of cell proliferation and also the molecular target for the anthracycline class of chemotherapy drugs commonly used in breast cancer treatment. Assessment of topoIIα expression by IHC has been shown to highly significantly correlate with tumour proliferation rate measured by SPF (Jarvinen et al. 1996) or by Ki67 labelling (Depowski et al. 2000; Misell et al. 2005), giving the information on the number of cycling tumour cells. High topoIIα expression is associated with an aggressive tumour phenotype, however the topoIIα IHC assay has not been developed for clinical use.
- **Thymidine kinase 1** (TK1) is an enzyme involved in phosphorylation of deoxy-thymidine during DNA synthesis. TK1 is expressed in the cytoplasm and activated at late G1 phase of the cell cycle. TK1 can be detected by IHC or ELISA; its expression is high in proliferating and malignant cells, but low or absent in quiescent cells. High levels of TK1 activity are associated with poor prognosis of breast cancer (Spyratos et al. 2002). This marker is currently used only for research approaches; the IHC assays for in vitro diagnostic use (IVD) are not developed.

7.5 Ki67

- **Background**: Ki67 index is the most developed and popular marker of proliferation, although with obvious flaws. Ki67 is a non-histone nuclear cortex protein, involved in the early steps of polymerase I-dependent ribosomal RNA synthesis. It was first identified by Gerdes et al in 1983 in a Hodgkin lymphoma cell line (Gerdes et al. 1983), then named Ki after Kiel University and 67 after the clone number of the antibody able to detect it. The gene coding for Ki67 (*MKI67*) is located on chromosome 10q25-ter and organized in 15 exons and 14 introns. Exon 13 contains sixteen Ki67 repeats including a highly conserved motif of 66 bp, named the Ki67 motif (Duchrow et al. 1996). The Ki67 protein is expressed in the cell nucleus during the G1, S, G2 and M phase of the cell cycle, but not in the G0 cell quiescent state. In the interphase the Ki67 protein is localized in the dense fibrillary components of the nucleolus. During mitosis it gets associated with the periphery of the condensed chromosomes. The Ki67 protein expression varies throughout the different phases of the cell cycle, being at the peak level during mitosis. While the function of the Ki67 protein is not completely elucidated, there is evidence that it has a role in cell division and ribosomal RNA synthesis. Ki67 index represents a percentage of tumour cells labelled with an anti-Ki67 antibody, in a IHC assay. It can serve as an

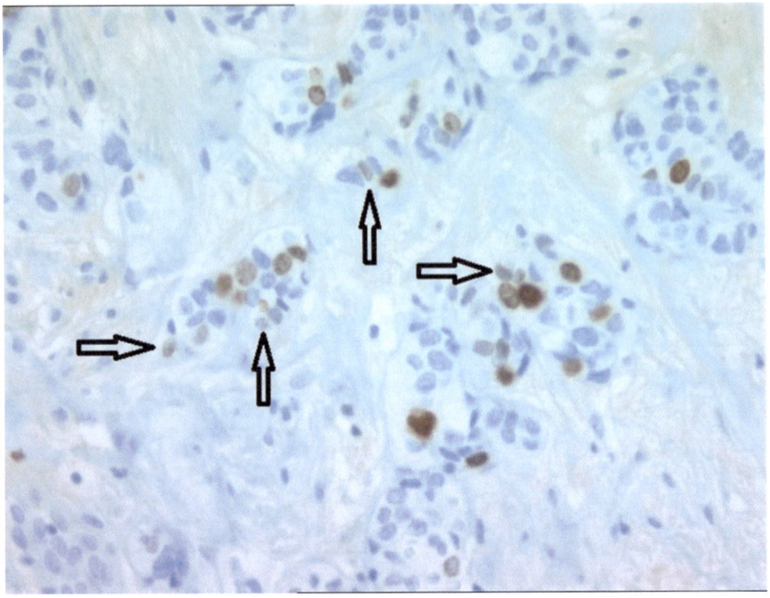

Fig. 7.1 Immunohistochemical detection of Ki67 using the MIB-1 clone (X400). Any intensity of nuclear staining indicates a Ki67-positive cell (*black arrows* show light brown positive nuclei)

alternative to mitotic index and correlates with increasing tumour grade. But Ki67 does not correlate well with PhH3 (r = 0.79) or mitotic score (r = 0.83) as reported by Lee et al. (2014) in a series of breast cancers. This confirms that PhH3 and Ki67 express distinct biological information and should be treated separately.

Despite massive literature addressing the caveats of Ki67 as an accurate biomarker for prognostication in early breast cancer (reviewed in de Azambuja et al. 2007; Yerushalmi et al. 2010; Dowsett et al. 2011; Luporsi et al. 2012), Ki67 is a popular and cheap biomarker in breast cancer, widely used to assess proliferation, and especially in segregating luminal A from luminal B tumours.

7.5.1 Analytical Validity

Lack of standardization impacts the analytical validity of Ki67. An international group of pathologists, clinicians and biologists was convened to examine data available upon Ki67 as a biomarker in early breast cancer and to propose guidelines (Dowsett et al. 2011). Several antibody clones, like MIB-1, MM-1, Ki-S5 and SP6, have been tested for Ki67 detection by IHC on FFPE tissue sections. The most popular and most widely used antibody is the MIB-1 clone.

As for any immunodetection, several **pre-analytical issues** such as time to fixation, type of fixative, duration of fixation and storage of slides with unstained tissue sections might adversely affect Ki67 expression assessment (reviewed in Dowsett et al. 2011). Eventually, the guidelines for tissue handling, which are already in place for ER immunohistochemical assessment (8–72 h of neutral buffered formalin fixation) (Hammond et al. 2010), can be considered for Ki67 IHC. Fortunately, Ki67 is one of the most robust biomarkers assessed by IHC, showing relatively consistent signals in tissue specimens across a range of conditions used in routine fixation, tissue processing, and IHC staining procedures.

Analytical steps are quite classical. Of note, protease and low pH methods for antigen retrieval should be avoided. Immunohistochemistry for Ki67 results in a nuclear staining. Any intensity of nuclear staining indicates a Ki67-positive cell (Fig. 7.1). Therefore it is important to have the counterstaining optimized, because, if it is weak, might result in an overestimation of the Ki-67 index.

How to count? The post-analytical phase of Ki67 IHC assay is the most critical one. The poor reproducibility reported for Ki67 scoring mainly resulted from a lack of consensus about which area of the tumour should be assessed, i.e. tumour invasive edge, a whole tumour section, or the hot spots (i.e. the areas of the highest proliferative activity). The international Ki67 in Breast Cancer Working Group provided guidelines covering also the Ki67 scoring (Dowsett et al. 2011) (Box 7.1). In brief, it is recommended to assess Ki67 either on core biopsies or on full-face tumour tissue sections. At least three HPFs should be selected to represent the spectrum of staining seen on the initial overview of the entire section. The invasive edge of the tumour should be counted and hot spots included in the overall score (Fig. 7.2). The Ki67 score or index should be expressed as the percentage of positively stained cells among the total number of invasive cancer cells in the area scored.

Overall, the International Ki67 in Breast Cancer Working Group concluded that measurements of proliferation could be important

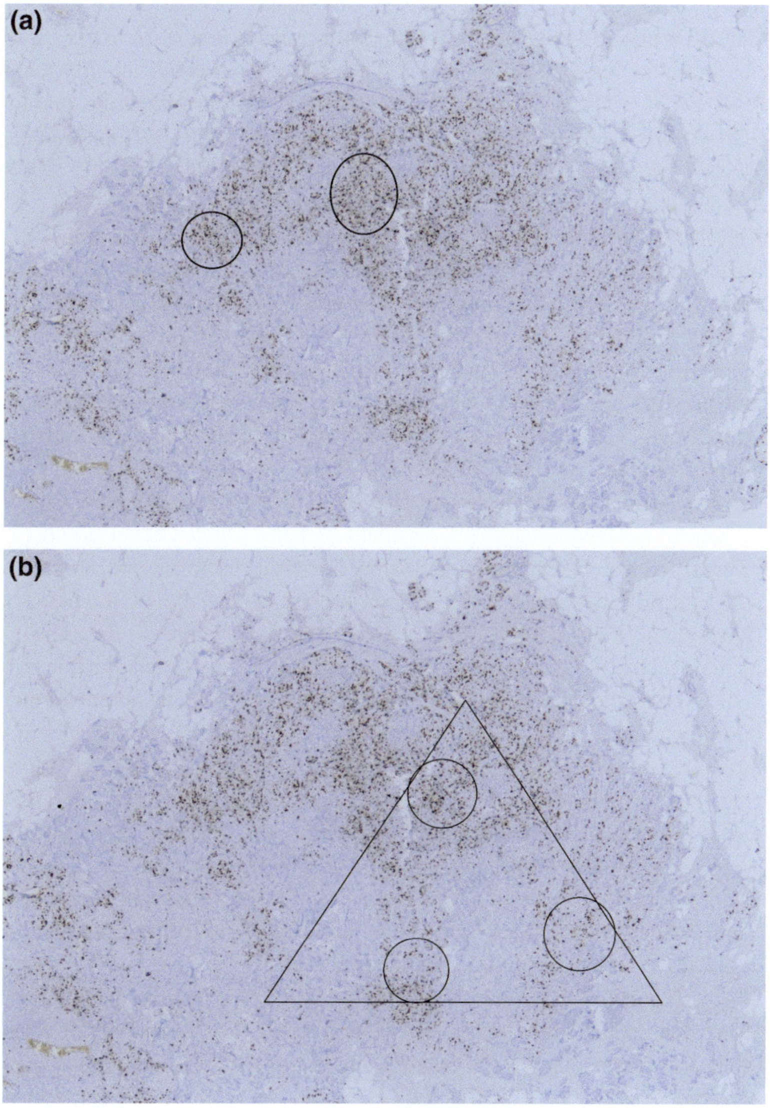

Fig. 7.2 Ki67 scoring. **a** Hot spots method: the evaluation is performed in the area with the highest number of positive nuclei (hot spot) (*black circle*). **b** Three high power fields including a hot spot: at least three HPFs should be selected to represent the spectrum of staining seen on the initial overview of the entire section. The invasive edge of the tumour should be counted and hot spots included in the overall score

both in standard clinical practice and, particularly, in clinical trials. Ki67 assessed by IHC using monoclonal antibody MIB-1 has the largest body of literature support. Standardization efforts have recently been made to improve the reproducibility of quantitative IHC assessment of Ki67 between different laboratories and observers, particularly with regards to the intermediate levels of Ki67 expression (Polley et al. 2013, 2015). The intra-class correlation coefficient (ICC) corresponding to the percentage of variance that is derived from the biomarker (i.e. Ki67) has to be as high (close to 1) as possible (otherwise the variance is due to the variation in interpretation). The International Ki67 in Breast Cancer Working Group showed that, with training and guidelines, the ICC for Ki67 went from 0.71 (95 % CI 0.47–0.78) to 0.92 (95 % CI 0.88–0.96). A quality assurance study from the Swiss working group of breast and gynaecological pathologists (Varga et al. 2012) evaluated the Ki67-based proliferative fraction in grade II breast carcinomas by different methods, for example, by eyeballing or by counting in self-selected versus the preselected areas. The reproducibility was good for low and high Ki67 indexes, but assessment of mid-range Ki67 was impaired by high inter- and intra-observer variability (Varga et al. 2012). The use of computer-assisted automated scoring proved to be helpful to standardize the assessment of Ki67 in breast cancer specimens in the GeparTrio trial and was well correlated with clinical endpoints (Klauschen et al. 2015). Finally, for the intermediate levels of Ki67 index, validated multigene assays could be a good re-test option (Goldhirsch et al. 2013; Coates et al. 2015).

7.5.2 Clinical Validity—Prognostic or Predictive?

Various meta-analyses (reviewed in de Azambuja et al. 2007; Yerushalmi et al. 2010; Dowsett et al. 2011; Luporsi et al. 2012; Andre et al. 2015) showed an independent prognostic value of Ki67 index for node-negative, ER-positive breast cancer [and to a lesser extent for the node-positive one (Andre et al. 2015)]. A study from the European Institute of Oncology showed that high Ki67 values (≥ 32 %) predict the benefit from cytotoxic chemotherapy addition in 1241 patients with luminal breast cancer and 1–3 axillary lymph nodes (Criscitiello et al. 2014). Nevertheless, other studies showed either a modest predictive value for chemotherapy benefit in node-positive patients [in PACS01 trial, for docetaxel addition (Penault-Llorca et al. 2009)], if any [such as in the BCIRG001 trial (Dumontet et al. 2010)]. In the neoadjuvant setting, high Ki67 index predicted for complete pathological response (pCR) in a large number of studies (de Azambuja et al. 2007; Luporsi et al. 2012; Denkert et al. 2013). Furthermore, Ki67 evaluation showed an important clinical utility as a pharmacodynamic or clinical endpoint for neoadjuvant treatment, namely for endocrine therapy (Jones et al. 2009). The largest study of post-neoadjuvant chemotherapy Ki67 index prognostic value in breast cancer, GeparTrio, distinguished three patient groups according to the Ki67 index level (0–15 vs. 15.1–35 vs. >35.1 %) (von Minckwitz et al. 2013). The low Ki67 group had an outcome comparable to the pCR group, while the high Ki67 group had a significantly higher recurrence and death risk compared to the low or intermediate Ki67 group. Taken together, the post-therapy Ki67 index level could provide additional prognostic information in the ER-positive breast cancer where pCR shows a limited prognostic value, whereas in the ER-negative cancer the post-neoadjuvant Ki67 does not have a stronger prognostic power than pCR (von Minckwitz et al. 2013). Decrease in Ki67 index is now being explored as the primary endpoint for pre-surgical trials with CDK4/6 inhibitors, like the Monaleesa-1 trial (NCT01919229).

- **Biomarkers combining Ki67 index with other parameters**: Ki67 index has been integrated into several mathematically derived parameters, which were tested as predictors of various features in breast cancer. In the following text we will highlight the most important ones:

Preoperative Endocrine Prognostic Index (PEPI) (Ellis et al. 2008) was generated using data of the P024 neoadjuvant endocrine breast cancer therapy trial in which prognostic relevance for recurrence-free survival (RFS) and overall survival (OS) was independently evaluated for five post-therapy tumour features: pathological size, pathological node status, ER status, histological grade and Ki67 index. The levels of Ki67 index were expressed in the form of natural logarithm-transformed intervals. PEPI was further constructed as a score representing an arithmetic sum of risk points assigned to each mentioned feature, according to its hazard risk estimate (Ellis et al. 2008). That way PEPI score distinguished three categories of significantly different risk for breast cancer-induced death. The PEPI score was independently validated on 203 patients included in the neoadjuvant IMPACT trial (Ellis et al. 2008) and is now being prospectively tested in the on-going ALTERNATE trial, conducted by The Alliance of Clinical Trials in Oncology, to identify patients with a very low recurrence risk after neoadjuvant endocrine therapy (Suman et al. 2015).

Residual Proliferative Cancer Burden (RPCB) (Sheri et al. 2015) was obtained by applying a formula that generates a sum of relative event rates for post-therapy Ki67 index and the Residual Cancer Burden (RCB) developed by Symmans et al. (2007). Its prognostic value for time to recurrence was evaluated in a cohort of 220 breast cancer patients treated by neoadjuvant chemotherapy. RPCB, classified into tertiles, was able to distribute the patients into groups with significantly different RFS and OS rates after a 5-year median follow-up (Sheri et al. 2015).

IHC4 is an IHC-based assay of four markers including Ki67, which has been shown to predict residual risk of distant recurrence in patients on adjuvant endocrine therapy in the ATAC trial as robustly as the recurrence score from OncotypeDX® (Cuzick et al. 2011). Recently, Engelberg and colleagues published a web-based pathologist training tool named "Score the Core" to improve the reproducibility of IHC4 scoring and thus eventually increase its clinical use (Engelberg et al. 2015).

MAGEE equation-based recurrence score (MS) is based on tumour pathological characteristics (SBR grade, H-scores for ER and PR, HER2, Ki67 index and tumour size) and can be used to estimate the Oncotype DX® recurrence score (RS), using the Magee equation (http://path.upmc.edu/onlineTools/ptvr.html) (Klein et al. 2013). The concordance between MS (tiered score) and RS was 98.6 %, when the intermediate category of MS was eliminated, but dropped to 54.3 % when the total populations were included in the comparison. Consequently, MS may be used instead of the actual Oncotype DX® RS, if the estimated MS is clearly high or low.

To summarize the complexities in evaluating the clinical utility of Ki67 in breast cancer, Denkert et al. (2015) have highlighted three different groups of tumours (quoted):

(a) Low proliferating tumours are not responding to chemotherapy but have a good prognosis anyway (low Ki67 linked to good outcome)
(b) In those high proliferating tumours that are therapy sensitive, high Ki67 is linked to an increased chance of pCR and improved survival (high Ki67 linked to good outcome)
(c) In contrast, in high proliferating tumours that are chemotherapy or hormone therapy resistant, increased Ki67 is linked to reduced survival (high Ki67 linked to poor outcome).

This suggests that, in the adjuvant setting, it is always very difficult to separate prognostic from predictive value of the Ki67 index. However, in the neoadjuvant setting, the pre-treatment Ki67 index is predictive and the post-treatment one is prognostic.

- **Clinical utility of the Ki67 index**: In breast cancer, Ki67 index is mainly used to discriminate luminal A from luminal B tumours in the ER-positive, HER2-negative breast cancers and consequently to guide the choice of chemotherapy, versus hormonotherapy alone. As mentioned by the St. Gallen expert Panel in 2015, "the distinction between strongly endocrine responsive, low proliferation, good prognosis 'luminal A-like' and less endocrine responsive, higher proliferation, poorer prognosis 'luminal B-like'

(HER2-negative) tumours could be derived from IHC tests for ER, PgR and Ki67, though the use of Ki67 required knowledge of local laboratory values" (Coates et al. 2015).

Does an ideal cut-off exist for Ki67? Despite all the lack of standardization and the variability in the cutpoints used to define a high Ki67 index (from 5 to 34 % or more), prognostic or predictive value of Ki67 index has been demonstrated in a majority of studies (Denkert et al. 2015). The St. Gallen consensus 2009 (Goldhirsch et al. 2009) proposed three categories: low (≤ 15 %), intermediate (16–30 %) and high (>30); St. Gallen 2011 (Goldhirsch et al. 2011) held for two categories with a cut-off of 14 % between luminal A and luminal B; St. Gallen 2013 (Goldhirsch et al. 2013) changed the cutpoint to 20 % with the option to use local laboratory values. In 2015, "a majority of the Panel was prepared to accept a threshold value of Ki67 within the range of 20–29 % to distinguish 'luminal B-like' disease" (Coates et al. 2015). Interestingly, a recent meta-analysis (Petrelli et al. 2015) of 41 studies, encompassing more than 64,000 patients, addressed specifically the major issue we have with the Ki67 clinical utility: which Ki67 cut-off provides the strongest prognostic information in early breast cancer (except in the neoadjuvant setting)? In 25 studies, available for analysis of the Ki67 cut-off significance for overall survival, the cut-off of 25 % was significant for prediction of OS (HR = 2.05, 95 % CI 1.66–2.53, $p < 0.00001$). Moreover, in the ER-positive population, this 25 % cut-off was also significant (HR = 1.51, 95 % CI 1.25–1.81, $p < 0.00001$). However, because of the complexity of the significance of Ki67 in different settings, reaching a unique cutpoint for Ki67 is likely idealistic.

- **Conclusion on Ki67**: Although not the most robust prognostic or predictive marker in breast cancer, Ki67 index is an additional piece of information that may be used in clinical decision making, provided the physician understands the limitations of the test and the test result. Ki67 IHC is widely available and less expensive than a multigene assay. Low Ki67 index (<15 %) is associated with good prognosis, whereas the high values (≥ 25 %) are likely predictive of chemosensitivity. The "grey zone" between 15 and 25 % might require either a second assessment by another pathologist, by image analysis, or use of multigene assays.

7.6 Molecular Signatures

In the early 2000s, several multigene signatures were developed [MammaPrint® (Agendia, the Netherlands), 76-gene signature (Veridex, USA), Oncotype DX® (Genomic Health, USA)] by searching, without a priori biologic assumption, for gene expression profiles associated with clinical outcome of breast cancer. Simultaneously, other signatures were developed in a "bottom-up" fashion by interrogating genes associated with a specific biologic process such as histologic grade [Genomic Grade Index or GGI® (Qiagen, the Netherlands)], wound healing, or invasiveness (reviewed in Wirapati et al. 2008). Although all demonstrate additional prognostic value, those gene expression signatures did not have many genes in common. They are described in details elsewhere in this book. The genes selected are implied in different biologic processes of breast cancer carcinogenesis e.g. cell cycle, invasion, metastasis, angiogenesis, immune response and, for some of them, in ER-, PR- and HER2-related pathways. The common denominator of all commercially available multigene assays are the proliferation genes, and it is believed that the group of proliferation-associated genes has the biggest impact on breast cancer prognosis (Mook et al. 2010). Proliferation-related (cell cycle) genes are highly represented in the available multigene assays: Oncotype Dx® has 5 proliferation-related genes, out of total 16: *MKI67*, *AURKA* (formerly *STK15*), *BIRC5* (coding for survivin), *CCNB1* and *MYBL2*; the 70-gene signature known as Mammaprint® contains 19 proliferation-related out of 70 total genes, the 76-gene signature (Rotterdam) has 16 out of 60 and the GG has 89 out of 98. Thus proliferation is the driving force of prognostic information provided by those signatures. When only proliferation genes were used, the overall performance of the mentioned signatures was not reduced. In contrast, when proliferation genes were removed, the non-proliferation partial signatures showed reduced performance in giving the prognostic information. Consequently, this important weight of proliferation genes implies a strong time dependence of the prognostic information provided by the signatures, informative mainly for early (<5 years) recurrences.

Then a second generation of gene expression signatures was developed, with Endopredict® (Myriad Genetics, USA) and Prosigna® (Nanostring technologies, USA) signatures. Like OncotypeDX®, those commercially available tests are dedicated to ER-positive, HER2-negative breast cancers, node-negative or positive for up to three nodes. Endopredict® is a RT PCR-based test of 12 genes, with three proliferation-related genes (*UBE2C*, *BIRC5*, *DHCR7*), 5 ER-related genes, 3 normalization genes and one DNA control gene (Filipits et al. 2011). The results are given in a binary fashion (high risk vs low risk) with the Endopredict score (EP) or the Endopredict Clinical score (EP Clin) by adding tumour size and nodal status. Proliferation gene module predicts for early distant recurrence and oestrogen-related gene module for late (>5 years) recurrence). Prosigna® test provides the PAM50 profile (50 target genes plus eight normalization genes) of the intrinsic classification plus a 19 proliferation-associated gene expression module (*CCNE1, KIF2C, PTTG1, TYMS, KNTC2, CDCA1, MELK, CEP55, HSPC150, EX01 CCNB1, RRM2, UBE2C, CDC6, PHGDH, MYBL2, MKI67, CDC20, ORC6L, MYC*) along with tumour size (Nielsen et al. 2014). The test gives a risk of recurrence (ROR) score (with two different scales depending upon the nodal status), risk category (low, intermediate and high), and intrinsic subtype (luminal A/B, HER2-enriched, basal-like).

The capacity of gene signatures to predict late relapse in ER-positive breast cancer has been evaluated for Oncotype DX®, Prosigna®, and EndoPredict®, and all of them demonstrated independent correlation with late relapses, but the association was weaker than with early relapses. Thus, if proliferation-based gene expression signatures are strongly prognostic for early relapses, in ER-positive, HER2-negative breast cancers, they are suboptimal to predict late relapses, although that capacity is strong for PAM50 (Sestak et al. 2015) and encouraging data have been published for EndoPredict® and Oncotype DX® in post-menopausal women treated by hormonal treatment (Sestak et al. 2015; Tang et al. 2011; Alvarado et al. 2015).

7.7 Conclusion

Proliferation is a major biomarker in breast cancer, used for prognosis, prediction of treatment response, or both. Proliferation assessment is of paramount importance in ER-positive, HER2-negative breast cancers for guiding the choice of treatment. The most important methods for proliferation assessment in breast cancer are summarized in Table 7.1. In summary, mitotic index gives an insight into proliferation while S-phase and other biomarkers are not routinely used. Ki67 is a popular and cheap biomarker in breast cancer, widely used for measuring and monitoring tumour proliferation in breast specimens, despite poor agreement on its precise clinical utility, analytical approaches, scoring methods, cut-offs, use as a continuous variable for decision making, and data handling approaches. Ki67 appears to be a marker of the continuous variable type, reflecting tumour biology. Coordinated international efforts have provided rules to standardize Ki67 assessment and enhance its reproducibility. The clinical utility of very low and very high Ki67 indexes is good. Ki67 index cut-off of 25 % has shown significance for prediction of overall survival. For the "grey zone" Ki67 index, multigene assays might provide useful information to guide patient management in the ER-positive, HER2-negative breast cancers.

Table 7.1 Most frequently used proliferation markers in breast cancer

Marker	Specimen	Method	Reporting	Clinical utility
Mitotic index (MI)	FFPE tissue, undissociated	H&E staining	Count per 10 HPF	Prognosis (RFS, OS) (Beresford et al. 2006; Rakha et al. 2008)
Tritiated thymidine labeling index (3HTdR LI)	Fresh viable tissue, (undissociated or in a single cell suspension)	Autoradiography or measurement of radioactivity (counter)	Fraction (% of labelled tumour cells) or counts per minute	Prognosis (RFS) (Paradiso et al. 1990; Nio et al. 1999)
5-bromodeoxyuridine labeling index (BrdU LI)	Fresh viable tissue, (in a single cell suspension or undissociated)	Flow cytometry or IHC	Fraction (% of labelled tumour cells)	Prognosis (RFS) (Meyer and Province 1994)
DNA content (DNA index, DI)	FFPE or fresh, in a single cell suspension	Flow cytometry	Ratio between DNA content of normal and the examined population	Prognosis (RFS); reviewed in Danielsen et al. (2015)
Phosphorylated histone 3	Any, most frequently FFPE undissociated	IHC	Count per 10 HPF	Putative prognostic marker (complement to MI)
Proliferating cell nuclear antigen (PCNA)	Any	IHC	Fraction (% of labelled cells)	Prognosis (RFS, OS) (Tahan et al. 1993; Haerslev and Jacobsen 1994; Stuart-Harris et al. 2008)
Cyclins (D1, E, A)	Any, most frequently FFPE undissociated	IHC or ISH	Histoscore (IHC), number of copies (ISH)	Prognosis (RFS, OS) (Lundgren et al. 2012; Xu et al. 2013; Roy et al. 2010; Gao et al. 2013; Klintman et al. 2013)
Topoisomerase 2α	FFPE tissue, undissociated	ISH	Number of copies	Prediction of response to anthracyclines (Press et al. 2011; Du et al. 2011)
Ki67	Any	IHC	Fraction (% of labelled tumour cells)	Prediction of response to taxane-based chemotherapy (de Azambuja et al. 2007; Luporsi et al. 2012; Criscitiello et al. 2014; Denkert et al. 2013), pharmacodynamic marker for neoadjuvant endocrine therapy (Jones et al. 2009), prognosis (RFS and OS) (Denkert et al. 2013; von Minckwitz et al. 2013)
Ki67-based mathematically-derived markers (PEPI, RPCB, IHC4)	FFPE tissue, undissociated	IHC and H&E staining	Scores	Prognosis (RFS) (Ellis et al. 2008; Sheri et al. 2015; Cuzick et al. 2011)

(continued)

Table 7.1 (continued)

Marker	Specimen	Method	Reporting	Clinical utility
Multigene assays (Mammaprint®, OncotypeDX®, EndoPredict®, PAM50/Prosigna®)	Fresh or FFPE, undissociated	RT-pCR, "digital" pCR (Nanostring technology)	Scores	Prognosis (RFS) (Filipits et al. 2011; Dubsky et al. 2013; Saghatchian et al. 2013; Sgroi et al. 2013; Gnant et al. 2014, 2015; Filipits et al. 2014; Sestak et al. 2015), benefit from adjuvant chemotherapy (Oncotype DX®) (Tang et al. 2011)

FFPE formalin-fixed, paraffin-embedded; *H&E* haematoxylin-eosin; *HPF* high power field, *RFS* recurrence-free survival; *OS* overall survival; *IHC* immunohistochemistry, *ISH* in situ hybridization

BOX 7.1: Recommendations for Ki67 assessment in breast cancer from the International Ki67 in Breast Cancer Working Group (Dowsett et al. 2011)

Preanalytical

- Core-cut biopsies and whole sections from excision biopsies are acceptable specimens; when comparative scores are to be made it is preferable to use the same type for both samples (e.g. in presurgical studies).
- Tissue micro-arrays are acceptable for clinical trial evaluation or epidemiological studies of Ki67.
- Fixation in neutral buffered formalin should follow the same guidelines as published for steroid receptors.
- Once prepared, tissue sections should not be stored at room temperature for longer than 14 days. Results after longer storage must be viewed with caution.

Analytical

- Known positive and negative controls should be included in all batches; positive nuclei of non-malignant cells and positive nuclei with mitotic figures provide evidence of the quality of an individual section.
- Antigen retrieval procedures are required. The best evidence supports the use of heat-induced retrieval most frequently by microwave processing.
- The MIB-1 antibody is currently endorsed for Ki67.

Interpretation and Scoring

- In full sections, at least 3 high-power (×40 objective) fields should be selected to represent the spectrum of staining seen on initial overview of the whole section.
- For the purpose of prognostic evaluation the invasive edge of the tumour should be scored.
- If pharmacodynamic comparisons must be made between core-cuts and sections from the excision, assessment of the latter should be across the whole tumour.
- If there are clear hot-spots, data from these should be included in the overall score.
- Only nuclear staining is considered positive. Staining intensity is not relevant.
- Scoring should involve the counting of at least 500 malignant invasive cells (and preferably at least 1000 cells) unless a protocol clearly states reasons for fewer being acceptable.
- Image analysis methods for Ki67 remain to be proven for use in clinical practice.

Data Handling

- The Ki67 score or index should be expressed as the percentage of positively staining cells among the total number of invasive cells in the area scored.
- Statistical analysis should take account of the log-normal distribution generally followed by Ki67 measurement.
- The most appropriate end-point in comparative studies of treatment efficacy or response is the percentage suppression of Ki67-positive cells.
- The most appropriate end-point for assessing residual risk of recurrence is the on-treatment proportion of Ki67-positive cells.
- Cut-points for prognosis, prediction and monitoring should only be applied if the results from local practice have been validated against those in studies that have defined the cut-off for the intended use of the Ki67 result.

References

Aleskandarany MA, Green AR, Benhasouna AA, Barros FF, Neal K, Reis-Filho JS, Ellis IO, Rakha EA (2012) Prognostic value of proliferation assay in the luminal, HER2-positive, and triple-negative biologic classes of breast cancer. Breast Cancer Res 14(1):R3. doi:10.1186/bcr3084

Alvarado MD, Prasad C, Rothney M, Cherbavaz DB, Sing AP, Baehner FL, Svedman C, Markopoulos CJ (2015) A prospective comparison of the 21-gene recurrence score and the PAM50-based prosigna in estrogen receptor-positive early-stage breast cancer. Adv Ther. doi:10.1007/s12325-015-0269-2

Andre F, Arnedos M, Goubar A, Ghouadni A, Delaloge S (2015) Ki67—no evidence for its use in node-positive breast cancer. Nat Rev Clin Oncol 12(5):296–301. doi:10.1038/nrclinonc.2015.46

Beresford MJ, Wilson GD, Makris A (2006) Measuring proliferation in breast cancer: practicalities and applications. Breast Cancer Res 8(6):216. doi:10.1186/bcr1618

Canepa M, Gambini C, Sementa AR, Borgiani L, Rovida S (1990) Nucleolar organizer regions and Ki-67 immunostaining in ductal breast cancer: a comparative study. Pathologica 82(1078):125–132

Carey LA, Perou CM (2015) Palbociclib-taking breast-cancer cells out of gear. N Engl J Med 373 (3):273–274. doi:10.1056/NEJMe1506680

Catzavelos C, Bhattacharya N, Ung YC, Wilson JA, Roncari L, Sandhu C, Shaw P, Yeger H, Morava-Protzner I, Kapusta L, Franssen E, Pritchard KI, Slingerland JM (1997) Decreased levels of the cell-cycle inhibitor p27Kip1 protein: prognostic implications in primary breast cancer. Nat Med 3(2):227–230

Clark GM, Allred DC, Hilsenbeck SG, Chamness GC, Osborne CK, Jones D, Lee WH (1997) Mitosin (a new proliferation marker) correlates with clinical outcome in node-negative breast cancer. Cancer Res 57 (24):5505–5508

Coates AS, Winer EP, Goldhirsch A, Gelber RD, Gnant M, Piccart-Gebhart M, Thurlimann B, Senn HJ, Panel M (2015) Tailoring therapies-improving the management of early breast cancer: St. Gallen international expert consensus on the primary therapy of early breast cancer 2015. Ann Oncol 26(8):1533–1546. doi:10.1093/annonc/mdv221

Criscitiello C, Disalvatore D, De Laurentiis M, Gelao L, Fumagalli L, Locatelli M, Bagnardi V, Rotmensz N, Esposito A, Minchella I, De Placido S, Santangelo M, Viale G, Goldhirsch A, Curigliano G (2014) High Ki-67 score is indicative of a greater benefit from adjuvant chemotherapy when added to endocrine therapy in luminal B HER2 negative and node-positive breast cancer. Breast 23(1):69–75. doi:10.1016/j.breast.2013.11.007

Cuzick J, Dowsett M, Pineda S, Wale C, Salter J, Quinn E, Zabaglo L, Mallon E, Green AR, Ellis IO, Howell A, Buzdar AU, Forbes JF (2011) Prognostic value of a combined estrogen receptor, progesterone receptor, Ki-67, and human epidermal growth factor receptor 2 immunohistochemical score and comparison with the genomic health recurrence score in early breast cancer. J Clin Oncol 29(32):4273–4278. doi:10.1200/JCO.2010.31.2835

Danielsen HE, Pradhan M, Novelli M (2015) Revisiting tumour aneuploidy—the place of ploidy assessment in the molecular era. Nat Rev Clin Oncol. doi:10.1038/nrclinonc.2015.208

de Azambuja E, Cardoso F, de Castro G Jr, Colozza M, Mano MS, Durbecq V, Sotiriou C, Larsimont D, Piccart-Gebhart MJ, Paesmans M (2007) Ki-67 as prognostic marker in early breast cancer: a meta-analysis of published studies involving 12,155 patients. Br J Cancer 96(10):1504–1513. doi:10.1038/sj.bjc.6603756

Denkert C, Loibl S, Muller BM, Eidtmann H, Schmitt WD, Eiermann W, Gerber B, Tesch H, Hilfrich J, Huober J, Fehm T, Barinoff J, Jackisch C, Prinzler J, Rudiger T, Erbstosser E, Blohmer JU, Budczies J, Mehta KM, von Minckwitz G (2013) Ki67 levels as predictive and prognostic parameters in pretherapeutic breast cancer core biopsies: a translational investigation in the neoadjuvant GeparTrio trial. Ann Oncol 24 (11):2786–2793. doi:10.1093/annonc/mdt350

Denkert C, Budczies J, von Minckwitz G, Wienert S, Loibl S, Klauschen F (2015) Strategies for developing Ki67 as a useful biomarker in breast cancer. Breast 24 (Suppl 2):S67–S72. doi:10.1016/j.breast.2015.07.017

Depowski PL, Rosenthal SI, Brien TP, Stylos S, Johnson RL, Ross JS (2000) Topoisomerase II alpha expression in breast cancer: correlation with outcome variables. Mod Pathol 13(5):542–547. doi:10.1038/modpathol.3880094

Dessauvagie BF, Thomas C, Robinson C, Frost FA, Harvey J, Sterrett GF (2015) Validation of mitosis counting by automated phosphohistone H3 (PHH3) digital image analysis in a breast carcinoma tissue microarray. Pathology 47(4):329–334. doi:10.1097/PAT.0000000000000248

Dowsett M, Nielsen TO, A'Hern R, Bartlett J, Coombes RC, Cuzick J, Ellis M, Henry NL, Hugh JC, Lively T, McShane L, Paik S, Penault-Llorca F, Prudkin L, Regan M, Salter J, Sotiriou C, Smith IE, Viale G, Zujewski JA, Hayes DF, International Ki-67 in Breast Cancer Working G (2011) Assessment of Ki67 in breast cancer: recommendations from the International Ki67 in Breast Cancer working group. J Natl Cancer Inst 103(22):1656–1664. doi:10.1093/jnci/djr393

Du Y, Zhou Q, Yin W, Zhou L, Di G, Shen Z, Shao Z, Lu J (2011) The role of topoisomerase II alpha in predicting sensitivity to anthracyclines in breast cancer patients: a meta-analysis of published literatures. Breast Cancer Res Treat 129(3):839–848. doi:10.1007/s10549-011-1694-9

Dubsky P, Filipits M, Jakesz R, Rudas M, Singer CF, Greil R, Dietze O, Luisser I, Klug E, Sedivy R, Bachner M, Mayr D, Schmidt M, Gehrmann MC, Petry C, Weber KE, Kronenwett R, Brase JC, Gnant M, Austrian B, Colorectal Cancer Study G (2013) EndoPredict improves the prognostic classification derived from common clinical guidelines in ER-positive, HER2-negative early breast cancer. Ann Oncol 24(3):640–647. doi:10.1093/annonc/mds334

Duchrow M, Schluter C, Wohlenberg C, Flad HD, Gerdes J (1996) Molecular characterization of the gene locus of the human cell proliferation-associated nuclear protein defined by monoclonal antibody Ki-67. Cell Prolif 29(1):1–12

Dumontet C, Krajewska M, Treilleux I, Mackey JR, Martin M, Rupin M, Lafanechere L, Reed JC (2010) BCIRG 001 molecular analysis: prognostic factors in node-positive breast cancer patients receiving adjuvant chemotherapy. Clin Cancer Res 16(15):3988–3997. doi:10.1158/1078-0432.CCR-10-0079

Ellis MJ, Tao Y, Luo J, A'Hern R, Evans DB, Bhatnagar AS, Chaudri Ross HA, von Kameke A, Miller WR, Smith I, Eiermann W, Dowsett M (2008) Outcome prediction for estrogen receptor-positive breast cancer based on postneoadjuvant endocrine therapy tumor characteristics. J Natl Cancer Inst 100(19):1380–1388. doi:10.1093/jnci/djn309

Engelberg JA, Retallack H, Balassanian R, Dowsett M, Zabaglo L, Ram AA, Apple SK, Bishop JW, Borowsky AD, Carpenter PM, Chen YY, Datnow B, Elson S, Hasteh F, Lin F, Moatamed NA, Zhang Y, Cardiff RD (2015) "Score the Core" web-based pathologist training tool improves the accuracy of breast cancer IHC4 scoring. Hum Pathol 46(11):1694–1704. doi:10.1016/j.humpath.2015.07.008

Filipits M, Rudas M, Jakesz R, Dubsky P, Fitzal F, Singer CF, Dietze O, Greil R, Jelen A, Sevelda P, Freibauer C, Muller V, Janicke F, Schmidt M, Kolbl H, Rody A, Kaufmann M, Schroth W, Brauch H, Schwab M, Fritz P, Weber KE, Feder IS, Hennig G, Kronenwett R, Gehrmann M, Gnant M, Investigators EP (2011) A new molecular predictor of distant recurrence in ER-positive, HER2-negative breast cancer adds independent information to conventional clinical risk factors. Clin Cancer Res 17 (18):6012–6020. doi:10.1158/1078-0432.CCR-11-0926

Filipits M, Nielsen TO, Rudas M, Greil R, Stoger H, Jakesz R, Bago-Horvath Z, Dietze O, Regitnig P, Gruber-Rossipal C, Muller-Holzner E, Singer CF, Mlineritsch B, Dubsky P, Bauernhofer T, Hubalek M, Knauer M, Trapl H, Fesl C, Schaper C, Ferree S, Liu S, Cowens JW, Gnant M, Austrian B, Colorectal Cancer Study G (2014) The PAM50 risk-of-recurrence score predicts risk for late distant recurrence after endocrine therapy in postmenopausal women with endocrine-responsive early breast cancer. Clin Cancer Res 20(5):1298–1305. doi:10.1158/1078-0432.CCR-13-1845

Finn RS, Crown JP, Lang I, Boer K, Bondarenko IM, Kulyk SO, Ettl J, Patel R, Pinter T, Schmidt M, Shparyk Y, Thummala AR, Voytko NL, Fowst C, Huang X, Kim ST, Randolph S, Slamon DJ (2015) The cyclin-dependent kinase 4/6 inhibitor palbociclib in combination with letrozole versus letrozole alone as first-line treatment of oestrogen receptor-positive, HER2-negative, advanced breast cancer (PALOMA-1/TRIO-18): a randomised phase 2 study. Lancet Oncol 16(1):25–35. doi:10.1016/S1470-2045(14)71159-3

Gao S, Ma JJ, Lu C (2013) Prognostic value of cyclin E expression in breast cancer: a meta-analysis. Tumour Biol 34(6):3423–3430. doi:10.1007/s13277-013-0915-8

Gatza ML, Silva GO, Parker JS, Fan C, Perou CM (2014) An integrated genomics approach identifies drivers of proliferation in luminal-subtype human breast cancer. Nat Genet 46(10):1051–1059. doi:10.1038/ng.3073

Gerdes J, Schwab U, Lemke H, Stein H (1983) Production of a mouse monoclonal antibody reactive with a human nuclear antigen associated with cell proliferation. Int J Cancer 31(1):13–20

Gnant M, Filipits M, Greil R, Stoeger H, Rudas M, Bago-Horvath Z, Mlineritsch B, Kwasny W, Knauer M, Singer C, Jakesz R, Dubsky P, Fitzal F, Bartsch R, Steger G, Balic M, Ressler S, Cowens JW, Storhoff J, Ferree S, Schaper C, Liu S, Fesl C, Nielsen TO, Austrian B, Colorectal Cancer Study G (2014) Predicting distant recurrence in receptor-positive breast cancer patients with limited clinicopathological risk: using the PAM50 Risk of Recurrence score in 1478 postmenopausal patients of the ABCSG-8 trial treated with adjuvant endocrine therapy alone. Ann Oncol 25(2):339–345. doi:10.1093/annonc/mdt494

Gnant M, Sestak I, Filipits M, Dowsett M, Balic M, Lopez-Knowles E, Greil R, Dubsky P, Stoeger H, Rudas M, Jakesz R, Ferree S, Cowens JW, Nielsen T, Schaper C, Fesl C, Cuzick J (2015) Identifying clinically relevant prognostic subgroups of post-menopausal women with node-positive hormone receptor-positive early-stage breast cancer treated with endocrine therapy: a combined analysis of ABCSG-8 and ATAC using the PAM50 risk of recurrence score and intrinsic subtype. Ann Oncol 26(8):1685–1691. doi:10.1093/annonc/mdv215

Goldhirsch A, Ingle JN, Gelber RD, Coates AS, Thurlimann B, Senn HJ, Panel Members (2009) Thresholds for therapies: highlights of the St. Gallen International Expert Consensus on the primary therapy of early breast cancer 2009. Ann Oncol 20(8):1319–1329. doi:10.1093/annonc/mdp322

Goldhirsch A, Wood WC, Coates AS, Gelber RD, Thurlimann B, Senn HJ, Panel Members (2011) Strategies for subtypes—dealing with the diversity of breast cancer: highlights of the St. Gallen International Expert Consensus on the Primary Therapy of Early Breast Cancer 2011. Ann Oncol 22(8):1736–1747. doi:10.1093/annonc/mdr304

Goldhirsch A, Winer EP, Coates AS, Gelber RD, Piccart-Gebhart M, Thurlimann B, Senn HJ, Panel Members (2013) Personalizing the treatment of women with early breast cancer: highlights of the St Gallen International Expert Consensus on the Primary Therapy of Early Breast Cancer 2013. Ann Oncol 24 (9):2206–2223. doi:10.1093/annonc/mdt303

Gratzner HG (1982) Monoclonal antibody to 5-bromo- and 5-iododeoxyuridine: a new reagent for detection of DNA replication. Science 218(4571):474–475

Haerslev T, Jacobsen GK (1994) Proliferating cell nuclear antigen in breast carcinomas. An immunohistochemical study with correlation to histopathological features and prognostic factors. Virchows Arch 424 (1):39–46

Hammond ME, Hayes DF, Dowsett M, Allred DC, Hagerty KL, Badve S, Fitzgibbons PL, Francis G, Goldstein NS, Hayes M, Hicks DG, Lester S, Love R, Mangu PB, McShane L, Miller K, Osborne CK, Paik S, Perlmutter J, Rhodes A, Sasano H, Schwartz JN, Sweep FC, Taube S, Torlakovic EE, Valenstein P, Viale G, Visscher D, Wheeler T, Williams RB, Wittliff JL, Wolff AC, American Society of Clinical Oncology, College of American Pathologists (2010) American Society of Clinical Oncology/College of American Pathologists guideline recommendations for immunohistochemical testing of estrogen and progesterone receptors in breast cancer (unabridged version). Arch Pathol Lab Med 134(7): e48–e72. doi:10.1043/1543-2165-134.7.e48

Hanahan D, Weinberg RA (2011) Hallmarks of cancer: the next generation. Cell 144(5):646–674. doi:10.1016/j.cell.2011.02.013

Jarvinen TA, Kononen J, Pelto-Huikko M, Isola J (1996) Expression of topoisomerase II alpha is associated with rapid cell proliferation, aneuploidy, and c-erbB2 overexpression in breast cancer. Am J Pathol 148 (6):2073–2082

Jones RL, Salter J, A'Hern R, Nerurkar A, Parton M, Reis-Filho JS, Smith IE, Dowsett M (2009) The prognostic significance of Ki67 before and after neoadjuvant chemotherapy in breast cancer. Breast Cancer Res Treat 116(1):53–68. doi:10.1007/s10549-008-0081-7

Klauschen F, Wienert S, Schmitt WD, Loibl S, Gerber B, Blohmer JU, Huober J, Rudiger T, Erbstosser E, Mehta K, Lederer B, Dietel M, Denkert C, von Minckwitz G (2015) Standardized Ki67 diagnostics using automated scoring-clinical validation in the GeparTrio Breast Cancer Study. Clin Cancer Res 21 (16):3651–3657. doi:10.1158/1078-0432.CCR-14-1283

Klein ME, Dabbs DJ, Shuai Y, Brufsky AM, Jankowitz R, Puhalla SL, Bhargava R (2013) Prediction of the Oncotype DX recurrence score: use of pathology-generated equations derived by linear regression analysis. Mod Pathol 26(5):658–664. doi:10.1038/modpathol.2013.36

Klintman M, Strand C, Ahlin C, Beglerbegovic S, Fjallskog ML, Grabau D, Gudlaugsson E, Janssen EA, Lovgren K, Skaland I, Bendahl PO, Malmstrom P, Baak JP, Ferno M (2013) The prognostic value of mitotic activity index (MAI), phosphohistone H3 (PPH3), cyclin B1, cyclin A, and Ki67, alone and in combinations, in node-negative premenopausal breast cancer. PLoS ONE 8(12): e81902. doi:10.1371/journal.pone.0081902

Kuhling H, Alm P, Olsson H, Ferno M, Baldetorp B, Parwaresch R, Rudolph P (2003) Expression of cyclins E, A, and B, and prognosis in lymph node-negative breast cancer. J Pathol 199(4):424–431. doi:10.1002/path.1322

Lakhani SR, Ellis IO, Schnitt SJ, Tan PH, van de Vijver MJ (eds) (2012) WHO classification of tumours of the breast. IARC WHO classification of tumours, vol 4, 4th edn. IARC Press, Lyon

Lee LH, Yang H, Bigras G (2014) Current breast cancer proliferative markers correlate variably based on decoupled duration of cell cycle phases. Sci Rep 4:5122. doi:10.1038/srep05122

Leonardi E, Girlando S, Serio G, Mauri FA, Perrone G, Scampini S, Dalla Palma P, Barbareschi M (1992) PCNA and Ki67 expression in breast carcinoma: correlations with clinical and biological variables. J Clin Pathol 45(5):416–419

Lundgren K, Brown M, Pineda S, Cuzick J, Salter J, Zabaglo L, Howell A, Dowsett M, Landberg G, Ai Trans (2012) Effects of cyclin D1 gene amplification and protein expression on time to recurrence in postmenopausal breast cancer patients treated with anastrozole or tamoxifen: a TransATAC study. Breast Cancer Res 14(2):R57. doi:10.1186/bcr3161

Luporsi E, Andre F, Spyratos F, Martin PM, Jacquemier J, Penault-Llorca F, Tubiana-Mathieu N, Sigal-Zafrani B, Arnould L, Gompel A, Egele C, Poulet B, Clough KB, Crouet H, Fourquet A, Lefranc JP, Mathelin C, Rouyer N, Serin D, Spielmann M, Haugh M, Chenard MP, Brain E, de Cremoux P, Bellocq JP (2012) Ki-67: level of evidence and methodological considerations for its role in the clinical management of breast cancer: analytical and critical review. Breast Cancer Res Treat 132(3):895–915. doi:10.1007/s10549-011-1837-z

Meyer JS, Province MA (1994) S-phase fraction and nuclear size in long term prognosis of patients with breast cancer. Cancer 74(8):2287–2299

Misell LM, Hwang ES, Au A, Esserman L, Hellerstein MK (2005) Development of a novel method for measuring in vivo breast epithelial cell proliferation in humans. Breast Cancer Res Treat 89(3):257–264. doi:10.1007/s10549-004-2228-5

Mook S, Schmidt MK, Weigelt B, Kreike B, Eekhout I, van de Vijver MJ, Glas AM, Floore A, Rutgers EJ, van't Veer LJ (2010) The 70-gene prognosis signature predicts early metastasis in breast cancer patients between 55 and 70 years of age. Ann Oncol 21 (4):717–722. doi:10.1093/annonc/mdp388

Nielsen T, Wallden B, Schaper C, Ferree S, Liu S, Gao D, Barry G, Dowidar N, Maysuria M, Storhoff J (2014) Analytical validation of the PAM50-based Prosigna Breast Cancer Prognostic Gene Signature Assay and nCounter Analysis System using formalin-fixed paraffin-embedded breast tumor specimens. BMC Cancer 14:177. doi:10.1186/1471-2407-14-177

Nio Y, Tamura K, Kan N, Inamoto T, Ohgaki K, Kodama H (1999) In vitro DNA synthesis in freshly separated human breast cancer cells assessed by tritiated thymidine incorporation assay: relationship to the long-term outcome of patients. Br J Surg 86(11):1463–1469. doi:10.1046/j.1365-2168.1999.01248.x

Paradiso A, Tommasi S, Mangia A, Lorusso V, Simone G, De Lena M (1990) Tumor-proliferative activity, progesterone receptor status, estrogen receptor level, and clinical outcome of estrogen receptor-positive advanced breast cancer. Cancer Res 50(10):2958–2962

Penault-Llorca F, Andre F, Sagan C, Lacroix-Triki M, Denoux Y, Verriele V, Jacquemier J, Baranzelli MC, Bibeau F, Antoine M, Lagarde N, Martin AL, Asselain B, Roche H (2009) Ki67 expression and docetaxel efficacy in patients with estrogen receptor-positive breast cancer. J Clin Oncol 27(17):2809–2815. doi:10.1200/JCO.2008.18.2808

Perou CM, Sorlie T, Eisen MB, van de Rijn M, Jeffrey SS, Rees CA, Pollack JR, Ross DT, Johnsen H, Akslen LA, Fluge O, Pergamenschikov A, Williams C, Zhu SX, Lonning PE, Borresen-Dale AL, Brown PO, Botstein D (2000) Molecular portraits of human breast tumours. Nature 406(6797):747–752. doi:10.1038/35021093

Petrelli F, Viale G, Cabiddu M, Barni S (2015) Prognostic value of different cut-off levels of Ki-67 in breast cancer: a systematic review and meta-analysis of 64,196 patients. Breast Cancer Res Treat 153(3):477–491. doi:10.1007/s10549-015-3559-0

Pich A, Chiusa L, Margaria E (2000) Prognostic relevance of AgNORs in tumor pathology. Micron 31(2):133–141

Polley MY, Leung SC, McShane LM, Gao D, Hugh JC, Mastropasqua MG, Viale G, Zabaglo LA, Penault-Llorca F, Bartlett JM, Gown AM, Symmans WF, Piper T, Mehl E, Enos RA, Hayes DF, Dowsett M, Nielsen TO, International Ki67 in Breast Cancer Working Group of the Breast International Group, North American Breast Cancer Group (2013) An international Ki67 reproducibility study. J Natl Cancer Inst 105(24):1897–1906. doi:10.1093/jnci/djt306

Polley MY, Leung SC, Gao D, Mastropasqua MG, Zabaglo LA, Bartlett JM, McShane LM, Enos RA, Badve SS, Bane AL, Borgquist S, Fineberg S, Lin MG, Gown AM, Grabau D, Gutierrez C, Hugh JC, Moriya T, Ohi Y, Osborne CK, Penault-Llorca FM, Piper T, Porter PL, Sakatani T, Salgado R, Starczynski J, Laenkholm AV, Viale G, Dowsett M, Hayes DF, Nielsen TO (2015) An international study to increase concordance in Ki67 scoring. Mod Pathol. doi:10.1038/modpathol.2015.38

Press MF, Sauter G, Buyse M, Bernstein L, Guzman R, Santiago A, Villalobos IE, Eiermann W, Pienkowski T, Martin M, Robert N, Crown J, Bee V, Taupin H, Flom KJ, Tabah-Fisch I, Pauletti G, Lindsay MA, Riva A, Slamon DJ (2011) Alteration of topoisomerase II-alpha gene in human breast cancer: association with responsiveness to anthracycline-based chemotherapy. J Clin Oncol 29 (7):859–867. doi:10.1200/JCO.2009.27.5644

Rakha EA, El-Sayed ME, Lee AH, Elston CW, Grainge MJ, Hodi Z, Blamey RW, Ellis IO (2008) Prognostic significance of Nottingham histologic grade in invasive breast carcinoma. J Clin Oncol 26 (19):3153–3158. doi:10.1200/JCO.2007.15.5986

Raymond WA, Leong AS (1989) Nucleolar organizer regions relate to growth fractions in human breast carcinoma. Hum Pathol 20(8):741–746

Roberts PJ, Bisi JE, Strum JC, Combest AJ, Darr DB, Usary JE, Zamboni WC, Wong KK, Perou CM, Sharpless NE (2012) Multiple roles of cyclin-dependent kinase 4/6 inhibitors in cancer therapy. J Natl Cancer Inst 104(6):476–487. doi:10.1093/jnci/djs002

Roy PG, Pratt N, Purdie CA, Baker L, Ashfield A, Quinlan P, Thompson AM (2010) High CCND1 amplification identifies a group of poor prognosis women with estrogen receptor positive breast cancer. Int J Cancer 127(2):355–360. doi:10.1002/ijc.25034

Saghatchian M, Mook S, Pruneri G, Viale G, Glas AM, Guerin S, Cardoso F, Piccart M, Tursz T, Delaloge S, van't Veer L (2013) Additional prognostic value of the 70-gene signature (MammaPrint((R))) among breast

cancer patients with 4–9 positive lymph nodes. Breast 22(5):682–690. doi:10.1016/j.breast.2012.12.002
Sestak I, Cuzick J, Dowsett M, Lopez-Knowles E, Filipits M, Dubsky P, Cowens JW, Ferree S, Schaper C, Fesl C, Gnant M (2015) Prediction of late distant recurrence after 5 years of endocrine treatment: a combined analysis of patients from the Austrian breast and colorectal cancer study group 8 and arimidex, tamoxifen alone or in combination randomized trials using the PAM50 risk of recurrence score. J Clin Oncol 33(8):916–922. doi:10.1200/JCO.2014.55.6894
Sgroi DC, Sestak I, Cuzick J, Zhang Y, Schnabel CA, Schroeder B, Erlander MG, Dunbier A, Sidhu K, Lopez-Knowles E, Goss PE, Dowsett M (2013) Prediction of late distant recurrence in patients with oestrogen-receptor-positive breast cancer: a prospective comparison of the breast-cancer index (BCI) assay, 21-gene recurrence score, and IHC4 in the TransATAC study population. Lancet Oncol 14(11):1067–1076. doi:10.1016/S1470-2045(13)70387-5
Sheri A, Smith IE, Johnston SR, A'Hern R, Nerurkar A, Jones RL, Hills M, Detre S, Pinder SE, Symmans WF, Dowsett M (2015) Residual proliferative cancer burden to predict long-term outcome following neoadjuvant chemotherapy. Ann Oncol 26(1):75–80. doi:10.1093/annonc/mdu508
Spyratos F, Ferrero-Pous M, Trassard M, Hacene K, Phillips E, Tubiana-Hulin M, Le Doussal V (2002) Correlation between MIB-1 and other proliferation markers: clinical implications of the MIB-1 cutoff value. Cancer 94(8):2151–2159. doi:10.1002/cncr.10458
Stuart-Harris R, Caldas C, Pinder SE, Pharoah P (2008) Proliferation markers and survival in early breast cancer: a systematic review and meta-analysis of 85 studies in 32,825 patients. Breast 17(4):323–334. doi:10.1016/j.breast.2008.02.002
Suman VJ, Ellis MJ, Ma CX (2015) The ALTERNATE trial: assessing a biomarker driven strategy for the treatment of post-menopausal women with ER+/Her2-invasive breast cancer. Chin Clin Oncol 4(3):34. doi:10.3978/j.issn.2304-3865.2015.09.01
Symmans WF, Peintinger F, Hatzis C, Rajan R, Kuerer H, Valero V, Assad L, Poniecka A, Hennessy B, Green M, Buzdar AU, Singletary SE, Hortobagyi GN, Pusztai L (2007) Measurement of residual breast cancer burden to predict survival after neoadjuvant chemotherapy. J Clin Oncol 25(28):4414–4422. doi:10.1200/JCO.2007.10.6823
Tahan SR, Neuberg DS, Dieffenbach A, Yacoub L (1993) Prediction of early relapse and shortened survival in patients with breast cancer by proliferating cell nuclear antigen score. Cancer 71(11):3552–3559
Tang G, Shak S, Paik S, Anderson SJ, Costantino JP, Geyer CE Jr, Mamounas EP, Wickerham DL, Wolmark N (2011) Comparison of the prognostic and predictive utilities of the 21-gene recurrence score assay and adjuvant! for women with node-negative, ER-positive breast cancer: results from NSABP B-14 and NSABP B-20. Breast Cancer Res Treat 127 (1):133–142. doi:10.1007/s10549-010-1331-z
Tsuchiya A, Zhang GJ, Kanno M (1999) Prognostic impact of cyclin-dependent kinase inhibitor p27kip1 in node-positive breast cancer. J Surg Oncol 70 (4):230–234
Van Poznak C, Somerfield MR, Bast RC, Cristofanilli M, Goetz MP, Gonzalez-Angulo AM, Hicks DG, Hill EG, Liu MC, Lucas W, Mayer IA, Mennel RG, Symmans WF, Hayes DF, Harris LN (2015) Use of biomarkers to guide decisions on systemic therapy for women with metastatic breast cancer: American Society of Clinical Oncology Clinical Practice Guideline. J Clin Oncol 33(24):2695–2704. doi:10.1200/JCO.2015.61.1459
Varga Z, Diebold J, Dommann-Scherrer C, Frick H, Kaup D, Noske A, Obermann E, Ohlschlegel C, Padberg B, Rakozy C, Sancho Oliver S, Schobinger-Clement S, Schreiber-Facklam H, Singer G, Tapia C, Wagner U, Mastropasqua MG, Viale G, Lehr HA (2012) How reliable is Ki-67 immunohistochemistry in grade 2 breast carcinomas? A QA study of the Swiss Working Group of Breast- and Gynecopathologists. PLoS ONE 7(5):e37379. doi:10.1371/journal.pone.0037379
Varughese RK, Lind-Landstrom T, Habberstad AH, Salvesen O, Haug CS, Sundstrom S, Torp SH (2016) Mitosin and pHH3 predict poorer survival in astrocytomas WHO grades II and III. J Clin Pathol 69 (1):26–34. doi:10.1136/jclinpath-2015-202983
von Minckwitz G, Schmitt WD, Loibl S, Muller BM, Blohmer JU, Sinn BV, Eidtmann H, Eiermann W, Gerber B, Tesch H, Hilfrich J, Huober J, Fehm T, Barinoff J, Rudiger T, Erbstoesser E, Fasching PA, Karn T, Muller V, Jackisch C, Denkert C (2013) Ki67 measured after neoadjuvant chemotherapy for primary breast cancer. Clin Cancer Res 19(16):4521–4531. doi:10.1158/1078-0432.CCR-12-3628
Winzer KJ, Bellach J, Hufnagl P (2013) Long-term analysis to objectify the tumour grading by means of automated microscopic image analysis of the nucleolar organizer regions (AgNORs) in the case of breast carcinoma. Diagn Pathol 8:56. doi:10.1186/1746-1596-8-56
Wirapati P, Sotiriou C, Kunkel S, Farmer P, Pradervand S, Haibe-Kains B, Desmedt C, Ignatiadis M, Sengstag T, Schutz F, Goldstein DR, Piccart M, Delorenzi M (2008) Meta-analysis of gene expression profiles in breast cancer: toward a unified understanding of breast cancer subtyping and prognosis signatures. Breast Cancer Res 10(4):R65. doi:10.1186/bcr2124
Xu XL, Chen SZ, Chen W, Zheng WH, Xia XH, Yang HJ, Li B, Mao WM (2013) The impact of cyclin D1 overexpression on the prognosis of ER-positive breast cancers: a meta-analysis. Breast Cancer Res Treat 139 (2):329–339. doi:10.1007/s10549-013-2563-5
Yerushalmi R, Woods R, Ravdin PM, Hayes MM, Gelmon KA (2010) Ki67 in breast cancer: prognostic and predictive potential. Lancet Oncol 11(2):174–183. doi:10.1016/S1470-2045(09)70262-1

Novel Immunohistochemical Based Biomarkers in Breast Cancer

8

Emad A. Rakha and Ian O. Ellis

Abstract

There is increasing use of immunohistochemistry (IHC) in the breast pathology work up. Although most diagnoses in breast pathology can be made with H&E sections, IHC plays a useful supplementary role in several situations and is the only diagnostic aid in certain situations including diagnosing low-nuclear grade spindle cell lesions and identification of tissue of origin in metastatic lesions. While the predictive and prognostic role of estrogen receptor and HER2 status in breast cancer is well established, several other IHC-based biomarkers are currently used individually and in combination to predict the outcome of breast cancer (IHC-based prognostic gene signatures). This chapter focuses on the value of IHC biomarkers analysis for diagnosis, prognosis, and prediction of outcomes in patients with breast cancer. The limitations of some antibodies, the use of diagnostic and prognostic panels of biomarkers and the importance of quality control and interpretation of IHC results in combination with morphology are also emphasized.

Keywords

Breast cancer · Immunohistochemistry · Diagnosis · Prognosis and prediction

8.1 Introduction

Generally speaking, a prognostic factor is any measurable parameter capable of providing information on patient clinical outcome, i.e. assessing the risk of disease recurrence at the time of primary diagnosis, independent of therapy. Prognostic factors are usually indicators of tumor growth, invasiveness, and metastatic potential. A predictive factor is any measurable

E.A. Rakha (✉) · I.O. Ellis
Division of Cancer and Stem Cells, Department of Histopathology, School of Medicine, The University of Nottingham, Nottingham, UK
e-mail: Emad.Rakha@nottingham.ac.uk

E.A. Rakha · I.O. Ellis
Nottingham City Hospital, Nottingham University Hospitals NHS Trust, Nottingham NG5 1PB, UK

S. Badve and Y. Gökmen-Polar (eds.), *Molecular Pathology of Breast Cancer*, DOI 10.1007/978-3-319-41761-5_8

parameter capable of providing information on the likelihood of response to a particular therapeutic modality (Gasparini et al. 1993; Hayes et al. 1998). A Prognostic/predictive factor could be either a single trait or signature of traits that can stratify patients into different population. Although prognostic and predictive factors could be separately classified, several factors in breast cancer provide both prognostic and predictive information (e.g. ER expression and HER2 overexpression). Biological molecular prognostic and predictive variables are primary tumor molecular characteristics that reflect the underlying genetic abnormalities and their assessment, using different platforms, can be used to determine tumor behavior and response to therapy.

Estrogen receptor (ER), progesterone receptor (PR), human epidermal growth factor receptors 2 (HER2), tumor size, lymph node stage and histological grade are the existing practical prognostic and predictive parameters (Pathology Reporting of Breast Disease 2005a). The last three prognostic parameters are combinatorially incorporated into the Nottingham Prognostic Index (NPI) (Galea et al. 1992); a well-recognized prognostic tool in breast cancer because of its simplicity and clinical utility (Elston et al. 1999). However, there are increasing concerns that these parameters are not sufficient to assess prognosis and response to therapy in view of the diversity and heterogeneity of breast cancer behavior. In addition, although positivity of hormonal receptors and over-expression of HER2 in breast cancer provide prognostic information and act as predictive parameters for the response of hormonal therapy and anti-HER2 targeted agents respectively (Early Breast Cancer Trialists' Collaborative Group 1998, 2005; Mauri et al. 2006), there remains a need for further refinement of management decision. In recent years, personalized systemic therapy has become an increasingly required in patient management, especially in early stage breast cancer. Accordingly, there is a need to develop or update the existing prognostic and predictive classifiers.

Gene-expression profiling studies have attracted attention by demonstrating the presence of different molecular classes with clinical relevance and that breast cancer morphologic heterogeneity can be linked to specific molecular profiles. Most of these molecular profiling studies have identified at least four distinctive molecular/biological subgroups: two luminal subtypes; namely luminal A and luminal B, the HER2-enriched, and the basal-like types (Perou et al. 2000; Sorlie et al. 2001).

Despite the prognostic relevance of molecular taxonomies and the well-documented prognostic power of certain gene signatures, there remain technical and cost effectiveness issues regarding their incorporation into routine practice. Previous studies have demonstrated that the behavior of well-established clinical parameters varies in the different molecular classes. Therefore, performance of current clinical prognostic indices may not provide the same information within the different molecular classes. Adjustment of the performance of the clinical parameters and prognostic indices to the most recent advancement in molecular classification of breast cancer is considered a way forward for personalized patient management. An additional problem with this approach is the cost and feasibility of microarray and chip gene expression technology for routine management of breast cancer. Alternatively, immunohistochemistry (IHC) is considered a practical, cost-effective, reliable technique for molecular classification and the gold standard in the routine assessment of the essential predictive molecular biomarkers; ER, PR and HER2 (Badve and Nakshatri 2009; Park et al. 2007).

8.2 Diagnostic Use of Immunohistochemistry

Apart from the predictive and prognostic use of hormone receptor and HER2 in breast cancer, currently the most routine use of IHC in breast pathology is in the diagnosis and differential diagnosis of often morphologically challenging breast lesions. Although most diagnoses in breast pathology can be made with H&E sections, IHC plays an important role in the following situations:

A. Differential diagnosis of:

   (i) Invasive versus in situ carcinoma,
   (ii) Usual type hyperplasia (HUT) versus atypical ductal hyperplasia (ADH),
   (iii) Lobular versus ductal carcinoma (in situ and invasive), and
   (iv) Radial scar versus tubular carcinoma and low grade adenosquamous carcinoma

B. Diagnosis and differential diagnosis of:

   (i) Papillary lesions (Collins and Schnitt 2008),
   (ii) Bland-looking spindle cell lesions,
   (iii) Certain special type carcinomas including metaplastic carcinoma, secretory carcinoma, neuroendocrine carcinoma, salivary gland like carcinomas and myoepithelial tumors,
   (iv) Paget disease of the nipple, and
   (v) Determination of tissue/cell or origin of certain malignant lesions and to exclude the possibility of metastatic carcinoma, melanoma, lymphoma in the breast.

In addition, IHC can be used in other situation such as assessment of lymphovascular invasion in morphologically indeterminate cases, diagnosis of scanty/suspicious cells of uncertain nature (such as after neoadjuvant therapy and isolated tumor cells in the lymph nodes).

Although several antibodies are available and used in routine diagnostic practice of breast pathology, these can be classified broadly into few categories: myoepithelial and epithelial specific biomarkers, cadherins, hormone and growth factor receptors and proliferation markers. More than one biomarker is typically used in the diagnostic work up of breast lesions and a large panel of antibodies are often used in challenging cases.

8.2.1 Myoepithelial Markers

Myoepithelial cells are present around normal ducts and lobules and at the epithelial stroma interface of hyperplastic and benign lesions and carcinoma in situ, but in invasive carcinoma. Myoepithelial cells can be difficult to identify on H&E sections and IHC can be of crucial importance. Myoepithelial cells are contractile cells exhibiting a combined epithelial and smooth muscle immunoprofile. The epithelial immunoprofile of myoepithelial cells are often called basal epithelial phenotype with expression of high molecular weight/basal-type cytokeratins (CK) and p-cadherin and lack of expression of low molecular weight/luminal-type CK, E-cadherin, EMA and hormone receptor. Several myoepithelial antibodies are available and show variable degree of specificity and sensitivities. Myoepithelial specific markers in breast pathology include contractile proteins such as smooth muscle actin (SMA), muscle specific actin, smooth muscle myosin heavy chain (SMMHC), and calponin, the p53 homologue p63, p75, CD10, S100, P-cadherin, maspin, caveolin 1 and 2, podoplanin, nestin, 14-3-3 sigma (stratifin), and basal-type CK such as CK5, CK5/6, CK14 and CK17 (Dewar et al. 2011). Broadly, myoepithelial makers can be classified into nuclear and cytoplasmic: P63 is the only marker exclusively expressed in the nuclei while S100 and maspin are expressed in the nuclei and cytoplasm. Other markers show pure cytoplasmic expression.

SMA and p63 are robust myoepithelial markers with a high sensitivity. SMA is often positive even in suboptimally fixed or infarcted tissue but its specificity is low as it is expressed in stromal myofibroblasts, vascular smooth muscle and pericytes, as well as subsets of invasive ductal carcinomas (Dewar et al. 2011). p63 shows good specificity with no staining of myofibroblasts or

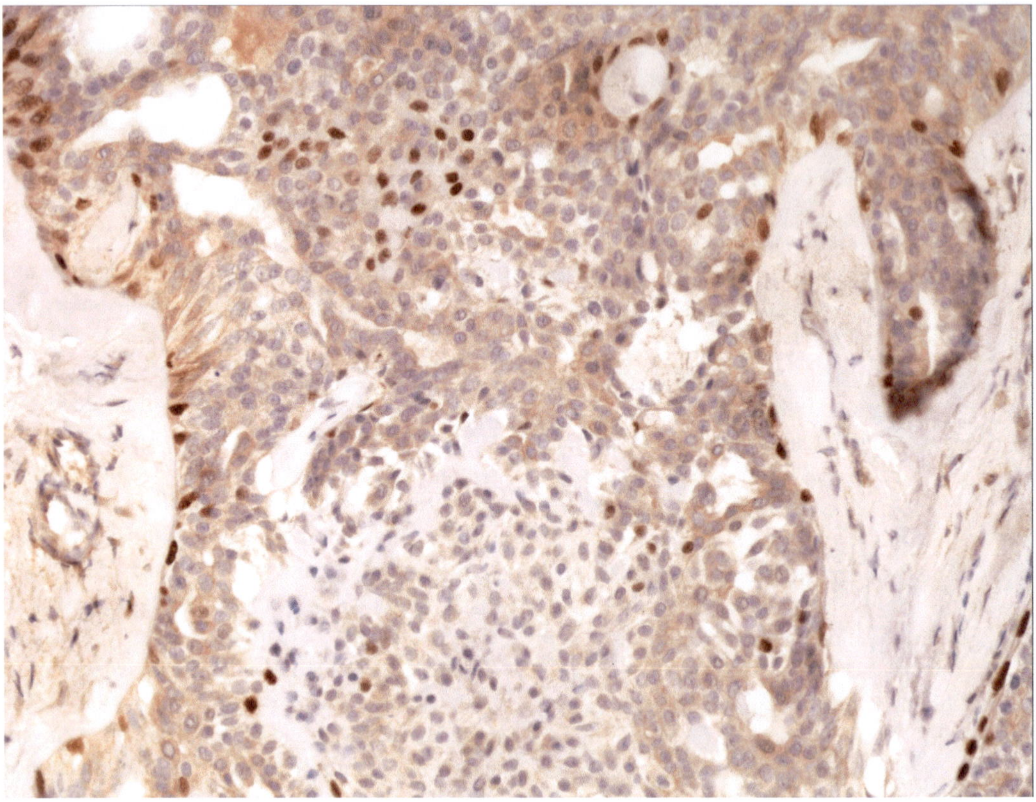

Fig. 8.1 Papillary lesion of the breast showing positive p63 nuclear staining in myoepithelial cells and in scattered epithelial cells which sometimes makes it difficult to comment of the presence of benign myoepithelial cells at the epithelial stromal interface

(a) (b)

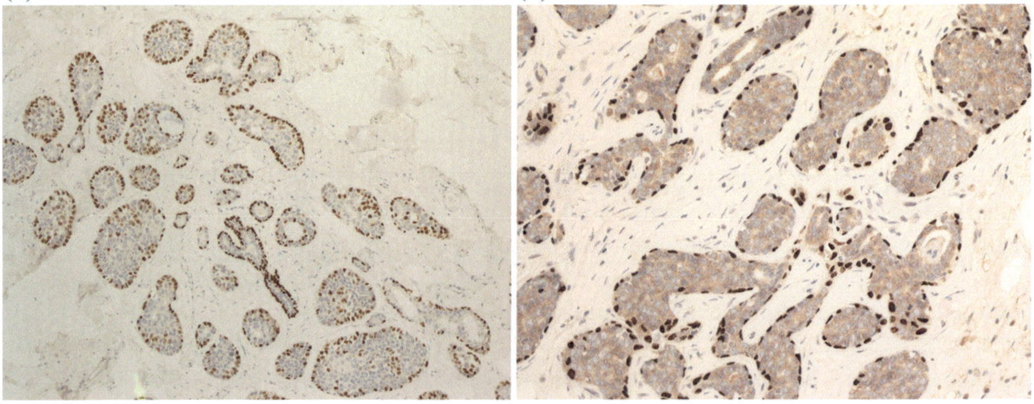

Fig. 8.2 A case of adenoid cystic carcinoma of the breast showing positive p63 nuclear staining in proliferating neoplastic cells (**a**). Some clusters show p63 positivity at the periphery mimicking benign myoepithelial cells seen in the in situ lesions (**b**)

blood vessels, but it may be expressed by papillary (Fig. 8.1) and salivary gland-like breast lesions (Fig. 8.2) some proliferating epithelial cells in papillary and salivary gland-like breast lesions and in some metaplastic breast carcinoma (Dewar et al. 2011). As p63 is a nuclear marker, interpretation of staining can be difficult in some sclerosing lesions, particularly if the myoepithelial layer is attenuated or discontinuous. SMMHC and calponin show good sensitivity for myoepithelial cells with less staining of myofibroblasts and they are easier to interpret than SMA. CD10 and calponin are specific than SMA but less sensitive. Basal CK such as CK5/6 and CK14 stain myoepithelial cells with no cross reactivity in stromal cells or blood vessels, but are not reliable markers as they are frequently expressed at low levels and may be expressed in the epithelial cells which can hamper interpretation. Pan CK 34βE12 (which recognizes CK1, CK5, CK10, and CK14) exhibits considerably lower sensitivity to myoepithelial cells (Dewar et al. 2011). None of the available myoepithelial markers provide absolute sensitivity and specificity and typically two or more myoepithelial markers should be used in combination to avoid false negative or false positive diagnosis. It is most effective to use a panel of antibodies. We routinely use a combination of the sensitive marker SMA, and two more specific markers such as p63 and SMMHC. It should also be noted that many of the myoepithelial markers show a variable degree of reduction in staining of myoepithelial cells around DCIS relative to normal myoepithelial cells with least reduction in SMA and p63 while the most reduction is observed with SMMHC. Finally, myoepithelial markers may be expressed in a subset breast carcinoma including metaplastic carcinomas, salivary gland-like breast carcinomas as well as ductal carcinomas displaying myoepithelial or basal-like differentiation (Rakha et al. 2005). Therefore, the diagnostic significance of myoepithelial marker staining should be interpreted in the right morphologic and immunophenotypic context of the given lesion. Absence of myoepithelial cell staining is also seen in some benign lesions including microglandular adenosis and infiltrating epitheliosis (Yamaguchi et al. 2012).

Myoepithelial markers are used in breast pathology to distinguish between DCIS, particularly those involving sclerosing adenosis, and invasive carcinoma, between cribriform DCIS and invasive cribriform carcinoma and to differentiate between microinvasive carcinomas and tiny foci of cancerization of lobules by DCIS. Myoepithelial markers are useful in the classification of papillary lesions (Collins and Schnitt 2008). The presence of myoepithelial cells at the epithelial stroma interface within the papillary cores and at the periphery can be used to distinguish benign papilloma, papilloma involved by DCIS, papillary DCIS, solid and encapsulated papillary carcinoma and invasive papillary carcinoma (Collins and Schnitt 2008). Preservation of myoepithelial cells within the cores and at the periphery indicates benign papilloma. Focal absence within a papilloma associated with evidence of a monoclonal epithelial proliferation is a feature of papilloma involved by ADH/DCIS based on the size of the atypia area. Papillary DCIS shows preservation of myoepithelial cells at the periphery but lacks them within the cores. Solid and encapsulated papillary carcinoma lacks myoepithelial cells within the cores in 100 % of cases and at the periphery in 70–90 % of cases (Rakha et al. 2011) (Fig. 8.3). An important pitfall is staining of stromal myofibroblasts and blood vessels for SMA and occasional epithelial cells for p63, which can be mistaken for myoepithelial cells. Myoepithelial markers can be used to differentiate between pure tubular carcinomas and entrapped glands in a radial scar/complex sclerosing lesion and between adenoid cystic carcinoma and mimics including collagenous spherulosis particularly in needle core biopsies. Myoepithelial markers can also be used in combination with epithelial specific markers to determine the amount of myoepithelial cell proliferation in a papillary lesion and to delineate the myoepithelial component of adenomyoepitheliomas. However, it should be noted that some reactive benign lesions lack expression of myoepithelial markers namely Microglandular adenosis and infiltrating epitheliosis and absence of myoepithelial cells in these specific entities

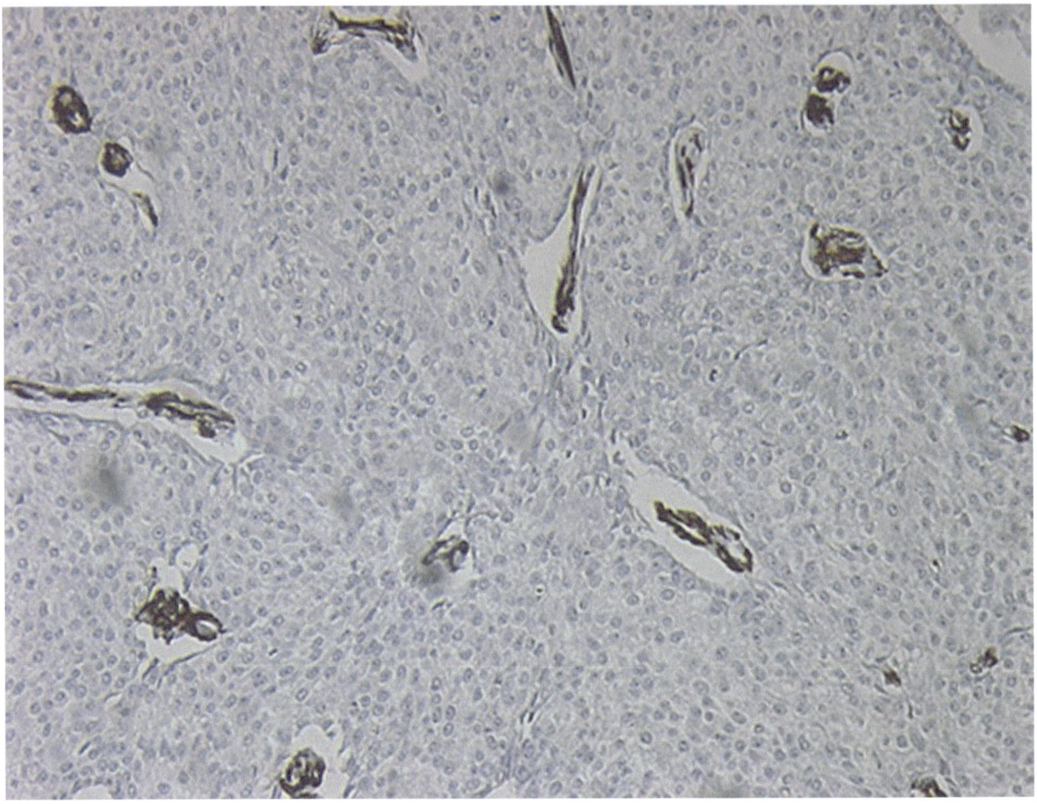

Fig. 8.3 A case of solid papillary carcinoma in situ of the breast showing absence of expression of smooth muscle actin (SMA) in the cores and at the periphery

does not mean invasive carcinoma. Both microglandular adenosis and secretory carcinoma express the myoepithelial marker S100 in a strong diffuse pattern (Fig. 8.4).

8.2.2 Epithelial Markers

In human mammary glands, the ductal and lobular units are composed of the luminal epithelium, and the myoepithelial cells. Luminal cells express low-molecular-weight luminal-type CKs (CK7, CK8, CK18, and CK19) and other luminal enriched markers including ER, progesterone receptor (PR), GATA binding protein 3 (GATA3), E-cadherin, epithelial membrane antigen (EMA), gross cystic disease fluid protein 15 (GCDFP-15), muc-1 and other epithelial markers. A subset of luminal cells express markers characteristic of both luminal and myoepithelial cells called “basal cells”. These “basal cells” express basal-type CKs, EGFR and P-cadherin but often lack expression of myoid markers characteristic of end differentiated myoepithelial cells and markers characteristic of luminal end-differentiated cells such as ER and EMA. Epithelial IHC markers are used in routine practice in the following:

A. *Diagnosis of an intraductal epithelial proliferation*: The demonstration of basal and luminal cells in an intraductal proliferative breast lesion indicate hyperplastic process while pure luminal epithelial cell proliferation is consistent with a clonal neoplastic process. Apart from myoepithelial lesions and metaplastic carcinomas, benign and malignant proliferative process typically lack myoepithelial cell component and lack the expression of myoepithelial myoid

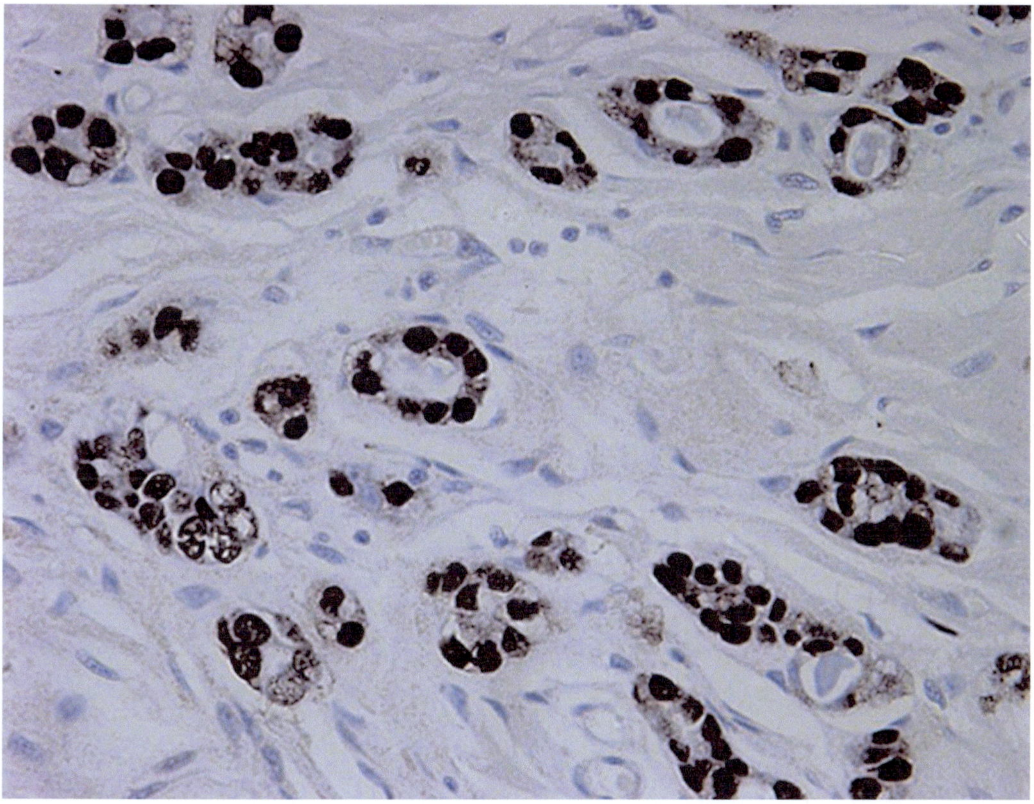

Fig. 8.4 Microglandular adenosis is characterised by diffuse strong nuclear S100 expression in the proliferating epithelial cells with absence of peripheral myoepithelial cells as demonstrated by morphology and other myoepithelial markers

markers and p63 apart from normal myoepithelial cells at the epithelial stroma interface. Therefore differential pattern of expression of basal cytokeratins and luminal end differentiated marker ER can differentiate hyperplasia of usual-type (HUT) from atypical ductal hyperplasia (ADH). HUT exhibits a mosaic staining pattern while ADH shows negative basal CKs staining together with diffuse strong nuclear ER staining (Otterbach et al. 2000; Shoker et al. 1999). We routinely use a combination of CK14, CK5/6 and ER. If the results are concordant it strengthens the interpretation. However, flat epithelial atypia (FEA) and columnar cell change (CCC) may show the same immunoprofile of ADH with negative basal CKs and strong diffuse nuclear ER staining and that nuclear features and architecture are used to differentiate CCC and FEA from ADH. Lobular neoplasia (lobular carcinoma in situ (LCIS) and atypical lobular hyperplasia (ALH)) displays the same immunoprofile but shows cell discohesive, lacks micropapillary or cribriform pattern of ADH, express cytoplasmic p120 and lacks membrane expression of E-cadherin and β-catenin expression (Fig. 8.5). Hyperplastic and neoplastic apocrine cells lack expression of ER, PR, and basal CKs but express GCDFP-15 and androgen receptor and exhibit apocrine cytomorphology. A small proportion of DCIS express basal cytokeratins, but these are usually of high grade, so the diagnosis can be made on morphology. Basal CKs expression in such a situation can be used to indicate the molecular class of DCIS rather

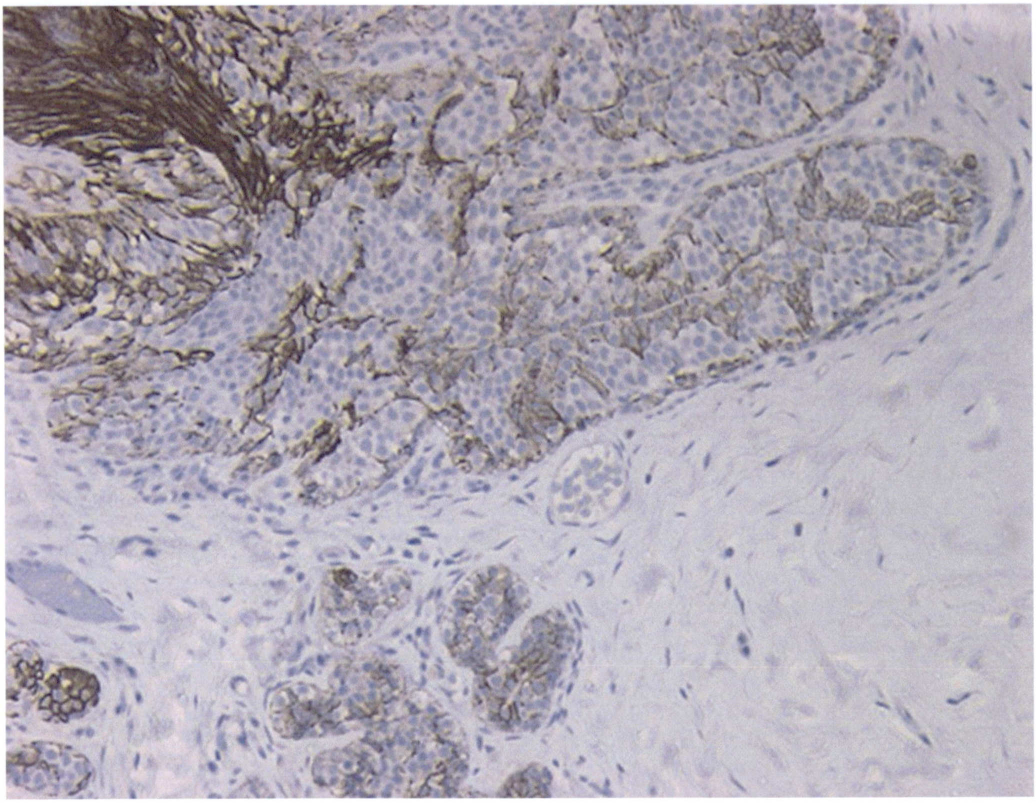

Fig. 8.5 Absent E-cadherin membrane expression is seen in lobular cells in a case of lobular neoplasia (LCIS). Positive staining seen in some cells denotes expression in the residual ductal cells

than differentiating it from hyperplasia. Therefore, IHC results must be interpreted in the light of the morphology.

B. *Detection of subtle invasive carcinomas*: epithelial markers can be used to diagnose malignant epithelial cells that are difficult to identify on H&E sections such as low volume nodal metastasis, residual low cellular invasive tumor following neoadjuvant therapy and bland-looking hypocellular invasive lobular carcinoma. In such situations it may be difficult to recognise malignant cells or to differentiate malignant cells from other cells such as histiocytes. It may be appropriate to apply IHC if there are groups of suspicious cells on routine H&E sections rather than routinely stain sections of axillary nodes or post-neoadjuvant cases with CKs. We routinely use pan-CK AE1/AE3 but CK7 can be used. ER is helpful for confirming ER+ carcinomas such as invasive lobular carcinoma which is positive in over 95 % of cases. CKs together with myoepithelial markers are also helpful in crushed biopsies of carcinoma and in some cases with infarction.

C. *Spindle cell lesions*: Spindle cell lesions of the breast comprise a heterogeneous group of disease which ranges from reactive, benign to highly malignant lesions. Broadly speaking spindle cell lesion can be classified into bland-looking and malignant looking spindle cell. The diagnosis of malignant spindle cell metaplastic carcinoma is usually straightforward if there is conventional invasive carcinoma or DCIS. Also the presence of entrapped epithelial element with specific architecture helps to indicate the spindle cell lesion is fibroepithelial lesion including phyllodes. IHC expression of epithelial differentiation markers in malignant spindle cells breast lesions lacking coexisting conventional mammary-type carcinoma or DCIS and lacking architecture features of phyllodes tumor is used to indicate metaplastic carcinoma rather than sarcoma. Low grade spindle cell metaplastic carcinoma can resemble fibromatosis but typically express CK particularly basal CK and p63. Other differential diagnoses of bland-looking spindle cell lesions include scar, nodular fasciitis, myofibroblastoma and pseudoangiomatous stromal hyperplasia. No marker is expressed by all spindle cell carcinomas so it is important to use a panel of antibodies including luminal and basal CK, p63 in addition to markers characteristic of other entities in the differential diagnosis such as ER, CD34 and desmin. Myofibroblastoma is typically ER, CD34 and desmin positive, pseudoangiomatous stromal hyperplasia and phyllodes tumor are positive for CD34 while low grade metaplastic breast carcinoma is typically ER, CD34 and desmin negative. Nuclear expression of β-catenin is seen in about 80 % of fibromatoses of the breast. However it is of limited diagnostic value in such situations as it is also expressed in up to 20 % of spindle cell carcinoma and in a high proportion of phyllodes tumors (Lacroix-Triki et al. 2010). It is important to note that CK expression in spindle cell lesion per se does not exclude other diagnoses. Focal patchy expression of some CKs can be seen in the stromal cells of phyllodes tumors (Chia et al. 2012). Leiomyosarcoma and angiosarcoma can also express CKs but morphology and other immunoprofiles of these cases are characteristic.

D. *Paget disease of the breast*: IHC is useful not only in the diagnosis of the Paget disease but also in differentiating it from other entities included in the differential diagnosis. Paget cells show similar IHC staining pattern as that of mammary adenocarcinomas. They show overexpression with luminal CKs including CK7 (in almost all cases) and typically do not express basal CKs that stain the neoplastic cells of epidermoid carcinoma or Bowen disease, CK20 or melanocytic markers (Karakas 2011). Paget cells also express other glandular antigens such as epithelial membrane antigen (EMA), carcinoembryonic antigen (CEA), gross cystic disease fluid protein 15 (GCDFP-15) and several mucins, Paget disease often is ER and PR negative, p53 positive. The majority of Paget disease is HER2 positive. Toker cells are consistently positive for CK7 and ER but negative for HER2.

8.2.3 Distinction of Lobular and Ductal Carcinoma

Lobular lesions are characterized by E-cadherin dysfunction in the majority of cases and E-cadherin is considered as a tumor suppressor gene in lobular but not in ductal carcinomas. Therefore E-cadherin IHC is a good marker for distinguishing lobular and ductal lesions. Ductal carcinomas and DCIS usually show membrane expression which is diffuse and strong in low grade lesion and may be patchy and weak in high grade lesion. Very few cases of high-grade ductal carcinoma completely lack membrane expression of E-cadherin IHC (Rakha et al. 2013). Invasive lobular carcinoma and lobular neoplasia (LCIS and ALH) are typically negative. About 10 % of invasive lobular carcinomas show some membrane staining, but this is usually patchy and weak (Rakha et al. 2010). E-cadherin positive invasive lobular carcinomas typically show aberrant cytoplasmic expression of other members of the cadherin-catenin membrane complex namely β-catenin and p120 consistent with the central role of loss of function of the E-cadherin–catenin complex in lobular morphology. Membranous expression of E-cadherin can also be seen occasionally in LCIS but in contrast to invasive lobular carcinoma, staining is usually focal, incomplete and reduced compared to adjacent normal control or ductal lesions. A combination of E-cadherin, β-catenin and p120 IHC together with morphology can distinguish lobular from ductal lesion in the vast majority of cases however, cases with indeterminate features and cases with mixed ductolobular nature exist. These cases are often considered as of ductal origin for management purpose. We use E-cadherin IHC for assessment of solid low grade intra-acinar proliferations in which the distinction of LCIS and low grade solid DCIS is difficult, but clinically important. Also in core biopsy distinction of ductal versus lobular lesions is crucial for further management decision. It is essential to ensure that there is membrane expression in normal breast epithelium and that IHC is interpreted in combination with the H&E sections.

8.2.4 Metastases to the Breast

Accurate distinction of primary mammary carcinoma from metastases to the breast is clinically important. Patients with metastases to the breast often require different systemic therapy and can be saved therapeutic breast or nodal surgery. IHC is often useful if there is no history of extramammary tumor, the morphology is not distinctive or to confirm the diagnosis. As with much IHC, it is important to use a panel of antibodies and not place too much emphasis on any individual result. No marker is completely sensitive or specific for any tumor type (Lee 2007). Useful antibodies in identifying the common tumors that metastasize to the breast include markers expressed in breast carcinomas including hormone receptor, HER2, GCDFP-15, lactoferrin, lactalbumin, mammaglobin, GATA3, in addition to the epithelial markers CK7 and EMA and negative expression of markers characteristic of other malignancy from non-breast primary including TTF1, CDX2, CK20, PAX8, melanoma and lymphoid markers. Primary carcinomas of the breast are usually CK7 positive (>95 %), CK20 negative (>95 %), ER positive (70–90 %), PR positive (60–70 %) and GCDFP-15 positive (40–70 %). Hormone receptor positivity in primary or metastatic carcinoma is considered as strong diagnostic clue to breast origin. ER is expressed in both breast carcinomas and tumors of gynecological origin. Although aberrant ER expression may be observed in other tissues such as lung carcinoma and colorectal carcinoma, the expression is usually weak and focal. For a diagnostic purpose ER is often combined with other biomarkers based on initial assessment of the index tumor. Markers that can be used to determine origin of carcinoma with ER expression include PAX8 (gynecological tumors), CDX2 (colorectal), TTF1 (lung and thyroid carcinoma), S100 and HMB45 (Melanoma). Interpretation of these markers is usually considered in combination with morphology of the tumors. Gross cystic disease fluid protein-15 (GCDFP-15) is a marker of apocrine differentiation that is considered to be specific to the breast but it has low sensitivity. Mammaglobin, a mammary-specific member of the uteroglobin family that is known to be overexpressed in human breast cancer; however it is also expressed in some non-breast cancer sites such as endometrioid carcinomas, endocervical adenocarcinoma in situ and sweat gland carcinomas. GATA3 is a sensitive and relatively specific marker for breast and urothelial carcinomas. However, data are emerging, reporting GATA3 expression in other tumors including salivary gland tumors, pheochromocytoma, benign Brenner tumors of the ovary, and parathyroid tumors. Although Serous papillary carcinoma of the ovary is CK7+/CK20—and may be ER+ but it is PAX8+, WT1+ and shows strong diffuse p53 positivity together with absence of GCDFP-15 expression. S100 is a very sensitive marker for malignant melanoma, but is also expressed in about 50 % of breast cancers. It is therefore important to use other markers such as melan-A and HMB45. Distinction of primary and metastatic neuroendocrine tumors of the breast can be difficult on routine sections if there is no DCIS. Primary mammary neuroendocrine tumors are typically ER and GCDFP-15 positive, whereas most neuroendocrine tumors metastatic to the breast are negative for these markers. Lymphoid markers are needed for the diagnosis of

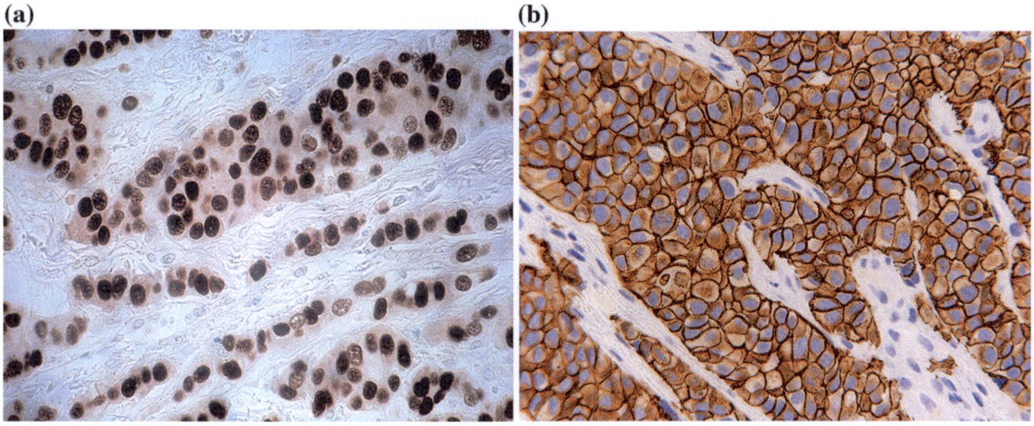

Fig. 8.6 A case of breast cancer showing strong positive nuclear expression of estrogen receptor (**a**) and strong complete membrane expression of HER2 (**b**)

lymphomas. Clinical criteria are used to differentiate primary and secondary lymphomas.

For the diagnostic use of IHC, it is important to be sure that the technique has worked by looking at internal controls, and if necessary, external controls. This is particularly important if the marker of interest is absent. It is also important to be aware nonspecific expression of certain IHC. The use of a panel of IHC marker is recommended in most situations in which IHC results are needed for interpretation of a specific breast lesion.

8.3 Predictive and Prognostic IHC Based Markers

IHC markers are used in breast pathology for predicting response to treatment and to stratify patients according to their predicted clinical outcome. IHC, which detects protein expression of genes of interest, can be considered as a measure of the biological features of the tumors and IHC expression or lack of expression of certain genes can be used as surrogate marker of tumor behavior, aggressiveness or response to specific therapy. Prediction of response to specific therapeutic agent is typically based on IHC assessment of individual genes such as ER for predicting response to hormone therapy and HER2 overexpression for predicting response to Herceptin treatment. However, multiple genes when used individually or in combination can refine the predictive value. For prognostic purposes, IHC is used to either assess the expression of an individual gene with independent prognostic significance such as Ki67, ER and HER2 or assess the combinatorial expression of a group of relevant genes (IHC gene sets) that can be used to generate a score or a prognostic index to stratify patients into specific prognostic groups. IHC gene sets can also be used to stratify BC into molecularly distinct groups akin to those produced by microarray gene expression (transcriptomic) profiling (GEP) and the result of this molecular classification can be used to predict behavior and help guide further treatment options or be subsequently utilized by combination with clinical variables to accurately predict outcome such as the novel NPI+ approach (discussed below). The most important predictive and prognostic IHC biomarkers in breast carcinoma include hormone receptor (ER and PR) and HER2 (Fig. 8.6) and these are discussed in details in Chaps. 4 and 5.

The expression of the hormone receptor ER acts as a predictive and prognostic parameter and IHC assessment of its expression is an established standard procedure in breast pathology. The current gold standard to assess ER and PR status is IHC performed on formalin-fixed, paraffin-embedded cancer tissue. Although a score of >1 % is used to define ER positivity for management purpose and patients with ER expression in >1 % of invasive tumor cells are candidate for hormone therapy, a higher cutoff is preferred for diagnostic ER staining (i.e., determination of breast origin of a tumor). Although gene amplification is the main target, the standard HER2 assessment in breast cancer starts with IHC assessment to determine negative and overexpressing tumors while indeterminate tumors (IHC borderline) undergo genetic testing for HER2 gene copy number measurement using in situ hybridization (ISH) technique. Details of the methodology and interpretation of IHC HER2 assessment in breast cancer have been published (Rakha et al. 2015; Wolff et al. 2013). HER2 IHC in breast cancer is also used to diagnose Paget disease of the breast in which it is expressed in more than 90 % of Paget cells therefore it is used to differentiate Paget disease from melanocytic lesion and Bowen disease of the nipple. HER2 overexpression in indeterminate benign/malignant breast epithelial lesion favors malignancy. In addition HER2 IHC overexpression in breast tumors can be used to provide further evidence of malignancy as benign tumors do not show HER expression or show weak to moderate staining not associated with gene amplification. To emphasize the importance of their assessment in breast cancer and to ensure the highest degree of test accuracy, reproducibility and precision of IHC assessment of ER, PR and HER2 in breast cancer, national guideline recommendation addressing IHC assessment of ER, PR and HER2 have been published including that of the ASCO/CAP (Hammond et al. 2010; Wolff et al. 2013), the UK RCPath NHSBSP (Pathology Reporting of Breast Disease 2005b) and others (Rakha et al. 2015). These guidelines not only provide recommendation to standardize and improve the quality of technical aspects such as assay performance, validation, proficiency testing and accreditation but also recommend testing all newly diagnosed cases as well as any local or distant recurrence whenever appropriate.

Ki67 expression levels are determined as the percentage of tumor cell nuclei positively stained. Ki67 IHC expression has long been reported as a prognostic marker in breast cancer (Trihia et al. 2003; Domagala et al. 1996; de Azambuja et al. 2007; Viale et al. 2008a) and several studies and meta-analysis involving several thousands of patients demonstrated that the Ki-67 positivity confers a higher risk of recurrence and a worse survival rate in patients with early breast cancer (Inwald et al. 2013; Petrelli et al. 2015; Aleskandarany et al. 2012; Stuart-Harris et al. 2008). The addition of Ki67 into the definition of intrinsic subtype of breast cancer has been enforced by several authors (Goldhirsch et al. 2011; Senkus et al. 2015). Ki67 when combined with HER2 and hormone receptor can provide addition prognostic information similar to multiparameter prognostic gene signatures (Dowsett et al. 2013). IHC expression of Ki67 is now widely used as an objective molecular measure of proliferation to overcome problems related to tumor fixation and mitotic figures identification (Colozza et al. 2005; Viale et al. 2008b). Ki67 expression in breast cancer is discussed in details in Chap. 7.

In addition to ER, PR, HER2 and Ki67, several prognostic biomarkers have been investigated in breast cancer to improve risk stratification. Despite this, most candidate-based prognostic markers, with the exception of urokinase plasminogen activator (uPA) and plasminogen activator inhibitor 1 (PAI-1), have not succeeded in making the transition from the laboratory to clinical practice (Harris et al. 2007). IHC for uPA and PAI-1 is not accurate. Apart from Ki67, present data are insufficient to recommend IHC assessment of other proliferation and cell cycle associated markers including cyclin D, cyclin E, p27, p21, thymidine kinase, histone-H3, surviving, aurora-A or topoisomerase II to assign patients to prognostic groups (Harris et al. 2007). Expression of BCL2, an antiapoptotic protein, is associated with features of good prognosis including ER-positive low-grade and slowly proliferating tumors (Dawson et al. 2010). Several authors have reported that IHC expression of BCL2 is associated with improved survival from breast cancer when used individually (Dawson et al. 2010; Callagy et al. 2008), or when combined with other variable including Ki67 particularly in the luminal ER-positive tumors (Chen et al. 2015; Ali et al. 2012) or p53 (Abdel-Fatah et al. 2010a; Rolland et al. 2007). Ali et al. (2012) have reported that the Ki67/BCL2 index is significantly associated with survival at 10 years in ER-positive disease and its prognostic value remained in the multivariate analysis. They validated this finding in an independent cohort of 3992 tumors containing 2761 ER-positive tumors (Ali et al. 2012). In a previous study, we hypothesized that the interaction between BCL2 and mitotic index (M) could accurately discriminate between low- and high-grade breast cancers. Tumors were classified according to the combined BCL2/M profile showed prognostic value that remained significant in multivariate analyses and performed better than lymph node status and tumor size in the model. Importantly, when BCL2/M profile was incorporated into the Nottingham Prognostic Index, it reclassified twice as many patients into the excellent prognosis group. Therefore we concluded that a grading system defined by BCL2 IHC expression combined with mitotic counting accurately reclassified patients with grade 2 tumors, improving prognosis and therapeutic planning (Abdel-Fatah et al. 2010b).

8.4 Novel Biomarkers in Breast Cancer Research

Several other novel IHC biomarkers are under investigation in breast cancer but currently have not been validated for clinical use. For instance our group in Nottingham are investigating members of the DNA damage repair pathways namely base excision repair, homologous recombination and nonhomologous endjoining (Abdel-Fatah et al. 2015; Rakha et al. 2008b; Alshareeda et al. 2013) and related proteins such as those involved in check points control and SUMOylation (Alshareeda et al. 2014). Although most of these biomarkers have limited clinical utility, they can provide important information regarding identification of tumors with deficient BRCA1 function and therefore candidate for genetic testing (Aleskandarany et al. 2015) and tumors that are candidate for synthetic lethality approach that target other DNA damage repair pathway in sporadic tumors (Albarakati et al. 2015). Although the number of genes involved in DNA damage repair mechanisms is large, with complex interaction between them and none of the individual genes assessed can reflect fully the underlying genetic alterations, there is a potential that they, when used individually or in combination, can refine breast cancer prognosis and therapeutic response prediction. Other markers under investigation include nuclear receptor superfamily and ER-related proteins such as The coactivator-associated arginine methyltransferase-1 (CARM1) (Habashy et al. 2013), Forkhead box O3a (FOXO3a) transcription factor (Habashy et al. 2011b), the RAS-Like, Estrogen-Regulated, Growth Inhibitor (RERG) and the Forkhead Box A1 (FOXA1) (Habashy et al. 2011a), the androgen receptor (AR), the transferrin receptor (CD71) and the proline, glutamate and leucine rich protein 1 (PELP1) (Habashy et al. 2010), the Peroxisome proliferator-activated receptor-gamma (PPARγ) (Abduljabbar et al. 2015a) and the glucocorticoid receptor (GR) (Abduljabbar et al. 2015b). These markers are not only associated with other prognostic parameters and outcome but also can potentially refine stratification of tumor for hormone therapy when used individually or in combination in ER-positive tumors or identify a subset of ER-negative tumors that are likely to respond to specific systemic therapy. We have also investigated members of the AKT/PI3K pathway (Aleskandarany et al. 2011), the mitogen activated protein kinase (MAPK) and the mammalian target of rapamycin (mTOR) pathways family members (Jerjees et al. 2015), stem cell makers such as CD24/CD44 (Ahmed et al. 2012), global histone modification proteins (Elsheikh et al. 2009) and the nuclear transport protein KPNA2 (Alshareeda et al. 2015). Several other proteins related to prognosis or biological interaction with other established molecules such as ER and HER2 or biological function such as invasion, metastasis and lymphovascular invasion have been investigated or currently under investigation by our group and others (for details see https://www.nottingham.ac.

uk/research/groups/pathology/nottingham-breast-pathology-research-group.aspx).

8.5 IHC-Based Prognostic Gene Signatures

Due to the technical, cost, and reproducibility issues of gene expression microarrays or even RT-PCR, complex IHC biomarkers assessment has been used to provide a surrogate technique for molecular profiling of breast cancer and prognostic stratification of patients. Many studies, using surrogate IHC panels of markers, have recapitulated the intrinsic molecular classes of GEP with considerable success and reproducibility (Rakha et al. 2009; Nielsen et al. 2004; Abd El-Rehim et al. 2005; Blows et al. 2010; Senkus et al. 2015). The feature common to GEP and their IHC surrogates is the use of a group of gene transcripts in the former, and protein products in the latter to define classes which has proven to be prognostically more informative than using these genes/markers individually. The choice of these biomarker panels was essentially based on the realization that the GEP-derived molecular subtypes are a reflection of the ER status, HER2 status and proliferation status in breast cancer (Rakha et al. 2008a). Accordingly, the IHC expression of ER, PR, HER2, basal CKs and Ki67 was used to devise a robust molecular classification of breast cancer. The resulting subtypes were the luminal, the HER2-over-expressing, and the triple-negative/basal-like breast cancers. The luminal subtype was subsequently subdivided into at least two subtypes; luminal A and luminal B. However, the criteria of defining luminal breast cancer subtypes are still based on different views; whether taking Ki67, PR expression, and HER2 expression along with ER status into account. It was initially proposed that those ER+ cancers overexpressing HER2 and being Ki67 high expressers (≥14 %) as luminal B, while the ER+, HER2 negative, Ki67 low as luminal A (Cheang et al. 2009). Later on, the international expert panel gathered in the St Gallen International Breast Cancer Conference in 2013, have endorsed the use of PR expression in defining luminal A breast cancer for those cases having substantial PR expression (≥20 %). Moreover, they have recommended a Ki67 threshold of ≥20 % as an indicative of high Ki67 status in defining luminal B cancers (Goldhirsch et al. 2013). In a recent publication by the European Society for Medical Oncology (ESMO) (Senkus et al. 2015), they defined luminal A (Luminal A-like tumors) as being ER-positive, HER2-negative, Ki67 low (≤10 %) and PR high (>20 %). Luminal B (Luminal B-like) was subclassified into HER2-negative and HER2-positive. Luminal B HER2 negative class is characterized by ER-positive, HER2-negative and either Ki67 high (≥30 %) or PR low while luminal B HER2-positive tumors is characterized by ER-positive and HER2-positive regardless of Ki67 or PR. They recommended that all luminal cancers should be treated with endocrine therapy. Most luminal A tumors, except those with the highest risk of relapse such as tumors with extensive nodal involvement, require no chemotherapy. Indications for chemotherapy within luminal B HER2-negative cancers subtype depend on the individual's risk of relapse, taking into account the tumor extent and features suggestive of its aggressiveness and patient preferences. The defined features associated with lower endocrine responsiveness include low ER expression, lack of PR expression, and high expression of Ki67 in addition to high tumor grade.

The HER2 overexpressing/enriched breast cancers are those which showed evident unequivocal IHC expression of HER2 (3+) as assessed by IHC, or those proven as *HER2/neu* amplified as assessed by ISH. Because *HER2* is an oncogene with the known impact of dismal outcome, based on the oncogene addiction theory (Weinstein and Joe 2008), it has been proposed by some authorities that HER2 over-expressing breast cancers should be allocated into the HER2 class irrespective of hormone receptor status (Rakha et al. 2009). Probably the most intensively debated issue within the topic IHC-defined breast cancer subtypes basal-like breast cancer. Although a consensus agreement exists for considering breast cancer lacking the expression of ER, PR, and HER2 to be triple negative, to-date, there is no consensus definition, using IHC surrogate markers, for the basal-like cancer. Both triple negative and basal-like cancer have poor clinical outcome, and lack any modality of specific targeted therapy as those possessed by the HER2 over-expressing breast cancers. Different IHC markers have been used in defining the basal phenotype including: lack of ER, PR, HER2 expression (i.e., TN), and expressing one or more of the basal CKs (CK5/6, CK14, or CK17) and/or EGFR (Cheang et al. 2008; Nielsen et al. 2004). This subtype is reported in the 15–20 % within most of the studied series. This relatively low frequency has hindered the development of consensus IHC panel that can define basal-like tumors. However, in their seminal meta-analysis of more than 10,000 breast cancer cases, Blows et al. reported the superior advantage of using five markers in definition of different molecular subtypes of breast cancer including the basal-like class (Blows et al. 2010).

In a different approach some authorities have utilized unsupervised clustering methodology and IHC expression data of a number of relevant biomarkers to classify breast cancer patients into distinct subtypes based on similarity of immunoprofile (Abd El-Rehim et al. 2005; Callagy et al. 2003). These IHC defined classes were comparable to the intrinsic subtypes defined by GEP and they often showed difference in prognosis and hence clinical significance. For instance, in a previous study we have assessed the expression of a selective panel of 25 BC-related biomarkers using IHC on tissue microarray (TMA) and data were analyzed using unsupervised classification approaches and artificial neuronal network. Markers were related to epithelial cell lineage, differentiation, hormone and growth factor receptors and gene products known to be altered in some forms of breast cancer. Six groups or breast cancer classes were identified which were significantly different in clinicopathological parameters and patient outcome in terms of overall and disease-free survival, independent of standard prognostic parameters; grade, tumor size and lymph node stage (Abd El-Rehim et al. 2005). Of note, is the HER2 group was only 7 % of the studied patient population, which is below those reported in literature and in other studies. A minimized panel of ten biomarkers was subsequently identified that can be used to identify those molecular classes with high level of accuracy and those classes was used to develop the novel NPI+ prognostic index (see below) (Rakha et al. 2014a).

Despite the biological and clinical significance of the intrinsic subtype approach, the development of prognostic gene signatures using RNA expression of a selected genes chosen based on the association with clinical outcome has attracted more attention. As a surrogate technique, IHC has been applied using a panel of IHC markers (Fig. 8.7) that have been chosen based on their prognostic significance and the collect IHC expression of these genes was used to generate a score or index which can be divided using cutoff(s) to stratify patients in distinct risk groups. Several authors now believe that using a panel of IHC markers to predict prognosis and responses to specific therapy is more robust and potentially powerful than using a single marker approach and has the potential for implementation in routine pathology assessment of breast cancers. Examples of IHC-based assays include Mammostrat, IHC4 and Nottingham Prognostic Index (NPI+).

8.5.1 Mammostrat

Ring et al. (2006) have combined the novel information emerged from GEP with conventional IHC technology to design IHC prognostic assay. They used three breast cancer cohorts; one cohort (n = 466) was used as a discovery cohort while the other two (n = 299 and 344 patients, respectively) were used as independent validating cohorts. They have identified target genes and applied IHC to FFPE samples to calculate the relative risk of recurrence. This IHC based test is currently commercially available as the Mammostrat assay (Ring et al. 2006). Further validation of Mammostrat had been conducted by other investigators (Ross et al. 2008; Bartlett et al. 2010; Bartlett et al. 2012). Mammostrat uses five IHC markers: P53, SLC7A5 (solute carrier family 7 cationic amino acid transporter), NDRG1 (N-myc downstream-regulated

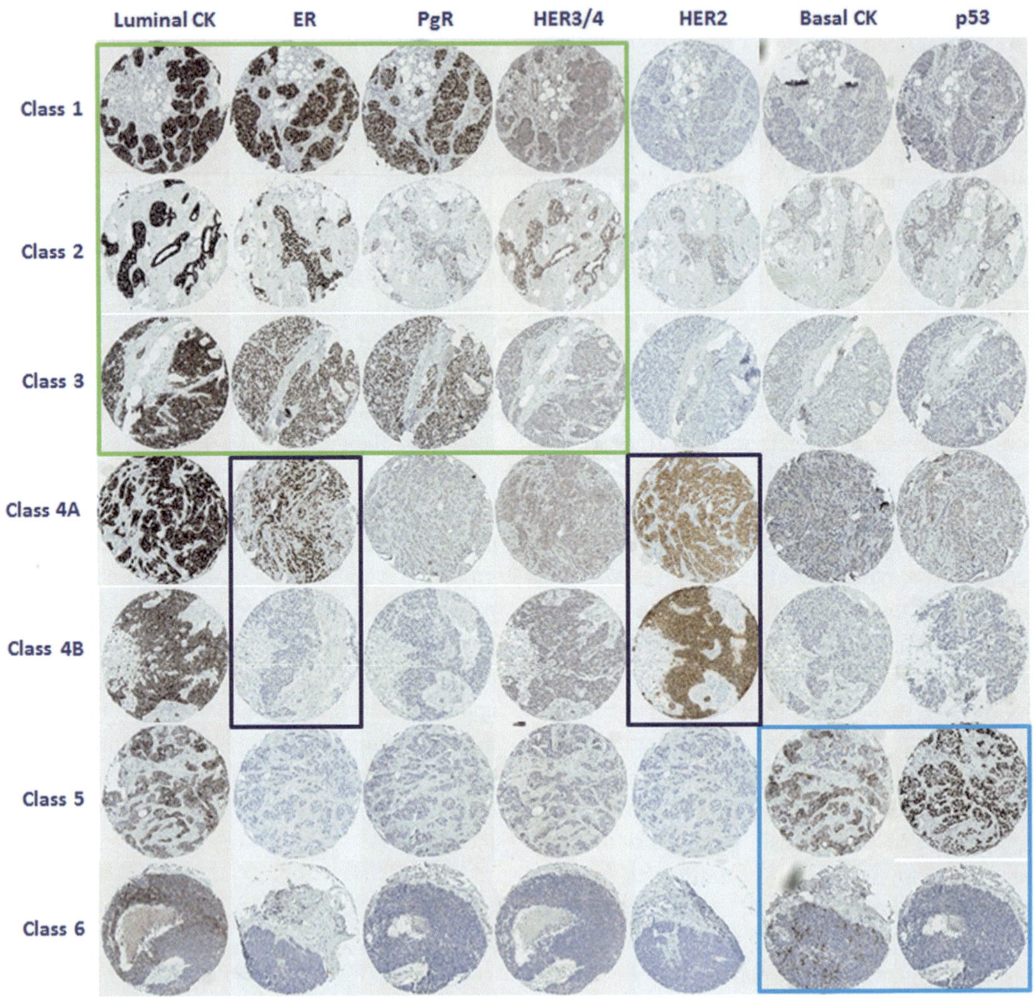

Fig. 8.7 This panel represents tissue microarray (TMA) cores from 7 invasive breast cancers (*rows*) stained with different antibodies (*columns*) to produce molecular clusters. In this panel each case represents a distinct molecular cluster characterised by a specific pattern of expression of the *different markers*

gene 1), CEACAM5 (carcinoembryonic antigen cell adhesion molecule 5) and HTF9C (HpaII tiny fragments locus 9C). These five biomarkers are independent of one another and do not directly measure either hormone receptor or HER2 status or proliferation. Mammostrat can stratify early-stage ER-positive tamoxifen-treated breast cancer patients into three risk groups. Prognostic index = 0 represents the low risk group; prognostic index >0 and ≤0.7 represents the moderate-risk group; and prognostic index >0.7 represents the high-risk group (Ring et al. 2006; Ross et al. 2008). In principle, Mammostrat results could be interpreted in conjunction with conventional histopathological information about the proliferation and hormone receptor status of a tumor. Mammostrat Plus is a modified assay that incorporate four other markers (Mammostrat, ER, PR, Ki67, HER2 by IHC and FISH). Cost-effectiveness analysis of Mammostrat compared with Oncotype DX to inform the treatment of breast cancer have revealed that both tests resulted in similar life years and quality-adjusted life years but Mammostrat is cost saving (Mislick et al. 2014).

8.5.2 IHC4 Score

IHC4 is a prognostic score that assesses the levels of the four widely measured proteins in breast cancer (ER, PR, HER2 and Ki67). Cuzick et al. developed IHC4 and compared it to the Oncotype DX to assess its utility on 1,125 ER-positive cases that had GHI-RS data and whether it can add a prognostic and predictive value to the classical prognostic parameters (tumor size, lymph node status and histological grade) in early stage breast cancer patients. The IHC4 score proved to be an independent prognostic factor in addition to the existing classical variables. Importantly, the result provided by the IHC4 score were found to be identical to that presented by Oncotype DX. In addition, the IHC4 prognostic value was validated on an independent cohort of 786 patients with their outcome were equal as assessed by both Oncotype DX and IHC4 assay (Cuzick et al. 2011). The IHC4 score can be combined with clinical parameters (tumor grade, size, nodal burden, patient age, and treatment with aromatase inhibitor or tamoxifen) to produce IHC4+ Clinical (IHC4+C) score. IHC4+C has been tested to estimate the residual risk of distant recurrence at 10 years in post-menopausal women with ER-positive breast cancer who have received 5 years of endocrine therapy. However, although IHC4 is inexpensive and can be performed in local laboratories, it uses the four markers in a different way to that used in routine practice; as continuous variables, and requires an algorithm for calculation of the score. In addition, standardization of IHC4 and quality assurance programs are required before its widespread use (Dowsett et al. 2013).

8.5.3 *Nottingham Prognostic Index plus (NPI+)*

The Nottingham Prognostic Index (NPI) is an approved and widely accepted method for prognosis as well as survival prediction in operable cases of primary breast cancer (Blamey et al. 2007). It was one of the earliest indices to be developed. In 1982, it was applied throughout a retrospective study of 387 women with primary operable breast cancer using multivariate regression analysis; (Haybittle et al. 1982) and in 1991, the prognostic importance of NPI in breast cancer was initially expressed (Elston and Ellis 1991). Then, after the long-term follow-up (Galea et al. 1992) and independent validation in different centers (Balslev et al. 1994; D'Eredita et al. 2001; Brown et al. 1993). As the performance of clinicopathological factors varies among the molecular classes, the concept of refining the traditional NPI Plus (NPI+) was introduced. NPI+ was based on classifying breast carcinoma into seven distinct molecular classes using those 10 biomarkers followed by incorporation of clinicopathological variables to identify distinct prognostic groups with each of the seven classes (Rakha et al. 2014c). Using the NPI+ formulae, through incorporating molecular features and clinicopathological parameters, an improved patients' outcome stratification was achieved superior to the traditional NPI (Rakha et al. 2014c; Green et al. 2013; Rakha et al. 2014b). Studies for further refinement, standardization of the techniques and clinical validation of NPI+ are undergoing.

8.6 Conclusion

IHC can play a helpful role in the diagnosis of problematic breast lesions, prognosis and prediction of response to therapy. IHC markers can be used individually or in combination. It is important to be aware of the limitations of individual antibodies. Quality control is also essential. When IHC is used in diagnosis, it must be interpreted in combination with the morphology seen on H&E sections.

References

Abd El-Rehim DM, Ball G, Pinder SE et al (2005) High-throughput protein expression analysis using tissue microarray technology of a large well-characterised series identifies biologically distinct classes of breast cancer confirming recent cDNA expression analyses. Int J Cancer 116(3):340–350

Abdel-Fatah TM, Powe DG, Agboola J et al (2010a) The biological, clinical and prognostic implications of p53 transcriptional pathways in breast cancers. J Pathol 220(4):419–434

Abdel-Fatah TM, Powe DG, Ball G et al (2010b) Proposal for a modified grading system based on mitotic index and Bcl2 provides objective determination of clinical outcome for patients with breast cancer. J Pathol 222 (4):388–399

Abdel-Fatah TM, Arora A, Moseley PM et al (2015) DNA repair prognostic index modelling reveals an essential role for base excision repair in influencing clinical outcomes in ER negative and triple negative breast cancers. Oncotarget 6(26):21964–21978

Abduljabbar R, Al-Kaabi MM, Negm OH et al (2015a) Prognostic and biological significance of peroxisome proliferator-activated receptor-gamma in luminal breast cancer. Breast Cancer Res Treat 150(3):511–522

Abduljabbar R, Negm OH, Lai CF et al (2015b) Clinical and biological significance of glucocorticoid receptor (GR) expression in breast cancer. Breast Cancer Res Treat 150(2):335–346

Ahmed MA, Aleskandarany MA, Rakha EA et al (2012) A CD44(−)/CD24(+) phenotype is a poor prognostic marker in early invasive breast cancer. Breast Cancer Res Treat 133(3):979–995

Albarakati N, Abdel-Fatah TM, Doherty R et al (2015) Targeting BRCA1-BER deficient breast cancer by ATM or DNA-PKcs blockade either alone or in combination with cisplatin for personalized therapy. Mol Oncol 9(1):204–217

Aleskandarany MA, Rakha EA, Ahmed MA, Powe DG, Ellis IO, Green AR (2011) Clinicopathologic and molecular significance of phospho-Akt expression in early invasive breast cancer. Breast Cancer Res Treat 127(2):407–416

Aleskandarany MA, Green AR, Benhasouna AA et al (2012) Prognostic value of proliferation assay in the luminal, HER2-positive, and triple-negative biologic classes of breast cancer. Breast Cancer Res 14(1):R3

Aleskandarany M, Caracappa D, Nolan CC et al (2015) DNA damage response markers are differentially expressed in BRCA-mutated breast cancers. Breast Cancer Res Treat 150(1):81–90

Ali HR, Dawson SJ, Blows FM et al (2012) A Ki67/BCL2 index based on immunohistochemistry is highly prognostic in ER-positive breast cancer. J Pathol 226(1):97–107

Alshareeda AT, Negm OH, Albarakati N et al (2013) Clinicopathological significance of KU70/KU80, a key DNA damage repair protein in breast cancer. Breast Cancer Res Treat 139(2):301–310

Alshareeda AT, Negm OH, Green AR et al (2014) SUMOylation proteins in breast cancer. Breast Cancer Res Treat 144(3):519–530

Alshareeda AT, Negm OH, Green AR et al (2015) KPNA2 is a nuclear export protein that contributes to aberrant localisation of key proteins and poor prognosis of breast cancer. Br J Cancer 112(12):1929–1937

Badve S, Nakshatri H (2009) Oestrogen-receptor-positive breast cancer: towards bridging histopathological and molecular classifications. J Clin Pathol 62(1):6–12

Balslev I, Axelsson CK, Zedeler K, Rasmussen BB, Carstensen B, Mouridsen HT (1994) The Nottingham Prognostic Index applied to 9149 patients from the studies of the Danish Breast Cancer Cooperative Group (DBCG). Breast Cancer Res Treat 32(3):281–290

Bartlett JM, Thomas J, Ross DT et al (2010) Mammostrat as a tool to stratify breast cancer patients at risk of recurrence during endocrine therapy. Breast Cancer Res 12(4):R47. doi:10.1186/bcr2604 (England)

Bartlett JM, Bloom KJ, Piper T et al (2012) Mammostrat as an immunohistochemical multigene assay for prediction of early relapse risk in the tamoxifen versus exemestane adjuvant multicenter trial pathology study. J Clin Oncol 30(36):4477–4484

Blamey RW, Pinder SE, Ball GR et al (2007) Reading the prognosis of the individual with breast cancer. Eur J Cancer 43(10):1545–1547

Blows FM, Driver KE, Schmidt MK et al (2010) Subtyping of breast cancer by immunohistochemistry to investigate a relationship between subtype and short and long term survival: a collaborative analysis of data for 10,159 cases from 12 studies. PLoS Med 7(5): e1000279

Brown J, Jones M, Benson EA (1993) Comment on the Nottingham Prognostic Index. Breast Cancer Res Treat 25(3):283

Callagy G, Cattaneo E, Daigo Y et al (2003) Molecular classification of breast carcinomas using tissue microarrays. Diagn Mol Pathol 12(1):27–34

Callagy GM, Webber MJ, Pharoah PD, Caldas C (2008) Meta-analysis confirms BCL2 is an independent prognostic marker in breast cancer. BMC Cancer 8:153

Cheang MC, Voduc D, Bajdik C et al (2008) Basal-like breast cancer defined by five biomarkers has superior prognostic value than triple-negative phenotype. Clin Cancer Res 14(5):1368–1376

Cheang MC, Chia SK, Voduc D et al (2009) Ki67 index, HER2 status, and prognosis of patients with luminal B breast cancer. J Natl Cancer Inst 101(10):736–750

Chen LY, Tsang JY, Ni YB et al (2015) Bcl2 and Ki67 refine prognostication in luminal breast cancers. Breast Cancer Res Treat 149(3):631–643

Chia Y, Thike AA, Cheok PY, Chong LY-Z, Man-Kit Tse G, Tan PH (2012) Stromal keratin expression in phyllodes tumours of the breast: a comparison with other spindle cell breast lesions. J Clin Pathol 65 (4):339–347

Collins LC, Schnitt SJ (2008) Papillary lesions of the breast: selected diagnostic and management issues. Histopathology 52(1):20–29

Colozza M, Azambuja E, Cardoso F, Sotiriou C, Larsimont D, Piccart MJ (2005) Proliferative markers as prognostic and predictive tools in early breast cancer: where are we now? Ann Oncol 16(11):1723–1739

Cuzick J, Dowsett M, Pineda S et al (2011) Prognostic value of a combined estrogen receptor, progesterone receptor, Ki-67, and human epidermal growth factor receptor 2 immunohistochemical score and comparison with the Genomic Health recurrence score in early breast cancer. J Clin Oncol 29(32):4273–4278

D'Eredita G, Giardina C, Martellotta M, Natale T, Ferrarese F (2001) Prognostic factors in breast cancer: the predictive value of the Nottingham Prognostic Index in patients with a long-term follow-up that were treated in a single institution. Eur J Cancer 37(5):591–596

Dawson SJ, Makretsov N, Blows FM et al (2010) BCL2 in breast cancer: a favourable prognostic marker across molecular subtypes and independent of adjuvant therapy received. Br J Cancer 103(5):668–675

de Azambuja E, Cardoso F, de Castro G, Jr. et al (2007) Ki-67 as prognostic marker in early breast cancer: a meta-analysis of published studies involving 12,155 patients. Br J Cancer 96(10):1504–1513

Dewar R, Fadare O, Gilmore H, Gown AM (2011) Best practices in diagnostic immunohistochemistry: myoepithelial markers in breast pathology. Arch Pathol Lab Med 135(4):422–429

Domagala W, Markiewski M, Harezga B, Dukowicz A, Osborn M (1996) Prognostic significance of tumor cell proliferation rate as determined by the MIB-1 antibody in breast carcinoma: its relationship with vimentin and p53 protein. Clin Cancer Res 2(1):147–154

Dowsett M, Sestak I, Lopez-Knowles E et al (2013) Comparison of PAM50 risk of recurrence score with oncotype DX and IHC4 for predicting risk of distant recurrence after endocrine therapy. J Clin Oncol 31 (22):2783–2790

Early Breast Cancer Trialists' Collaborative Group (1998) Tamoxifen for early breast cancer: an overview of the randomised trials. Lancet 351(9114):1451–1467

Early Breast Cancer Trialists' Collaborative Group (2005) Effects of chemotherapy and hormonal therapy for early breast cancer on recurrence and 15-year survival: an overview of the randomised trials. Lancet 365 (9472):1687–1717

Elsheikh SE, Green AR, Rakha EA et al (2009) Global histone modifications in breast cancer correlate with tumor phenotypes, prognostic factors, and patient outcome. Cancer Res 69(9):3802–3809

Elston CW, Ellis IO (1991) Pathological prognostic factors in breast cancer. I. The value of histological grade in breast cancer: experience from a large study with long-term follow-up. Histopathology 19(5):403–410

Elston CW, Ellis IO, Pinder SE (1999) Pathological prognostic factors in breast cancer. Crit Rev Oncol Hematol 31(3):209–223

Galea MH, Blamey RW, Elston CE, Ellis IO (1992) The Nottingham Prognostic Index in primary breast cancer. Breast Cancer Res Treat 22(3):207–219

Gasparini G, Pozza F, Harris AL (1993) Evaluating the potential usefulness of new prognostic and predictive indicators in node-negative breast cancer patients. J Natl Cancer Inst 85(15):1206–1219

Goldhirsch A, Wood WC, Coates AS et al (2011) Strategies for subtypes—dealing with the diversity of breast cancer: highlights of the St. Gallen International Expert Consensus on the Primary Therapy of Early Breast Cancer 2011. Ann Oncol 22(8): 1736–1747. doi:10.1093/annonc/mdr304 (England)

Goldhirsch A, Winer EP, Coates AS et al (2013) Personalizing the treatment of women with early breast cancer: highlights of the St Gallen International Expert Consensus on the Primary Therapy of Early Breast Cancer 2013. Ann Oncol 24(9):2206–2223

Green AR, Powe DG, Rakha EA et al (2013) Identification of key clinical phenotypes of breast cancer using a reduced panel of protein biomarkers. Br J Cancer 109 (7):1886–1894

Habashy HO, Powe DG, Rakha EA et al (2010) The prognostic significance of PELP1 expression in invasive breast cancer with emphasis on the ER-positive luminal-like subtype. Breast Cancer Res Treat 120 (3):603–612

Habashy HO, Powe DG, Glaab E et al (2011a) RERG (Ras-like, oestrogen-regulated, growth-inhibitor) expression in breast cancer: a marker of ER-positive luminal-like subtype. Breast Cancer Res Treat 128 (2):315–326

Habashy HO, Rakha EA, Aleskandarany M et al (2011b) $FOXO_{3a}$ nuclear localisation is associated with good prognosis in luminal-like breast cancer. Breast Cancer Res Treat 129(1):11–21

Habashy HO, Rakha EA, Ellis IO, Powe DG (2013) The oestrogen receptor coactivator CARM1 has an oncogenic effect and is associated with poor prognosis in breast cancer. Breast Cancer Res Treat 140(2):307–316

Hammond ME, Hayes DF, Dowsett M et al (2010) American Society of Clinical Oncology/College Of American Pathologists guideline recommendations for immunohistochemical testing of estrogen and progesterone receptors in breast cancer. J Clin Oncol 28 (16):2784–2795

Harris L, Fritsche H, Mennel R et al (2007) American Society of Clinical Oncology 2007 update of recommendations for the use of tumor markers in breast cancer. J Clin Oncol 25(33):5287–5312

Haybittle JL, Blamey RW, Elston CW et al (1982) A prognostic index in primary breast cancer. Br J Cancer 45(3):361–366

Hayes DF, Trock B, Harris AL (1998) Assessing the clinical impact of prognostic factors: when is "statistically significant" clinically useful? Breast Cancer Res Treat 52(1–3):305–319

Inwald EC, Klinkhammer-Schalke M, Hofstadter F et al (2013) Ki-67 is a prognostic parameter in breast cancer patients: results of a large population-based cohort of a cancer registry. Breast Cancer Res Treat 139(2):539–552

Jerjees DA, Negm OH, Alabdullah ML et al (2015) The mammalian target of rapamycin complex 1 (mTORC1) in breast cancer: the impact of oestrogen receptor and HER2 pathways. Breast Cancer Res Treat 150(1):91–103

Karakas C (2011) Paget's disease of the breast. J Carcinog 10:31

Lacroix-Triki M, Geyer FC, Lambros MB et al (2010) Beta-catenin/Wnt signalling pathway in fibromatosis, metaplastic carcinomas and phyllodes tumours of the breast. Mod Pathol 23(11):1438–1448

Lee AH (2007) The histological diagnosis of metastases to the breast from extramammary malignancies. J Clin Pathol 60(12):1333–1341

Mauri D, Pavlidis N, Polyzos NP, Ioannidis JP (2006) Survival with aromatase inhibitors and inactivators versus standard hormonal therapy in advanced breast cancer: meta-analysis. J Natl Cancer Inst 98 (18):1285–1291

Mislick K, Schonfeld W, Bodnar C, Tong KB (2014) Cost-effectiveness analysis of Mammostrat(R) compared with Oncotype DX(R) to inform the treatment of breast cancer. ClinicoEcon Outcomes Res 6:37–47

Nielsen TO, Hsu FD, Jensen K et al (2004) Immunohistochemical and clinical characterization of the basal-like subtype of invasive breast carcinoma. Clin Cancer Res 10(16):5367–5374

Otterbach F, Bankfalvi A, Bergner S, Decker T, Krech R, Boecker W (2000) Cytokeratin 5/6 immunohistochemistry assists the differential diagnosis of atypical proliferations of the breast. Histopathology 37(3):232–240

Park D, Karesen R, Noren T, Sauer T (2007) Ki-67 expression in primary breast carcinomas and their axillary lymph node metastases: clinical implications. Virchows Arch 451(1):11–18

Pathology Reporting of Breast Disease (2005a) A Joint Document Incorporating the Third Edition of the NHS Breast Screening Programme's Guidelines for Pathology Reporting in Breast Cancer Screening and the Second Edition of The Royal College of Pathologists' Minimum Dataset for Breast Cancer Histopathology. NHSBSP Pub. No 58

Pathology Reporting of Breast Disease (2005b) A Joint Document Incorporating the Third Edition of the NHS Breast Screening Programme's Guidelines for Pathology Reporting in Breast Cancer Screening and the Second Edition of The Royal College of Pathologists' Minimum Dataset for Breast Cancer Histopathology. (January 2005)

Perou CM, Sorlie T, Eisen MB et al (2000) Molecular portraits of human breast tumours. Nature 406 (6797):747–752

Petrelli F, Viale G, Cabiddu M, Barni S (2015) Prognostic value of different cut-off levels of Ki-67 in breast cancer: a systematic review and meta-analysis of 64,196 patients. Breast Cancer Res Treat 153(3):477–491

Rakha E, Putti T, Abd El-Rehim D, Paish EC, Ellis I (2005) Breast carcinomas with basal/myoepithelial differentiation: a review of morphology and immunophenotypical analysis. J Pathol 207:5

Rakha EA, El-Sayed ME, Reis-Filho JS, Ellis IO (2008a) Expression profiling technology: its contribution to our understanding of breast cancer. Histopathology 52 (1):67–81

Rakha EA, El-Sheikh SE, Kandil MA, El-Sayed ME, Green AR, Ellis IO (2008b) Expression of BRCA1 protein in breast cancer and its prognostic significance. Hum Pathol 39(6):857–865

Rakha EA, Elsheikh SE, Aleskandarany MA et al (2009) Triple-negative breast cancer: distinguishing between basal and nonbasal subtypes. Clin Cancer Res 15 (7):2302–2310

Rakha EA, Patel A, Powe DG et al (2010) Clinical and biological significance of E-cadherin protein expression in invasive lobular carcinoma of the breast. Am J Surg Pathol 34(10):1472–1479

Rakha EA, Gandhi N, Climent F et al (2011) Encapsulated papillary carcinoma of the breast: an invasive tumor with excellent prognosis. Am J Surg Pathol 35 (8):1093–1103

Rakha EA, Teoh TK, Lee AH, Nolan CC, Ellis IO, Green AR (2013) Further evidence that E-cadherin is not a tumour suppressor gene in invasive ductal carcinoma of the breast: an immunohistochemical study. Histopathology 62(5):695–701

Rakha EA, Soria D, Green AR et al (2014a) Nottingham Prognostic Index Plus (NPI+): a modern clinical decision making tool in breast cancer. Br J Cancer 110(7):1688–1697

Rakha EA, Soria D, Green AR et al (2014b) Nottingham Prognostic Index Plus (NPI+): a modern clinical decision making tool in breast cancer. Br J Cancer

Rakha EA, Soria D, Green AR et al (2014c) Nottingham Prognostic Index Plus (NPI+): a modern clinical decision making tool in breast cancer. Br J Cancer 1532–1827 (Electronic)

Rakha EA, Pinder SE, Bartlett JM et al (2015) Updated UK recommendations for HER2 assessment in breast cancer. J Clin Pathol 68(2):93–99

Ring BZ, Seitz RS, Beck R et al (2006) Novel prognostic immunohistochemical biomarker panel for estrogen receptor-positive breast cancer. J Clin Oncol 24 (19):3039–3047

Rolland P, Spendlove I, Madjd Z et al (2007) The p53 positive Bcl-2 negative phenotype is an independent marker of prognosis in breast cancer. Int J Cancer 120 (6):1311–1317

Ross DT, Kim CY, Tang G et al (2008) Chemosensitivity and stratification by a five monoclonal antibody immunohistochemistry test in the NSABP B14 and B20 trials. Clin Cancer Res 14(20):6602–6609. doi:10.1158/1078-0432.ccr-08-0647 (United States)

Senkus E, Kyriakides S, Ohno S et al (2015) Primary breast cancer: ESMO Clinical Practice Guidelines for diagnosis, treatment and follow-up. Ann Oncol 26 (Suppl 5):v8–v30

Shoker BS, Jarvis C, Sibson DR, Walker C, Sloane JP (1999) Oestrogen receptor expression in the normal and pre-cancerous breast. J Pathol 188(3):237–244

Sorlie T, Perou CM, Tibshirani R et al (2001) Gene expression patterns of breast carcinomas distinguish tumor subclasses with clinical implications. Proc Natl Acad Sci U S A 98(19):10869–10874

Stuart-Harris R, Caldas C, Pinder SE, Pharoah P (2008) Proliferation markers and survival in early breast cancer: a systematic review and meta-analysis of 85 studies in 32,825 patients. Breast 17(4):323–334

Trihia H, Murray S, Price K et al (2003) Ki-67 expression in breast carcinoma: its association with grading systems, clinical parameters, and other prognostic factors–a surrogate marker? Cancer 97(5):1321–1331

Viale G, Giobbie-Hurder A, Regan MM et al (2008a) Prognostic and predictive value of centrally reviewed Ki-67 labeling index in postmenopausal women with endocrine-responsive breast cancer: results from Breast International Group Trial 1-98 comparing adjuvant tamoxifen with letrozole. J Clin Oncol 26 (34):5569–5575

Viale G, Regan MM, Mastropasqua MG et al (2008b) Predictive value of tumor Ki-67 expression in two randomized trials of adjuvant chemoendocrine therapy for node-negative breast cancer. J Natl Cancer Inst 100 (3):207–212

Weinstein IB, Joe A (2008) Oncogene addiction. Cancer Res 68(9):3077–3080

Wolff AC, Hammond ME, Hicks DG et al (2013) Recommendations for human epidermal growth factor receptor 2 testing in breast cancer: American Society of Clinical Oncology/College of American Pathologists clinical practice guideline update. J Clin Oncol 31(31):3997–4013

Yamaguchi R, Maeshiro K, Ellis IO et al (2012) Infiltrative epitheliosis of the breast. J Clin Pathol 65(8):766–768

Tumor Heterogeneity in Breast Cancer

9

Sunil Badve

Abstract

Traditional teachings state that monoclonality is a sine qua non of malignancy. *Tumor heterogeneity* at first glance flies in the face of clonal origin of tumors. However, heterogeneity represents clonal evolution and adaption to adverse environment and is a cardinal feature of all life forms including tumors. The major concern is that these adaptations could interfere with therapies and affect patient outcomes. Variability in clinical presentation, tumor histology, response to treatment and outcomes have been long recognized by clinicians and pathologists. In this review, we revisit this old friend (or, perhaps more correctly, a foe) and document that heterogeneity that exists at all, clinical, histological and molecular, levels and briefly outline the strategies that have been used by clinicians and pathologists to tackle this complicated issue.

Keywords

Breast cancer · Tumor heterogeneity

9.1 Introduction

To even the most casual observer of human cancer, it is obvious that there is a marked variability in clinical outcomes. Some patients have very aggressive disease while others manage to outlive their cancers and die of other causes. These observations raise fundamental questions regarding why some patients can be successfully treated while others are not so fortunate and develop recurrences in spite of appropriate therapy. A closer look at the histology of chemotherapy treated cancers has shown that there are often pockets of surviving tumor cells in the midst of dead/nonviable areas of tumor. It follows the cancer cells in these pockets are different from the rest of the tumor; i.e., tumor heterogeneity is the cause of recurrences and metastases. Needless to say that better understanding of tumor heterogeneity will assist us in better treating our patients.

S. Badve (✉)
Department of Pathology and Laboratory Medicine, Indiana University School of Medicine, 350 West 11th Street, IUHPL 4050, Indianapolis, IN 46202, USA
e-mail: sbadve@iupui.edu

S. Badve and Y. Gökmen-Polar (eds.), *Molecular Pathology of Breast Cancer*, DOI 10.1007/978-3-319-41761-5_9

9.2 Extent of Tumor Heterogeneity?

There is a wide variation in the clinical presentation of patients with cancers. The tumors can be small or large tumors and progress at different speeds and result in different outcomes after getting the standard therapies. Some cancers are associated with calcifications and can be easily detected by mammographic screening while others are radiologically invisible in spite of being palpable. Similarly, the presence and extent of nodal involvement at presentation can be completely variable in patients with similarly sized primary tumors. Histologically, the tumor heterogeneity is evident in all tumors (Fig. 9.1a, b). It has also been recognized by the approximately 17 different histological types in the WHO classification as well as in parameters such as tumor grade. The latter is a well-established prognostic factor even in this era of molecular predictors and gene signatures. Foci that have distinct morphological features can be frequently identified within tumors. For example, small foci of tubular/glandular differentiation are commonly noted in lobular carcinomas. The presence of higher grade foci within tumors in large excision specimens is well recognized.

The development of high throughput technologies has enabled assessment of thousands to millions of markers simultaneously. These analyses have shown that no two tumors are alike. A number of classifications using expression patterns of mRNA have been proposed, of which the intrinsic classification is most commonly used. Perou et al. divided breast cancers into ER^+ subtypes (luminal A and luminal B) and ER^- subtypes (basal-like, HER2-enriched, and normal-like carcinomas) (Perou et al. 2000). The 21-gene recurrence score, an assay commonly used in clinical practice, uses qRT-PCR to classify ER+ tumors into prognostic categories (see Chap. 4 and 18). These types of assays has been shown to predict outcomes in patients treated with chemo- and endocrine therapies (Gnant et al. 2014; Liu et al. 2015; Sestak et al. 2015).

The Cancer Genome Atlas (TCGA) project analysis over 1000 tumors using multiple "-omics" technologies (Cancer Genome Atlas 2012) has documented a plethora of mutations; some of these are specific to a single tumor. These studies also document that ER^- tumors harbor a significantly higher number of mutations compared to ER^+ tumors (Cancer Genome Atlas 2012). It is difficult to determine which of these mutations are driving the oncogenic process (driver mutations) and which are incidental to the disturbed DNA replication processes (passenger mutations) present within cancers. Recent studies seem to suggest that the designation of driver and passenger mutations is probably contextual in nature. Passenger mutations might to be important for adapting to the stresses induced by hypoxia and other factors involved in the metastatic process.

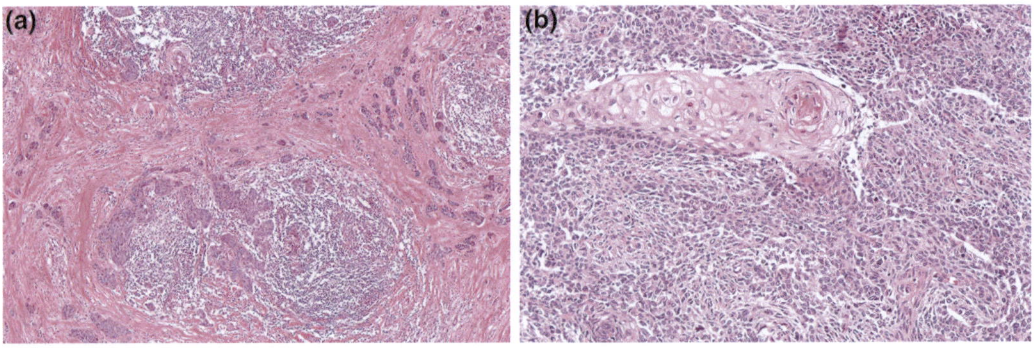

Fig. 9.1 Histological evidence of tumor heterogeneity. **a** Tumor composed of solid ness of epithelial cells as well as cords separated by stroma (tumor microenvironment) containing stromal cells, blood vessels, and immune cells. **b** A high grade carcinoma with a predominantly spindle cell component exhibiting focal squamous differentiation

The roles of BRCA1 and BRCA2 genes in the causation of breast cancer are well documented. It appears that these tumors are particularly vulnerable to agents that target the DNA pathway (Turner et al. 2008; Fong et al. 2009). The mutations commonest in breast cancer are TP53 and PIK3CA genes. Therapeutic targeting of TP53 is difficult. The presence of PI3 kinase mutations would possibly sensitize the cancers to mTOR inhibitors such as Everolimus. However, in the BOLERO-2 clinical trial, all patients showed benefit from the addition of Everolimus in irrespective of the PI3 kinase mutations status (Beck et al. 2014).

The high incidence of low frequency mutations in cancer has led some investigators to concentrate on an alternative approach that focuses on the type of mutation (e.g., C > T) rather than the gene in which the mutation occurs (Alexandrov et al. 2013). The APOBEC enzymes (1 and 3), which have been casually implicated in multiple cancers including breast cancer (Cescon et al. 2015; Nik-Zainal et al. 2014; Swanton et al. 2015) have been targeted for drug development.

Lastly, from the treatment standpoint it was hoped that cancer would be just one condition in which all cells are identical in their genetic content. More importantly, the cells would be sensitive to therapeutic agent(s) and use of this treatment would result in complete destruction of the entire population effecting a "cure". Anyone who has ever come in touch with cancer knows that this is far from the truth. This intratumoral heterogeneity is the focus of the remainder of this chapter. We will include discussions on tumor cell genetic heterogeneity but details of tumor microenvironment and immune cell infiltrates are covered elsewhere in this book.

9.3 Origins of Tumor

Prior to understanding the origins of TH in cancers, it is important to understand the mechanisms that could lead to the development of cancers. It is presumed that cancers arise from the malignant transformation of a single normal cell. Whether this hypothesis is true is not clear. It is equally possible that cancers arise from (perhaps, near simultaneous) transformation of multiple stem or differentiated cells. Most studies based on single cell sequencing of tumors seem to support a single cell origin (Hou et al. 2012; Li et al. 2012; Navin 2014; Navin and Hicks 2010; Xu et al. 2012). However, Yu et al. were able to demonstrate a bi-clonal origin of tumor in a case of colon cancer (Yu et al. 2014).

The process of transformation could be gradual accumulation of multiple insults/injuries or a single cataclysmic event (Fig. 9.2). A gradual development could allow expansion of a clone (i.e., benign tumor) from which a malignant clone could arise; the process contributing to TH. A classic example of this could be the adenoma-carcinoma progression model, first proposed in colon cancer. The genomic instability that contributed to the development of cancer continues within the cancer cells and gives rise to heterogeneity.

It appears (as in human evolution) that tumor cell evolution might be impacted by the pattern or sequence of prior mutations. Ortmann et al. (2015) have documented that the sequence of JAK2 and TET2 mutations are important in myeloproliferative disorders. Patients in whom JAK2 mutations occur first tend to be younger, have polycythemia vera and the progenitor cells are more sensitive to JAK2 inhibition (Swanton 2015). In the context of breast cancer the mice models have suggested that loss of Brca1 by itself results in cell-cycle arrest (Hakem et al. 1997). The presence of antecedent TP53 mutation rescues the cell and is critical for the development of tumors.

The "Big Bang" theory of cancer proposes that a single event such as karyotypic chaos, stress- induced mutational burst and chromothrypsis could lead to a rapid transformation of normal cells and development of cancer (Sottoriva et al. 2015). This rapid transformation leads to a single clone, which has all the characteristics of cancer cells. As the original insult was time limited and may have been removed, the processes to develop additional mutations contributing to progressive increase in heterogeneity are limited. The subsequent subclones

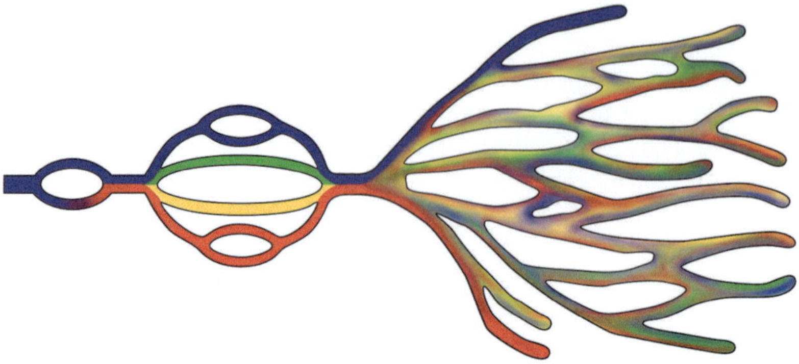

Fig. 9.2 Origin of tumors: It is commonly believed that tumors arise from the transformation of a single cell (*blue*). This may undergo additional changes to form diverse clones (*red/green/yellow*), which together contribute to the bulk of the tumor (*mixed colors*)

arise have only minor survival advantages over the parent clone and do not have the capacity to form the dominant clone within the tumor. The development of additional mutations is believed to be due to increased error rates/mutation rates in tumor cells. It was believed that this might be as high as 200 times of normal cells (Bielas et al. 2006; Bielas and Loeb 2005). Recent studies using single nucleus sequencing (NUC-SEQ) suggest that the mutation rate in TNBCs might be around 13 times the normal cells (Wang et al. 2014). On the other hand, the mutation rates in ER^+ tumors appear to be similar to that observed in normal cells (Wang et al. 2014).

Lastly, one always presumes that mutations are the direct cause of DNA damage. However, it is also possible that alterations in the DNA are secondary to other intra-cellular alterations. Recently Lee et al., have shown that the loss of NORAD, a lincRNA, results in unregulated action of PUMILIO proteins (Lee et al. 2016) The PUMILIO proteins drive chromosomal instability by hyperactively repressing mitotic, DNA repair, and DNA replication factors.

9.3.1 Origins of Intratumor Heterogeneity

Two distinct models have been proposed to explain the heterogeneity of cancer cells. The Cancer stem cell (CSC) theory posits that cancers arise from stem cells, which have the capacity for unequal division giving rise to undifferentiated (CSC) and differentiated (non-CSC) progeny. The later have the capacity to proliferate rapidly and constitute the bulk of the tumor, while the former constitute the slow growing inert population that resists chemo- and/or radiotherapy. The alternative hypothesis is termed "Clonal Evolution" model. In this model, heterogeneity develops from accumulating additional mutations in the single mutated cancer cell. These additional mutations give rise to subpopulations, each of which retain the ability to divide and mutate further. The resultant subclones possess an evolutionary advantage over the others within the tumor environment, and may become dominant in the tumor over time.

9.3.2 Cancer Stem Cells

Elegant work by Michael Clarke's group has documented that tumor cells that have $CD44^{high}$/$CD24^{low/-}$ phenotype have a significantly greater ability to give rise to metastasis in animal models (Al-Hajj et al. 2003). Of note, these studies were performed in a triple negative (MDA-231) cell line model and it was unclear whether the findings could be generalizable. Our group (Sheridan et al. 2006) analyzed a number of establish cell lines using flow cytometry for the presence of these markers. Surprisingly, $CD44^+$/$CD24^{low/-}$

cells were identified only in cell lines that had a mesenchymal phenotype and not in any of the luminal cell lines. Further work by Wicha's group showed that the expression of aldehyde dehydrogenase 1 (ALDH1) might be a better marker for CSCs (Ginestier et al. 2007). Although number of studies have corroborated these findings (see Chap. 10 by Cheng and colleagues), some groups, including ours, remain yet to be convinced (Neumeister and Rimm 2010; Tan et al. 2013; Zhong et al. 2013, 2014; Resetkova et al. 2010). ALDH1 expression is not restricted to the tumor cells but can be also noted in tumor associated fibroblasts and/or myoepithelial cells. Indeed, our group has documented its role as a prognostic factor when expression within stromal cells was analyzed but did not find a prognostic relevance for ALDH1 expression within tumor cells. Needless to say, the topic is controversial with excellent review articles highlighting the pros and the cons of the concept (Azizi and Wicha 2013; Badve and Nakshatri 2012; Gokmen-Polar and Badve 2013; Gokmen-Polar et al. 2011).

One of the related issues is whether cancer arises from stem cells within the breast. Our group identified pluripotent cells in cultures of explants of normal breast tissue obtained from the Susan G Komen normal tissue bank (Sauder et al. 2014). These cells from normal nontransformed epithelium could differentiate along multiple lineages including but not limited to melanocytes, neural, chondrocytes, and osteocytes (i.e., both ectodermal and mesodermal lineages). Data such as these show the degree of plasticity that exists within both normal and tumor cell populations. Similarly, Roy et al. identified pluripotent cells using cell surface markers associated with repression of p16INK4a/cyclin-dependent kinase inhibitor 2A (CDKN2A) (Roy et al. 2013). Similar to human embryonic stem cells and inducible pluripotent stem cells (iPSCs) (Takahashi et al. 2007), these cells express OCT3/4, SOX2, and NANOG at high levels. It also raises the possibility that neoplastic transformation in differentiated cells could lead to "de-differentiation" and acquisition of stem cell characteristics.

9.3.3 Clonal Evolution

The basic principle of Darwinian clonal evolution is that seemly purposeless genetic variations in individuals arising from a common descendent and that these variations could in the long-run provide for a survival advantage. Cancers can show similar evolution. It is currently believed (as discussed previously) that cancers arise from a single cell, which could be a differentiated cell or a stem cell. Over time these cancer initiating cells accumulate increasing mutational load and undergo a Darwinian "*survival of the fittest*" evolution model (Fig. 9.2). In this context, the terms driver and passenger can be explained as driver mutations are ones that sustain cancer growth while passenger mutations provide for a better adaptation to the cellular environment.

Clonal evolution can occur in linear manner or in a branched manner similar to that described by Charles Darwin during his work on evolution of species. In the linear model, the clones in addition to acquiring new mutation, continue to bear all the mutations in the parent cells. In the branched evolution model any expansion occurs in a splitting manner in which many distinct progeny arise, due to genetic instability, from a single "root" clone. This process might make it hard to decipher the common origin of the tumor clones. A number of studies exist to support both of these hypothesis and a possibility of a mixed model incorporating elements of both the models of evolution cannot be excluded.

The net result of these processes is to provide a pool of mutations that help improve adaptation of the tumor cells to the environment as well as escape immune surveillance. These can be further influenced by therapy as well as changes in tissue environment (Voss et al. 2014; Misale et al. 2012; Diaz et al. 2012). Therapy might not only select for mutations but also lead to acquisition of additional ones shaping the evolutionary trajectory of the tumor (McGranahan and Swanton 2015). Cis-platinum treatment in *C. elegans*, has been shown to cause a striking increase in C > A transversions—as well as an elevated rate of dinucleotide substitutions indels, and structural variations (Meier et al. 2014).

9.3.4 Codependency of Clones

Similar to any ecological habitat, the presence of divergent clones could impact the behavior of the tumor cells in different manner (see Tabassum and Polyak (2015) for review). A dominant clone may suppress the growth of other clones. Recent studies in colon cancer by Sottoriva et al. (2015) have shown that at least in some tumors, there is a single dominant clone (arising due to Big Bang) with very little divergence of clones. This dominance could be due to a variety of factors including growth advantage, availability of nutrients and oxygen as well as diffusible secreted factors. The latter has been documented in insulinomas (Archetti et al. 2015). From the therapeutic standpoint, the lack of bio-diversity could make the tumor susceptible to extinction.

Cooperation between clones can take many forms; these have been described as commensalism, synergism and mutualism. This has been classically shown in mouse models of non-small cell lung cancer, where the presence of two distinct populations together can lead to disease progression and metastases, while neither of the populations alone is able to do so (Calbo et al. 2011). Cleary et al. (2014) in the MMTV-Wnt1 model have demonstrated cooperative interactions between different clones. Similarly, Zhang et al. have documented that cytokines secreted by $C29^{hi}CD24^{low}$ cells stimulated renewal and tumor initiating capacity of $C29^{hi}CD24^{hi}$ cells through a feedback loop (Zhang et al. 2015). In human breast cancers, the expression of ER is seen in a variable number of tumor cells ranging from 1 to 100 %. This heterogeneity is preserved even in cell lines and PDX models. Treatment with anti-estrogenic agents can control the growth of the tumors suggesting the necessity of ER+ population for the growth of the ER− subpopulation.

9.4 Heterogeneity in Primary and Metastatic Tumors

Tumors by and large retain their morphological features even at metastatic sites. However, alterations in protein expression have been noted. For example, up to 10 % of metastatic lesions can be $HER2^{+}$ even when the primary tumor has been shown to be negative for HER2 expression/amplification (Liedtke et al. 2009; Niikura et al. 2012). Analyses of matched primary and metastatic tumors using NGS methods have shown significant differences (Shah et al. 2009; Stephens et al. 2012; Thomas et al. 2007). In these studies, clones that are barely detectable (or undetectable) in primary tumors have been shown to predominate at the metastatic sites (Shah et al. 2009). Ding et al. performed the genomic analyses of four DNA samples (peripheral blood, the primary tumor, a brain metastasis and a xenograft derived from the primary tumor) from an African-American patient with basal-like breast cancer to identify two de novo mutations and a large deletion not present in the primary tumor, in addition to significant enrichment in 20 shared mutations. They suggest that secondary tumors may arise from a minority of cells within the primary tumor. Navin et al. have used a single nucleus sequencing (SNS) approach to study TNBCs. Using data from 100 single cell copy-number analyses from 2 patients, they describe that copy number alterations (CNAs) evolved in punctuated bursts of evolution followed by stable clonal expansions. They also identified rare populations that had more than 50-fold amplification of KRAS; this could not be detected in major tumor subpopulations. This suggests that the most malignant populations in the tumor might be also the rarest (Navin and Hicks 2010). In data presented at the European Cancer Congress meeting (2015), Yates et al. analyzed the 839 primary tumors and 161 metastatic/recurrence tissue samples (66 matched samples) for 365 genes. They found that 11 genes including TP53 and ARID1A were significantly increased in metastatic samples. Furthermore, JAK-STAT pathway was downregulated in the metastatic tissues.

The differences in the primary and metastatic tumor population is a subject of extensive research. Analyses of the circulating tumors cells and DNA (see Chaps. 14 and 15 for details) have been very useful in documenting the development of new mutations/clones following targeted therapies. More recently, the Breast International Group (BIG) has launched the AURORA initiative—Aiming to Understand the Molecular Aberrations in Metastatic Breast Cancer (Zardavas et al. 2014, 2015). The goal is to collect samples from over 1300 patients who have not received more than one line of systemic treatment for advanced disease. Primary tumor, metastases, whole blood, plasma and serum with analyzed by multiple "omics" technologies to better understand the changes associated with progression of breast cancer.

9.5 Implications of Tumor Heterogeneity

Inter and intratumor heterogeneity has been recognized for a prolonged period of time and used for classifying tumors. Heterogeneity exists at all levels—clinical, histopathological, and molecular within primary tumors and between primary and metastatic tumors. It has important implications for treating patients.

1. In glioblastomas, four subtypes, classical, neural, proneural and mesenchymal, have been described. It has been suggested that recognition of these subtypes would result in development of more effective patient stratification, targeted therapeutics, and prediction of patient outcome (Aldape et al. 2015). However, in single cell sequencing study, all the subtypes could be seen in the same tumor (Patel et al. 2014; Verhaak et al. 2010). This raises concerns about molecular classification of tumors.
2. Tumors are composed of variable number of mutations, some of which might be necessary growth and proliferation while others may have no significant value to the tumor. Targeting of any and every mutation within a tumor may not be beneficial. There is a possibility that this might result in development/emergence of more resistant clones. The presence of V600E BRAF mutations in melanoma indicates sensitivity to vemurafenib (PLX4032) (Flaherty et al. 2010), however the identical mutation when observed in colo-rectal cancer is not associated with response to this agent (Kopetz et al. 2015).
3. The sequence of acquisition of mutations has been suggested in myelodysplastic studies to be important for treatment. If this is also true for breast cancer, the current mutation detection and treatment approaches may not be as effective as originally conceived. Dissection of molecular pathways will prove to be extremely critical. Single cell sequencing technologies could provide better understanding of the underlying processes.
4. Clonal diversity and interdependence of clones could be exploited for therapeutic purposes. The identification of molecular basis of these relationships is critical.
5. Tumors that have prominent heterogeneity might be better able to adapt to the changing environment caused by therapy and give rise to recurrences. Almendro et al. (2014) analyzed intratumor genetic diversity and found that it was tumor-subtype specific. More importantly, it did not change during treatment in tumors. However, lower pretreatment genetic diversity was significantly associated with pathologic complete response. In contrast, Swanton's group, have shown that extreme chromosomal instability was associated with improved outcomes in the TACT trial (Issa-Nummer et al. 2013; Jamal-Hanjani et al. 2015).
6. Most treatment decisions are made on the basis of primary tumors and not the basis of metastatic tumors. Gene signatures and other types of molecular analyses using whole

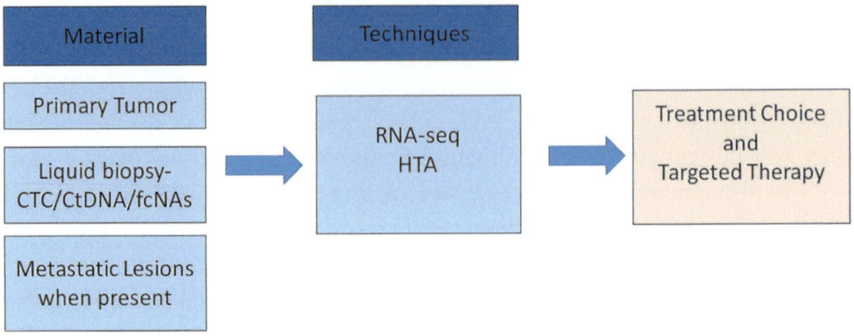

Fig. 9.3 Clinical monitoring to target spatial and temporal tumor heterogeneity in breast cancer

tumors may not accurately reflect the metastatic potential of the tumor. As discussed earlier the most malignant clone may not be represented in the analysis of the bulk tumor.

7. Do we accept that primary tumors and metastatic tumors could have completely different biological processes? If so, could this be the reason why some drugs (combinations) that are effective in metastatic settings are not so efficient in treating adjuvant tumors.
8. Lastly, what are the tools to monitor the tumor heterogeneity. As illustrated in Fig. 9.3, analysis of primary and metastatic tumors could provide some leads to appropriate targeting of tumors. The more recent, liquid biopsy technique, could provide for continuous monitoring of patients. This could be done for early identification of recurrence. But importantly, it could identify novel mutations in patients with metastatic cancer and provide the first evidence of development of resistance to targeted therapies.

9.6 Summary and Future Directions

Heterogeneity is common in tumors and has been documented in every analysis that has been performed. This is at first shocking because mono-clonality has been considered the hallmark of neoplastic proliferations. However, by virtue of the epithelial nature of carcinomas, tumor cells need to have interactions with stromal elements, which provide nutrition to the cells. Obviously not all cells can be located in the prime real-estate next to blood vessels; this will undoubtedly result in well-nourished and poorly nourished cells leading to heterogeneity. Poorly nourished clones will need/try to muscle in on the blood stream and this could perhaps be the driving force for additional mutations. Similarly, different regions of the tumor might acquire additional mutations and try to establish dominance. All of this contributes to intra-tumor heterogeneity.

Tumor heterogeneity is undoubtedly important in the treatment of cancer. Whether in the form of "cancer stem cells" or emerging "clonal evolution", heterogeneity is essential for survival of tumor cells in increasing adverse environments in the surgical bed and created by chemo- and radio-therapies. However, we currently lack the understanding and the tools to effectively combat the heterogeneity. The current tools essentially consist of recognizing the heterogeneity and documenting it in details so that one can develop effective strategies in the future.

Disclosure The authors disclose no potential conflicts of interest or NIH funding to disclose.

References

Aldape K, Zadeh G, Mansouri S, Reifenberger G, von Deimling A (2015) Glioblastoma: pathology, molecular mechanisms and markers. Acta Neuropathol 129 (6):829–848. doi:10.1007/s00401-015-1432-1

Alexandrov LB, Nik-Zainal S, Wedge DC, Aparicio SA, Behjati S, Biankin AV, Bignell GR, Bolli N, Borg A, Borresen-Dale AL, Boyault S, Burkhardt B, Butler AP, Caldas C, Davies HR, Desmedt C, Eils R, Eyfjord JE, Foekens JA, Greaves M, Hosoda F, Hutter B, Ilicic T, Imbeaud S, Imielinski M, Jager N, Jones DT, Jones D, Knappskog S, Kool M, Lakhani SR, Lopez-Otin C, Martin S, Munshi NC, Nakamura H, Northcott PA, Pajic M, Papaemmanuil E, Paradiso A, Pearson JV, Puente XS, Raine K, Ramakrishna M, Richardson AL, Richter J, Rosenstiel P, Schlesner M, Schumacher TN, Span PN, Teague JW, Totoki Y, Tutt AN, Valdes-Mas R, van Buuren MM, van 't Veer L, Vincent-Salomon A, Waddell N, Yates LR, Australian Pancreatic Cancer Genome I, Consortium IBC, Consortium IM-S, PedBrain I, Zucman-Rossi J, Futreal PA, McDermott U, Lichter P, Meyerson M, Grimmond SM, Siebert R, Campo E, Shibata T, Pfister SM, Campbell PJ, Stratton MR (2013) Signatures of mutational processes in human cancer. Nature 500 (7463):415–421. doi:10.1038/nature12477

Al-Hajj M, Wicha MS, Benito-Hernandez A, Morrison SJ, Clarke MF (2003) Prospective identification of tumorigenic breast cancer cells. Proc Natl Acad Sci U S A 100(7):3983–3988. doi:10.1073/pnas.0530291100

Almendro V, Cheng YK, Randles A, Itzkovitz S, Marusyk A, Ametller E, Gonzalez-Farre X, Munoz M, Russnes HG, Helland A, Rye IH, Borresen-Dale AL, Maruyama R, van Oudenaarden A, Dowsett M, Jones RL, Reis-Filho J, Gascon P, Gonen M, Michor F, Polyak K (2014) Inference of tumor evolution during chemotherapy by computational modeling and in situ analysis of genetic and phenotypic cellular diversity. Cell Rep 6(3):514–527. doi:10.1016/j.celrep.2013.12.041

Archetti M, Ferraro DA, Christofori G (2015) Heterogeneity for IGF-II production maintained by public goods dynamics in neuroendocrine pancreatic cancer. Proc Natl Acad Sci U S A 112(6):1833–1838. doi:10.1073/pnas.1414653112

Azizi E, Wicha MS (2013) Point: cancer stem cells—the evidence accumulates. Clin Chem 59(1):205–207. doi:10.1373/clinchem.2012.195990

Badve S, Nakshatri H (2012) Breast-cancer stem cells-beyond semantics. Lancet Oncol 13(1):e43–48. doi:10.1016/S1470-2045(11)70191-7

Beck JT, Hortobagyi GN, Campone M, Lebrun F, Deleu I, Rugo HS, Pistilli B, Masuda N, Hart L, Melichar B, Dakhil S, Geberth M, Nunzi M, Heng DY, Brechenmacher T, El-Hashimy M, Douma S, Ringeisen F, Piccart M (2014) Everolimus plus exemestane as first-line therapy in HR(+), HER2 (−) advanced breast cancer in BOLERO-2. Breast Cancer Res Treat 143(3):459–467. doi:10.1007/s10549-013-2814-5

Bielas JH, Loeb LA (2005) Mutator phenotype in cancer: timing and perspectives. Environ Mol Mutagen 45(2–3):206–213. doi:10.1002/em.20111

Bielas JH, Loeb KR, Rubin BP, True LD, Loeb LA (2006) Human cancers express a mutator phenotype. Proc Natl Acad Sci U S A 103(48):18238–18242. doi:10.1073/pnas.0607057103

Calbo J, van Montfort E, Proost N, van Drunen E, Beverloo HB, Meuwissen R, Berns A (2011) A functional role for tumor cell heterogeneity in a mouse model of small cell lung cancer. Cancer Cell 19 (2):244–256. doi:10.1016/j.ccr.2010.12.021

Cancer Genome Atlas N (2012) Comprehensive molecular portraits of human breast tumours. Nature 490 (7418):61–70. doi:10.1038/nature11412

Cescon DW, Haibe-Kains B, Mak TW (2015) APOBEC3B expression in breast cancer reflects cellular proliferation, while a deletion polymorphism is associated with immune activation. Proc Natl Acad Sci U S A 112(9):2841–2846. doi:10.1073/pnas.1424869112

Cleary AS, Leonard TL, Gestl SA, Gunther EJ (2014) Tumour cell heterogeneity maintained by cooperating subclones in Wnt-driven mammary cancers. Nature 508(7494):113–117. doi:10.1038/nature13187

Diaz LA Jr, Williams RT, Wu J, Kinde I, Hecht JR, Berlin J, Allen B, Bozic I, Reiter JG, Nowak MA, Kinzler KW, Oliner KS, Vogelstein B (2012) The molecular evolution of acquired resistance to targeted EGFR blockade in colorectal cancers. Nature 486 (7404):537–540. doi:10.1038/nature11219

Flaherty KT, Puzanov I, Kim KB, Ribas A, McArthur GA, Sosman JA, O'Dwyer PJ, Lee RJ, Grippo JF, Nolop K, Chapman PB (2010) Inhibition of mutated, activated BRAF in metastatic melanoma. N Engl J Med 363(9):809–819. doi:10.1056/NEJMoa1002011

Fong PC, Boss DS, Yap TA, Tutt A, Wu P, Mergui-Roelvink M, Mortimer P, Swaisland H, Lau A, O'Connor MJ, Ashworth A, Carmichael J, Kaye SB, Schellens JH, de Bono JS (2009) Inhibition of poly(ADP-ribose) polymerase in tumors from BRCA mutation carriers. N Engl J Med 361(2):123–134. doi:10.1056/NEJMoa0900212

Ginestier C, Hur MH, Charafe-Jauffret E, Monville F, Dutcher J, Brown M, Jacquemier J, Viens P, Kleer CG, Liu S, Schott A, Hayes D, Birnbaum D, Wicha MS, Dontu G (2007) ALDH1 is a marker of normal and malignant human mammary stem cells and a predictor of poor clinical outcome. Cell Stem Cell 1 (5):555–567. doi:10.1016/j.stem.2007.08.014

Gnant M, Filipits M, Greil R, Stoeger H, Rudas M, Bago-Horvath Z, Mlineritsch B, Kwasny W, Knauer M, Singer C, Jakesz R, Dubsky P, Fitzal F, Bartsch R, Steger G, Balic M, Ressler S, Cowens JW, Storhoff J, Ferree S, Schaper C, Liu S, Fesl C, Nielsen TO, Austrian B, Colorectal Cancer Study G (2014) Predicting distant recurrence in receptor-positive breast cancer patients with limited clinicopathological risk: using the PAM50 Risk of Recurrence score in 1478 postmenopausal patients of the ABCSG-8 trial treated with adjuvant endocrine therapy alone. Ann Oncol 25(2):339–345. doi:10.1093/annonc/mdt494

Gokmen-Polar Y, Badve SS (2013) Counterpoint: cancer stem cells: nonbelievers' viewpoint. Clin Chem 59 (1):208–210. doi:10.1373/clinchem.2012.185637

Gokmen-Polar Y, Nakshatri H, Badve S (2011) Biomarkers for breast cancer stem cells: the challenges ahead. Biomark Med 5(5):661–671. doi:10.2217/bmm.11.57

Hakem R, de la Pompa JL, Elia A, Potter J, Mak TW (1997) Partial rescue of Brca1 (5–6) early embryonic lethality by p53 or p21 null mutation. Nat Genet 16 (3):298–302. doi:10.1038/ng0797-298

Hou Y, Song L, Zhu P, Zhang B, Tao Y, Xu X, Li F, Wu K, Liang J, Shao D, Wu H, Ye X, Ye C, Wu R, Jian M, Chen Y, Xie W, Zhang R, Chen L, Liu X, Yao X, Zheng H, Yu C, Li Q, Gong Z, Mao M, Yang X, Yang L, Li J, Wang W, Lu Z, Gu N, Laurie G, Bolund L, Kristiansen K, Wang J, Yang H, Li Y, Zhang X, Wang J (2012) Single-cell exome sequencing and monoclonal evolution of a JAK2-negative myeloproliferative neoplasm. Cell 148(5):873–885. doi:10.1016/j.cell.2012.02.028

Issa-Nummer Y, Darb-Esfahani S, Loibl S, Kunz G, Nekljudova V, Schrader I, Sinn BV, Ulmer HU, Kronenwett R, Just M, Kuhn T, Diebold K, Untch M, Holms F, Blohmer JU, Habeck JO, Dietel M, Overkamp F, Krabisch P, von Minckwitz G, Denkert C (2013) Prospective validation of immunological infiltrate for prediction of response to neoadjuvant chemotherapy in HER2-negative breast cancer—a substudy of the neoadjuvant GeparQuinto trial. PLoS ONE 8(12):e79775. doi:10.1371/journal.pone.0079775

Jamal-Hanjani M, A'Hern R, Birkbak NJ, Gorman P, Gronroos E, Ngang S, Nicola P, Rahman L, Thanopoulou E, Kelly G, Ellis P, Barrett-Lee P, Johnston SR, Bliss J, Roylance R, Swanton C (2015) Extreme chromosomal instability forecasts improved outcome in ER-negative breast cancer: a prospective validation cohort study from the TACT trial. Ann Oncol 26(7):1340–1346. doi:10.1093/annonc/mdv178

Kopetz S, Desai J, Chan E, Hecht JR, O'Dwyer PJ, Maru D, Morris V, Janku F, Dasari A, Chung W, Issa JP, Gibbs P, James B, Powis G, Nolop KB, Bhattacharya S, Saltz L (2015) Phase II pilot study of vemurafenib in patients with metastatic BRAF-mutated colorectal cancer. J Clin Oncol 33 (34):4032–4038. doi:10.1200/JCO.2015.63.2497

Lee S, Kopp F, Chang TC, Sataluri A, Chen B, Sivakumar S, Yu H, Xie Y, Mendell JT (2016) Noncoding RNA NORAD regulates genomic stability by sequestering PUMILIO proteins. Cell 164(1–2):69–80. doi:10.1016/j.cell.2015.12.017

Li Y, Xu X, Song L, Hou Y, Li Z, Tsang S, Li F, Im KM, Wu K, Wu H, Ye X, Li G, Wang L, Zhang B, Liang J, Xie W, Wu R, Jiang H, Liu X, Yu C, Zheng H, Jian M, Nie L, Wan L, Shi M, Sun X, Tang A, Guo G, Gui Y, Cai Z, Li J, Wang W, Lu Z, Zhang X, Bolund L, Kristiansen K, Wang J, Yang H, Dean M, Wang J (2012) Single-cell sequencing analysis characterizes common and cell-lineage-specific mutations in a muscle-invasive bladder cancer. Gigascience 1(1):12. doi:10.1186/2047-217X-1-12

Liedtke C, Broglio K, Moulder S, Hsu L, Kau SW, Symmans WF, Albarracin C, Meric-Bernstam F, Woodward W, Theriault RL, Kiesel L, Hortobagyi GN, Pusztai L, Gonzalez-Angulo AM (2009) Prognostic impact of discordance between triple-receptor measurements in primary and recurrent breast cancer. Ann Oncol 20(12):1953–1958. doi:10.1093/annonc/mdp263

Liu S, Chapman JA, Burnell MJ, Levine MN, Pritchard KI, Whelan TJ, Rugo HS, Albain KS, Perez EA, Virk S, Barry G, Gao D, O'Brien P, Shepherd LE, Nielsen TO, Gelmon KA (2015) Prognostic and predictive investigation of PAM50 intrinsic subtypes in the NCIC CTG MA.21 phase III chemotherapy trial. Breast Cancer Res Treat 149 (2):439–448. doi:10.1007/s10549-014-3259-1

McGranahan N, Swanton C (2015) Biological and therapeutic impact of intratumor heterogeneity in cancer evolution. Cancer Cell 27(1):15–26. doi:10.1016/j.ccell.2014.12.001

Meier B, Cooke SL, Weiss J, Bailly AP, Alexandrov LB, Marshall J, Raine K, Maddison M, Anderson E, Stratton MR, Gartner A, Campbell PJ (2014) *C. elegans* whole-genome sequencing reveals mutational signatures related to carcinogens and DNA repair deficiency. Genome Res 24(10):1624–1636. doi:10.1101/gr.175547.114

Misale S, Yaeger R, Hobor S, Scala E, Janakiraman M, Liska D, Valtorta E, Schiavo R, Buscarino M, Siravegna G, Bencardino K, Cercek A, Chen CT, Veronese S, Zanon C, Sartore-Bianchi A, Gambacorta M, Gallicchio M, Vakiani E, Boscaro V, Medico E, Weiser M, Siena S, Di Nicolantonio F, Solit D, Bardelli A (2012) Emergence of KRAS mutations and acquired resistance to anti-EGFR therapy in colorectal cancer. Nature 486(7404):532–536. doi:10.1038/nature11156

Navin NE (2014) Cancer genomics: one cell at a time. Genome Biol 15(8):452. doi:10.1186/s13059-014-0452-9

Navin NE, Hicks J (2010) Tracing the tumor lineage. Mol Oncol 4(3):267–283. doi:10.1016/j.molonc.2010.04.010

Neumeister V, Rimm D (2010) Is ALDH1 a good method for definition of breast cancer stem cells? Breast Cancer Res Treat 123(1):109–111. doi:10.1007/s10549-009-0656-y

Niikura N, Liu J, Hayashi N, Mittendorf EA, Gong Y, Palla SL, Tokuda Y, Gonzalez-Angulo AM, Hortobagyi GN, Ueno NT (2012) Loss of human epidermal growth factor receptor 2 (HER2) expression in metastatic sites of HER2-overexpressing primary breast tumors. J Clin Oncol 30(6):593–599. doi:10.1200/JCO.2010.33.8889

Nik-Zainal S, Wedge DC, Alexandrov LB, Petljak M, Butler AP, Bolli N, Davies HR, Knappskog S, Martin S, Papaemmanuil E, Ramakrishna M,

Shlien A, Simonic I, Xue Y, Tyler-Smith C, Campbell PJ, Stratton MR (2014) Association of a germline copy number polymorphism of APOBEC3A and APOBEC3B with burden of putative APOBEC-dependent mutations in breast cancer. Nat Genet 46(5):487–491. doi:10.1038/ng.2955

Ortmann CA, Kent DG, Nangalia J, Silber Y, Wedge DC, Grinfeld J, Baxter EJ, Massie CE, Papaemmanuil E, Menon S, Godfrey AL, Dimitropoulou D, Guglielmelli P, Bellosillo B, Besses C, Dohner K, Harrison CN, Vassiliou GS, Vannucchi A, Campbell PJ, Green AR (2015) Effect of mutation order on myeloproliferative neoplasms. N Engl J Med 372 (7):601–612. doi:10.1056/NEJMoa1412098

Patel AP, Tirosh I, Trombetta JJ, Shalek AK, Gillespie SM, Wakimoto H, Cahill DP, Nahed BV, Curry WT, Martuza RL, Louis DN, Rozenblatt-Rosen O, Suva ML, Regev A, Bernstein BE (2014) Single-cell RNA-seq highlights intratumoral heterogeneity in primary glioblastoma. Science 344(6190):1396–1401. doi:10.1126/science.1254257

Perou CM, Sorlie T, Eisen MB, van de Rijn M, Jeffrey SS, Rees CA, Pollack JR, Ross DT, Johnsen H, Akslen LA, Fluge O, Pergamenschikov A, Williams C, Zhu SX, Lonning PE, Borresen-Dale AL, Brown PO, Botstein D (2000) Molecular portraits of human breast tumours. Nature 406(6797):747–752. doi:10.1038/35021093

Resetkova E, Reis-Filho JS, Jain RK, Mehta R, Thorat MA, Nakshatri H, Badve S (2010) Prognostic impact of ALDH1 in breast cancer: a story of stem cells and tumor microenvironment. Breast Cancer Res Treat 123(1):97–108. doi:10.1007/s10549-009-0619-3

Roy S, Gascard P, Dumont N, Zhao J, Pan D, Petrie S, Margeta M, Tlsty TD (2013) Rare somatic cells from human breast tissue exhibit extensive lineage plasticity. Proc Natl Acad Sci U S A 110(12):4598–4603. doi:10.1073/pnas.1218682110

Sauder CA, Koziel JE, Choi M, Fox MJ, Grimes BR, Badve S, Blosser RJ, Radovich M, Lam CC, Vaughan MB, Herbert BS, Clare SE (2014) Phenotypic plasticity in normal breast derived epithelial cells. BMC Cell Biol 15:20. doi:10.1186/1471-2121-15-20

Sestak I, Cuzick J, Dowsett M, Lopez-Knowles E, Filipits M, Dubsky P, Cowens JW, Ferree S, Schaper C, Fesl C, Gnant M (2015) Prediction of late distant recurrence after 5 years of endocrine treatment: a combined analysis of patients from the Austrian Breast and Colorectal Cancer Study Group 8 and arimidex, tamoxifen alone or in combination randomized trials using the PAM50 Risk of recurrence score. J Clin Oncol 33(8):916–922. doi:10.1200/JCO.2014.55.6894

Shah SP, Morin RD, Khattra J, Prentice L, Pugh T, Burleigh A, Delaney A, Gelmon K, Guliany R, Senz J, Steidl C, Holt RA, Jones S, Sun M, Leung G, Moore R, Severson T, Taylor GA, Teschendorff AE, Tse K, Turashvili G, Varhol R, Warren RL, Watson P, Zhao Y, Caldas C, Huntsman D, Hirst M, Marra MA, Aparicio S (2009) Mutational evolution in a lobular breast tumour profiled at single nucleotide resolution. Nature 461(7265):809–813. doi:10.1038/nature08489

Sheridan C, Kishimoto H, Fuchs RK, Mehrotra S, Bhat-Nakshatri P, Turner CH, Goulet R Jr, Badve S, Nakshatri H (2006) CD44+/CD24− breast cancer cells exhibit enhanced invasive properties: an early step necessary for metastasis. Breast Cancer Res 8(5):R59. doi:10.1186/bcr1610

Sottoriva A, Kang H, Ma Z, Graham TA, Salomon MP, Zhao J, Marjoram P, Siegmund K, Press MF, Shibata D, Curtis C (2015) A Big Bang model of human colorectal tumor growth. Nat Genet 47(3):209–216. doi:10.1038/ng.3214

Stephens PJ, Tarpey PS, Davies H, Van Loo P, Greenman C, Wedge DC, Nik-Zainal S, Martin S, Varela I, Bignell GR, Yates LR, Papaemmanuil E, Beare D, Butler A, Cheverton A, Gamble J, Hinton J, Jia M, Jayakumar A, Jones D, Latimer C, Lau KW, McLaren S, McBride DJ, Menzies A, Mudie L, Raine K, Rad R, Chapman MS, Teague J, Easton D, Langerod A, Oslo Breast Cancer C, Lee MT, Shen CY, Tee BT, Huimin BW, Broeks A, Vargas AC, Turashvili G, Martens J, Fatima A, Miron P, Chin SF, Thomas G, Boyault S, Mariani O, Lakhani SR, van de Vijver M, van 't Veer L, Foekens J, Desmedt C, Sotiriou C, Tutt A, Caldas C, Reis-Filho JS, Aparicio SA, Salomon AV, Borresen-Dale AL, Richardson AL, Campbell PJ, Futreal PA, Stratton MR (2012) The landscape of cancer genes and mutational processes in breast cancer. Nature 486(7403):400–404. doi:10.1038/nature11017

Swanton C (2015) Cancer evolution constrained by mutation order. N Engl J Med 372(7):661–663. doi:10.1056/NEJMe1414288

Swanton C, McGranahan N, Starrett GJ, Harris RS (2015) APOBEC enzymes: mutagenic fuel for cancer evolution and heterogeneity. Cancer Discov 5(7):704–712. doi:10.1158/2159-8290.CD-15-0344

Tabassum DP, Polyak K (2015) Tumorigenesis: it takes a village. Nat Rev Cancer 15(8):473–483. doi:10.1038/nrc3971

Takahashi K, Tanabe K, Ohnuki M, Narita M, Ichisaka T, Tomoda K, Yamanaka S (2007) Induction of pluripotent stem cells from adult human fibroblasts by defined factors. Cell 131(5):861–872. doi:10.1016/j.cell.2007.11.019

Tan EY, Thike AA, Breast Surgical Team at Outram, Tan PH (2013) ALDH1 expression is enriched in breast cancers arising in young women but does not predict outcome. Br J Cancer 109(1):109–113. doi:10.1038/bjc.2013.297

Thomas RK, Baker AC, Debiasi RM, Winckler W, Laframboise T, Lin WM, Wang M, Feng W, Zander T, MacConaill L, Lee JC, Nicoletti R, Hatton C, Goyette M, Girard L, Majmudar K, Ziaugra L, Wong KK, Gabriel S, Beroukhim R, Peyton M,

Barretina J, Dutt A, Emery C, Greulich H, Shah K, Sasaki H, Gazdar A, Minna J, Armstrong SA, Mellinghoff IK, Hodi FS, Dranoff G, Mischel PS, Cloughesy TF, Nelson SF, Liau LM, Mertz K, Rubin MA, Moch H, Loda M, Catalona W, Fletcher J, Signoretti S, Kaye F, Anderson KC, Demetri GD, Dummer R, Wagner S, Herlyn M, Sellers WR, Meyerson M, Garraway LA (2007) High-throughput oncogene mutation profiling in human cancer. Nat Genet 39(3):347–351. doi:10.1038/ng1975

Turner NC, Lord CJ, Iorns E, Brough R, Swift S, Elliott R, Rayter S, Tutt AN, Ashworth A (2008) A synthetic lethal siRNA screen identifying genes mediating sensitivity to a PARP inhibitor. EMBO J 27(9):1368–1377. doi:10.1038/emboj.2008.61

Verhaak RG, Hoadley KA, Purdom E, Wang V, Qi Y, Wilkerson MD, Miller CR, Ding L, Golub T, Mesirov JP, Alexe G, Lawrence M, O'Kelly M, Tamayo P, Weir BA, Gabriel S, Winckler W, Gupta S, Jakkula L, Feiler HS, Hodgson JG, James CD, Sarkaria JN, Brennan C, Kahn A, Spellman PT, Wilson RK, Speed TP, Gray JW, Meyerson M, Getz G, Perou CM, Hayes DN, Cancer Genome Atlas Research N (2010) Integrated genomic analysis identifies clinically relevant subtypes of glioblastoma characterized by abnormalities in PDGFRA, IDH1, EGFR, and NF1. Cancer Cell 17(1):98–110. doi:10.1016/j.ccr.2009.12.020

Voss MH, Hakimi AA, Pham CG, Brannon AR, Chen YB, Cunha LF, Akin O, Liu H, Takeda S, Scott SN, Socci ND, Viale A, Schultz N, Sander C, Reuter VE, Russo P, Cheng EH, Motzer RJ, Berger MF, Hsieh JJ (2014) Tumor genetic analyses of patients with metastatic renal cell carcinoma and extended benefit from mTOR inhibitor therapy. Clin Cancer Res 20(7):1955–1964. doi:10.1158/1078-0432.CCR-13-2345

Wang Y, Waters J, Leung ML, Unruh A, Roh W, Shi X, Chen K, Scheet P, Vattathil S, Liang H, Multani A, Zhang H, Zhao R, Michor F, Meric-Bernstam F, Navin NE (2014) Clonal evolution in breast cancer revealed by single nucleus genome sequencing. Nature 512(7513):155–160. doi:10.1038/nature13600

Xu X, Hou Y, Yin X, Bao L, Tang A, Song L, Li F, Tsang S, Wu K, Wu H, He W, Zeng L, Xing M, Wu R, Jiang H, Liu X, Cao D, Guo G, Hu X, Gui Y, Li Z, Xie W, Sun X, Shi M, Cai Z, Wang B, Zhong M, Li J, Lu Z, Gu N, Zhang X, Goodman L, Bolund L, Wang J, Yang H, Kristiansen K, Dean M, Li Y, Wang J (2012) Single-cell exome sequencing reveals single-nucleotide mutation characteristics of a kidney tumor. Cell 148(5):886–895. doi:10.1016/j.cell.2012.02.025

Yu C, Yu J, Yao X, Wu WK, Lu Y, Tang S, Li X, Bao L, Li X, Hou Y, Wu R, Jian M, Chen R, Zhang F, Xu L, Fan F, He J, Liang Q, Wang H, Hu X, He M, Zhang X, Zheng H, Li Q, Wu H, Chen Y, Yang X, Zhu S, Xu X, Yang H, Wang J, Zhang X, Sung JJ, Li Y, Wang J (2014) Discovery of biclonal origin and a novel oncogene SLC12A5 in colon cancer by single-cell sequencing. Cell Res 24(6):701–712. doi:10.1038/cr.2014.43

Zardavas D, Maetens M, Irrthum A, Goulioti T, Engelen K, Fumagalli D, Salgado R, Aftimos P, Saini KS, Sotiriou C, Campbell P, Dinh P, von Minckwitz G, Gelber RD, Dowsett M, Di Leo A, Cameron D, Baselga J, Gnant M, Goldhirsch A, Norton L, Piccart M (2014) The AURORA initiative for metastatic breast cancer. Br J Cancer 111(10):1881–1887. doi:10.1038/bjc.2014.341

Zardavas D, Irrthum A, Swanton C, Piccart M (2015) Clinical management of breast cancer heterogeneity. Nat Rev Clin Oncol 12(7):381–394. doi:10.1038/nrclinonc.2015.73

Zhang M, Tsimelzon A, Chang CH, Fan C, Wolff A, Perou CM, Hilsenbeck SG, Rosen JM (2015) Intratumoral heterogeneity in a Trp53-null mouse model of human breast cancer. Cancer Discov 5(5):520–533. doi:10.1158/2159-8290.CD-14-1101

Zhong Y, Lin Y, Shen S, Zhou Y, Mao F, Guan J, Sun Q (2013) Expression of ALDH1 in breast invasive ductal carcinoma: an independent predictor of early tumor relapse. Cancer Cell Int 13(1):60. doi:10.1186/1475-2867-13-60

Zhong Y, Shen S, Zhou Y, Mao F, Guan J, Lin Y, Xu Y, Sun Q (2014) ALDH1 is a better clinical indicator for relapse of invasive ductal breast cancer than the CD44+/CD24− phenotype. Med Oncol 31(3):864. doi:10.1007/s12032-014-0864-0

Breast Cancer Stem Cells

10

Dong Soon Choi, Roberto R. Rosato and Jenny C. Chang

Abstract

Cancer stem cells (CSCs) represent a heterogeneous subpopulation of cancer cells within tumors. CSCs divide asymmetrically to generate daughter cells that either have CSC characteristics including self-renewal, or differentiation potential to form neoplastic cells which constitute most of the tumor. These characteristics suggest that the cells may play an important role in tumor initiation, and development of chemo-resistance. These characteristics are evident in the ability of CSCs to seed new tumors upon transplantation in experimental animal models. In this chapter, we describe the evidence around the role of CSCs in breast cancer. A brief overview of the methods and markers used to identify these cells is also provided. More importantly, we present the data regarding the signaling pathways that are implicated in the aggressiveness associated with CSCs. Lastly, we discuss the strategies that can be used for targeting these pathways for therapeutic purposes.

Keywords

Cscs · CD24 · CD44 · ALDH1 · Chemo-resistance

10.1 Cancer Stem Cells

Cancer stem cells (CSCs) represent a special, heterogeneous subpopulation of cancer cells within tumors that display a marked capacity of self-renewal, multi-lineage differentiation, tumor initiation, and chemoresistance. These characteristics are evident in the ability of CSCs to seed new tumors upon transplantation in experimental animal models. When transplanted into an orthotopic site (xenograft), CSCs can initiate tumor formation because of their self-renewal

D.S. Choi
Houston Methodist Hospital, Houston Methodist Cancer Center, Houston, TX 77030, USA

R.R. Rosato
Weill Cornell Medical College, New York, NY 10065, USA

J.C. Chang (✉)
Department of Oncology, Houston Methodist Hospital, Houston Methodist Cancer Center, Houston, TX 77030, USA
e-mail: jcchang@houstonmethodist.org

S. Badve and Y. Gökmen-Polar (eds.), *Molecular Pathology of Breast Cancer*, DOI 10.1007/978-3-319-41761-5_10

and differentiation capacities which are similar to those of normal stem cells. The bulk of the remaining tumor-forming cells undergo a more differentiated process since they lack CSC characteristics (Pattabiraman and Weinberg 2014; Rosen and Jordan 2009; Vlashi and Pajonk 2015). In other words, CSCs divide asymmetrically to generate daughter cells that either have CSC characteristics including self-renewal, or differentiation potential to form neoplastic cells which constitute most of the tumor. In fact, it is interesting to note that while normal stem cells have the ability to differentiate into multiple distinct cell types, most of the currently known CSCs differentiate into a single cell type which compose the majority of the tumor.

Suggestions of the existence of a small set of cells having stem cell-like characteristics in tumors can be found from studies dating from the end of the 1800s (Vlashi and Pajonk 2015), but it was the seminal work of Dick et al. that became the paradigm of later studies (Lapidot et al. 1994). The observation that most human acute myeloid leukemia (AML) cells have limited proliferative capacity suggested that the leukemia clone was maintained by a rare population of stem cells. Based on this premise, and also overcoming some of the technical limitations in the identification of these cells in, the authors were able to characterize the leukemia progenitor cells by transplanting AML-initiating cells in immunocompromised mice. Further studies showed that the frequency of these leukemia-initiating cells in the peripheral blood of AML patients was one engraftment unit in 250,000 cells. The authors identified these cells as $CD34^+/CD38^-$ by using fluorescence-activated cell sorting (FACS) analysis (Lapidot et al. 1994).

10.2 Discovery of Breast Cancer Stem Cells

Similar approaches led to the identification of CSCs in breast (Al-Hajj et al. 2003). Based on the observation that breast tumors are a phenotypically diverse population of cells, Al-Hajj et al. isolated a minority of cells harboring the ability to form new tumors (Al-Hajj et al. 2003). They were able to distinguish these tumor-initiating cells by the cell surface markers $CD44^+/CD24^{-/low}$ in eight of the nine patients investigated (Al-Hajj et al. 2003). Concordant with earlier studies by Dick et al. (Lapidot et al. 1994), $CD44^+/CD24^{-/low}$ cells formed tumors in mice, whereas tens of thousands of cells not having the $CD44^+/CD24^{-/low}$ phenotype failed to do so (Al-Hajj et al. 2003).

Other proteins, such as the intracellular detoxifying enzyme aldehyde dehydrogenase 1 (ALDH1), have been used in addition to the cell-surface markers for studying both normal and cancer stem cells. ALDH1 is a protein that may identify CSCs in several types of cancers including leukemia (Cheung et al. 2007), breast (Ginestier et al. 2007), lung (Jiang et al. 2009), colon (Carpentino et al. 2009), liver (Ma et al. 2008), pancreas (Rasheed et al. 2010). ALDH1 activity can be evaluated by using the ALDEFLUOR assay, a method based on its ability to oxidize intracellular aldehydes. In primary breast xenografts, $CD44^+CD24^-$ and ALDH1 identified overlapping but nonidentical cell populations, each capable of initiating tumors in NOD/SCID mice (Ginestier et al. 2007). Moreover, cells coexpressing $CD44^+CD24^-$ and ALDH1 displayed the greatest tumorigenic activity, generating tumors from as few as 20 cells in xenograft experiments (Ginestier et al. 2007). Interestingly, $CD44^+CD24^-$ expression is highest in cells located at the tumor edge near the stroma, whereas ALDH1 expression is most prominent in more centrally-localized tumor cells (Angeloni et al. 2015). These data are consistent with other observations showing increased ALDH1 activity under hypoxic conditions, a state known to occur near the tumor center (Conley et al. 2012).

As described for hematopoietic, breast and other cancer models, the presence of CSCs is reflected by an increased tumorigenicity and pluripotency of a subset of cancer cells which can be isolated from the bulk of the tumor; in fact, the in vivo limiting dilution assay of generating xenografts in immune-compromised mice represents the reference standard method to demonstrate a CSC phenotype (see Section Methods for details). It is important to note that, while the examples described above revealed low frequencies of CSC populations within tumors, additional studies in several other cancers have shown that CSCs need not to be rare and can constitute as much as 25 % of the tumor cellular composition, depending on the tumor type (Krivtsov et al. 2006; Quintana et al. 2008). Genetically engineered mouse models (GEMMs) have also helped to demonstrate the presence of CSCs in certain leukemia and breast cancers, providing additional and direct support for the CSC model in syngeneic mice (Cho et al. 2008; Deshpande et al. 2006). These studies have been important in addressing the potential concerns that have arisen due to the use of immune-compromised mice as the standard model to demonstrate and support the CSC theory.

10.3 The Epithelial-to-Mesenchymal Transition (EMT) and Breast Cancer Stemness

The EMT biological program was initially observed to occur during the interconversions underlying normal organogenesis throughout development. During EMT, epithelial cells lose their differentiated characteristics including cell-cell adhesion and lack of motility, and acquire mesenchymal cell migratory and invasive features as well as stem cell properties (Mani et al. 2008; Oft et al. 1996). EMT is characterized by the disappearance of epithelial marker genes including CD24 and E-cadherin, and upregulation of the mesenchymal markers CD44, vimentin, and N-cadherin, providing the characteristic $CD44^{+}CD24^{-}$ markers that are used to identify CSCs (Pattabiraman and Weinberg 2014; Polyak and Weinberg 2009). During EMT, the expression of a vast number of additional genes help tumor cells circumvent apoptosis, anoikis, oncogene addiction and cellular senescence, providing a way for tumor cells to escape immune surveillance and generate chemotherapy resistance (Thiery 2002; Tiwari et al. 2012). In terms of cancer pathogenesis, EMT confers cancer cells the ability to invade locally and disseminate to distant sites, initiating the process of metastasis (Nieto 2011).

Recent studies have shown the plasticity of BCSCs, which may exist in distinct mesenchymal-like (epithelial-to-mesenchymal transition, EMT) and epithelial-like (mesenchymal-to-epithelial transition, MET) states characterized by the expression of distinct CSC markers (Liu et al. 2014b). Furthermore, gene expression profiles have shown that EMT BCSCs resemble those of basal stem cells, whereas the MET profiles were closer to those of luminal stem cells in normal breast tissue. Based on these studies, a theory was proposed in which reversible transitions between mesenchymal-like and epithelial-like stem cell states are necessary for tumor invasion and metastasis at distant sites, a process that appeared to be regulated by the tumor microenvironment (Liu et al. 2014b). Furthermore, these observations have helped to address controversies claiming that CSCs and EMT states are mutually exclusive (Tsuji et al. 2008). In fact, Liu et al. proposed the mesenchymal-like state as being associated with the expression of mesenchymal markers, relative quiescence and high invasive capacity while the epithelial-like state is characterized by the expression of epithelial markers, establishment of cell polarity, and extensive proliferation (Liu et al. 2014b). They concluded that the plasticity of BCSCs allows them to undergo microenvironment-regulated reversible EMT/MET transitions, which are needed for successful metastatic colonization. Importantly, these observations represent critical factors to be considered at the moment of designing new drugs or therapeutic interventions.

10.4 CSCs and the Development of Resistance to Conventional Therapies

One of the most relevant features of CSCs is the challenge they pose from a therapeutic point of view. Induction of an EMT phenotype gives CSCs the ability to acquire chemotherapy and radiotherapy resistance, a phenomenon that is well documented in breast and ovarian cancer

(Farmer et al. 2009; Kurrey et al. 2009). Resistance to cytotoxic treatments may be attributable in part to the lower proliferative rate resulting from the mesenchymal properties (Anjomshoaa et al. 2009; Moore and Lyle 2011). In addition, there is evidence supporting other factors associated with CSC chemoresistance including high expression of the anti-apoptotic (pro-survival) Bcl-2 protein family, proteins involved in efflux pumping, ALDH1 (see below) and enhanced DNA damage response pathways (Abdullah and Chow 2013; Angeloni et al. 2015; Cojoc et al. 2015). Other mechanisms contributing to chemoresistance involve the activation of autophagy, developmental pathways and stimuli from the CSC microenvironment (Cojoc et al. 2015; Mitra et al. 2015).

The EMT phenotype, as mentioned, helps to spare slow growing cells, most notably $CD44^+/CD24^{-/low}$ cells, by inducing them into quiescence and delayed metastasis (Brabletz 2012). In fact, a link between cancer treatment resistance and CSCs has been shown due to the presence of increased numbers of $CD44^+/CD24^{-/low}$ cells both before and after chemotherapy (Lee et al. 2011; Li et al. 2008). Patients showing increased levels of $CD44^+/CD24^{-/low}$ and $ALDH1^+$ cells after primary systemic therapy displayed significantly shorter disease-free survival time than those with no change or reduced CSC number (Lee et al. 2011). Importantly, $CD44^+/CD24^{-/low}$ cells have been shown to express higher levels of anti-apoptotic proteins of the Bcl-2 family, notably Bcl-xL (Keitel et al. 2014; Madjd et al. 2009). Recently, Keitel et al. showed that key players of the intrinsic apoptotic pathway are downregulated in these cells (Keitel et al. 2014). Thus, while expression of anti-apoptotic Bcl-xL is increased in $CD44^+/CD24^{-/low}$ cells, pro-apoptotic genes coding for Puma and Bim are downregulated, further enhancing their drug resistant phenotype and cell survival. On the other hand, high levels of ALDH1 activity, a biomarker used to identify CSCs by the Aldefluor assay, in breast carcinomas correlate with tumorigenic cell fractions having increased self-renewal capacity; ALDH1 also serves as a marker of poor prognosis (Ginestier et al. 2007). ALDH1 enzymatic activity plays a critical role in chemoresistance, since it acts as an oxidative stress scavenger of radiation-induced free radicals and produces the antioxidant NAD(P)H (Singh et al. 2013). Furthermore, increased activity of ALDH1 may also help cancer cells in metabolizing chemotherapeutic agents and their intermediate products (Cojoc et al. 2015; Magni et al. 1996; Parajuli et al. 2014). In fact, some very well established anti-cancer therapies rely on ALDH1 inhibition to increase the efficacy of the treatments, as is the case in regimes against acute promyelocytic leukemia (APL) (Fenaux et al. 1993, 1999; Tallman et al. 1997), ovarian (Formelli and Cleris 1993), breast, pancreatic and lung cancers (Bertrand et al. 2014; Croker and Allan 2012; Grunt et al. 1998; Kalemkerian and Ou 1999; Pettersson et al. 2001).

10.5 Signaling Pathways Involved in Breast Cancer Stem Cells

Cancer stem cells rely on critical signaling pathways for self-renewal and differentiation to progenitor populations similar to normal stem cells. Although there are substantial physiological differences between CSCs and normal stem cells, CSCs use the same pathways that regulate normal stem cells including STAT3, Notch, Wnt, Hhh, and transcriptional regulatory machinery used for embryonic stem cells.

10.5.1 JAK2-STAT3 Signaling Pathway

The Janus kinase (JAK)–signal transducer and acti-vator of transcription (STAT) pathway was first discovered as a mediator of cytokines such as interferon alpha, interferon gamma and interleukin 6, but was later found to be involved in a plethora of cascades governing a wide range of physiological processes in animals, humans, and flies (Rawlings et al. 2004; Wagner and Schmidt 2011; Chen et al. 2014). The JAK/STAT pathway regulates cell proliferation, apoptosis, cell differentiation, and cell migration, all of which are critical for homeostasis, immune development, mammary gland development and lactation, adipogenesis, and fate determination (Kamakura et al. 2004; Rawlings et al. 2004; Ivashkiv 2000; Ivashkiv and Hu 2004; Li et al. 2004). There are four Jak family members, and 7 members of STATs (Rawlings et al. 2004). Upon activation of Jak families, STATs are recruited to Jak for activation by phosphorylation and dimerization. The STAT dimer complex enters the nucleus to initiate transcription of multiple genes. STAT3 and STAT5 are frequently implicated in cancer progression, and mutations and amplifications in Jak1, Jak2, and Jak3 are commonly found in various cancer types (Kolosenko et al. 2014; Kim et al. 2015; Tefferi and Gilliland 2005; Harrison 2012; Amoyel et al. 2014; Vainchenker and Constantinescu 2013; Rawlings et al. 2004). Among the JAK/STAT interactions, the JAK2/STAT3 pathway is critical for stem cell maintenance in embryos and breast mammary glands (Hughes and Watson 2012; Constantinescu 2003; Cavaleri and Scholer 2003; Niwa et al. 1998). Zhou et al. reported that STAT3 activation was required for the viability and maintenance of breast cancer stem-like cells in the breast cancer cell line MCF7 (Zhou et al. 2007). Later, Marotta et al. found that the IL-6/JAK2/STAT3 pathway was preferentially active in $CD44^{+}/CD24^{-}$ breast cancer cells compared with other tumor cell types by studying clinical patient samples (Marotta et al. 2011). Similarly, the JAK2/STAT3 pathway seems to be important for cancer stem cell function in colon, ovary, or lung cancers (Zhu et al. 2014; Stechishin et al. 2013; Hsu et al. 2012; Abubaker et al. 2014). These findings have clinically relevant implications in targeting minimal residual disease, since chronic inflammation within the tumor microenvironment provides nourishing conditions to keep the JAK2/STAT3 pathway constitutively active in BCSCs. Recently, new biological roles of JAK2/STAT3 have been identified in tumorigenesis and formation of pre-metastatic niches, and also in cancer cell metabolism, drug resistance, and epigenetics (Alderton 2012; O'Brien et al. 2010; Choi et al. 2014; Martinez-Revollar et al. 2015). Additionally, STAT3 has been shown to cross-talk with various signaling molecules other than JAK2, including G-protein coupled receptors, Src, EGFR, mTOR, or MAPK family members (Rawlings et al. 2004; Harrison 2012; Li et al. 2004; Ivashkiv and Hu 2004; Kamakura et al. 2004; Ivashkiv 2000). Consistently, we identified a small molecule STAT3 inhibitor which reduced BCSCs in triple negative breast cancer (Dave et al. 2012). Similarly, others have confirmed our finding that selective targeting of STAT3 reduces BCSC populations and sensitizes drug-resistant BCSCs to chemotherapies, inhibiting cancer recurrence and metastasis (Chung and Vadgama 2015; Thakur et al. 2015).

10.5.2 Wnt/Beta-Catenin Pathway

Wnt-1 (*Wingless-related integration site 1*) was first identified as *Int-1* in 1982 by Roel Nusse and Harold Varmus as a proto-oncogene through gene mutagenesis to induce tumors in breast tissue using mouse mammary tumor viruses (Nusse and Varmus 1982). Later, *Int-1* was found to be a homolog of the Drosophila *Wingless* (*wg*) gene known to regulate segment polarity during larval development (Nusslein-Volhard and Wieschaus 1980; Rijsewijk et al. 1987). Currently, nineteen different Wnt genes have been identified both for humans and mouse, which regulate embryonic development, tissue regeneration, cell fate determination, cell proliferation, cell movement, and insulin sensitivity (Clevers 2006; Clevers and Nusse 2012; van Amerongen and Nusse 2009; Clevers et al. 2014; Nusse 2008; Abiola et al. 2009; Bilir et al. 2013; Mentink et al. 2014; Kimura-Yoshida et al. 2005). In order to initiate signaling cascades, Wnt family ligands bind to a Frizzled (Fz) family receptor, a GPCR, and often require co-receptors such as lipoprotein receptor-related protein (LRP)-5/6, receptor tyrosine kinases (RTKs), and receptor tyrosine kinase-like orphan receptor 2 (Komiya and Habas 2008; Clevers et al. 2014; Nusse 2008; Van Camp et al. 2014; van Amerongen and Nusse 2009; Clevers and Nusse 2012). The canonical Wnt signaling pathway involves β-catenin, a protein involved in cell-cell adhesion and other processes. In the absence of the Wnt-Fz interaction, β-catenin is destined for proteasomal degradation through interaction with a destruction complex that contains Axin, adenomatosis polyposis coli (APC), protein phosphatase 2A (PP2A), glycogen synthase kinase 3 (GSK3) and casein kinase 1α (CK1α) (Nusse and Varmus 1982; Clevers and Nusse 2012; Nusse 2008). The binding of Wnt to its receptor Fz phosphorylates and activates Disheveled (DVL), which subsequently phosphorylates LRP-5/6 (Clevers and Nusse 2012). Phosphorylated LRP-5/6 recruits and inhibits the destruction complex, allowing β-catenin to accumulate and translocate into the nucleus (Clevers and Nusse 2012). β-catenin then interacts with TCF/LEF to regulate gene expression for a variety of physiological processes (Behrens et al. 1996; Molenaar et al. 1996). Wnt pathways not involving β-catenin are classified as non-canonical pathways which activate various downstream signaling kinases and regulate planar cell polarity, calcium signaling, cell fate determination, and cell migration (Clevers and Nusse 2012; Behari 2010; Van Camp et al. 2014). Oncogenic roles of Wnt in human breast cancer have been extensively studied and were first discussed in 1995 (Bergstein et al. 1995; Wang et al. 2015). Previously, we analyzed gene expression array data and discovered that EMT in tumor-initiating cells takes advantage of the Wnt signaling pathway for proliferation and drug resistance. Supporting our data, others have found similar regulatory roles of Wnt in BCSC maintenance and disease progression by promoting EMT and tumor heterogeneity (Li et al. 2003; Williams et al. 2015; Creighton et al. 2010; Wang et al. 2015; Cleary et al. 2014; Martinez-Revollar et al. 2015). The Wnt pathway has been of particular interest for triple negative breast cancer, which is known to contain a large population of cancer stem cells (Martinez-Revollar et al. 2015; Yin et al. 2013; Akalay et al. 2015; Xu et al. 2015).

Furthermore, Vadakkhan et al. suggested biological differences between Wnt-responsive and non-responsive BCSCs, as the Wnt-responsive BCSCs localized near tumor blood vessels (Vadakkan et al. 2014) while a large population of BCSCs are found in hypoxic tumor areas (Kazi et al. 2014; Schwab et al. 2012; Xing et al. 2011). Despite good preclinical results on Wnt-targeting therapies against breast cancer and substantial knowledge about Wnt signaling, therapeutic inhibitors against the Wnt pathway have not been available and a few inhibitors have only recently entered clinical trials (Kahn 2014). Nevertheless, we found preliminary preventive effects of extracted olive oil on women with a high risk of breast cancer by targeting the Wnt pathway, especially in basal cell populations (unpublished data). Although this study is not yet completed not conclusive, our data suggest that targeting the Wnt pathway may be an effective therapy and may also help to prevent cancer.

10.5.3 Autophagy

Autophagy, meaning "self-eating", is a physiological salvage mechanism for damaged, redundant or dysfunctional proteins or cellular components (Mizushima and Komatsu 2011; Glick et al. 2010; Wang et al. 2011; Mizushima 2007). During this process, an array of protein complexes sequesters cellular components into double-membrane vesicles known as autophagosomes (Glick et al. 2010; Mizushima 2007; Mizushima and Komatsu 2011). The autophagosomes then form autolysosomes by fusing with lysosomes, where the engulfed organelles and proteins are degraded and recycled (Mentink et al. 2014; Kimura-Yoshida et al. 2005; Komiya and Habas 2008). Hence, autophagy is considered to be a normal housekeeping activity or an adaptive survival mechanism under stress conditions such as starvation, injuries, or inflammation (Mentink et al. 2014; Kimura-Yoshida et al. 2005; Komiya and Habas 2008). Autophagy can also be associated with diseases, cell death, or morbidity (Bilir et al. 2013; Mentink et al. 2014; Kimura-Yoshida et al. 2005; Komiya and Habas 2008). Indeed, although autophagy is considered as a tumor-suppressing process by eliminating harmful components and inducing cell death in defective cells (Wang et al. 2011), autophagy can also be considered carcinogenic as it protects cancer cells from cytotoxic stress (Bilir et al. 2013; Kimura-Yoshida et al. 2005). Autophagy can be subdivided into three different processes: macroautophagy, microautophagy, and chaperone-mediated autophagy (CMA) (Glick et al. 2010; Mizushima 2007; Mizushima and Komatsu 2011; Cuervo and Wong 2014). Autophagy is generally thought to be a bulky and non-selective process unlike ubiquitin-mediated protein degradation, but it can also be very selective for degradation of cytoplasmic organelles including peroxisomes, mitochondria, endoplasmic reticulum, lysosomes, and micronuclei (Glick et al. 2010; Mizushima 2007). Autophagy has been implicated in various aspects of cancer including survival, drug resistance, tumor dormancy, and metastasis (Janku et al. 2011; Kenific et al. 2010). Moreover, autophagy-mediated metabolic coupling between cancer cells and neighboring stromal cells has been shown to support cancer survival, growth, and resistance to cancer therapies (Martinez-Outschoorn et al. 2011; Sanchez et al. 2011). In 2006, Sotelo et al. demonstrated that inhibition of autophagy improved the survival of patients with an aggressive brain tumor, glioblastoma multiforme (Sotelo et al. 2006). Similarly, inhibition of autophagy sensitized cancer cells to conventional therapies and improved patient survival in various types of cancers (Firat et al. 2012; Livesey et al. 2009; Amaravadi et al. 2007; Janku et al. 2011; Rangwala et al. 2014; Liu et al. 2014a). Recently, we repurposed chloroquine (CQ), an anti-malarial drug, to target breast cancer stem cells through in silico analysis of our previously published cancer stem cell gene signatures identified from patients with recurrent breast cancer (Choi et al. 2014). We found that combination therapy of CQ and paclitaxel efficiently sensitized drug resistant TNBC cells to chemotherapy and inhibited recurrence and pleural metastasis by decreasing $CD44^+/CD24^-$ or $ALDH^+$ BCSC populations in TNBC in both preclinical and clinical settings (Choi et al. 2014). Similar to our findings, independent studies have confirmed the autophagy-dependency of BCSCs (Cufi et al. 2011; Gong et al. 2013). More importantly, we reported autophagy-independent drug mechanisms of CQ in regulating the JAK2/STAT3 pathway, DNA methylation, and mitochondrial function (data not shown) (Choi et al. 2014). Maes et al. (2014) reported another autophagy-independent activity of CQ which sensitizes tumors to chemotherapy by normalizing tumor vessel. Despite fifty years of CQ use and good patient responses from many clinical trials on various cancer types, retina and heart toxicity are major side effects of CQ and its derivatives (Finbloom et al. 1985; Taylor and White 2004). Hence, development of more potent and safer autophagy inhibitors and tumor-specific delivery systems for the inhibitors will potentiate the clinical application of anti-autophagy agents.

10.5.4 Induced Nitric Oxide Synthase (INOS) Pathway

Nitric Oxide (NO) is produced from L-arginine by the activity of Nitric Oxide Synthase (NOS), which has three isoforms: neuronal NOS (nNOS or NOS1), endothelial NOS (eNOS or NOS3), and an inducible calcium-independent form (iNOS or NOS2) (Ignarro 1990; Rosselli et al. 1998). As a cellular signaling molecule, NO is involved in numerous physiological processes including reproductive processes, vasodilation, immune system function, and neurotransmission (Rosselli et al. 1998; Hopper and Garthwaite 2006; Ignarro 1990). iNOS is a cytokine-inducible enzyme that is upregulated in settings of acute and chronic inflammation where it plays a fundamental role in innate host-defense and wound-healing processes (Nathan and Xie 1994; Yamasaki et al. 1998). Upregulation of iNOS results in increased NO production and affects the redox state of cells (Wink et al. 1998). Increased iNOS expression has been found in breast cancer (Bulut et al. 2005; Glynn et al. 2010; Loibl et al. 2005; Thomsen et al. 1995) and other cancers such as lung (Okayama et al. 2013), colon (Ambs et al. 1998), melanoma (Massi et al. 2001), and glioblastoma (Eyler et al.

2011). In breast cancer patients, we and others have demonstrated a correlation between high iNOS levels and aggressiveness and poor prognosis (Bulut et al. 2005; Glynn et al. 2010; Granados-Principal et al. 2015; Thomsen et al. 1995). More recently, increased iNOS expression has also been postulated as a prognostic factor for reduced survival in patients with basal-like ERα-negative breast cancer through the induction of interleukin-8 (*IL-8*), *CD44* and *c-Myc* (Glynn et al. 2010). These effects that may be partially due to the activation of the transcription factor Ets-1 (Switzer et al. 2012). Together, these observations strongly suggest that strategies targeting the NOS pathway may offer potential therapeutic advantages in cancer treatment. This possibility, with additional supporting evidence, is further addressed below.

10.6 CSCs and the Development of Mechanistically-Based Therapies

In earlier studies, we provided strong clinical evidence showing that chemotherapy treatment increased the percentage of $CD44^+/CD24^{-/low}$ cells and mammosphere formation efficiency (MSFE; see Section Methods), an in vitro surrogate assay of self-renewal capacity, from primary breast cancer biopsies obtained before and after treatment (Li et al. 2008). We derived a gene signature from both the $CD44^+/CD24^{-/low}$ lineage and cancer mammosphere (MS) cells by performing global gene expression analysis on human breast cancers. This signature was used to characterize the subpopulation of residual, chemoresistant tumor cells and to define the regulatory pathways involved in the survival of these cells (Creighton et al. 2009). The gene signature was compared to previously defined intrinsic subtypes of breast cancer to determine whether the expression pattern was similar to a specific cancer subtype. Furthermore, to determine the signature's clinical and therapeutic significance, we evaluated it in breast tumors before and after therapy (letrozole or docetaxel) to test the hypothesis that the tumor cells surviving after treatment have an increased expression of the $CD44^+/CD24^{-/low}$ MS signature. We found that the $CD44^+/CD24^{-/low}$ MS signature was detectable mainly in human breast tumors corresponding to the "claudin-low" molecular subtype, which is characterized by the expression of many EMT-associated genes (Herschkowitz et al. 2007). $CD44^+/CD24^{-/low}$ MS and claudin-low signatures were more pronounced in tumor tissue remaining after either endocrine therapy (letrozole) or chemotherapy (docetaxel), consistent with the selective survival of tumor-initiating cells post-treatment. In fact, an increased expression of mesenchymal markers, including vimentin (*VIM*) in cytokeratin-positive epithelial cells and metalloproteinase 2 (*MMP2*) was confirmed in two separate sets of post-letrozole versus pretreatment specimens (Herschkowitz et al. 2007).

Once the genes that were differentially expressed in BCSCs were identified (Creighton et al. 2009; Li et al. 2008), shRNA knockdown-based studies identified the candidates that affected BCSC self-renewal. Two of the top candidates were genes encoding ribosomal protein L39 (RPL39) and myeloid leukemia factor 2 (MLF2) (Dave et al. 2014). Furthermore, siRNA nanoparticles specifically targeting either RPL39 or MLF2 reduced both tumor volume and lung metastases in breast cancer patient-derived (PDX) and established cell line xenografts, concomitantly decreasing the BCSC population. These data supported the critical role of both proteins in the survival and expansion of this cell population (Dave et al. 2014). Furthermore, RNA deep sequencing identified damaging gain-of-function mutations in both genes from patient lung metastases, which were statistically associated with shorter median time to pulmonary metastasis. Also, both genes were mechanistically linked to the NOS pathway (see the iNOS section above), and appeared modified in their expression levels by hypoxia. The discovery of a BCSC gene signature and its association with NO signaling has led to important clinical investigations. Firstly, mutations of these genes are being investigated as they may serve as important biomarkers for diagnosis or treatment evaluation of breast cancer, especially for treatment-resistant TNBC. Secondly, the preclinical discovery of NO signaling as a key element in BCSC function, tumor growth and metastasis has fueled new therapeutic options. For example, we tested whether iNOS inhibition could decrease TNBC aggressiveness by reducing tumor initiation and metastasis through modulation of epithelial-mesenchymal transition (EMT)-inducing factors. Indeed, as we recently showed (Granados-Principal et al. 2015), either selective iNOS inhibitors or pan-NOS inhibitors perturbed cell proliferation, CSC self-renewal, and cell migration in vitro and also decreased the expression of EMT transcription factors (Snail, Slug, Twist1, and Zeb1). Moreover, iNOS inhibition significantly reduced tumor growth, the number of lung metastases, tumor initiation, and self-renewal in vivo xenografts models. New studies are currently being conducted to determine whether iNOS inhibitors, notably the pan-NOS inhibitor N^G-Monomethyl-L-arginine (L-NMMA), in combination with standard chemotherapies, improves therapeutic response by simultaneously targeting the bulk of the tumor (i.e. chemosensitive cells) and the chemoresistant CSCs.

10.7 Heterogeneity of Cancer or CSCs and Clinical Significance

Tumor heterogeneity describes differences in the same types of tumors among different patients and cellular diversity within a tumor of a cancer patient (Heppner and Miller 1989; Heppner 1984; Jamal-Hanjani et al. 2015; Skibinski and Kuperwasser 2015). Tumor heterogeneity not only causes drug response variation but also makes patient prognosis unpredictable. Importantly, intra-tumor heterogeneity poses additional problems for targeted-therapy since only a subset of the tumor cell population expressing the target would be affected, leaving other populations untouched (Chen et al. 2013; Natarajan et al. 2010) Conventional cancer therapy induces multiple drug resistant mechanisms within a tumor due to the intra-tumoral heterogeneity (Jamal-Hanjani et al. 2015; Skibinski and Kuperwasser 2015). Also, it is impossible to differentiate which set of gene mutations is present in a bulk population since the current gene-mutation data only represent the sum of detectable gene mutations in multiple different cell populations. Moreover, tumor-host mediated tumor heterogeneity is another major contributor to the complexity of tumors (Heppner et al. 1989). Similarly, BCSCs have not been well defined despite the diverse molecular or biochemical markers available to define them (Pinto et al. 2013; Giuliano et al. 2011). Additionally, BCSC plasticity places more emphasis on the need to find definitive characteristics of BCSC populations (Pinto et al. 2013; Giuliano et al. 2011). Given the importance of CSCs in cancer initiation and progression, a handful of therapeutic strategies targeting CSCs have been developed (Chen et al. 2013; Natarajan et al. 2010). Several clinical trials have recently started to evaluate the effectiveness of targeting CSCs using a variety of approaches. These include cancer vaccines or inhibitors against FAK, PI3K/mTOR, CXCR1, and autophagy for patients with cancers of the pancreas (NCT02074046), lung (NCT02115958, NCT01951690), breast (NCT01440127, NCT02001974, NCT01446016), and brain (NCT01171469). Although it is currently unknown whether targeting CSCs will have a strong clinical impact, there is much optimism that this type of therapy will improve the overall survival of patients with aggressive cancers. As advancements in CSC detection and mutation sequencing from bulk and single cells within tumors using parallel data acquisition and processing occur, the development of more potent and targeted therapeutics against CSCs is an exciting future endeavor.

10.8 Methods Used to Determine Cancer Stem Cells

10.8.1 Sphere-Forming Assay

In order to identify stem cells, investigators have developed both in vitro and in vivo methods to test key characteristics of stem cells. The sphere-forming assay is an in vitro culture technique to evaluate potential stem-like cells for their capacity of self-renewal and differentiation even at the single-cell level (Pastrana et al. 2011). This method has been utilized for the last two decades to identify stem cells in fully differentiated tissues such as brain, breast, and skin (Pastrana et al. 2011). For sphere-forming assays, both tumor-initiating and non-initiating tumor cells are cultured into spheres typically under non-adherent conditions, specifically defined two-dimensional, or 3D-assisted culture conditions, which allows the tumors cells to self-renew through proliferation and differentiation. Typically, serially diluted cells or single cells are cultured so that sphere formation solely depends on innate tumorigenic ability.

10.8.2 In Vivo Limiting Dilution Assay

True stem cells should be able to reconstitute an entire organism or a differentiated tissue or organ. Typically, different populations of embryonic, neuronal or hematopoietic stem cells have been challenged to give rise to an identical organism from a single embryonic cell or to reconstitute compromised neuronal or hematopoietic systems in vivo, respectively (Porrata et al. 2001; Anglani et al. 2010; Blau et al. 2001; Moore et al. 2006; Lin et al. 2003; Smith 2001; Odorico et al. 2001). Similar to this concept, mammary stem cells have been evaluated in vivo for their ability to reconstitute mouse mammary glands from a cleared mammary fat pad in vivo (Van Keymeulen et al. 2011; Visvader and Smith 2011). Similar to these assays, the in vivo limiting dilution assay (LDA) is a "mandatory" assay to test the stemness of a given subpopulation of tumor cells (Illa-Bochaca et al. 2010; O'Brien et al. 2010). For LDA, cell viability and tumor cellularity are critical because it would be difficult to determine the tumor-initiating capacity if only 10 % of the injected cells are tumor cells composed of a mixed population of cancer stem cells and stromal cells. The goal of this assay is to measure and compare tumor forming frequencies and tumor-initiating potentials to estimate CSC frequencies within serially-diluted cells from tumor-initiating or non-tumor-initiating populations in mice (Hu and Smyth 2009; O'Brien et al. 2010). An equally vital aim of an LDA is to determine if there are cooperating effects between tumor cells by testing multiple cell effects rather than a single CSC to generate a tumor using the goodness-of-fit statistical test, and to calculate the CSC frequency in a given population (Kimura-Yoshida et al. 2005). Thus, LDA requires a wide range of dilutions and a large number of replicates per dose to determine the goodness of fit of the data. In addition, it is ideal to include doses of cells which give both positive and negative results. Although the mammosphere forming assay is a surrogate in vitro LDA model, an in vivo LDA is a standard requirement for CSC research.

10.8.3 Lineage Tracing

Lineage tracing is a direct functional assay which allows researchers to trace a single cell or a group of cells to their progeny in vivo or in vitro in a spatiotemporal manner by detecting genetically or chemically inherited makers (Schepers et al. 2012; Kretzschmar and Watt 2012; Hsu 2015). Dr. Charles O Whitman was the first researcher to introduce the concept of lineage tracing in the early 19th century by observing the cleavage pattern of early leech embryos, following the fate of individual cells from the egg to germ layer stages (Hsu 2015). Since then, lineage tracing methods have evolved along with the discovery of fluorescent proteins and advancements of genetic engineering. Additionally, lineage tracing has provided important advantages for the identification of stem cells and their direct progenies regardless of the specific molecular marker used to detect the stem cells (Walther and Alison 2015; Gil-Sanz et al. 2015; Kretzschmar and Watt 2012; Schepers et al. 2012). Recently, three independent research groups traced CSCs in vivo using tamoxifen-inducible Cre–Lox technologies to express fluorescent proteins in different tissues (Baker 2012). They demonstrated the propagation of labeled CSCs into progenitor tumor cells having limited proliferative ability and their establishment of heterogenic tumor architecture within glioma, epidermal benign papilloma and squamous cell carcinomas, and intestinal adenomas. Kretzchmar and Watt (2012) comprehensively reviewed current methods of lineage tracing. Briefly, cell labeling methods for lineage tracing can be subcategorized into two large groups (Hsu 2015): (1) non-selective and transient cell labeling and (2) selective and permanent genetic labeling. The non-selective and transient cell labeling methods have been developed for labeling cell membranes, nuclei, and other cell organelles such as mitochondria, lysosomes, and endosomes. Additionally, cells can be pulsed with thymidine analogues such as 3H-thymidine, BrdU, or EdU for allowing incorporation of the analogues into DNA for a short period of time (Kretzschmar and Watt 2012; Maes et al. 2014). Actively proliferating cells will dilute out the initial amount of the thymidine analogues during the chase period, while relatively slowly growing cells will retain high levels in their DNA. These non-selective and transient cell labeling methods are most useful and convenient when genetic permanent labeling is not feasible.

Selective and permanent labeling depends on lineage-dependent expression of fluorescent proteins or enzymes (beta-galatosidase and alkaline phosphatase) in tissue, cell, or time-specific manners (Kretzschmar and Watt 2012; Gong et al. 2013). This allows researchers to trace the fate of tissue-specific stem cells that are analogues of human counterparts for longer time periods compared to transient labeling techniques. Permanent lineage tracing systems mainly utilize inducible genetic promoter systems, which are tightly regulated by endogenous or exogenous transcription factors or repressors. The Cre-Lox method is a widely used inducible system (Kretzschmar and Watt 2012; Cufi et al. 2011; Sauer 1998). In order to label stem cells or cancer stem cells, a mouse line carrying a *Cre* recombinase gene cassette under the control of a cell or tissue-specific promoter must be crossed with syngeneic mice carrying a reporter gene cassette under the control of ubiquitously expressed promoters with a stop codon flanked by two LoxP sites (Sauer 1998). Upon mating, the tissue and cell-specific promoter allows the expression of the Cre recombinase which, in turn, excises out the stop codon marked by the LoxP sites, allowing the expression of the reporter gene which can be a fluorescent protein or enzyme (Sauer 1998; Kretzschmar and Watt 2012; Hsu 2015). However, the constitutive expression system may cause a *confounding* effect as the reporter genes are continually expressed in either stem cells or progenitor cells. To overcome this perplexity, the expression of Cre or its access to the nucleus can be regulated by joining an inducible promoter behind the tissue-specific promoter or by creating fusion Cre constructs such as CreER (Reinert et al. 2012), which only functions in the presence of Tamoxifen.

10.8.4 Patient-Derived Xenografts (PDXs) as Preclinical Small Animal Models

In order to overcome some of the difficulties encountered in obtaining and studying primary human breast cancer tissues, as well as the lack of in vivo preclinical models that more accurately reflect tumor biology, we have established a cohort of human breast tumors grown in the epithelium-free mammary fat pad of SCID/Beige and NOD/SCID/IL2γ-receptor null (NSG) mice, under a series of transplant conditions (Zhang et al. 2013). The patient-derived xenograft (PDX) models developed in mice are becoming critical tools in replicating the diversity of human tumor biology in a preclinical setting as they are a renewable, quality-controlled tissue resource for studies investigating treatment responses and metastasis (Hidalgo et al. 2014; Rosfjord et al. 2014; Siolas and Hannon 2013; Tentler et al. 2012; Zhang et al. 2013). In our laboratory, more than 30 individual human breast cancer tumor lines, each representing a single patient, are currently being used for a range of studies. These studies include essential pre-clinical trials, where tumor responses to new experimental therapeutics and novel treatment combinations, among others, are being tested. These groups of human breast cancer PDXs are representative of many subtypes including "triple-negative" ($ER^-PR^-HER2^-$), $ER^-PR^-HER2^+$, $ER^+PR^-HER2^-$, $ER^+PR^+HER2^-$ and "triple-positive" ($ER^+PR^+HER2^+$) tumors (Zhang et al. 2013). Serially passaged xenografts have shown biological consistency with the tumor of origin, are phenotypically stable across multiple transplant generations at the histologic, transcriptomic, proteomic, and genomic levels, and present comparable treatment responses in breast cancer patients. Importantly, PDX models often reproduce the same characteristics observed in patients such as metastasis to the mouse lung. In summary, PDX mouse models serve as a renewable, quality-controlled tissue resource for preclinical studies investigating cancer cell responses to therapy and also metastasis, the stage of cancer which is often most lethal.

10.9 Conclusions

The knowledge regarding the role of CSCs in breast cancer is still evolving. It is undoubted that these in part contribute to tumor heterogeneity. Accumulating evidence also suggests that these cells play a key role in the development of recurrence and metastases and should be targeted for therapeutic purposes. Recent studies have elucidated a number of key pathways are critical for CSC function and for contributing to therapeutic resistance. Concerted efforts are required as to apply this knowledge to develop novel therapeutics and overcome chemoresistance.

References

Abdullah LN, Chow EK (2013) Mechanisms of chemoresistance in cancer stem cells. Clin Transl Med 2(1):3. doi:10.1186/2001-1326-2-3

Abiola M, Favier M, Christodoulou-Vafeiadou E, Pichard AL, Martelly I, Guillet-Deniau I (2009) Activation of Wnt/beta-catenin signaling increases insulin sensitivity through a reciprocal regulation of Wnt10b and SREBP-1c in skeletal muscle cells. PLoS ONE 4(12):e8509. doi:10.1371/journal.pone.0008509

Abubaker K, Luwor RB, Zhu H, McNally O, Quinn MA, Burns CJ, Thompson EW, Findlay JK, Ahmed N (2014) Inhibition of the JAK2/STAT3 pathway in ovarian cancer results in the loss of cancer stem cell-like characteristics and a reduced tumor burden. BMC Cancer 14:317. doi:10.1186/1471-2407-14-317

Akalay I, Tan TZ, Kumar P, Janji B, Mami-Chouaib F, Charpy C, Vielh P, Larsen AK, Thiery JP, Sabbah M, Chouaib S (2015) Targeting WNT1-inducible signaling pathway protein 2 alters human breast cancer cell susceptibility to specific lysis through regulation of KLF-4 and miR-7 expression. Oncogene 34(17):2261–2271. doi:10.1038/onc.2014.151

Al-Hajj M, Wicha MS, Benito-Hernandez A, Morrison SJ, Clarke MF (2003) Prospective identification of tumorigenic breast cancer cells. Proc Natl Acad Sci U S A 100(7):3983–3988. doi:10.1073/pnas.0530291100

Alderton GK (2012) Metastasis: STAT3 promotes premetastatic niche formation. Nat Rev Cancer 12(7):453. doi:10.1038/nrc3313

Amaravadi RK, Yu D, Lum JJ, Bui T, Christophorou MA, Evan GI, Thomas-Tikhonenko A, Thompson CB (2007) Autophagy inhibition enhances therapy-induced apoptosis in a Myc-induced model of lymphoma. J Clin Investig 117(2):326–336. doi:10.1172/JCI28833

Ambs S, Merriam WG, Bennett WP, Felley-Bosco E, Ogunfusika MO, Oser SM, Klein S, Shields PG, Billiar TR, Harris CC (1998) Frequent nitric oxide synthase-2 expression in human colon adenomas: implication for tumor angiogenesis and colon cancer progression. Cancer Res 58(2):334–341

Amoyel M, Anderson AM, Bach EA (2014) JAK/STAT pathway dysregulation in tumors: a Drosophila perspective. Semin Cell Dev Biol 28:96–103. doi:10.1016/j.semcdb.2014.03.023

Angeloni V, Tiberio P, Appierto V, Daidone MG (2015) Implications of stemness-related signaling pathways in breast cancer response to therapy. Semin Cancer Biol 31:43–51. doi:10.1016/j.semcancer.2014.08.004

Anglani F, Mezzabotta F, Ceol M, Cristofaro R, Del Prete D, D'Angelo A (2010) The regenerative potential of the kidney: what can we learn from developmental biology? Stem Cell Rev 6(4):650–657. doi:10.1007/s12015-010-9186-6

Anjomshoaa A, Nasri S, Humar B, McCall JL, Chatterjee A, Yoon HS, Mcnoe L, Black MA, Reeve AE (2009) Slow proliferation as a biological feature of colorectal cancer metastasis. Br J Cancer 101(5):822–828. doi:10.1038/sj.bjc.6605229

Baker M (2012) Cancer stem cells tracked. Nature 488(7409):13–14. doi:10.1038/488013a

Behari J (2010) The Wnt/beta-catenin signaling pathway in liver biology and disease. Expert Rev Gastroenterol Hepatol 4(6):745–756. doi:10.1586/egh.10.74

Behrens J, von Kries JP, Kuhl M, Bruhn L, Wedlich D, Grosschedl R, Birchmeier W (1996) Functional interaction of beta-catenin with the transcription factor LEF-1. Nature 382(6592):638–642. doi:10.1038/382638a0

Bergstein I, Schultz R, Osborne MP, Welcsh PL, Bowcock AM, Brown AM (1995) Investigation of the possible role of WNT genes in human breast cancer. Ann N Y Acad Sci 768:257

Bertrand G, Maalouf M, Boivin A, Battiston-Montagne P, Beuve M, Levy A, Jalade P, Fournier C, Ardail D, Magne N, Alphonse G, Rodriguez-Lafrasse C (2014) Targeting head and neck cancer stem cells to overcome resistance to photon and carbon ion radiation. Stem Cell Rev 10(1):114–126. doi:10.1007/s12015-013-9467-y

Bilir B, Kucuk O, Moreno CS (2013) Wnt signaling blockage inhibits cell proliferation and migration, and induces apoptosis in triple-negative breast cancer cells. J Trans Med 11:280. doi:10.1186/1479-5876-11-280

Blau HM, Brazelton TR, Weimann JM (2001) The evolving concept of a stem cell: entity or function? Cell 105(7):829–841

Brabletz T (2012) To differentiate or not—routes towards metastasis. Nat Rev Cancer 12(6):425–436. doi:10.1038/nrc3265

Bulut AS, Erden E, Sak SD, Doruk H, Kursun N, Dincol D (2005) Significance of inducible nitric oxide synthase expression in benign and malignant breast epithelium: an immunohistochemical study of 151 cases. Virchows Archiv: Int J Pathol 447(1):24–30. doi:10.1007/s00428-005-1250-2

Carpentino JE, Hynes MJ, Appelman HD, Zheng T, Steindler DA, Scott EW, Huang EH (2009) Aldehyde dehydrogenase-expressing colon stem cells contribute to tumorigenesis in the transition from colitis to cancer. Cancer Res 69(20):8208–8215. doi:10.1158/0008-5472.CAN-09-1132

Cavaleri F, Scholer HR (2003) Nanog: a new recruit to the embryonic stem cell orchestra. Cell 113(5):551–552

Chen K, Huang YH, Chen JL (2013) Understanding and targeting cancer stem cells: therapeutic implications and challenges. Acta Pharmacol Sin 34(6):732–740. doi:10.1038/aps.2013.27

Chen Q, Giedt M, Tang L, Harrison DA (2014) Tools and methods for studying the Drosophila JAK/STAT pathway. Methods 68(1):160–172. doi:10.1016/j.ymeth.2014.03.023

Cheung AM, Wan TS, Leung JC, Chan LY, Huang H, Kwong YL, Liang R, Leung AY (2007) Aldehyde dehydrogenase activity in leukemic blasts defines a subgroup of acute myeloid leukemia with adverse prognosis and superior NOD/SCID engrafting potential. Leukemia 21(7):1423–1430. doi:10.1038/sj.leu.2404721

Cho RW, Wang X, Diehn M, Shedden K, Chen GY, Sherlock G, Gurney A, Lewicki J, Clarke MF (2008) Isolation and molecular characterization of cancer stem cells in MMTV-Wnt-1 murine breast tumors. Stem Cells 26(2):364–371. doi:10.1634/stemcells.2007-0440

Choi DS, Blanco E, Kim YS, Rodriguez AA, Zhao H, Huang TH, Chen CL, Jin G, Landis MD, Burey LA, Qian W, Granados SM, Dave B, Wong HH, Ferrari M, Wong ST, Chang JC (2014) Chloroquine eliminates cancer stem cells through deregulation of Jak2 and DNMT1. Stem Cells 32(9):2309–2323. doi:10.1002/stem.1746

Chung SS, Vadgama JV (2015) Curcumin and epigallocatechin gallate inhibit the cancer stem cell phenotype via down-regulation of STAT3-NFkappaB signaling. Anticancer Res 35(1):39–46

Cleary AS, Leonard TL, Gestl SA, Gunther EJ (2014) Tumour cell heterogeneity maintained by cooperating subclones in Wnt-driven mammary cancers. Nature 508(7494):113–117. doi:10.1038/nature13187

Clevers H (2006) Wnt/beta-catenin signaling in development and disease. Cell 127(3):469–480. doi:10.1016/j.cell.2006.10.018

Clevers H, Loh KM, Nusse R (2014) Stem cell signaling. An integral program for tissue renewal and regeneration: Wnt signaling and stem cell control. Science 346(6205):1248012. doi:10.1126/science.1248012

Clevers H, Nusse R (2012) Wnt/beta-catenin signaling and disease. Cell 149(6):1192–1205. doi:10.1016/j.cell.2012.05.012

Cojoc M, Mabert K, Muders MH, Dubrovska A (2015) A role for cancer stem cells in therapy resistance: cellular and molecular mechanisms. Semin Cancer Biol 31:16–27. doi:10.1016/j.semcancer.2014.06.004

Conley SJ, Gheordunescu E, Kakarala P, Newman B, Korkaya H, Heath AN, Clouthier SG, Wicha MS (2012) Antiangiogenic agents increase breast cancer stem cells via the generation of tumor hypoxia. Proc Natl Acad Sci U S A 109(8):2784–2789. doi:10.1073/pnas.1018866109

Constantinescu S (2003) Stemness, fusion and renewal of hematopoietic and embryonic stem cells. J Cell Mol Med 7(2):103–112

Creighton CJ, Chang JC, Rosen JM (2010) Epithelial-mesenchymal transition (EMT) in tumor-initiating cells and its clinical implications in breast cancer. J Mamm Gland Biol Neoplasia 15(2):253–260. doi:10.1007/s10911-010-9173-1

Creighton CJ, Li XX, Landis M, Dixon JM, Neumeister VM, Sjolund A, Rimm DL, Wong H, Rodriguez A, Herschkowitz JI, Fan C, Zhang XM, He XP, Pavlick A, Gutierrez MC, Renshaw L, Larionov AA, Faratian D, Hilsenbeck SG, Perou CM, Lewis MT, Rosen JM, Chang JC (2009) Residual breast cancers after conventional therapy display mesenchymal as well as tumor-initiating features. Proc Natl Acad Sci U S A 106(33):13820–13825. doi:10.1073/pnas.0905718106

Croker AK, Allan AL (2012) Inhibition of aldehyde dehydrogenase (ALDH) activity reduces chemotherapy and radiation resistance of stem-like ALDHhiCD44(+) human breast cancer cells. Breast Cancer Res Treat 133(1):75–87. doi:10.1007/s10549-011-1692-y

Cuervo AM, Wong E (2014) Chaperone-mediated autophagy: roles in disease and aging. Cell Res 24(1):92–104. doi:10.1038/cr.2013.153

Cufi S, Vazquez-Martin A, Oliveras-Ferraros C, Martin-Castillo B, Vellon L, Menendez JA (2011) Autophagy positively regulates the CD44(+) CD24(−/low) breast cancer stem-like phenotype. Cell Cycle 10 (22):3871–3885. doi:10.4161/cc.10.22.17976

Dave B, Granados-Principal S, Zhu R, Benz S, Rabizadeh S, Soon-Shiong P, Yu KD, Shao Z, Li X, Gilcrease M, Lai Z, Chen Y, Huang TH, Shen H, Liu X, Ferrari M, Zhan M, Wong ST, Kumaraswami M, Mittal V, Chen X, Gross SS, Chang JC (2014) Targeting RPL39 and MLF2 reduces tumor initiation and metastasis in breast cancer by inhibiting nitric oxide synthase signaling. Proc Natl Acad Sci U S A 111(24):8838–8843. doi:10.1073/pnas.1320769111

Dave B, Landis MD, Tweardy DJ, Chang JC, Dobrolecki LE, Wu MF, Zhang X, Westbrook TF, Hilsenbeck SG, Liu D, Lewis MT (2012) Selective small molecule Stat3 inhibitor reduces breast cancer tumor-initiating cells and improves recurrence free survival in a human-xenograft model. PLoS ONE 7 (8):e30207. doi:10.1371/journal.pone.0030207

Deshpande AJ, Cusan M, Rawat VPS, Reuter H, Krause A, Pott C, Quintanilla-Martinez L, Kakadia P, Kuchenbauer F, Ahmed F, Delabesse E, Hahn M, Lichter P, Kneba M, Hiddemann W, Macintyre E, Mecucci C, Ludwig WD, Humphries RK, Bohlander SK, Feuring-Buske M, Buske C (2006) Acute myeloid leukemia is propagated by a leukemic stem cell with lymphoid characteristics in a mouse model of CALM/AF10-positive leukemia. Cancer Cell 10 (5):363–374. doi:10.1016/j.ccr.2006.08.023

Eyler CE, Wu Q, Yan K, MacSwords JM, Chandler-Militello D, Misuraca KL, Lathia JD, Forrester MT, Lee J, Stamler JS, Goldman SA, Bredel M, McLendon RE, Sloan AE, Hjelmeland AB, Rich JN (2011) Glioma stem cell proliferation and tumor growth are promoted by nitric oxide synthase-2. Cell 146(1):53–66. doi:10.1016/j.cell.2011.06.006

Farmer P, Bonnefoi H, Anderle P, Cameron D, Wirapati P, Becette V, Andre S, Piccart M, Campone M, Brain E, Macgrogan G, Petit T, Jassem J, Bibeau F, Blot E, Bogaerts J, Aguet M, Bergh J, Iggo R, Delorenzi M (2009) A stroma-related gene signature predicts resistance to neoadjuvant chemotherapy in breast cancer. NatMed 15(1):68–74. doi:10.1038/nm.1908. (nm.1908 [pii])

Fenaux P, Chastang C, Chevret S, Sanz M, Dombret H, Archimbaud E, Fey M, Rayon C, Huguet F, Sotto JJ, Gardin C, Makhoul PC, Travade P, Solary E, Fegueux N, Bordessoule D, Miguel JS, Link H, Desablens B, Stamatoullas A, Deconinck E, Maloisel F, Castaigne S, Preudhomme C, Degos L (1999) A randomized comparison of all transretinoic acid (ATRA) followed by chemotherapy and ATRA plus chemotherapy and the role of maintenance therapy in newly diagnosed acute promyelocytic leukemia. The European APL Group. Blood 94(4):1192–1200

Fenaux P, Le Deley MC, Castaigne S, Archimbaud E, Chomienne C, Link H, Guerci A, Duarte M, Daniel MT, Bowen D (1993) Effect of all transretinoic acid in newly diagnosed acute promyelocytic leukemia. Results of a multicenter randomized trial. European APL 91 Group. Blood 82(11):3241–3249

Finbloom DS, Silver K, Newsome DA, Gunkel R (1985) Comparison of hydroxychloroquine and chloroquine use and the development of retinal toxicity. J Rheumatol 12(4):692–694

Firat E, Weyerbrock A, Gaedicke S, Grosu AL, Niedermann G (2012) Chloroquine or chloroquine-PI3 K/Akt pathway inhibitor combinations strongly promote gamma-irradiation-induced cell death in primary stem-like glioma cells. PLoS ONE 7 (10):e47357. doi:10.1371/journal.pone.0047357

Formelli F, Cleris L (1993) Synthetic retinoid fenretinide is effective against a human ovarian-carcinoma xenograft and potentiates cisplatin activity. Cancer Res 53(22):5374–5376

Gil-Sanz C, Espinosa A, Fregoso SP, Bluske KK, Cunningham CL, Martinez-Garay I, Zeng H, Franco SJ, Muller U (2015) Lineage Tracing Using Cux2-Cre and Cux2-CreERT2 Mice. Neuron 86(4):1091–1099. doi:10.1016/j.neuron.2015.04.019

Ginestier C, Hur MH, Charafe-Jauffret E, Monville F, Dutcher J, Brown M, Jacquemier J, Viens P, Kleer CG, Liu SL, Schott A, Hayes D, Birnbaum D, Wicha MS, Dontu G (2007) ALDH1 is a marker of normal and malignant human mammary stem cells and a predictor of poor clinical outcome. Cell Stem Cell 1 (5):555–567. doi:10.1016/j.stem.2007.08.014

Giuliano M, Schifp R, Osborne CK, Trivedi MV (2011) Biological mechanisms and clinical implications of endocrine resistance in breast cancer. Breast 20(Suppl 3):S42–49. doi:10.1016/S0960-9776(11)70293-4

Glick D, Barth S, Macleod KF (2010) Autophagy: cellular and molecular mechanisms. J Pathol 221(1):3–12. doi:10.1002/path.2697

Glynn SA, Boersma BJ, Dorsey TH, Yi M, Yfantis HG, Ridnour LA, Martin DN, Switzer CH, Hudson RS, Wink DA, Lee DH, Stephens RM, Ambs S (2010) Increased NOS2 predicts poor survival in estrogen receptor-negative breast cancer patients. J Clin Invest 120(11):3843–3854. doi:10.1172/JCI42059

Gong C, Bauvy C, Tonelli G, Yue W, Delomenie C, Nicolas V, Zhu Y, Domergue V, Marin-Esteban V, Tharinger H, Delbos L, Gary-Gouy H, Morel AP, Ghavami S, Song E, Codogno P, Mehrpour M (2013) Beclin 1 and autophagy are required for the tumorigenicity of breast cancer stem-like/progenitor cells. Oncogene 32(18):2261–2272, 2272e, 2261–2211. doi:10.1038/onc.2012.252

Granados-Principal S, Liu Y, Guevara ML, Blanco E, Choi DS, Qian W, Patel T, Rodriguez AA, Cusimano J, Weiss HL, Zhao H, Landis MD, Dave B, Gross SS, Chang JC (2015) Inhibition of iNOS as a novel effective targeted therapy against triple-negative breast cancer. Breast Cancer Res 17:25. doi:10.1186/s13058-015-0527-x. ARTN 25

Grunt ThW, Dittrich E, Offterdinger M, Schneider SM, Dittrich C, Huber H (1998) Effects of retinoic acid and

fenretinide on the c-erbB-2 expression, growth and cisplatin sensitivity of breast cancer cells. Br J Cancer 78(1):79–87
Harrison DA (2012) The Jak/STAT pathway. Cold Spring Harb Perspect Biol 4(3). doi:10.1101/cshperspect.a011205
Heppner GH (1984) Tumor heterogeneity. Cancer Res 44 (6):2259–2265
Heppner GH, Chong YC, Fulton AM (1989) Host-mediated induction of tumor heterogeneity. Ann N Y Acad Sci 567:234–242
Heppner GH, Miller BE (1989) Therapeutic implications of tumor heterogeneity. Semin Oncol 16(2):91–105
Herschkowitz JI, Simin K, Weigman VJ, Mikaelian I, Usary J, Hu Z, Rasmussen KE, Jones LP, Assefnia S, Chandrasekharan S, Backlund MG, Yin Y, Khramtsov AI, Bastein R, Quackenbush J, Glazer RI, Brown PH, Green JE, Kopelovich L, Furth PA, Palazzo JP, Olopade OI, Bernard PS, Churchill GA, Van Dyke T, Perou CM (2007) Identification of conserved gene expression features between murine mammary carcinoma models and human breast tumors. Genome Biol 8(5):R76. doi:10.1186/gb-2007-8-5-r76. (gb-2007-8-5-r76 [pii])
Hidalgo M, Amant F, Biankin AV, Budinska E, Byrne AT, Caldas C, Clarke RB, de Jong S, Jonkers J, Maelandsmo GM, Roman-Roman S, Seoane J, Trusolino L, Villanueva A (2014) Patient-derived xenograft models: an emerging platform for translational cancer research. Cancer Discovery 4(9):998–1013. doi:10.1158/2159-8290.CD-14-0001
Hopper RA, Garthwaite J (2006) Tonic and phasic nitric oxide signals in hippocampal long-term potentiation. J Neurosci 26(45):11513–11521. doi:10.1523/JNEUROSCI.2259-06.2006
Hsu HS, Lin JH, Hsu TW, Su K, Wang CW, Yang KY, Chiou SH, Hung SC (2012) Mesenchymal stem cells enhance lung cancer initiation through activation of IL-6/JAK2/STAT3 pathway. Lung Cancer 75(2):167–177. doi:10.1016/j.lungcan.2011.07.001
Hsu YC (2015) Theory and practice of lineage tracing. Stem Cells 33(11):3197–3204. doi:10.1002/stem.2123
Hu Y, Smyth GK (2009) ELDA: extreme limiting dilution analysis for comparing depleted and enriched populations in stem cell and other assays. J Immunol Methods 347(1–2):70–78. doi:10.1016/j.jim.2009.06.008
Hughes K, Watson CJ (2012) The spectrum of STAT functions in mammary gland development. Jakstat 1 (3):151–158. doi:10.4161/jkst.19691
Ignarro LJ (1990) Nitric oxide. A novel signal transduction mechanism for transcellular communication. Hypertension 16(5):477–483
Illa-Bochaca I, Fernandez-Gonzalez R, Shelton DN, Welm BE, Ortiz-de-Solorzano C, Barcellos-Hoff MH (2010) Limiting-dilution transplantation assays in mammary stem cell studies. Methods Mol Biol 621:29–47. doi:10.1007/978-1-60761-063-2_2
Ivashkiv LB (2000) Jak-STAT signaling pathways in cells of the immune system. Rev Immunogenet 2(2):220–230
Ivashkiv LB, Hu X (2004) Signaling by STATs. Arthritis Res Ther 6(4):159–168. doi:10.1186/ar1197
Jamal-Hanjani M, Quezada SA, Larkin J, Swanton C (2015) Translational implications of tumor heterogeneity. Clin Cancer Res 21(6):1258–1266. doi:10.1158/1078-0432.CCR-14-1429
Janku F, McConkey DJ, Hong DS, Kurzrock R (2011) Autophagy as a target for anticancer therapy. Nat Rev Clin Oncol 8(9):528–539. doi:10.1038/nrclinonc.2011.71
Jiang F, Qiu Q, Khanna A, Todd NW, Deepak J, Xing LX, Wang HJ, Liu ZQ, Su Y, Stass SA, Katz RL (2009) Aldehyde dehydrogenase 1 is a tumor stem cell-associated marker in lung cancer. Mol Cancer Res 7(3):330–338. doi:10.1158/1541-7786.Mcr-08-0393
Kahn M (2014) Can we safely target the WNT pathway? Nat Rev Drug Discov 13(7):513–532. doi:10.1038/nrd4233
Kalemkerian GP, Ou X (1999) Activity of fenretinide plus chemotherapeutic agents in small-cell lung cancer cell lines. Cancer Chemother Pharmacol 43(2):145–150. doi:10.1007/s002800050875
Kamakura S, Oishi K, Yoshimatsu T, Nakafuku M, Masuyama N, Gotoh Y (2004) Hes binding to STAT3 mediates crosstalk between Notch and JAK-STAT signalling. Nat Cell Biol 6(6):547–554. doi:10.1038/ncb1138
Kazi AA, Gilani RA, Schech AJ, Chumsri S, Sabnis G, Shah P, Goloubeva O, Kronsberg S, Brodie AH (2014) Nonhypoxic regulation and role of hypoxia-inducible factor 1 in aromatase inhibitor resistant breast cancer. Breast Cancer Res 16(1):R15. doi:10.1186/bcr3609
Keitel U, Scheel A, Thomale J, Halpape R, Kaulfuss S, Scheel C, Dobbelstein M (2014) Bcl-xL mediates therapeutic resistance of a mesenchymal breast cancer cell subpopulation. Oncotarget 5(23):11778–11791. doi:10.18632/oncotarget.2634
Kenific CM, Thorburn A, Debnath J (2010) Autophagy and metastasis: another double-edged sword. Curr Opin Cell Biol 22(2):241–245. doi:10.1016/j.ceb.2009.10.008
Kim MS, Lee WS, Jeong J, Kim SJ, Jin W (2015) Induction of metastatic potential by TrkB via activation of IL6/JAK2/STAT3 and PI3 K/AKT signaling in breast cancer. Oncotarget 6(37):40158–40171. doi:10.18632/oncotarget.5522
Kimura-Yoshida C, Nakano H, Okamura D, Nakao K, Yonemura S, Belo JA, Aizawa S, Matsui Y, Matsuo I (2005) Canonical Wnt signaling and its antagonist regulate anterior-posterior axis polarization by guiding cell migration in mouse visceral endoderm. Dev Cell 9 (5):639–650. doi:10.1016/j.devcel.2005.09.011
Kolosenko I, Grander D, Tamm KP (2014) IL-6 activated JAK/STAT3 pathway and sensitivity to Hsp90

inhibitors in multiple myeloma. Curr Med Chem 21 (26):3042–3047
Komiya Y, Habas R (2008) Wnt signal transduction pathways. Organogenesis 4(2):68–75
Kretzschmar K, Watt FM (2012) Lineage tracing. Cell 148(1–2):33–45. doi:10.1016/j.cell.2012.01.002
Krivtsov AV, Twomey D, Feng Z, Stubbs MC, Wang Y, Faber J, Levine JE, Wang J, Hahn WC, Gilliland DG, Golub TR, Armstrong SA (2006) Transformation from committed progenitor to leukaemia stem cell initiated by MLL-AF9. Nature 442(7104):818–822. doi:10.1038/nature04980
Kurrey NK, Jalgaonkar SP, Joglekar AV, Ghanate AD, Chaskar PD, Doiphode RY, Bapat SA (2009) Snail and slug mediate radioresistance and chemoresistance by antagonizing p53-mediated apoptosis and acquiring a stem-like phenotype in ovarian cancer cells. Stem Cells 27(9):2059–2068. doi:10.1002/stem.154
Lapidot T, Sirard C, Vormoor J, Murdoch B, Hoang T, Cacerescortes J, Minden M, Paterson B, Caligiuri MA, Dick JE (1994) A cell initiating human acute myeloid-leukemia after transplantation into SCID mice. Nature 367(6464):645–648. doi:10.1038/367645a0
Lee HE, Kim JH, Kim YJ, Choi SY, Kim SW, Kang E, Chung IY, Kim IA, Kim EJ, Choi Y, Ryu HS, Park SY (2011) An increase in cancer stem cell population after primary systemic therapy is a poor prognostic factor in breast cancer. Br J Cancer 104 (11):1730–1738. doi:10.1038/bjc.2011.159
Li X, Lewis MT, Huang J, Gutierrez C, Osborne CK, Wu MF, Hilsenbeck SG, Pavlick A, Zhang X, Chamness GC, Wong H, Rosen J, Chang JC (2008) Intrinsic resistance of tumorigenic breast cancer cells to chemotherapy. J Natl Cancer Inst 100(9):672–679. doi:10.1093/jnci/djn123
Li Y, Welm B, Podsypanina K, Huang S, Chamorro M, Zhang X, Rowlands T, Egeblad M, Cowin P, Werb Z, Tan LK, Rosen JM, Varmus HE (2003) Evidence that transgenes encoding components of the Wnt signaling pathway preferentially induce mammary cancers from progenitor cells. Proc Natl Acad Sci U S A 100 (26):15853–15858. doi:10.1073/pnas.2136825100
Li YJ, Cui W, Tian ZJ, Hao YM, Du J, Liu F, Zhang H, Zu XG, Liu SY, Xie RQ, Yang XH, Wu YZ, Chen L, An W (2004) Crosstalk between ERK1/2 and STAT3 in the modulation of cardiomyocyte hypertrophy induced by cardiotrophin-1. Chin Med J (Engl) 117 (8):1135–1142
Lin H, Lei J, Wininger D, Nguyen MT, Khanna R, Hartmann C, Yan WL, Huang SC (2003) Multilineage potential of homozygous stem cells derived from metaphase II oocytes. Stem Cells 21(2):152–161. doi:10.1634/stemcells.21-2-152
Liu F, Shang Y, Chen SZ (2014a) Chloroquine potentiates the anti-cancer effect of lidamycin on non-small cell lung cancer cells in vitro. Acta Pharmacol Sin 35 (5):645–652. doi:10.1038/aps.2014.3
Liu S, Cong Y, Wang D, Sun Y, Deng L, Liu Y, Martin-Trevino R, Shang L, McDermott SP, Landis MD, Hong S, Adams A, D'Angelo R, Ginestier C, Charafe-Jauffret E, Clouthier SG, Birnbaum D, Wong ST, Zhan M, Chang JC, Wicha MS (2014b) Breast cancer stem cells transition between epithelial and mesenchymal states reflective of their normal counterparts. Stem Cell Reports 2(1):78–91. doi:10.1016/j.stemcr.2013.11.009
Livesey KM, Tang D, Zeh HJ, Lotze MT (2009) Autophagy inhibition in combination cancer treatment. Curr Opin Investig Drugs 10(12):1269–1279
Loibl S, Buck A, Strank C, von Minckwitz G, Roller M, Sinn HP, Schini-Kerth V, Solbach C, Strebhardt K, Kaufmann M (2005) The role of early expression of inducible nitric oxide synthase in human breast cancer. Eur J Cancer 41(2):265–271. doi:10.1016/j.ejca.2004.07.010
Ma S, Chan KW, Lee TK, Tang KH, Wo JY, Zheng BJ, Guan XY (2008) Aldehyde dehydrogenase discriminates the CD133 liver cancer stem cell populations. Mol Cancer Res 6(7):1146–1153. doi:10.1158/1541-7786.MCR-08-0035
Madjd Z, Mehrjerdi AZ, Sharifi AM, Molanaei S, Shahzadi SZ, Asadi-Lari M (2009) CD44+ cancer cells express higher levels of the anti-apoptotic protein Bcl-2 in breast tumours. Cancer Immun 9:4. (doi:090304 [pii])
Maes H, Kuchnio A, Peric A, Moens S, Nys K, De Bock K, Quaegebeur A, Schoors S, Georgiadou M, Wouters J, Vinckier S, Vankelecom H, Garmyn M, Vion AC, Radtke F, Boulanger C, Gerhardt H, Dejana E, Dewerchin M, Ghesquiere B, Annaert W, Agostinis P, Carmeliet P (2014) Tumor vessel normalization by chloroquine independent of autophagy. Cancer Cell 26(2):190–206. doi:10.1016/j.ccr.2014.06.025
Magni M, Shammah S, Schiro R, Mellado W, Dalla-Favera R, Gianni AM (1996) Induction of cyclophosphamide-resistance by aldehyde-dehydrogenase gene transfer. Blood 87(3):1097–1103
Mani SA, Guo W, Liao MJ, Eaton EN, Ayyanan A, Zhou AY, Brooks M, Reinhard F, Zhang CC, Shipitsin M, Campbell LL, Polyak K, Brisken C, Yang J, Weinberg RA (2008) The epithelial-mesenchymal transition generates cells with properties of stem cells. Cell 133(4):704–715. doi:10.1016/j.cell.2008.03.027
Marotta LL, Almendro V, Marusyk A, Shipitsin M, Schemme J, Walker SR, Bloushtain-Qimron N, Kim JJ, Choudhury SA, Maruyama R, Wu Z, Gonen M, Mulvey LA, Bessarabova MO, Huh SJ, Silver SJ, Kim SY, Park SY, Lee HE, Anderson KS, Richardson AL, Nikolskaya T, Nikolsky Y, Liu XS, Root DE, Hahn WC, Frank DA, Polyak K (2011) The JAK2/STAT3 signaling pathway is required for growth of CD44(+)CD24(−) stem cell-like breast cancer cells in human tumors. J Clin Investig 121 (7):2723–2735. doi:10.1172/JCI44745
Martinez-Outschoorn UE, Lin Z, Ko YH, Goldberg AF, Flomenberg N, Wang C, Pavlides S, Pestell RG, Howell A, Sotgia F, Lisanti MP (2011) Understanding the metabolic basis of drug resistance: therapeutic

induction of the Warburg effect kills cancer cells. Cell Cycle 10(15):2521–2528

Martinez-Revollar G, Garay E, Martin-Tapia D, Nava P, Huerta M, Lopez-Bayghen E, Meraz-Cruz N, Segovia J, Gonzalez-Mariscal L (2015) Heterogeneity between triple negative breast cancer cells due to differential activation of Wnt and PI3 K/AKT pathways. Exp Cell Res 339(1):67–80. doi:10.1016/j.yexcr.2015.10.006

Massi D, Franchi A, Sardi I, Magnelli L, Paglierani M, Borgognoni L, Maria Reali U, Santucci M (2001) Inducible nitric oxide synthase expression in benign and malignant cutaneous melanocytic lesions. J Pathol 194(2):194–200. doi:10.1002/1096-9896(200106)194:2<194:AID-PATH851>3.0.CO;2-S

Mentink RA, Middelkoop TC, Rella L, Ji N, Tang CY, Betist MC, van Oudenaarden A, Korswagen HC (2014) Cell intrinsic modulation of Wnt signaling controls neuroblast migration in *C. elegans*. Dev Cell 31(2):188–201. doi:10.1016/j.devcel.2014.08.008

Mitra A, Mishra L, Li S (2015) EMT, CTCs and CSCs in tumor relapse and drug-resistance. Oncotarget 6 (13):10697–10711. doi:10.18632/oncotarget.4037

Mizushima N (2007) Autophagy: process and function. Genes Dev 21(22):2861–2873. doi:10.1101/gad.1599207

Mizushima N, Komatsu M (2011) Autophagy: renovation of cells and tissues. Cell 147(4):728–741. doi:10.1016/j.cell.2011.10.026

Molenaar M, van de Wetering M, Oosterwegel M, Peterson-Maduro J, Godsave S, Korinek V, Roose J, Destree O, Clevers H (1996) XTcf-3 transcription factor mediates beta-catenin-induced axis formation in Xenopus embryos. Cell 86(3):391–399

Moore MA, Shieh JH, Lee G (2006) Hematopoietic cells. Methods Enzymol 418:208–242. doi:10.1016/S0076-6879(06)18013-1

Moore N, Lyle S (2011) Quiescent, slow-cycling stem cell populations in cancer: a review of the evidence and discussion of significance. J Oncol 2011. doi:10.1155/2011/396076

Natarajan TG, Ganesan N, Fitzgerald KT (2010) Cancer stem cells and markers: new model of tumorigenesis with therapeutic implications. Cancer Biomark 9(1–6):65–99. doi:10.3233/CBM-2011-0173

Nathan C, Xie QW (1994) Nitric oxide synthases: roles, tolls, and controls. Cell 78(6):915–918. doi:10.1016/0092-8674(94)90266-6. [pii]

Nieto MA (2011) The ins and outs of the epithelial to mesenchymal transition in health and disease. Annu Rev Cell Dev Biol 27:347–376. doi:10.1146/annurev-cellbio-092910-154036

Niwa H, Burdon T, Chambers I, Smith A (1998) Self-renewal of pluripotent embryonic stem cells is mediated via activation of STAT3. Genes Dev 12 (13):2048–2060

Nusse R (2008) Wnt signaling and stem cell control. Cell Res 18(5):523–527. doi:10.1038/cr.2008.47

Nusse R, Varmus HE (1982) Many tumors induced by the mouse mammary tumor virus contain a provirus integrated in the same region of the host genome. Cell 31(1):99–109

Nusslein-Volhard C, Wieschaus E (1980) Mutations affecting segment number and polarity in Drosophila. Nature 287(5785):795–801

O'Brien CA, Kreso A, Jamieson CH (2010) Cancer stem cells and self-renewal. Clin Cancer Res 16(12):3113–3120. doi:10.1158/1078-0432.CCR-09-2824

Odorico JS, Kaufman DS, Thomson JA (2001) Multilineage differentiation from human embryonic stem cell lines. Stem Cells 19(3):193–204. doi:10.1634/stemcells.19-3-193

Oft M, Peli J, Rudaz C, Schwarz H, Beug H, Reichmann E (1996) TGF-beta1 and Ha-Ras collaborate in modulating the phenotypic plasticity and invasiveness of epithelial tumor cells. Genes Dev 10(19):2462–2477

Okayama H, Saito M, Oue N, Weiss JM, Stauffer J, Takenoshita S, Wiltrout RH, Hussain SP, Harris CC (2013) NOS2 enhances KRAS-induced lung carcinogenesis, inflammation and microRNA-21 expression. Int J Cancer J Int du Cancer 132(1):9–18. doi:10.1002/ijc.27644

Parajuli B, Fishel ML, Hurley TD (2014) Selective ALDH3A1 inhibition by benzimidazole analogues increase mafosfamide sensitivity in cancer cells. J Med Chem 57(2):449–461. doi:10.1021/jm401508p

Pastrana E, Silva-Vargas V, Doetsch F (2011) Eyes wide open: a critical review of sphere-formation as an assay for stem cells. Cell Stem Cell 8(5):486–498. doi:10.1016/j.stem.2011.04.007

Pattabiraman DR, Weinberg RA (2014) Tackling the cancer stem cells—what challenges do they pose? Nat Rev Drug Discov 13(7):497–512

Pettersson F, Colston KW, Dalgleish AG (2001) Retinoic acid enhances the cytotoxic effects of gemcitabine and cisplatin in pancreatic adenocarcinoma cells. Pancreas 23(3):273–279

Pinto CA, Widodo E, Waltham M, Thompson EW (2013) Breast cancer stem cells and epithelial mesenchymal plasticity—Implications for chemoresistance. Cancer Lett 341(1):56–62. doi:10.1016/j.canlet.2013.06.003

Polyak K, Weinberg RA (2009) Transitions between epithelial and mesenchymal states: acquisition of malignant and stem cell traits. Nat Rev Cancer 9 (4):265–273. doi:10.1038/nrc2620

Porrata LF, Litzow MR, Markovic SN (2001) Immune reconstitution after autologous hematopoietic stem cell transplantation. Mayo Clin Proc 76(4):407–412. doi:10.4065/76.4.407

Quintana E, Shackleton M, Sabel MS, Fullen DR, Johnson TM, Morrison SJ (2008) Efficient tumour formation by single human melanoma cells. Nature 456(7222):593–598. doi:10.1038/nature07567

Rangwala R, Leone R, Chang YC, Fecher LA, Schuchter LM, Kramer A, Tan KS, Heitjan DF, Rodgers G, Gallagher M, Piao S, Troxel AB, Evans TL, DeMichele AM, Nathanson KL, O'Dwyer PJ, Kaiser J, Pontiggia L, Davis LE, Amaravadi RK (2014) Phase I trial of hydroxychloroquine with dose-intense temozolomide in patients with advanced solid tumors and melanoma. Autophagy 10(8):1369–1379. doi:10.4161/auto.29118

Rasheed ZA, Yang J, Wang Q, Kowalski J, Freed I, Murter C, Hong SM, Koorstra JB, Rajeshkumar NV, He X, Goggins M, Iacobuzio-Donahue C, Berman DM, Laheru D, Jimeno A, Hidalgo M, Maitra A, Matsui W (2010) Prognostic significance of tumorigenic cells with mesenchymal features in pancreatic adenocarcinoma. J Natl Cancer Inst 102(5):340–351. doi:10.1093/jnci/djp535

Rawlings JS, Rosler KM, Harrison DA (2004) The JAK/STAT signaling pathway. J Cell Sci 117(Pt 8):1281–1283. doi:10.1242/jcs.00963

Reinert RB, Kantz J, Misfeldt AA, Poffenberger G, Gannon M, Brissova M, Powers AC (2012) Tamoxifen-Induced Cre-loxP Recombination Is Prolonged in Pancreatic Islets of Adult Mice. PLoS ONE 7(3):e33529. doi:10.1371/journal.pone.0033529

Rijsewijk F, Schuermann M, Wagenaar E, Parren P, Weigel D, Nusse R (1987) The Drosophila homolog of the mouse mammary oncogene int-1 is identical to the segment polarity gene wingless. Cell 50(4):649–657

Rosen JM, Jordan CT (2009) The increasing complexity of the cancer stem cell paradigm. Science 324(5935):1670–1673. doi:10.1126/science.1171837

Rosfjord E, Lucas J, Li G, Gerber HP (2014) Advances in patient-derived tumor xenografts: from target identification to predicting clinical response rates in oncology. Biochem Pharmacol 91(2):135–143. doi:10.1016/j.bcp.2014.06.008

Rosselli M, Keller PJ, Dubey RK (1998) Role of nitric oxide in the biology, physiology and pathophysiology of reproduction. Hum Reprod Update 4(1):3–24

Sanchez CG, Penfornis P, Oskowitz AZ, Boonjindasup AG, Cai DZ, Dhule SS, Rowan BG, Kelekar A, Krause DS, Pochampally RR (2011) Activation of autophagy in mesenchymal stem cells provides tumor stromal support. Carcinogenesis 32(7):964–972. doi:10.1093/carcin/bgr029

Sauer B (1998) Inducible gene targeting in mice using the Cre/lox system. Methods 14(4):381–392. doi:10.1006/meth.1998.0593

Schepers AG, Snippert HJ, Stange DE, van den Born M, van Es JH, van de Wetering M, Clevers H (2012) Lineage tracing reveals Lgr5+ stem cell activity in mouse intestinal adenomas. Science 337(6095):730–735. doi:10.1126/science.1224676

Schwab LP, Peacock DL, Majumdar D, Ingels JF, Jensen LC, Smith KD, Cushing RC, Seagroves TN (2012) Hypoxia-inducible factor 1alpha promotes primary tumor growth and tumor-initiating cell activity in breast cancer. Breast Cancer Res 14(1):R6. doi:10.1186/bcr3087

Singh S, Brocker C, Koppaka V, Chen Y, Jackson BC, Matsumoto A, Thompson DC, Vasiliou V (2013) Aldehyde dehydrogenases in cellular responses to oxidative/electrophilic stress. Free Radic Biol Med 56:89–101. doi:10.1016/j.freeradbiomed.2012.11.010

Siolas D, Hannon GJ (2013) Patient-derived tumor xenografts: transforming clinical samples into mouse models. Cancer Res 73(17):5315–5319. doi:10.1158/0008-5472.Can-13-1069

Skibinski A, Kuperwasser C (2015) The origin of breast tumor heterogeneity. Oncogene 34(42):5309–5316. doi:10.1038/onc.2014.475

Smith AG (2001) Embryo-derived stem cells: of mice and men. Annu Rev Cell Dev Biol 17:435–462. doi:10.1146/annurev.cellbio.17.1.435

Sotelo J, Briceno E, Lopez-Gonzalez MA (2006) Adding chloroquine to conventional treatment for glioblastoma multiforme: a randomized, double-blind, placebo-controlled trial. Ann Intern Med 144(5):337–343

Stechishin OD, Luchman HA, Ruan Y, Blough MD, Nguyen SA, Kelly JJ, Cairncross JG, Weiss S (2013) On-target JAK2/STAT3 inhibition slows disease progression in orthotopic xenografts of human glioblastoma brain tumor stem cells. Neuro Oncol 15(2):198–207. doi:10.1093/neuonc/nos302

Switzer CH, Cheng RY, Ridnour LA, Glynn SA, Ambs S, Wink DA (2012) Ets-1 is a transcriptional mediator of oncogenic nitric oxide signaling in estrogen receptor-negative breast cancer. Breast Cancer Res 14(5):R125. doi:10.1186/bcr3319

Tallman MS, Andersen JW, Schiffer CA, Appelbaum FR, Feusner JH, Ogden A, Shepherd L, Willman C, Bloomfield CD, Rowe JM, Wiernik PH (1997) All-trans-retinoic acid in acute promyelocytic leukemia. New Engl J Med 337(15):1021–1028. doi:10.1056/NEJM199710093371501

Taylor WR, White NJ (2004) Antimalarial drug toxicity: a review. Drug Saf 27(1):25–61

Tefferi A, Gilliland DG (2005) The JAK2V617F tyrosine kinase mutation in myeloproliferative disorders: status report and immediate implications for disease classification and diagnosis. Mayo Clin Proc 80(7):947–958. doi:10.4065/80.7.947

Tentler JJ, Tan AC, Weekes CD, Jimeno A, Leong S, Pitts TM, Arcaroli JJ, Messersmith WA, Eckhardt SG (2012) Patient-derived tumour xenografts as models for oncology drug development. Nat Rev Clin Oncol 9(6):338–350. doi:10.1038/nrclinonc.2012.61

Thakur R, Trivedi R, Rastogi N, Singh M, Mishra DP (2015) Inhibition of STAT3, FAK and Src mediated signaling reduces cancer stem cell load, tumorigenic potential and metastasis in breast cancer. Sci Rep 5:10194. doi:10.1038/srep10194

Thiery JP (2002) Epithelial-mesenchymal transitions in tumour progression. Nat Rev Cancer 2(6):442–454. doi:10.1038/nrc822. (nrc822 [pii])

Thomsen LL, Miles DW, Happerfield L, Bobrow LG, Knowles RG, Moncada S (1995) Nitric oxide synthase activity in human breast cancer. Br J Cancer 72(1):41–44

Tiwari N, Gheldof A, Tatari M, Christofori G (2012) EMT as the ultimate survival mechanism of cancer cells. Semin Cancer Biol 22(3):194–207. doi:10.1016/

j.semcancer.2012.02.013. (S1044-579X(12)00049-1 [pii])

Tsuji T, Ibaragi S, Shima K, Hu MG, Katsurano M, Sasaki A, Hu GF (2008) Epithelial-mesenchymal transition induced by growth suppressor p12CDK2-AP1 promotes tumor cell local invasion but suppresses distant colony growth. Cancer Res 68 (24):10377–10386. doi:10.1158/0008-5472.CAN-08-1444

Vadakkan TJ, Landua JD, Bu W, Wei W, Li F, Wong ST, Dickinson ME, Rosen JM, Lewis MT, Zhang M (2014) Wnt-responsive cancer stem cells are located close to distorted blood vessels and not in hypoxic regions in a p53-null mouse model of human breast cancer. Stem Cells Transl Med 3(7):857–866. doi:10.5966/sctm.2013-0088

Vainchenker W, Constantinescu SN (2013) JAK/STAT signaling in hematological malignancies. Oncogene 32 (21):2601–2613. doi:10.1038/onc.2012.347

van Amerongen R, Nusse R (2009) Towards an integrated view of Wnt signaling in development. Development 136(19):3205–3214. doi:10.1242/dev.033910

Van Camp JK, Beckers S, Zegers D, Van Hul W (2014) Wnt signaling and the control of human stem cell fate. Stem Cell Rev 10(2):207–229. doi:10.1007/s12015-013-9486-8

Van Keymeulen A, Rocha AS, Ousset M, Beck B, Bouvencourt G, Rock J, Sharma N, Dekoninck S, Blanpain C (2011) Distinct stem cells contribute to mammary gland development and maintenance. Nature 479(7372):189–193. doi:10.1038/nature10573

Visvader JE, Smith GH (2011) Murine mammary epithelial stem cells: discovery, function, and current status. Cold Spring Harb Perspect Biol 3(2). doi:10.1101/cshperspect.a004879

Vlashi E, Pajonk F (2015) Cancer stem cells, cancer cell plasticity and radiation therapy. Semin Cancer Biol 31:28–35. doi:10.1016/j.semcancer.2014.07.001

Wagner KU, Schmidt JW (2011) The two faces of Janus kinases and their respective STATs in mammary gland development and cancer. J Carcinog 10:32. doi:10.4103/1477-3163.90677

Walther V, Alison MR (2015) Cell lineage tracing in human epithelial tissues using mitochondrial DNA mutations as clonal markers. Wiley Interdiscip Rev Dev Biol. doi:10.1002/wdev.203

Wang C, Wang Y, McNutt MA, Zhu WG (2011) Autophagy process is associated with anti-neoplastic function. Acta Biochim Biophys Sin (Shanghai) 43 (6):425–432. doi:10.1093/abbs/gmr028

Wang D, Cai C, Dong X, Yu QC, Zhang XO, Yang L, Zeng YA (2015) Identification of multipotent mammary stem cells by protein C receptor expression. Nature 517(7532):81–84. doi:10.1038/nature13851

Williams KE, Bundred NJ, Landberg G, Clarke RB, Farnie G (2015) Focal adhesion kinase and Wnt signaling regulate human ductal carcinoma in situ stem cell activity and response to radiotherapy. Stem Cells 33(2):327–341. doi:10.1002/stem.1843

Wink DA, Vodovotz Y, Laval J, Laval F, Dewhirst MW, Mitchell JB (1998) The multifaceted roles of nitric oxide in cancer. Carcinogenesis 19(5):711–721

Xing F, Okuda H, Watabe M, Kobayashi A, Pai SK, Liu W, Pandey PR, Fukuda K, Hirota S, Sugai T, Wakabayshi G, Koeda K, Kashiwaba M, Suzuki K, Chiba T, Endo M, Mo YY, Watabe K (2011) Hypoxia-induced Jagged2 promotes breast cancer metastasis and self-renewal of cancer stem-like cells. Oncogene 30(39):4075–4086. doi:10.1038/onc.2011.122

Xu J, Prosperi JR, Choudhury N, Olopade OI, Goss KH (2015) beta-Catenin is required for the tumorigenic behavior of triple-negative breast cancer cells. PLoS ONE 10(2):e0117097. doi:10.1371/journal.pone.0117097

Yamasaki K, Edington HD, McClosky C, Tzeng E, Lizonova A, Kovesdi I, Steed DL, Billiar TR (1998) Reversal of impaired wound repair in iNOS-deficient mice by topical adenoviral-mediated iNOS gene transfer. J Clin Investig 101(5):967–971. doi:10.1172/JCI2067

Yin S, Xu L, Bonfil RD, Banerjee S, Sarkar FH, Sethi S, Reddy KB (2013) Tumor-initiating cells and FZD8 play a major role in drug resistance in triple-negative breast cancer. Mol Cancer Ther 12(4):491–498. doi:10.1158/1535-7163.MCT-12-1090

Zhang X, Claerhout S, Prat A, Dobrolecki LE, Petrovic I, Lai Q, Landis MD, Wiechmann L, Schiff R, Giuliano M, Wong H, Fuqua SW, Contreras A, Gutierrez C, Huang J, Mao S, Pavlick AC, Froehlich AM, Wu MF, Tsimelzon A, Hilsenbeck SG, Chen ES, Zuloaga P, Shaw CA, Rimawi MF, Perou CM, Mills GB, Chang JC, Lewis MT (2013) A renewable tissue resource of phenotypically stable, biologically and ethnically diverse, patient-derived human breast cancer xenograft models. Cancer Res 73(15):4885–4897. doi:10.1158/0008-5472.CAN-12-4081

Zhou J, Wulfkuhle J, Zhang H, Gu P, Yang Y, Deng J, Margolick JB, Liotta LA, Petricoin E 3rd, Zhang Y (2007) Activation of the PTEN/mTOR/STAT3 pathway in breast cancer stem-like cells is required for viability and maintenance. Proc Natl Acad Sci U S A 104(41):16158–16163. doi:10.1073/pnas.0702596104

Zhu L, Cheng X, Ding Y, Shi J, Jin H, Wang H, Wu Y, Ye J, Lu Y, Wang TC, Yang CS, Tu SP (2014) Bone marrow-derived myofibroblasts promote colon tumorigenesis through the IL-6/JAK2/STAT3 pathway. Cancer Lett 343(1):80–89. doi:10.1016/j.canlet.2013.09.017

The Tumor Microenvironment as a Metastasis Biomarker in Breast Cancer

11

Joseph A. Sparano, Joan Jones, Thomas E. Rohan, Allison S. Harney, John Condeelis and Maja H. Oktay

Abstract

Distant metastasis is the primary cause of death in breast cancer, and metastasis often occurs despite potentially curative local therapy of the primary tumor. Prognostic factors for distant recurrence after local therapy are largely "tumor-centric". Defining the interactions between tumor cells and their microenvironment, and identifying the molecular mechanisms that define their interactions, provides a basis for development of metastasis biomarkers, and the ability to therapeutically target individual steps in the metastatic cascade. In vivo imaging modalities and other techniques have facilitated identification of the steps required for metastasis. These initial steps include streaming of tumor cells toward endothelial cells in collaboration with tumor-associated macrophages, formation of microanatomic structures consisting of tumor cells, macrophages, and endothelial cells, and transendothelial migration of tumor cells at these sites resulting in intravasation and dissemination to distant sites. Metastasis biomarkers that have been associated with distant recurrence in humans, and are based on observations of the tumor microenvironment, include a multiplex immunofluorescence assay that measures invasive isoforms of the actin regulatory protein Mena (a marker

J.A. Sparano (✉)
Department of Oncology, Montefiore Medical Center, Albert Einstein College of Medicine, 1300 Morris Park Avenue, Bronx, NY 10461, USA
e-mail: JSPARANO@montefiore.org

J. Jones · M.H. Oktay
Department of Pathology, Montefiore Medical Center, Albert Einstein College of Medicine, 1300 Morris Park Avenue, Bronx, NY 10461, USA

J. Jones · T.E. Rohan
Department of Epidemiology and Population Health, Montefiore Medical Center, Albert Einstein College of Medicine, 1300 Morris Park Avenue, Bronx, NY 10461, USA

J. Jones · A.S. Harney · J. Condeelis
Department of Anatomy and Structural Biology, Montefiore Medical Center, Albert Einstein College of Medicine, 1300 Morris Park Avenue, Bronx, NY 10461, USA

A.S. Harney · J. Condeelis
Gruss Lipper Biophotonics Center, Montefiore Medical Center, Albert Einstein College of Medicine, 1300 Morris Park Avenue, Bronx, NY 10461, USA

J. Jones · A.S. Harney · J. Condeelis
Integrated Imaging Program, Montefiore Medical Center, Albert Einstein College of Medicine, 1300 Morris Park Avenue, Bronx, NY 10461, USA

S. Badve and Y. Gökmen-Polar (eds.), *Molecular Pathology of Breast Cancer*, DOI 10.1007/978-3-319-41761-5_11

which we call "Mena^{calc}") that enable tumor cell streaming. Multiplex immunohistochemical assays that identify where Mena-expressing tumor cells, endothelial cells, and macrophages form microanatomic structures can serve as platforms for transendothelial migration, intravasation, and metastasis (which we call "TMEM" for tumor microenvironment of metastasis). An understanding of the signaling molecules that drive these interactions may provide a foundation for developing therapeutic strategies to prevent metastasis. There is potential for these biomarkers to both exhibit clinical utility by more accurately characterizing prognosis and thus the potential to benefit from standard therapies. They could also to predict benefit from novel interventions that prevent metastasis.

Keywords
Metastasis · Tumor microenvironment · Biomarker · Mena · TMEM · Breast cancer

11.1 Introduction

The development of distant metastasis is the primary cause of death in breast cancer. For those who present with localized breast cancer, prognostic factors for distant recurrence after local therapy and predictive factors for benefit from systemic adjuvant therapy are largely "tumor-centric". Classical clinicopathologic prognostic factors such as the number of positive axillary lymph nodes, tumor size, and tumor grade rely entirely on the histological characteristics and local burden of tumor cells rather than on the local microenvironment in which they reside or the local or distant microenvironmental niches from which they emanate from or metastasize to. Predictive factors for response to systemic therapies, such as estrogen receptor (ER) expression for endocrine therapy and HER2 overexpression for anti-HER2–directed therapy, also rely exclusively on biomarker expression in the tumor cells; the associated adjuvant systemic therapies are also largely "tumor-centric". The sole exception includes bone remodeling agents, such as bisphosphonates and inhibitors of receptor activator of nuclear factor kappa-B (RANK) ligand, which also have modest effects in reducing the risk of bone recurrence in older women with early stage disease or in treating established bone metastases. On the other hand, there are no predictive factors that identify which patients are likely to benefit from such therapy (Gralow 2012). New approaches are needed to identify biomarkers that reflect tumor-microenvironmental interactions, as are therapeutic approaches that target the interactions that drive tumor cell dissemination and their ability to seed distant organs, survive, and develop into clinically detectable metastases.

Several multiparameter gene expression assays provide prognostic information that is independent of classical clinicopathologic features (e.g., Oncotype DX, MammaPrint, Prosigna, Breast Cancer Index) (Sparano et al. 2010). Although these signatures include different genes, they provide similar prognostic information driven largely by proliferation genes and estrogen-dependent pathways, and not by the intrinsic propensity of a tumor to interact with its microenvironment, disseminate, and form metastases (Fan et al. 2006; Paik 2011; Sparano et al. 2010; Wirapati et al. 2008; Desmedt et al. 2008). Among the most widely used is the Oncotype DX Recurrence Score (RS), which is recommended by American Society of Clinical Oncology (ASCO) guidelines for use as a prognostic marker, and also as a predictive marker for chemotherapy benefit (Harris et al. 2007).

Although the RS provides a clear therapeutic direction for approximately 30 % of patients with a very low RS (endocrine therapy alone) or high RS (chemoendocrine therapy), for the remaining 70 % the benefit of chemotherapy is uncertain (Sparano and Paik 2008). This has prompted 3 large prospective trials that are now ongoing to evaluate the role of chemotherapy in patients with node-negative breast cancer and a mid-range RS of 11–25 (TAILORx), and in patients with positive axillary nodes and low to mid-range RS of less than 25 (RxPonder, OPTIMA) (Sparano and Solin 2010; Bartlett et al. 2013).

11.2 The Hallmarks of Cancer and the Tumor Microenvironment

Hanahan and Weinberg (2000) proposed "hallmarks of cancer" as an organizing principle to explain the complexities of neoplastic disease. They propose that genomic instability generates the somatic mutations and genetic diversity associated with specific "hallmarks" that classify biological capabilities of cancer cells acquired during the multistep development of human tumors. The "hallmarks" include sustained proliferative signaling, evading growth suppressors, resisting cell death, enabling replicative immortality, inducing angiogenesis, activating invasion and metastasis, reprogramming of energy metabolism and evading immune destruction. They have recently recognized that tumors also contain a repertoire of recruited non-cancer cells that contribute to the acquisition of hallmark traits by creating the "tumor microenvironment" (Hanahan and Weinberg 2011). Others have proposed that proliferation and motility are the default state of all cells, and reciprocal interactions among cells and between cells and their extracellular matrix, and thus the microenvironment, play a more central role in contributing to carcinogenesis and the acquisition of cancer hallmarks (Sonnenschein and Soto 2013; Pickup et al. 2014).

11.3 Epithelial-to-Mesenchymal Transition (EMT), Mena, and Metastasis

Epithelial-to-mesenchymal transition ("EMT") is a developmental regulatory program involved in normal embryogenesis, wound healing, and fibrosis that is also implicated in the development of tumor invasion and metastasis. EMT confers traits which characterize malignant cells, including motility, invasiveness, heightened resistance to apoptosis, and dissemination from primary tumor sites (Thiery et al. 2009). It is these metastatic colonies that are responsible for almost all carcinoma-associated mortality (Fidler and Poste 2008). The EMT program is thought to be initiated in neoplastic epithelial cells by a confluence of heterotypic signals received from the nearby stroma (Kalluri and Weinberg 2009). Activation of the EMT program is associated with shifts in the expression of thousands of mRNAs and accompanying changes in the expression levels of many of the corresponding proteins. The EMT-associated changes in epithelial and mesenchymal genes and proteins can be observed both in preclinical models and in cancer in humans.

Along with transcriptional control, post-transcriptional mechanisms also regulate mRNAs encoding EMT/metastasis-relevant proteins. One critical layer of post-transcriptional regulation during EMT and tumor progression involves the production of distinct mRNA isoforms through alternative splicing (Warzecha and Carstens 2012). The resulting mRNA isoforms encode distinct protein products that can have subtle or dramatically different functions (Ellis et al. 2012). For example, Mena, a molecule involved in regulation of actin dynamics and cell adhesion, undergoes EMT-dependent and tumor microenvironment-dependent changes in alternative splicing producing isoforms with distinct functions that influence tumor progression (Gertler and Condeelis 2011). Specifically, alternative splicing of Mena gives rise to multiple mRNAs that encode functionally distinct protein isoforms that are expressed in specific tissues and cell-types.

In the context of breast cancer, at least three Mena isoforms, each with distinct activities and sensitivities to epidermal growth factor (EGF), are expressed during tumor progression. An isoform containing only the constitutively-included Mena exons is expressed throughout tumor progression. Inclusion of the normally epithelial-specific 11a exon gives rise to "Mena11a", which is expressed in well-differentiated tumor cells and suppresses tumor cell motility and chemotaxis (Roussos et al. 2011a, c). In normal tissue and cells, the Mena11a isoform is expressed exclusively in epithelial cells, and inclusion of 11a in Mena is suppressed as cells undergo an EMT (Shapiro et al. 2011). Consistent with its cellular function, Mena11a has an apparent anti-metastatic effect as patients with relatively low Mena11a levels (as a proportion of total Mena) exhibit significantly poorer clinical outcome (Agarwal et al. 2012).

An isoform of Mena associated with tumor cell streaming and invasiveness (called "Mena^{INV}") is expressed in poorly differentiated, aggressive, and highly migratory and invasive tumor cells (Goswami et al. 2009). Upregulation of Mena^{INV} is associated with a migratory subpopulation of tumor cells that are chemotactic to EGF in vivo (Goswami et al. 2009). Mena^{INV} expression increases tumor cell motility and invasion, and potentiates chemotactic responses to epidermal growth factor (EGF) both in vitro and in vivo (Philippar et al. 2008; Roussos et al. 2011a).

11.4 Role of Mena and Cofilin in Promoting Tumor Cell Motility and Metastasis

Mena in the Rho/Cofilin/Mena signaling axis inhibits capping protein so as to amplify the effects of cofilin and N-WASP on actin polymerization (Gertler and Condeelis 2011; Roussos et al. 2011a, b). Mena^{INV} is a Mena isoform which promotes metastasis by sensitizing the EGF receptor to EGF thereby increasing the amount of active cofilin in protrusions, causing increased actin polymerization, protrusion and chemotaxis in response to EGF and other growth factors (Roussos et al. 2011a, b). This finding places Mena as a key regulator of actin polymerization and tumor cell migration in the Rho/Cofilin/Mena signaling axis. Mena knockout mice, crossbred with PyMT-oncogene carrying mice, develop primary mammary tumors that grow at the same rate as in wild type mice, but have dramatically fewer metastatic tumors. This is correlated with almost complete absence of dissemination of tumor cells from the primary tumor (Roussos et al. 2010).

Migrating tumor cells use two types of protrusions at the cell front, invadopods and locomotory protrusions, to invade and migrate in vivo (Desmarais et al. 2009; Bravo-Cordero et al. 2012). These two types of protrusions are regulated by cofilin and Mena during invasion as described in detail elsewhere (Bravo-Cordero et al. 2011, 2012, 2013a, b; Roussos et al. 2011b). Cofilin activity in locomotory protrusions generates localized increases in actin polymerization that is required for chemotactic sensing of EGF gradients (Mouneimne et al. 2006; van Rheenen et al. 2007; Oser and Condeelis 2009; Bravo-Cordero et al. 2011, 2012; Magalhaes et al. 2011; Wang et al. 2007a). Cofilin is activated locally in tumor cells by release from binding to PI(4,5)P2 in locomotory protrusions such as pseudopods, and release from binding to cortactin in invasive protrusions (invadopods) (van Rheenen et al. 2007; Oser and Condeelis 2009; Magalhaes et al. 2011). Regulation of cofilin activity by the regulatory G-proteins of the Rho/Cofilin/Mena signaling axis is required for chemotaxis to EGF, migration, intravasation and metastasis in vivo in mice, as well as chemotaxis, invadopod assembly and transendothelial migration in mouse and human breast tumor cells in vitro (Wang et al. 2006; Oser and Condeelis 2009; Bravo-Cordero et al. 2011; Magalhaes et al. 2011; Mouneimne et al. 2006). RhoC is responsible for determining the spatial distribution of cofilin activity in both locomotory and invasive protrusions, leading to amplification of actin polymerization and efficient chemotaxis and invasion (Bravo-Cordero et al. 2011). RhoA is required for macrophage-induced invadopod assembly and maturation during intravasation (Roh-Johnson et al. 2013; Sakurai-Yageta et al. 2008). Mena is key regulator of all of these pathways, including EGFR, cortactin and Rho-G protein signaling (Bravo-Cordero et al. 2013a). In addition, RhoA is activated by Mena in carcinoma cells (Lin et al. 2014).

11.5 Interaction Between Migratory Tumor Cells and the Microenvironment

As described above, Mena and cofilin are critical regulators of tumor cell motility. Multi-photon microscopy has been used to observe the behavior of motile tumor cells at single cell resolution in mammary tumors in living mice in real time. This has demonstrated the presence of a subpopulation of tumor cells that are discohesive and migratory, as demonstrated schematically in Fig. 11.1. In vitro these carcinoma cells form migratory streams when associated with macrophages on linear 2 μm diameter collagen-I fibers which have a coating of fibronectin (Sharma et al. 2012). The tumor cell-macrophage tropism results from EGF/CSF1-paracrine chemotaxis causing the formation of tumor cell-macrophage cell pairs and streams (Roussos et al. 2011b; Patsialou et al. 2013). The unidirectional streaming of tumor cell-macrophage

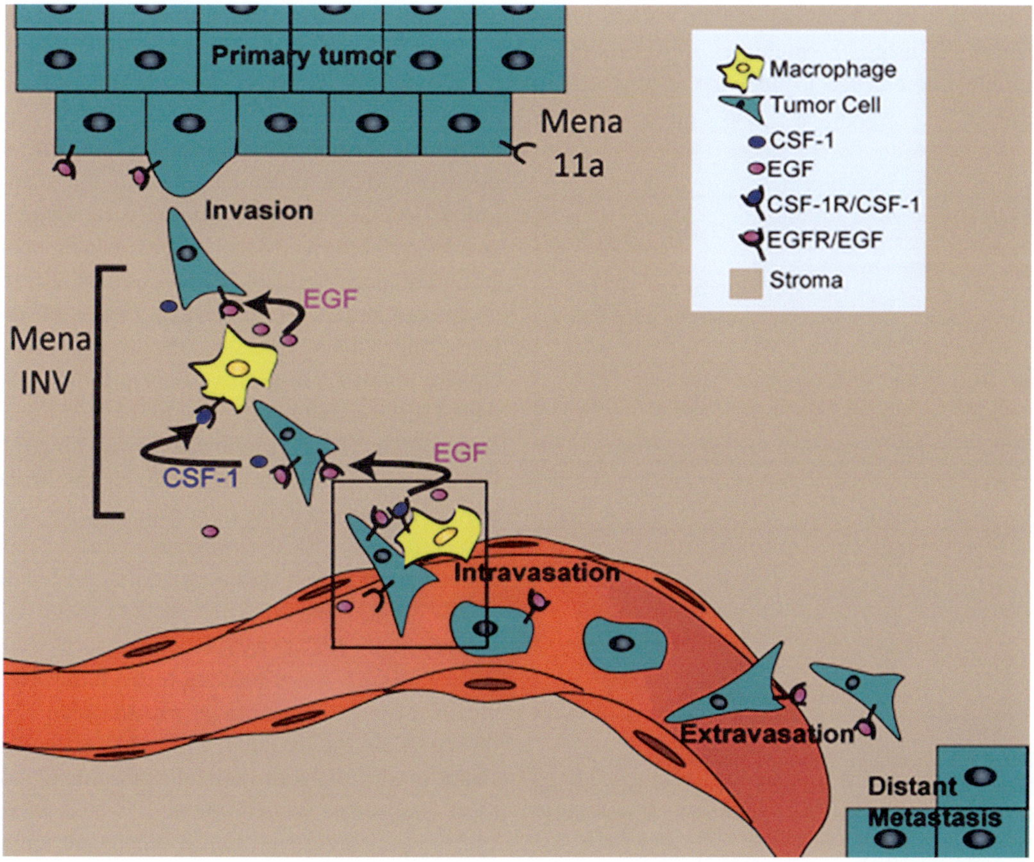

Fig. 11.1 Role of Mena in tumor cell streaming and formation of Tumor Microenvironment of Metastasis (TMEM) structures that serve as tumor cell intravasation sites. Cartoon depicting findings in mouse, rat and human mammary tumors. Alternative splicing of Mena 11a and Mena^{Inv}, in primary tumor results in a $\text{Mena}^{\text{INVHi}}$ and Mena 11a^{Lo} subpopulation of tumor cells capable of streaming migration toward blood vessels where they contribute to TMEM assembly and function

cell pairs is a spontaneously emergent phenomenon resulting not only from chemotactic signaling between macrophages and tumor cells in the paracrine loop, but also from an additional endothelial cell associated signals emanating from blood vessels. These signals result in endothelium directed streaming of the cell pairs and the formation of microanatomic structures consisting of a Mena-overexpressing tumor cell, endothelial cell, and macrophage in direct contact, which has been named "TMEM" (Tumor Microenvironment of Metastasis) (Robinson et al. 2009). TMEM are identifiable in human breast cancer (Fig. 11.2) and are associated with risk of distant recurrence. The tumor cells involved in migration toward and assembly of TMEM structures express invasive Mena isoforms that may be measured in human breast cancer using multiplex quantitative immunofluorescence to generate a score called "Mena^{calc}", which is also prognostic for recurrence and survival (Fig. 11.3) (Agarwal et al. 2012).

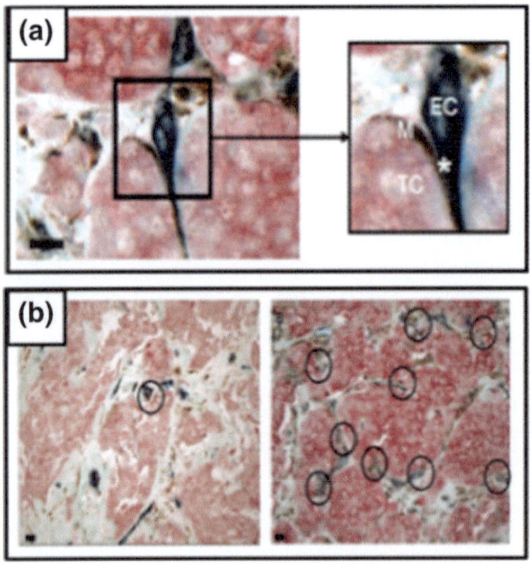

Fig. 11.2 Identifying TMEM structures in primary human breast cancer. **a** *TMEM* direct contact between an invasive tumor cell (anti-pan-Mena), a perivascular macrophage (anti-CD68), and an endothelia cell (anti-CD31).*TMEM score* number of TMEMs per 10 high power field (400× magnification). **b** Examples of a primary breast cancer with low TMEM score (*left*) and high TMEM score (*right*) (Robinson et al. 2009; Rohan et al. 2014)

11.6 Motility and Transendothelial Migration (TREM) Are Required for Development of Metastasis

Migratory tumor cells are also required to undergo transendothelial migration (TREM) in order to traverse the vascular endothelium and metastasize to distant sites. The migration and TMEM assembly phenotypes of disseminating tumor cells depend on the Rho/Cofilin/Mena signaling axis within a metastasis invasion signature (Roussos et al. 2011b; Patsialou et al. 2012) and involve switching from a migratory to a TREM competent phenotype at blood vessels (Gligorijevic et al. 2014). The activation of this pathway and the phenotype switching is supported by coordinated increased expression of invasive Mena isoforms (Mena^{Classic} and Mena^{INV}) and decreased expression of suppressive Mena isoforms (Mena 11A) (Patsialou et al. 2012; Philippar et al. 2008; Roussos et al. 2011a, c; Bravo-Cordero et al. 2011). Genes of the Rho/Cofilin/Mena signaling axis are also differentially regulated in primary human tumor cells with TREM activity compared to those in tumor cells without TREM activity (Shapiro et al. 2011; Patsialou et al. 2012; Pignatelli et al. 2014). Similar differential expression patterns have been observed in TREM-competent tumor cells derived from breast tumor cell lines, including MDA-MB-231 and MTLn3 cell lines (both "triple negative" lines), PyMT-derived met1 cells ($ER/PR^{+}HER2^{-}$), and primary breast tumor cells obtained from a breast cancer patient called TN1 (Wang et al. 2007b, 2004; Liu et al. 2010; Patsialou et al. 2012). In particular, the Mena isoform expression pattern Mena^{INVHi} and Mena 11a^{Lo} was observed in TREM competent tumor cells derived from both cell lines and primary tumor cells from breast cancer patients (Pignatelli et al. 2014).

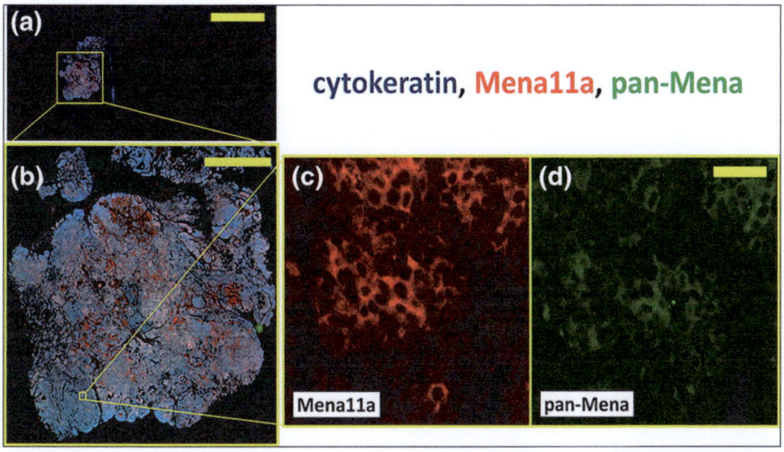

Fig. 11.3 Multiplex quantitative immunofluorescence for scoring of Mena^{Calc}. High-throughput automated analysis of fluorescence images performed on whole digital slides are used to score Mena^{Calc} for large cohorts. **a** Whole slide scan of a triple stained tumor section. *Bar* 10,000 um, **b** Zoom into just tumor tissue of interest. *Bar* 2000 um, **c** and **d** Single high power field of view showing individual sells stained with Mena11a (*Red*) and pan-Mena (*Green*) *Bar* 25 µm. Each case is scored for Mena^{Calc} (Pan-Mena minus Mena11a normalized intensity, on one slide [*pixel size* 1.0 µm (Agarwal et al. 2012)]. *Source* Reproduced with permission from Robinson et al. Clinical Cancer Research 2009

11.7 TREM and Intravasation Occur at TMEM Sites in Primary Tumors

We have used multiphoton intravital imaging to reveal the mechanism of TMEM assembly and function as schematically summarized below and in Fig. 11.4 (Harney et al. 2015). The key steps include: (1) initial streaming of cells which form pairs by CSF1/CSF1R and EGF/EGFR paracrine loop chemotactic signaling which contributes to their migration toward blood vessels, (2) TMEM assembly, which involves a direct heterotypic cell-cell interaction between the tumor cell and macrophage within the assembling TMEM resulting in the initiation of an invadopodium by the tumor cell which protrudes between endothelial cells in TMEM, (3) TMEM function, involving the local transient loss of endothelial cell junctions at TMEM caused by release of VEGF by the TMEM macrophage resulting in a transient opening between endothelial cells, and (4) TREM of tumor cells in the vicinity of TMEM.

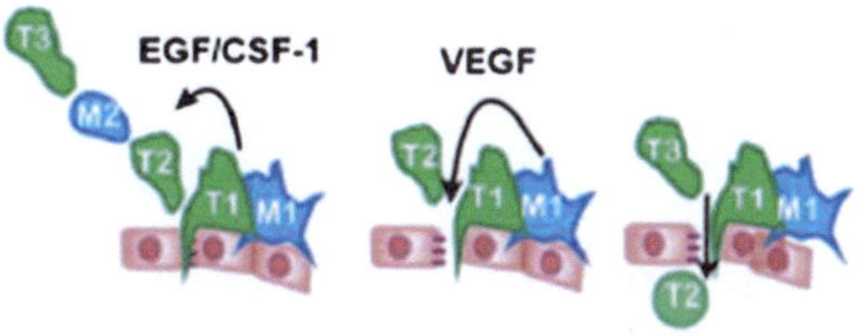

Fig. 11.4 Schematic of TMEM function. TMEM assemble with close association between the non-migratory TMEM Tumor Cell 1 (*green* T1) and Tie2^{Hi}/VEGFA^{Hi} macrophage (*blue* M1) on blood vessel endothelial cells (*red*). TMEM macrophage-released VEGFA destabilizes vascular junctions resulting in local vascular permeability at the TMEM Tumor Cell (*T1*) while Tumor Cell 2 (*T2*) intravasates. *Source* Reproduced with permission from Harney et al. Cancer Discovery 2015

Tumor cell lines (rat MTLn3 and human MDA-MB 231) and human primary breast carcinoma cells assemble TMEM in vitro after co-incubation of macrophages and tumor cells on a sealed endothelial monolayer for several hours (Roussos et al. 2011a; Roh-Johnson et al. 2013). The contact between the macrophage and tumor cell in TMEM initiates activation of RhoA in the

TMEM tumor cell. RhoA is required for macrophage-induced invadopodium assembly and maturation during intravasation (Roh-Johnson et al. 2013; Sakurai-Yageta et al. 2008). RhoA is activated by an unknown isoform of Mena in carcinoma cells (Lin et al. 2014).

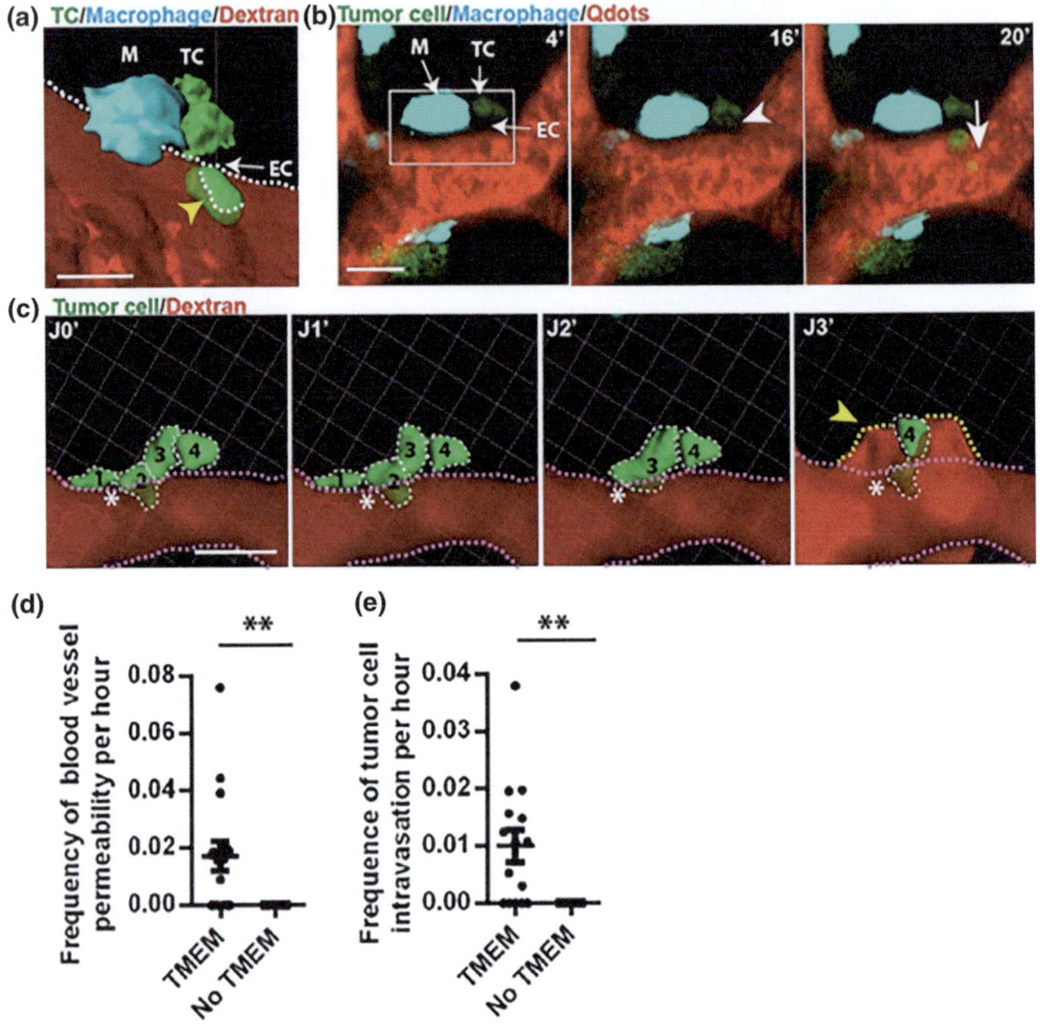

Fig. 11.5 Transient, local blood vessel permeability events accompany intravasation at TMEM. **a** 3D reconstruction of tumor cell (TC) intravasation (*yellow arrowhead*) at TMEM (luminal surface of the endothelium *dashed white line*). **b** Intravital microscopy (IVM) time lapse of tumor cell intravasation at TMEM [*white box* in 4′ panel containing stationary TMEM-Macrophage (*M*), -Tumor cell (*TC*) and -endothelial cell boundary (*EC*) (*arrows*)]. A non-TMEM tumor cell arrives at TMEM (*arrowhead* in panel 16′) and undergoes transendothelial migration (*arrow* in panel 20′) while TMEM-macrophage and TMEM-tumor cell remain immobile. *Scale bar* 10 μm. **c** 3D reconstruction of IVM time-lapse of tumor cell intravasation at TMEM (*white asterisk*). Transmigrating tumor cells (individually *numbered*, *dashed white lines*) are isolated from other cell types for clarity with time in minutes from start (*J0′*) to end of transmigration (*J3′*). The luminal endothelial surface is outlined in a *pink dashed line*. Extravascular dextran (*red*) leaking out of vessel at TMEM indicated with a *yellow arrowhead* and outlined in a *yellow dashed line*. **d** Frequency of blood vessel permeability events in the presence of TMEM or away from TMEM in 100 μm windows ($n = 16$, **, $P = 0.0034$). **e** Frequency of tumor cell intravasation events in the presence of TMEM or away from TMEM in 100 μm windows ($n = 16$, **, $P = 0.0012$). **d** and **e** show that vascular permeability and its associated intravasation of tumor cells occurs only at TMEM. *Source* Reproduced with permission from Harney et al. Cancer Discovery 2015

Use of high-resolution two-photon microscopy in the MMTV-PyMT mammary carcinoma cell lines and in patient-derived xenografts has shown that transient blood vessel permeability (bursting) and accompanying tumor cell intravasation occurs exclusively at TMEM sites (Fig. 11.5). Furthermore, the secretion of VEGFA from the pro-angiogenic $Tie2^{Hi}/VEGFA^{Hi}$ perivascular macrophage in TMEM leads to TMEM-associated transient blood vessel permeability and tumor cell intravasation (Harney et al. 2015). Tumor vasculature has been shown to be leaky, but it has not been appreciated from static studies that vessel leakiness is in fact a dynamic event that is regulated by TMEM-associated perivascular macrophages.

11.8 Invasive Mena Isoforms, TMEM Structures, and Recurrence in Human Breast Cancer

Based upon the preclinical data described above, it would be expected that higher expression of invasive Mena isoforms or higher TMEM counts in primary tumors would be associated with a higher rate of distant recurrence in early stage breast cancer. There have been four studies reported thus far evaluating these associations, as summarized in Table 11.1, including two studies evaluating invasive Mena isoform expression, and 2 studies evaluating TMEM counts (or TMEM "score").

Table 11.1 Evaluation of TMEM or $Mena^{Calc}$ in localized breast cancer

Marker	Method	Source	No.	Main findings (reference)
TMEM	Case: Control	Whole sections	60	• Higher median TMEM score in cases with distant recurrence compared with controls without distant recurrence (median TMEM density 150 vs. 50, $p = 0.00006$) • Odds ratio 1.9 (95 % confidence intervals 1.1–3.4) in the risk of distant recurrence for every 10 unit increase in TMEM density (Robinson et al. 2009)
TMEM	Nested case: Control	Whole sections	259 case control pairs	• TMEM score associated with distant recurrence in ER-positive, HER2 negative disease when evaluated in multivariate model including tumor size, nodal status, grade and IHC4 (odds ratio 2.67, $p = 0004$ for highest vs. lowest tertile) • TMEM score did not correlate with IHC4 (Spearman correlation 0.09) (Rohan et al. 2014)
$Mena^{calc}$	2 Cohorts	TMA	501/296	• $Mena^{calc}$ associated with higher risk of recurrence when evaluated as a dichotomous variable (hazard ratio 1.6, $p = 0.0015$ in comparison of highest quartile vs. lowest 3 quartiles) in multivariate model including age, nodal status, nuclear grade, and tumor size • $Mena^{calc}$ associated with higher risk of recurrence when evaluated as a continuous variable (hazard ratio 1.21, $p = 0.0016$) (Agarwal et al. 2012)
$Mena^{calc}$	Cohort	TMA	403	• In this cohort of node negative breast cancer patients, $Mena^{calc}$ was associated with decreased overall survival (odds ratio for risk of death = 2.0, $p = 0.0293$) in a multivariate model including HER2 status, tumor size, hormone receptor status, nuclear grade, age and lymphatic invasion • $Mena^{calc}$ was associated with decreased overall survival in a subset of patients who received no adjuvant hormone or chemotherapy (n = 143, odds ratio 3.77 $p = 0.0090$) (Forse et al. 2014)

Given the mechanistic roles of invasive isoforms Mena^{Classic} and Mena^{INV} and the invasion suppressive effects of Mena11a, a multiplex quantitative immunofluorescence (MQIF) method was used to evaluate formalin-fixed, paraffin-embedded (FFPE) tumor specimens in which the fraction of Mena protein that may promote invasion is inferred by subtraction of the non-invasive isoform (Mena11a) from the total Mena present in tumors containing Mena^{Classic} and Mena^{INV} (Agarwal et al. 2012). This biomarker, named "Mena^{calc}", was developed by subtracting the normalized automated quantitative analysis (AQUA) value of Mena11a from the normalized AQUA value of pan-Mena (i.e., subtract the mean Mena11a AQUA score for the study population from the AQUA score for the individual and divide by the standard deviation) (see Fig. 11.3). The association between Mena^{calc} and risk of death from breast cancer was studied in two cohorts of breast cancer patients (501 patients and 296 patients) who had surgery for breast cancer at Yale University Cancer Center (Agarwal et al. 2012). In both cohorts, relatively high Mena^{calc} levels were associated with poor outcome. In a multivariate analysis in which the 2 cohorts were combined, the hazard ratio for the highest quartile level of Mena^{calc} versus the lowest 3 quartiles was 1.60 (95 % confidence intervals [CI] 1.20–2.13) after adjusting for clinical variables. A second analysis was reported using tumor specimens prospectively collected from 403 axillary node negative breast cancer patients treated at eight Toronto hospitals between 1987 and 1996 (Forse et al. 2014). In this analysis, higher Mena^{calc} expression (in the upper two quartiles) was independently associated with decreased overall survival in multivariate analysis including HER2 overexpression, tumor size, hormone receptor expression, nuclear grade, patient age and lymphatic invasion (relative risk = 2.01, 95 % CI 0.07–3.77, $p = 0.0293$). Reduced overall survival was also observed when the multivariate model was applied to a subset 143 patients who did not receive adjuvant hormonal therapy or chemotherapy (RR = 3.77, 95 % CI 1.39–10.21 $p = 0.0090$).

There have been two reports evaluating the association between TMEM score and metastatic outcome. TMEM score was evaluated in FFPE primary breast cancers using a triple immunostain described in Fig. 11.2 that allows for simultaneous visualization of the macrophage (anti-CD68), endothelial cell (anti-CD31), and Mena overexpressing tumor cell (anti-pan Mena) that are in direct contact with one another in TMEM (Falini et al. 1993; Parums et al. 1990). The first report involved a case: control study including 60 patients with invasive ductal carcinoma, 30 of whom had developed subsequent distant metastasis (cases) and 30 who had not (controls)—the controls were individually matched to the cases based on standard prognostic variables (Robinson et al. 2009). A representative section of each patient's tumor was stained with the triple immunostain and examined by a pathologist blinded to outcome for assessment of TMEM score. The analysis indicated that the risk of metastasis nearly doubled (odds ratio (OR) = 1.9, 95 % CI 1.1–3.4) for every 10 unit increase in TMEM score. However, the study was small, and therefore the estimates of risk were imprecise. Furthermore, the inclusion criteria were rather restrictive (moderately or poorly differentiated tumors with ≥ 5 years of follow-up time), thereby limiting the generalizability of the findings. Given these limitations, we recently completed a population-based case-control study nested within a cohort of 3760 breast cancer patients diagnosed with invasive ductal carcinoma of the breast between 1980 and 2000 at Kaiser Permanente Northwest and followed through 2010 (Rohan et al. 2014). Cases were women who developed a subsequent distant metastasis; controls, selected using incidence density sampling, were matched (1:1) closely to cases on age at and calendar year of primary diagnosis. TMEM was assessed by triple immunostain and IHC4 by standard methods. IHC4 is an algorithm that integrates information derived from immunohistochemistry for ER, PR, HER2, and Ki67, and has been shown to correlate with multiparameter gene expression assays (e.g., recurrence score) and provide similar prognostic information (Cuzick et al. 2011). The stained slides were read by pathologists blinded to clinical outcomes. Odd ratios (ORs) and 95 % CI were estimated using logistic regression, with adjustment for clinical variables; also, a receiver operating characteristic (ROC) analysis was performed and the area under the curve (AUC) was estimated. TMEM score (the total number of TMEM sites in 10 high power fields) was associated with increased risk of distant metastasis in ER-positive/HER2-negative tumors (multivariate $OR_{\text{high vs. low tertile}} = 2.70$, 95 % CI 1.39–5.26), $P_{\text{trend}} = 0.004$), whereas IHC4 score had a borderline positive association ($OR_{\text{10 unit increase}} = 1.06$, 95 % CI 1.00–1.13); the association for TMEM score persisted after adjustment for IHC4 score. On ROC analysis, the AUC for a TMEM composite score (obtained from a multivariate logistic regression model with TMEM score and the clinical variables) was 0.78. The cross-validated ROC/AUC for the TMEM composite score (0.74) differed little from the ROC/AUC estimated using all of the data, indicating minimal overoptimism. Defining a low risk group as those with TMEM composite scores ≤ -0.94 (90 % sensitivity) and a high risk group as those with TMEM composite scores ≥ 0.70 (90 % specificity), we estimated that the absolute risks (95 % CI) of distant metastasis in the low, medium, and high risk groups were 5.9 % (95 % CI 5.1–6.9 %), 14.1 % (95 % CI 13.0–15.2 %), and 30.3 % (95 % CI 26.1–35.4 %), respectively. Neither TMEM score nor IHC4 score was independently associated with metastatic risk overall, or in the triple negative or HER2-negative subgroups. These findings indicate that TMEM score is positively associated with risk of distant metastasis in women with ER-positive/HER2-negative breast cancer and provides prognostic information that is independent of IHC4 score and other clinicopathologic risk factors.

11.9 Conclusions

The work described above suggests that the mechanism of hematogenous dissemination of breast cancer in humans is likely similar to that seen in mice and rats, where tumor cells expressing invasive Mena isoforms stream toward and intravasate in association with TMEM (Goswami et al. 2009; Wyckoff et al. 2007; Roussos et al. 2011a, b, c; Harney et al. 2015). The methodology for identifying and counting TMEM sites and for assessing the relative amount of invasive Mena isoforms is well developed and reproducible, and the association with distant recurrence and survival is robust, establishing both the analytic validity and clinical validity of these assays, respectively. Additional work is ongoing that will serve to strengthen the analytic validity and reproducibility of these assays and provide additional evidence supporting their clinical validity. The ultimate goal is to establish clinical utility of these assays by demonstrating that they impact therapeutic decision making, either by identifying patients at higher risk of recurrence and more likely to benefit from standard therapies (e.g., chemotherapy, endocrine therapy), or possibly by identify patients more likely to benefit from novel therapies which interfere with individual or sequential steps in the metastatic process.

References

Agarwal S, Gertler FB, Balsamo M et al (2012) Quantitative assessment of invasive mena isoforms (Menacalc) as an independent prognostic marker in breast cancer. Breast Cancer Res 14(5):R124

Bartlett J, Canney P, Campbell A et al (2013) Selecting breast cancer patients for chemotherapy: the opening of the UK OPTIMA trial. Clin Oncol (R Coll Radiol) 25(2):109–116

Bravo-Cordero JJ, Oser M, Chen X, Eddy R, Hodgson L, Condeelis J (2011) A novel spatiotemporal RhoC activation pathway locally regulates cofilin activity at invadopodia. Curr Biol 21(8):635–644

Bravo-Cordero JJ, Hodgson L, Condeelis J (2012) Directed cell invasion and migration during metastasis. Curr Opin Cell Biol 24(2):277–283

Bravo-Cordero JJ, Magalhaes MA, Eddy RJ, Hodgson L, Condeelis J (2013a) Functions of cofilin in cell locomotion and invasion. Nat Rev Mol Cell Biol 14 (7):405–415

Bravo-Cordero JJ, Sharma VP, Roh-Johnson M et al (2013b) Spatial regulation of RhoC activity defines protrusion formation in migrating cells. J Cell Sci 126 (Pt 15):3356–3369

Cuzick J, Dowsett M, Pineda S et al (2011) Prognostic value of a combined estrogen receptor, progesterone receptor, Ki-67, and human epidermal growth factor receptor 2 immunohistochemical score and comparison with the Genomic Health recurrence score in early breast cancer. J Clin Oncol 29(32):4273–4278

Desmarais V, Yamaguchi H, Oser M et al (2009) N-WASP and cortactin are involved in invadopodium-dependent chemotaxis to EGF in breast tumor cells. Cell Motil Cytoskeleton 66(6):303–316

Desmedt C, Haibe-Kains B, Wirapati P et al (2008) Biological processes associated with breast cancer clinical outcome depend on the molecular subtypes. Clin Cancer Res 14(16):5158–5165

Ellis JD, Barrios-Rodiles M, Colak R et al (2012) Tissue-specific alternative splicing remodels protein-protein interaction networks. Mol Cell 46 (6):884–892

Falini B, Flenghi L, Pileri S et al (1993) PG-M1: a new monoclonal antibody directed against a fixative-esistant epitope on the macrophage-restricted form of the CD68 molecule. Am J Pathol 142(5):1359–1372

Fan C, Oh DS, Wessels L et al (2006) Concordance among gene-expression-based predictors for breast cancer. N Engl J Med 355(6):560–569

Fidler IJ, Poste G (2008) The "seed and soil" hypothesis revisited. Lancet Oncol 9(8):808

Forse CL, Agarwal S, Pinnaduwage D et al (2014) Menacalc, a quantitative method of metastasis assessment, as a prognostic marker for axillary node-negative breast cancer. In: USCAP annual meeting, San Diego, 1–7 March 2014

Gertler F, Condeelis J (2011) Metastasis: tumor cells becoming MENAcing. Trends Cell Biol 21(2):81–90

Gligorijevic B, Bergman A, Condeelis J (2014) Multiparametric classification links tumor microenvironments with tumor cell phenotype. PLoS Biol 12(11): e1001995

Goswami S, Philippar U, Sun D et al (2009) Identification of invasion specific splice variants of the cytoskeletal protein Mena present in mammary tumor cells during invasion in vivo. Clin Exp Metastasis 26(2):153–159

Gralow J (2012) Can bone-targeted therapy reduce recurrence and improve survival in early-stage breast cancer? Oncology (Williston Park) 26(10):969–970

Hanahan D, Weinberg RA (2000) The hallmarks of cancer. Cell 100(1):57–70

Hanahan D, Weinberg RA (2011) Hallmarks of cancer: the next generation. Cell 144(5):646–674

Harney AS, Arwert EN, Entenberg D et al (2015) Perivascular macrophages regulate tumor cell intravasation by inducing localized transient blood vessel permeability through VEGF signaling. Cancer Discov 5(9):932–943

Harris L, Fritsche H, Mennel R et al (2007) American Society of Clinical Oncology 2007 update of recommendations for the use of tumor markers in breast cancer. J Clin Oncol 25(33):5287–5312

Kalluri R, Weinberg RA (2009) The basics of epithelial-mesenchymal transition. J Clin Invest 119 (6):1420–1428

Lin L, Yang XM, Li J, Zhang YL, Qin W, Zhang ZG (2014) Microfilament regulatory protein MENA increases activity of RhoA and promotes metastasis of hepatocellular carcinoma. Exp Cell Res 327 (1):113–132

Liu H, Patel MR, Prescher JA et al (2010) Cancer stem cells from human breast tumors are involved in spontaneous metastases in orthotopic mouse models. Proc Natl Acad Sci U S A 107(42):18115–18120

Magalhaes MA, Larson DR, Mader CC et al (2011) Cortactin phosphorylation regulates cell invasion through a pH-dependent pathway. J Cell Biol 195 (5):903–920

Mouneimne G, DesMarais V, Sidani M et al (2006) Spatial and temporal control of cofilin activity is required for directional sensing during chemotaxis. Curr Biol 16(22):2193–2205

Oser M, Condeelis J (2009) The cofilin activity cycle in lamellipodia and invadopodia. J Cell Biochem 108 (6):1252–1262

Paik S (2011) Is gene array testing to be considered routine now? Breast 20(Suppl 3):S87–91

Parums DV, Cordell JL, Micklem K, Heryet AR, Gatter KC, Mason DY (1990) JC70: a new monoclonal antibody that detects vascular endothelium associated antigen on routinely processed tissue sections. J Clin Pathol 43(9):752–757

Patsialou A, Wang Y, Lin J et al (2012) Selective gene-expression profiling of migratory tumor cells in vivo predicts clinical outcome in breast cancer patients. Breast Cancer Res 14(5):R139

Patsialou A, Bravo-Cordero JJ, Wang Y et al (2013) Intravital multiphoton imaging reveals multicellular streaming as a crucial component of in vivo cell migration in human breast tumors. IntraVital 2(2)

Philippar U, Roussos ET, Oser M et al (2008) A Mena invasion isoform potentiates EGF-induced carcinoma cell invasion and metastasis. Dev Cell 15(6):813–828

Pickup MW, Mouw JK, Weaver VM (2014) The extracellular matrix modulates the hallmarks of cancer. EMBO Rep 15(12):1243–1253

Pignatelli J, Goswami S, Jones JG et al (2014) Invasive breast carcinoma cells from patients exhibit MenaINV-and macrophage-dependent transendothelial migration. Sci Signal 7(353):ra112

Robinson BD, Sica GL, Liu YF et al (2009) Tumor microenvironment of metastasis in human breast carcinoma: a potential prognostic marker linked to hematogenous dissemination. Clin Cancer Res 15 (7):2433–2441

Rohan T, Xue X, Lin HM et al (2014) Tumor Microenvironment of metastasis and risk of distant metastasis of breast cancer. J Natl Cancer Inst 106(8)

Roh-Johnson M, Bravo-Cordero JJ, Patsialou A et al (2013) Macrophage contact induces RhoA GTPase signaling to trigger tumor cell intravasation. Oncogene 33(33):4203–4212

Roussos ET, Wang Y, Wyckoff JB et al (2010) Mena deficiency delays tumor progression and decreases metastasis in polyoma middle-T transgenic mouse mammary tumors. Breast Cancer Res 12(6):R101

Roussos ET, Balsamo M, Alford SK et al (2011a) Mena invasive (MenaINV) promotes multicellular streaming motility and transendothelial migration in a mouse model of breast cancer. J Cell Sci 124(Pt 13):2120–2131

Roussos ET, Condeelis JS, Patsialou A (2011b) Chemotaxis in cancer. Nat Rev Cancer 11(8):573–587

Roussos ET, Goswami S, Balsamo M et al (2011c) Mena invasive (Mena(INV)) and Mena11a isoforms play distinct roles in breast cancer cell cohesion and association with TMEM. Clin Exp Metastasis 28 (6):515–527

Sakurai-Yageta M, Recchi C, Le Dez G et al (2008) The interaction of IQGAP1 with the exocyst complex is required for tumor cell invasion downstream of Cdc42 and RhoA. J Cell Biol 181(6):985–998

Shapiro IM, Cheng AW, Flytzanis NC et al (2011) An EMT-driven alternative splicing program occurs in human breast cancer and modulates cellular phenotype. PLoS Genet 7(8):e1002218

Sharma VP, Beaty BT, Patsialou A et al (2012) Reconstitution of in vivo macrophage-tumor cell pairing and streaming motility on one-dimensional micropatterned substrates. Intravital 1(1):77–85

Sonnenschein C, Soto AM (2013) The aging of the 2000 and 2011 Hallmarks of cancer reviews: a critique. J Biosci 38(3):651–663

Sparano JA, Paik S (2008) Development of the 21-gene assay and its application in clinical practice and clinical trials. J Clin Oncol 26(5):721–728

Sparano JA, Solin LJ (2010) Defining the clinical utility of gene expression assays in breast cancer: the intersection of science and art in clinical decision making. J Clin Oncol 28(10):1625–1627

Sparano JA, Fazzari M, Kenny PA (2010) Clinical application of gene expression profiling in breast cancer. Surg Oncol Clin N Am 19(3):581–606

Thiery JP, Acloque H, Huang RY, Nieto MA (2009) Epithelial-mesenchymal transitions in development and disease. Cell 139(5):871–890

van Rheenen J, Song X, van Roosmalen W et al (2007) EGF-induced PIP2 hydrolysis releases and activates cofilin locally in carcinoma cells. J Cell Biol 179 (6):1247–1259

Wang W, Goswami S, Lapidus K et al (2004) Identification and testing of a gene expression signature of invasive carcinoma cells within primary mammary tumors. Cancer Res 64(23):8585–8594

Wang W, Mouneimne G, Sidani M et al (2006) The activity status of cofilin is directly related to invasion, intravasation, and metastasis of mammary tumors. J Cell Biol 173(3):395–404

Wang W, Eddy R, Condeelis J (2007a) The cofilin pathway in breast cancer invasion and metastasis. Nat Rev Cancer 7(6):429–440

Wang W, Wyckoff JB, Goswami S et al (2007b) Coordinated regulation of pathways for enhanced cell motility and chemotaxis is conserved in rat and mouse mammary tumors. Cancer Res 67(8):3505–3511

Warzecha CC, Carstens RP (2012) Complex changes in alternative pre-mRNA splicing play a central role in the epithelial-to-mesenchymal transition (EMT). Semin Cancer Biol 22(5–6):417–427

Wirapati P, Sotiriou C, Kunkel S et al (2008) Meta-analysis of gene expression profiles in breast cancer: toward a unified understanding of breast cancer subtyping and prognosis signatures. Breast Cancer Res 10(4):R65

Wyckoff JB, Wang Y, Lin EY et al (2007) Direct visualization of macrophage-assisted tumor cell intravasation in mammary tumors. Cancer Res 67 (6):2649–2656

Tumor Infiltrating Lymphocytes as a Prognostic and Predictive Biomarker in Breast Cancer

12

Murali Janakiram, Hina Khan, Susan Fineberg,
Xingxing Zang and Joseph A. Sparano

Abstract

Tumor infiltrating lymphocytes (TILs) have been recognized in various cancers and may reflect a host immune response to malignant cells. TILs are a heterogeneous population of various types of mononuclear cells, including CD8 or CD4 + T cells and their subsets, B cells, myeloid derived suppressor cells (MDSC), macrophages, and other cells. Immunosuppressive factors in the tumor microenvironment (TME) that inhibit recruitment and function of TILs include immunosuppressive cells, cytokines secreted by tumor or mesenchymal cells, and co-inhibitory ligands expressed by tumor cells. Despite this complex interplay of immune cells and the TME, higher TIL density is associated with favorable prognosis in certain breast cancer subtypes, including HER2 overexpressing cancers, and "triple negative" cancers that do not express the estrogen and progesterone receptors or overexpress HER2. TILs infiltrating the tumor stroma (sTILs) are associated with higher rates of complete pathologic response to neoadjuvant chemotherapy, decreased recurrence and improved survival in early stage triple negative and HER2-positive breast cancer treated with adjuvant systemic therapy. An international working group has published guidelines on reporting TILs in pathology specimens. In this chapter we review the composition of TILs, mechanisms of immune evasion, recommendations for TILs measurement,

Murali Janakiram and Hina Khan are contributed equally to this work.

M. Janakiram · H. Khan · X. Zang · J. A. Sparano (✉)
Department of Medicine, Montefiore Medical Center, Albert Einstein College of Medicine, 1695 Eastchester Road, Bronx, NY 10461, USA
e-mail: JSPARANO@montefiore.org

M. Janakiram · H. Khan · X. Zang · J.A. Sparano
Department of Oncology, Montefiore Medical Center, Albert Einstein College of Medicine, 1695 Eastchester Road, Bronx, NY 10461, USA

S. Fineberg
Department of Pathology, Montefiore Medical Center, Albert Einstein College of Medicine, 1695 Eastchester Road, Bronx, NY 10461, USA

M. Janakiram · X. Zang
Department of Microbiology and Immunology, Montefiore Medical Center, Albert Einstein College of Medicine, 1695 Eastchester Road, Bronx, NY 10461, USA

S. Badve and Y. Gökmen-Polar (eds.), *Molecular Pathology of Breast Cancer*, DOI 10.1007/978-3-319-41761-5_12

and data supporting use of TILs as a prognostic and predictive biomarker in breast cancer.

Keywords
Tumor infiltrating lymphocytes · CD8 · CD4 · MDSC

12.1 Introduction

It has been recognized for decades that some primary breast cancers are associated with infiltration by lymphocytes, often referred to as "tumor infiltrating lymphocytes", or "TILs". This phenomenon was first described in medullary carcinoma of the breast, an uncommon subtype of poorly differentiated invasive carcinoma characterized by dense lymphocytic infiltration, circumscription, syncytial growth and absence of estrogen receptor (ER), progesterone receptor (PR) expression and HER2 overexpression, and a relatively favorable prognosis (Moore and Foote 1949; Richardson 1956; Bloom et al. 1970). Recent reports have noted that lymphocytic infiltration to be more prevalent in HER2 overexpressing and "triple negative" invasive ductal carcinomas, and distinguished between lymphocytic infiltration of the tumor (iTILs) and stroma (sTILs) (Loi et al. 2013). In addition, there is a consistent body of evidence indicating a strong correlation between the presence of TILs, especially sTILs, in the primary tumor and a significantly reduced risk of breast cancer recurrence and mortality in both HER2 overexpressing (Dieci et al. 2015) and triple negative breast cancer (TNBC) (Loi et al. 2013; Dieci et al. 2015; Adams et al. 2014). An association between TILs in residual tumor after neoadjuvant chemotherapy and prognosis has also been reported (Dieci et al. 2014), and higher TIL density in diagnostic pre-treatment core biopsies is also predictive of pathologic complete response to neoadjuvant chemotherapy (Denkert et al. 2010, 2015; West et al. 2011; Ono et al. 2012; Mao et al. 2014). This strong association between TILs and clinical outcomes has led to an expert group providing guidelines for evaluating and scoring TILs in breast cancer, with the ultimate goal of capturing the prognostic information in an accurate and reproducible manner that provides sufficient analytic validity to permit further investigation and eventually clinical application (Salgado et al. 2015b). Although the infiltrating cells comprising the infiltrate have been dubbed "lymphocytes", they are identified morphologically as mononuclear cells, and hence actually consist of a mixed population of cells including not only cytotoxic and suppressor T lymphocyte and B lymphocyte populations, but also natural killer (NK) cells, plasma cells, macrophages, dendritic cells, and myeloid derived progenitor cells (Fig. 12.1). With the emergence of immune checkpoint blockade as a new strategy to treat a wide variety of cancers, there has also been interest in more precisely characterizing the composition of the TIL population with the ultimate goal of developing predictive biomarkers that identify tumors more susceptible to eradication by immune checkpoint blockade or other immunotherapeutic approaches.

12.2 Characterization of TILs in Breast Cancer

As described above, the International TILs Working Group is an expert panel that has provided recommendations for evaluation of TILs in breast cancer (Salgado et al. 2015b). The recommendations of the panel are summarized in Table 12.1, and several key recommendations are described herein. First, the panel recommended that all mononuclear cells within the border of the primary invasive tumor be identified as TILs in whole sections excluding areas with necrosis, crush artifact, or hyalinization; the panel did not recommend use of tissue

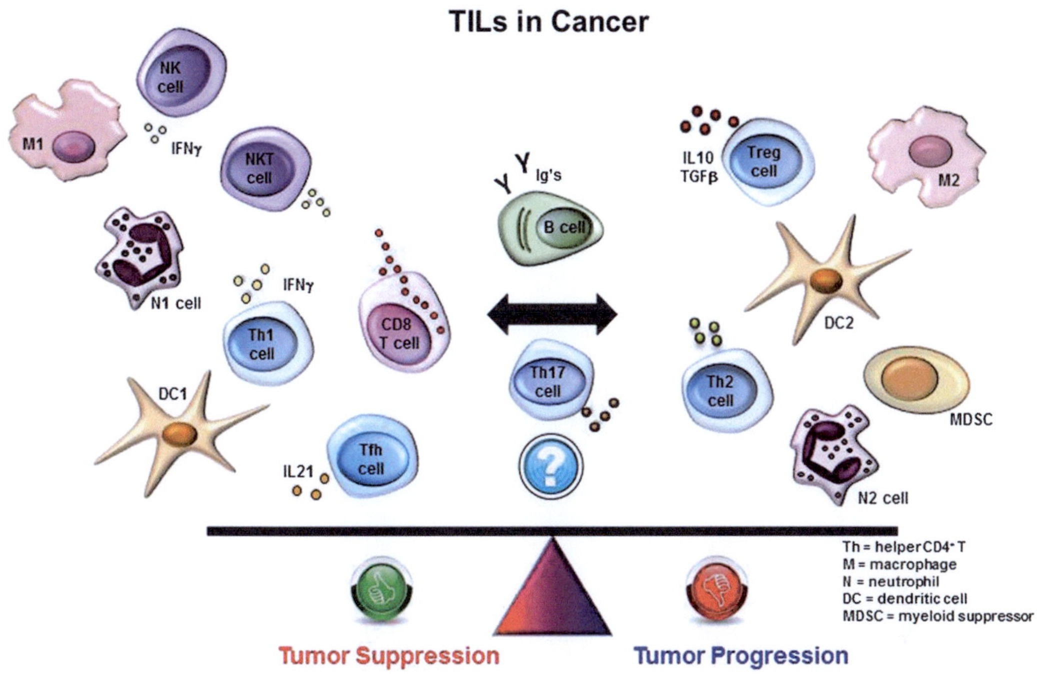

Fig. 12.1 TILs are composed of a heterogeneous population of cells that may promote or suppress the development of cancer [Reproduced with permission from Salgado et al. (2015b)]

microarrays (TMA) or evaluating only "hot spots" in either whole sections or TMAs. Although pretreatment core biopsies may also be used for TIL assessment prior to administration of neoadjuvant chemotherapy, there is limited information about analytic validity of assessing TILs in residual tumor after therapy. Second, the panel recommended distinguishing between iTILs and sTILs (Fig. 12.2), and to report primarily sTILs when assessing TIL status. The group defined iTILs as those in tumor nests having cell-to-cell contact with no intervening stroma and directly interacting with carcinoma cells. sTILs were defined as TILs dispersed in the stroma between the carcinoma cells that are not directly in contact with the malignant cells, and should be reported as percentage of stromal areas occupied by sTILs. The panel pointed out that trafficking between tumor and stromal microenvironment is likely a dynamic process captured in a static manner by histologic evaluation at a single time point, and hence distinguishing between iTILs and sTILs may be artifactual. Characterization of sTILs is more practical because of the greater abundance of sTILs relative to iTILs, greater ease in recognizing and enumerating sTILs, and no additional or more accurate prognostic information provided above and beyond that provided by sTILs enumeration. Third, the panel recommended that sTILs be characterized and reported in a continuous manner (ex. deciles of <10 %, 10–20 %, etc.), rather than a binary manner (ex. lymphocyte predominant breast cancer with at least 50 % sTILs), because very densely infiltrated tumors may be uncommon (<5–10 %). There is also a linear relationship between sTILs and prognosis without a prognostically relevant binary threshold.

The essential characteristics of a prognostic and/or predictive biomarker include analytic validity, clinical validity, and clinical utility. Although there is strong evidence supporting the association between sTILs and prognosis in early stage breast cancer treated with adjuvant chemotherapy and response to neoadjuvant cytotoxic therapy in TNBC, and hence clinical

Table 12.1 TIL working group recommendations for evaluating TILs in breast cancer

Specimen source
• Full sections are preferred over biopsies whenever possible. Cores can be used in the pre-therapeutic neoadjuvant setting; currently no validated methodology has been developed to score TILs after neoadjuvant treatment • One Section (4–5 μm, magnification Å ~ 200–400) per patient is currently considered to be sufficient
Methodology for characterizing TILs
• TILs should be evaluated within the borders of the invasive tumor • A full assessment of average TILs in the tumor area by the pathologist should be used. Do not focus on hotspots • Exclude TILs outside of the tumor border and around DCIS and normal lobules. Exclude TILs in tumor zones with crush artifacts, necrosis, regressive hyalinization as well as in the previous core biopsy site • All mononuclear cells (including lymphocytes and plasma cells) should be scored, but polymorphonuclear leukocytes are excluded • TILs should be reported for the stromal compartment (=% stromal TILs). The denominator used to determine the % stromal TILs is the area of stromal tissue (i.e. area occupied by mononuclear inflammatory cells over total intratumoral stromal area), not the number of stromal cells (i.e.fraction of total stromal nuclei that represent mononuclear inflammatory cell nuclei) • The percentage of stromal TILs is a semiquantitative parameter for this assessment, for example, 80 % stromal TILs means that 80 % of the stromal area shows a dense mononuclear infiltrate. For assessment of percentage values, the dissociated growth pattern of lymphocytes needs to be taken into account. Lymphocytes typically do not form solid cellular aggregates; therefore, the designation '100 % stromal TILs' would still allow some empty tissue space between the individual lymphocytes
Reporting results
• Pathologist should report their scores in as much detail as the pathologist feels comfortable with • The working group's consensus is that TILs may provide more biological relevant information when scored as a continuous variable, and thus should TILs should be assessed as a continuous parameter (as deciles) • Lymphocyte predominant breast cancer can be used as a descriptive term for tumors that contain 'more lymphocytes than tumor cells'. However, the thresholds vary between 50 % and 60 % stromal lymphocytes
Clinical implications of results
• No formal recommendation for a clinically relevant TIL threshold(s) can be given at this stage. The consensus was that a valid methodology is currently more important than issues of thresholds for clinical use, which will be determined once a solid methodology is in place

Adapted from Salgado et al. (2015b)

validity, the clinical utility of this information remains uncertain. For example, there is currently insufficient level of evidence to spare chemotherapy based on TIL assessment, or to select for patients most likely to benefit from immune checkpoint blockade. In addition, few studies have evaluated the intra and inter observer reproducibility, or analytic validity, of TILs assessment. For example, in the report by Adams et al., inter observer correlation was evaluated in a subset of 99 evaluable cases. Rates of agreement within 10 percentage points between two expert breast pathologists were 85 % (95 % confidence intervals [CI] 76–91 %) for sTILs and 97 % (95 % CI 91–99 %) for iTILs. If categorical cut points from the Kaplan-Meier analysis were used, the kappa statistic showed moderate agreement between the two pathologists (sTILs, 0.40; iTILs, 0.43) (Adams et al. 2014). Hence further studies or guidelines are required to study methods to improvise interobserver agreement in TIL evaluation in breast cancer.

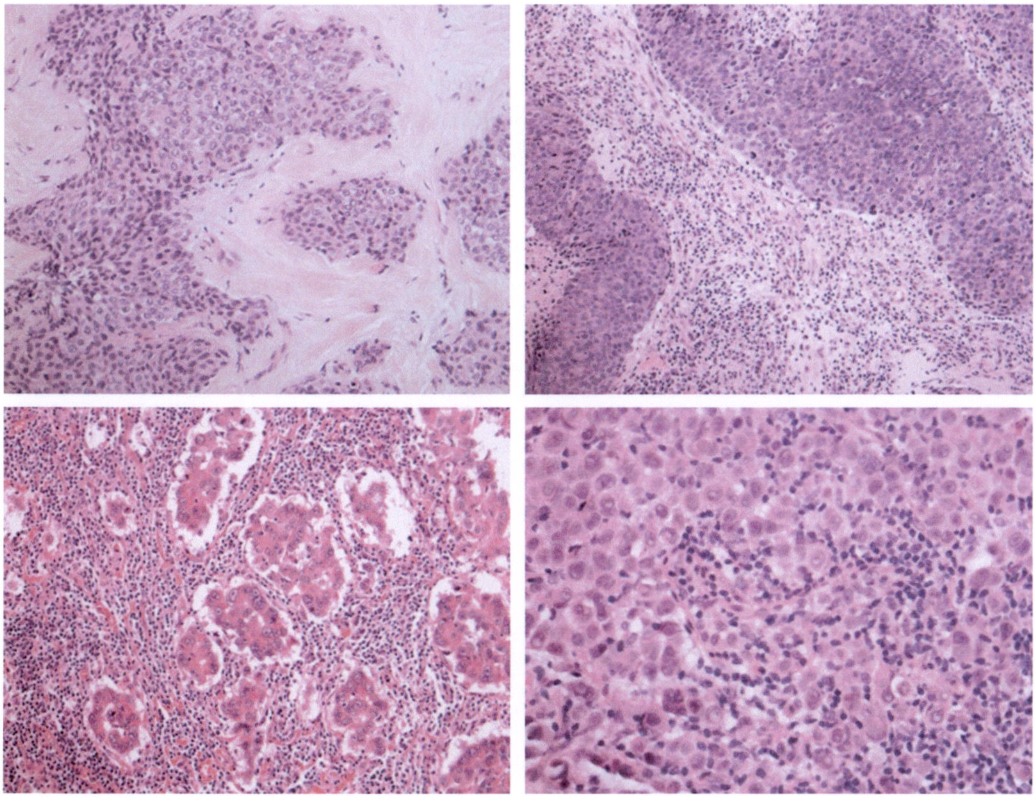

Fig. 12.2 Various levels of TIL infiltration in different breast cancer samples are shown. *Top left* sTILs < 1 % (20x)—The stroma is clearly visible in *pink* and is devoid of TILs, *Top right* sTILs—50 % (20x)—The stroma is visible and has a considerable infiltration of TILs, *Bottom left* sTILs—90 % (20x)—Intervening stroma is not seen and is nearly replaced by lymphocytes, *Bottom right* Intratumoral TILs (40x)—The lymphocytes are in direct contact with the tumor cells with no intervening stroma

12.3 TILs Are an Immunologic Response to Tumor Neoantigens

Tumors occurring in subjects harboring germ-line BRCA1 mutations are associated with more TILs than sporadic breast cancers (Lakhani et al. 1998). BRCA-mutation associated cancers have a higher mutational burden than sporadic cancers due to impaired homologous recombination and consequently less error free DNA repair. This results in a greater neoantigen burden and hence induces an immune response. Variability in the somatic mutational burden of cancer has been described, with tumors associated with exposure to tobacco and sunlight (e.g., lung cancer and melanoma, respectively) associated with the highest mutational burden, and breast cancer having a mutational burden in the intermediate range when considered in the context of all human cancers that have been characterized thus far (Alexandrov et al. 2013). Non-BRCA-associated TNBCs are also frequently characterized by defective DNA repair mechanisms due to germ-line defects in other DNA repair pathways (e.g., PALB2, RAD51) and BRCA1 promoter hypermethylation. Assays that identify tumors harboring "genomic scars" as a consequence of these deficiencies are likewise characterized by greater TIL density, providing additional evidence supporting the link between mutational burden and immune response (Telli et al. 2015). On the other hand, tumors harboring defective DNA repair mechanisms, whether due to germ-line or somatic alterations, are more sensitive to DNA damaging agents such as platinums, alkylating agents, and anthracyclines. Thus, it is unclear at this time as to whether the more favorable prognosis associated with TILs represents an effective immune response, greater sensitivity of tumors with high TILs to cytotoxic therapy, or both. Higher mutational burden has been shown to correlate with clinical response to anti-PD1 directed therapy in non-small cell lung cancer (Rizvi et al. 2015), suggesting that TILs may serve as a surrogate predictive biomarker for response to immune checkpoint blockade in a variety of cancers.

12.4 Composition of TILs and Subpopulations

The diagnosis of clinical cancer represents escape from cancer immunoediting, an immunologic process that reduces cancer burden through elimination or equilibrium (Dunn et al. 2004). Although the escape from or failure of this process results in the clinical detection of cancer, the association between TILs and prognosis suggests that host immunity is still relevant after cancer is diagnosed. TILs are composed of a heterogeneous population of cells having both immunostimulatory and immunosuppressive effects, and the balance of these effects contribute to tumor tolerance (Quezada et al. 2011).

The subpopulations of cells are shown in Fig. 12.1. Some cells in the TIL population suppress tumor progression, including CD8+ T cells, helper CD4+ T (Th1) cells, natural killer (NK) cells, whereas others promote tumor progression, including Th2 cells, myeloid derived stem cells, and T regulatory (Tregs) cells. Subpopulations of macrophage and dendritic cells can suppress (M1, DC1) or promote tumor (M2, DC2) tumors, while other cell populations may be either tumor suppressive or promoting, including B cells and Th17 cells (Salgado et al. 2015b). Although neutrophils are not considered in characterizing TILs, they may likewise have either tumor suppressing or promoting subpopulations (Sagiv et al. 2015).

TIL subpopulations may be evaluated using a variety of methodologies, including immunohistochemistry, RNA in situ hybridization, and flow cytometry. Gene expression profiling has identified tumor associated immune signatures that reflect the composition of the subpopulations. To date, classification of subpopulations has largely been described using immunohistochemistry including a panel of antibodies directed at CD4, CD8, CD25, and FOXP3+. Using this methodology, the major subtypes of immunosuppressive cells constituting TILs include T regs (CD4 + CD25+ FOXP3+) and myeloid derived suppressor cells (MDSC) (Jiang and Shapiro 2014). Tregs produce RANKL which binds to RANK on human breast cancer cell lines and promotes lung metastases in mouse models (Tan et al. 2011). Depletion of Tregs with a vaccine and low dose cyclophosphamide results in increased cytolytic activity of T cells in Her-2 Neu transgenic mice (Weiss et al. 2012). MDSC suppress T cell proliferation through production of reactive oxygen species, disrupt binding of antigen specific peptides to CD8 T cells by inactivating tyrosinases in the TCR-CD8 (T cell receptor-CD8) complexes, and inhibit antigen presentation by tumor cells via nitration of tumor MHC class I expression (Jiang and Shapiro 2014). Hence these cell populations through pleiotropic effects can prevent or suppress an effective immune response.

12.5 The Tumor Microenvironment and TIL Function

TILs comprise only one component of the tumor microenvironment (TME), which also includes mesenchymal cells, and extracellular matrix/stroma. The extracellular matrix functions as a scaffold for tissue architecture, and also provides biochemical and biomechanical signals that influence cell growth, survival, migration and differentiation, as well as vascular development and immune function, and hence modulates the hallmarks of cancer (Pickup et al. 2014). Thus, crosstalk between TIL subpopulations and other components of the TME, mediated in part by chemokines and cytokines, results in a complex interplay that can influence the balance between tumor promotion and suppression, as described below.

Cytokines and chemokines: The stromal cells and other immune cells secrete various cytokines that profoundly influence different subpopulations of immune effector cells. For example, TGF-beta induces transcriptional repression of genes in CD8+ T cells resulting in impaired cytolytic activity (Thomas and Massague 2005). Products of altered steroid metabolism can accumulate and inhibit CCR7 thus preventing dendritic cell maturation and translocation into the lymphoid organs (Villablanca et al. 2010). Tumors secrete soluble ligands such as MHC class I polypeptide-related sequence (MIC) that deplete T cell receptors and attenuate response of specific effector T cells in response to tumor antigens (Groh et al. 2002). Thus cytokines secreted in the TME can inhibit presentation of antigens to T cells and can also inhibit responses of T cells to the tumor. Other cytokines, most notably interferon-gamma, play an important role in enhancing cell immunity.

Co-inhibitory and co-stimulatory receptors and ligands: T cell activation depends on recognition of antigens on host antigen presenting cells (APCs) and the presence of a simultaneous co-stimulatory or co-inhibitory signal delivered through the CD28 –B7 family of receptor-ligand interaction between T cells and APC or malignant cells. Certain B7 ligands, including PD-L1, B7-H3, B7x and HHLA2 inhibit T cell responses when expressed on APCs or tumor cells. Expression of these ligands in breast cancer and other cancers has been associated with unfavorable clinical features (Janakiram et al. 2012; 2014). For example, PD-L1 expression on human pancreatic and ovarian cancers is inversely correlated with CD8 + TILs (Ohaegbulam et al. 2015). Several studies also show an inverse correlation of another co-inhibitory ligand B7x and TILs in various cancers. Tumor cell B7x expression is inversely correlated with the intensity of TILs in renal cell carcinoma (Zhang et al. 2013), with the number of CD3+ and CD8+ TILs in uterine endometrioid carcinoma (Miyatake et al. 2007) and with the densities of CD3+ TILs in tumor nest and CD8+ TILs in tumor stroma in esophageal carcinoma (Chen et al. 2011). These results suggest that tumor-expressed B7x may be important in limiting TILs infiltration. The expression of coinhibitory receptor PD-1 on TILs has also been shown to be associated with decreased overall survival in breast cancer (Sun et al. 2014; Muenst et al. 2013). In summary, TILs recruitment and function is influenced by a complex interplay of neoantigens and co-inhibitory ligands on the tumor, coinhibitory receptors on TILs, subpopulation of cells in the infiltrate and the tumor microenvironment.

12.6 Clinical Validity of TILs as a Prognostic Biomarker in Patients with Breast Cancer Treated with Adjuvant Chemotherapy

The results of studies evaluating the association between TILs and prognosis in operable breast cancer are summarized in Table 12.2.

Relationship between TILs and Breast Cancer Subtype: Loi et al. (2013) first described the variability of TILs by breast cancer subtype, and the strong association between TILs and prognosis in TNBC. TILs were evaluated independently by two expert pathologists in primary tumor specimens from 2009 patients with axillary node-positive breast cancer enrolled on the BIG 02-98 adjuvant phase III trial comparing anthracycline chemotherapy given without a taxane (doxorubicin followed by cyclophosphamide, methotrexate, and fluorouracil (CMF) or doxorubicin plus cyclophosphamide followed by CMF), concurrently or sequentially with a taxane (doxorubicin plus docetaxel followed by CMF or doxorubicin followed by docetaxel followed by CMF). iTILs and sTILs were found to be significantly higher in TNBC and HER2-positive breast cancer compared with ER-positive, HER2-negative breast cancer. In addition, there was no significant prognostic association in the entire population (n = 2009) or

Table 12.2 Clinical studies of TILs as a biomarker in adjuvant therapy of breast cancer

	Trial: author and reference	No. of samples analyzed	Method: H&E/IHC	TILs analyzed: i-TILs, s-TILs or t-TILs	Lymphocyte predominant breast cancer (LPBC)	Adjuvant Therapy used	Survival parameter in High TILs subgroup
TNBC	Loi et al. (2013)	256	H&E	s-TILs and i-TILs	High TILs (>50 %) were seen in 10.6 % patients	Anthracycline based combination regimens with taxanes	• Every 10 % increase in i-TILs and s-TILs were associated with 17 % ($p = 0.1$) and 15 % ($p = 0.025$) reduced risk of relapse, and 27 % ($p = 0.03$) and 17 % reduced risk of death ($p = 0.023$). • For high versus low TILs (>50 %) – DFS-HR: 0.30, 95 % CI: 0.11–0.81 – OS-HR: 0.29, 95 % CI: 0.091–0.92
	Adams et al. (2014)	481	H&E	s-TILs and i-TILs	High TILs (≥50 %) were seen in 4.4 % patients	AC, AC followed by taxane or CMF	• With every 10 % increase in s-TILs, a 14 % reduction of risk of recurrence or death ($p = 0.02$), 18 % reduction of risk of distant recurrence ($p = 0.04$), and 19 % reduction of risk of death ($p = 0.01$) was seen. sTILs were an independent prognostic marker of DFS, DRFI, and OS • For presence vs absence of sTILs – HR: 0.69, 95 % CI: 0.49–0.98 • For presence vs absence of iTILs – HR: 0.69; 95 % CI: 0.45–1.06
	Dieci et al. (2015)	199	H&E	s-TILs and i-TILs	High-TILs (>50 %) were seen in 5 % patients	FEC or FAC compared to no chemotherapy	• Each 10 % increase in i-TILs or s-TILs was associated with 14 and 13 % reduction in risk relapse in the high and low-TILs groups • For high versus low TILs (>50 %) – DFS-HR: 0.43, 95 % CI: 0.20–0.94 – 10 years DFS rate was 85 and 53 %
	Loi et al. (2014b)	134	H&E	s-TILs and i-TILs	TILs used as continuous variable, High TILs defined as ≥50 % for statistical analyses	Docetaxel or vinorelbine ×3 cycles, followed by three cycles of FEC	• For each 10 % increase in sTILs there was 13 % decrease in risk of distant recurrence in TNBC; and improvement in DFS. No difference in OS was observed • For high versus low TILs (≥50 %) – DFS-HR: 0.77, 95 % CI: 0.61–0.98

(continued)

Table 12.2 (continued)

	Trial: author and reference	No. of samples analyzed	Method: H&E/IHC	TILs analyzed: i-TILs, s-TILs or t-TILs	Lymphocyte predominant breast cancer (LPBC)	Adjuvant Therapy used	Survival parameter in High TILs subgroup
HER2 +	Loi et al. (2014b)	209	H&E	s-TILs and i-TILs	TILs used as continuous variable, High TILs defined as ≥50 % for statistical analyses	Docetaxel or vinorelbine ×3 cycles, followed by three cycles of FEC, with or without nine doses of weekly trastuzumab	• For each 10 % increase in lymphocytic infiltration, there was an 18 % decrease in relative risk of distant recurrence in patients randomized to the trastuzumab arm. Higher levels of TIL are associated with increased trastuzumab benefit in HER2+ disease • For High versus low TILs (≥50 %) – DFS-HR: 0.96, 95 % CI 0.82–1.3
	Perez et al. (2014)	945	H&E	s-TILs	High TILs (≥60 %) were seen in 9.9 % patients	AC followed by Taxol with or without Trastuzumab	• sTILs of ≥60 % was associated with RFS in chemotherapy only arm, but not in trastuzumab arm. The 10 year RFS was 90.9 % for high S-TILs group in the chemotherapy arm • 10 year RFS was not significantly different (80 %) in either groups in the trastuzumab arm • For High versus low TILs (≥60 %) – 10 year DFS HR: 0.23; 95 %CI: 0.073–0.73
	Dieci et al. (2015)	112	H&E	s-TILs and i-TILs	High-TILs (>50 %) were seen in 24 % patients	FEC or FAC compared to no chemotherapy	• 10 year DFS rate was higher in the high-TIL group • For high versus low TILs (>50 %) – DFS-HR: 0.48; 95 % CI: 0.21–1.07
	Liu et al. (2014)	498	IHC—FOXP3 cells	s-TILs and i-TILs	Median used to classify high and low TILs. FOXP3 TILs (≥2 IHC) were prevalent in 42.4 % samples	CMF, AC or FAC	• High FOXP3+ TILs were associated with improved survival in the HER2 +/ER—subgroup, with co-existent CD8+ T-cell infiltrates. In CD8+ group, the presence of high levels of FOXP3 + TILs was independent of standard clinical prognostic factors • For high versus low TILs (median) – OS-HR: 0.48, 95 % CI: 0.23–0.98
	Loi et al. (2013)	297	H&E	s-TILs and i-TILs	High TILs (>50 %) were seen in 11.1 % patients	Anthracycline based combination regimens with taxanes	• Each 10 % increase in sTILs was significantly associated with benefit with anthracycline-only regimen. In the LPBC (>50 % TILs) phenotype, a 5-year DFS of 78.6 % was seen in the anthracycline arm versus 57.9 % DFS in the anthracycline-docetaxel arm. • For high versus low TILs (>50 %) – 5 year DFS in LPBC–HR: 0.45; 95 % CI: 0.12–1.71 –5 year DFS in non-LPBC-HR: 2.05; 95 % CI: 1.41–2.97

(continued)

Table 12.2 (continued)

	Trial: author and reference	No. of samples analyzed	Method: H&E/IHC	TILs analyzed: i-TILs, s-TILs or t-TILs	Lymphocyte predominant breast cancer (LPBC)	Adjuvant Therapy used	Survival parameter in High TILs subgroup
ER+/PR+	Dieci et al. (2015)	463	H&E	s-TILs and i-TILs	High-TILs (>50 %) were seen in 15 % patients	FEC or FAC compared to no chemotherapy	• No prognostic effect was seen in the ER +/HER2— subgroup
	Liu et al. (2014)	2761	IHC—FOXP3 cells	s-TILs and i-TILs	Median used to classify high and low TILs. FOXP3 TILs (≥2 IHC) were prevalent in 27.2 % samples	CMF, AC or FAC	• High FOXP3 + TILs were associated with poor survival in ER+ breast cancers that lacked CD8+ T-cell infiltrates • For High versus low TILs [median] – OS HR: 1.30, 95 % CI: 1.02–1.66

TILs Tumor infiltrating lymphocytes; *s-TILs* Stromal tumor infiltrating lymphocytes; *i-TILs* Intratumoral tumor infiltrating lymphocytes; *t-TILs* Total tumor infiltrating lymphocytes; *H&E* Hematoxylin and eosin; *IHC* Immunohistochemistry; *TNBC* Triple negative breast cancer; *OS* Overall survival; *HR* Hazard ratio; *CI* Confidence interval; *DFS* Disease free survival; *RFS* Recurrence free survival; *DRFI* Disease recurrence free interval; *FOXP3* Forkhead box P3; *HER2* Human epidermal growth factor receptor 2; *CMF* Methotrexate, cyclophosphamide, 5-fluorouracil; *AC* Doxorubicin and Cyclophosphamide; *FEC* 5-Fluorouracil, Epirubicin and Cyclophosphamide; *FAC* Doxorubicin, cyclophosphamide, 5-fluorouracil

ER-positive, HER2-negative population (n = 1079).

Relationship between TILs and Prognosis in Triple Negative Breast Cancer: Although no association was found between TIL and prognosis in the overall population and in ER-positive, HER2-negative disease in analysis of the BIG 02-98 specimens reported by Loi et al. (Loi et al. 2013), each 10 % increase in iTILs and sTILs in the TNBC population was associated with 17 and 15 % reduced risk of relapse (adjusted $p = 0.1$ and $p = 0\ \ 0.025$), respectively, and 27 and 17 % reduced risk of death irrespective of chemotherapy type used (adjusted $p = 0.035$ and $p = 0.023$), respectively. This report therefore provided the first evidence indicating the strong associated between TILs and prognosis in TNBC. Adams et al. (2014) reported a confirmatory analysis that focused on 481 patients with stages I-III TNBC enrolled on two large adjuvant phase III trials (ECOG 2197 and ECOG 1199) in which all patients received anthracycline-cyclophosphamide-containing, usually in combination with a taxane. In contrast to the analysis by Loi et al., TILs were read independently rather than in tandem by two expert pathologists. Similar to the report by Loi et al., however, among the 481 tissue samples analyzed; for every 10 % increase in sTIL there was a 14 % reduction in risk of recurrence or death, 18 % reduction in risk of distant recurrence and a 19 % reduction in risk of death was seen. These two independent reports therefore demonstrated that sTILs were a strong and independent prognostic marker for disease-free survival (DFS) and overall survival (OS) in patients with stages I-III TNBC treated with adjuvant anthracycline-containing chemotherapy.

The relationship between TILs and prognosis was also evaluated retrospectively using breast cancer specimens obtained from two randomized trials comparing adjuvant chemotherapy with no chemotherapy in 817 patients with node-positive and node-negative breast cancer (Dieci et al. 2014). In the TNBC subgroup, both iTILs and sTILs were significantly associated with DFS, with each 10 % increase associated with 14 and 13 % reduction in risk of relapse (HR: 0.86,

95 % CI: 0.78–0.94 and HR: 0.87, 95 % CI: 0.80–0.94), respectively. TILs were prognostic in both the chemotherapy treated and untreated population, with no statistical interaction observed. The FinHer study was another phase III multicenter adjuvant trial that included 1010 patients with high-risk node-negative or node-positive breast cancer; in this cohort each 10 % increase in TILs was significantly associated with a 13 % decrease in risk of distant recurrence (HR: 0.77, 95 % CI: 0.61–0.98, $p = 0.02$) in 134 TIL evaluable primary TNBC cases (Loi et al. 2014b). Thus, several reports have confirmed the prognostic role of increased TIL in patients with operable TNBC treated with or without adjuvant chemotherapy.

HER2-Positive Breast Cancer: The association between TILs and prognosis was also demonstrated in HER2-positive operable breast cancer. As previously described, the FinHer study was a multicenter phase III trial that included not only patients with TNBC, but also patients with HER2 overexpressing breast cancer who received adjuvant chemotherapy alone or in combination with trastuzumab. In 209 patients with HER2-positive breast cancer treated with adjuvant trastuzumab in the FinHER study, a 10 % increase in sTILs was associated with an increase in distant disease free survival (HR = 0.77; 95 % CI: 0.61–0.98). The association between TILs and prognosis was also analyzed in the N9831 study, which compared adjuvant chemotherapy alone or in combination with trastuzumab in HER2 overexpressing operable breast cancer (Perez et al. 2014). Lymphocyte predominant breast cancers (LPBC) with high sTILs (>60 %), which accounted for 9.9 % (n = 94) of the population, was independently associated with improved recurrence-free survival (RFS) in patients treated with chemotherapy alone, but not in the chemotherapy plus trastuzumab group, and did not predict benefit from trastuzumab. In patients treated with chemotherapy alone, the 10 year RFS rates were 90.9% and 64.5 % for LPBC and non-LPBC groups, respectively (HR: 0.23; 95 % CI: 0.073–0.73). Subgroup analysis from the BIG-02-98 adjuvant phase III trial of lymph node positive breast cancer patients also showed a notable benefit of increasing TILs (10 % increments) in the HER2-positive cohort treated with anthracycline-only chemotherapy without trastuzumab, although this was not seen in anthracycline and docetaxel arm. It is unclear currently why such an interaction should be present with the type of chemotherapy regimen, although a higher dose of anthracycline could be responsible for the immune mediated response. Based on all these studies, a higher TILs infiltration is predictive of outcome in $HER2^+$ breast cancer especially in the anthracycline only treated subgroup.

ER-Positive, HER2-Negative Breast Cancer: Data on the prognostic effect of TIL in the hormone receptor positive breast cancer groups is limited. Recent preliminary data from two ongoing randomized adjuvant trials has shown that there is no prognostic impact of TIL in the $ER^+/HER2^-$ subgroup (Maria Vittoria Dieci et al. 2014).

12.7 Clinical Validity of TILs as a Prognostic and Predictive Biomarker in Patients with Breast Cancer Treated with Neoadjuvant Chemotherapy

Neoadjuvant chemotherapy of localized breast cancer leads to clinical responses in as many as 70–90 % of patients. However, pathological complete response (pCR), defined as a complete or near complete absence of residual tumor, is only seen in 10–25 % of patients (Fisher et al. 1998; Smith et al. 2002). pCR is a short term surrogate associated with a long-term favorable prognosis, especially in HER2-positive and TNBC (Cortazar and Geyer 2015), and is now accepted by regulatory agencies such as the United States Food and Drug Administration for accelerated approval of new agents in patients with localized breast cancer who are candidates for neoadjuvant chemotherapy (Prowell and

Pazdur 2012). Patients with residual disease have a variable prognosis, but extensive residual disease in patients with TNBC and HER-positive breast cancer appear to have a high risk of recurrence (Symmans et al. 2007). Hence there is an interest in determining the relationship between TILs in pretreatment core biopsies as a predictive biomarker for pCR in patients with neoadjuvant therapy, and as a prognostic biomarker in patients with residual disease after neoadjuvant therapy because of the variable prognosis for this population. The results of these reports are summarized in Table 12.3.

TILs and Predicting Response to Neoadjuvant Chemotherapy: Lymphocyte infiltration was analyzed in 1058 pre-treatment cancer tissues from the GeparDuo and GeparTrio cohorts, both of which were phase III, randomized trials assessing responses to combination neoadjuvant chemotherapy regimens. The presence of intratumoral lymphocytes, defined as >10 % stromal area infiltrated with lymphocytes, was an independent parameter for pCR in both the cohorts (Denkert et al. 2010). The pCR rates were 42 % and 40 %, respectively. Tumors with low TIL had pCR rates of 3 and 7 % respectively. In the GeparSixto neoadjuvant study assessing addition of carboplatin to an anthracycline-taxane combination in 580 patients, pCR rates were 76.2 % for LPBC (defined as >60 % of either intratumoral or stromal TILs) compared to 52.2 % for non-LPBC ($p = 0.01$) in those with TNBC (Denkert et al. 2015).

In a meta-analysis including 13 neoadjuvant studies and 3251 patients, TNBC with higher TILs in pretreatment biopsy correlated with higher pCR rates to neoadjuvant chemotherapy (Mao et al. 2014). Greater TIL density was associated with a higher pCR rate for neoadjuvant chemotherapy (OR: 3.93, 95 % CI: 3.26–4.73, $p < 0.001$), including iTILs (OR: 4.15, 95 % CI: 2.95–5.84, $p < 0.001$) or sTILs (OR: 3.58, 95 % CI: 2.50–5.13, $p < 0.001$). Pretreatment TILs had predictive values in ER negative, triple negative and HER2 positive breast cancer patients, but not in ER-positive disease. Therefore, TIL analysis on initial tumor samples serves as an important predicting factor for pathologic response in TNBC.

In a study of 180 stage II and III breast cancer patients, tumors with Foxp3 and CD8 infiltrates were associated with a high-pCR rate ($p < 0.001$ and $p = 0.007$, respectively) in those who received neo-adjuvant weekly paclitaxel followed by 5-fluourouracil, epirubicin and cyclophosphamide (Oda et al. 2012). Foxp3 infiltrate was a significant independent predictor of pCR ($p = 0.014$), but CD8 infiltrate was not. In another study with 153 tumor samples, high $CD8^+$ TILs in pretreatment biopsy was found to be an independent predictor of response to neoadjuvant chemotherapy (Seo et al. 2013). These results demonstrate that subpopulations of lymphocytes may also be predictive of response to neoadjuvant chemotherapy, although further studies in larger populations are needed in order to determine whether this provides more accurate prognostic and predictive information than simply evaluating sTILs by conventional hematoxylin and eosin staining.

TILs and Predicting Response to Trastuzumab: In the HER2-population, the response to trastuzumab and its association with TILs has been investigated in the neo-adjuvant setting. In the GeparQuattro trial, 156 patients with $HER2^+$ breast cancer received neoadjuvant trastuzumab with chemotherapy (4 cycles of epirubicin/cyclophosphamide with docetaxel with or without capecitabine); each 10 % increment in TILs was associated with higher rates of pCR (adjusted OR: 1.14, 95 % CI: 1.01–1.29) (Loi et al. 2014a). The neoadjuvant trial GeparSixto, investigated the effect of adding carboplatin to an neoadjuvant anthracycline-taxane combination in 580 patients with triple negative or $HER2^+$ breast cancer (Denkert et al. 2015); trastuzumab and lapatinib were also given in patients with $HER2^+$ disease, and bevacizumab to patients with TNBC, which included 25 % of patients who had LPBC (defined as >60 % of either iTILs or sILs). Overall, the pCR rate was significantly higher in the LPBC compared with the non-LPBC group (59.9 vs. 33.8 %, $p = 0.001$). pCR rate were significantly higher for the LPBC group in the

Table 12.3 Clinical studies of TILs as a biomarker in neoadjuvant therapy of breast cancer

	Trial-Author and reference	No. of samples	Method - H&E/IHC	TILs analyzed: i-TILs, s-TILs or t-TILs	Lymphocyte predominant breast cancer	Neoadjuvant Therapy	Survival parameter in High TILs subgroup
All types	Denkert et al. (2010)	1058	H&E	s-TILs and i-TILs	High TILs (>60 %) were seen in 9.5 % patients	GeparDuo cohort: docetaxel with doxorubicin vs doxorubicin/cyclophosphamide followed by docetaxel. GeparTrio cohort: TAC- 6-8 cycles vs four cycles of TAC followed by four cycles of vinorelbine and capecitabine	• High TILs/LPBC tumors had pCR of 40 %, compared to pCR of 5 % in tumors without any lymphocyte infiltrate (<0.0005)
	Oda et al. (2012)	180	IHC- FOXP3 and CD8	i-TILs	Median values used as cut-off, Intratumoral TILs used as continuous variable	Sequential weekly paclitaxel followed by FEC	• High pCR rate of 31.3 and 25.7 % was associated with tumors having FOXP3 and CD8 infiltrates ($p < 0.001$ and $p = 0.007$, respectively) • Breast tumors with both FOXP3 and CD8 infiltrates showed the highest pCR rate of 33.0 % when compared to those without lymphocyte infiltrate
	Yamaguchi et al. (2012)	68	H&E, IHC - CD3, CD20	s-TILs and i-TILs	High TIL defined as IHC 2 and 3 by visual grading, were seen in 38 % patients	Anthracycline- and taxane-based regimen (4 cycles of FEC and 4 cycles of docetaxel)	• High TILs was an independent predictor for pCR (OR: 4.7, 95 % CI: 2.2–10.06)
	Ladoire et al. (2008)	56	IHC - CD3 +, CD8+, FOXP3	i-TILs	Lymphocyte infiltrates were graded (0-3) per IHC	Anthracycline-based regimen: FEC or CEX; docetaxel was used sequentially with anthracyclines-based chemotherapy. Patients with HER-2–positive: treated with trastuzumab with docetaxel and carboplatin	• Higher CD8 infiltrate before and after chemotherapy was associated with pCR ($p = 0.037$ and $p = 0.026$, respectively) • After neoadjuvant therapy, FOXP3 + cells decreased in patients with pathologic complete responses (pCR), whereas these cells remained elevated in non-responders

(continued)

Table 12.3 (continued)

	Trial-Author and reference	No. of samples	Method - H&E/IHC	TILs analyzed: i-TILs, s-TILs or t-TILs	Lymphocyte predominant breast cancer	Neoadjuvant Therapy	Survival parameter in High TILs subgroup
	Lee et al. (2013)	175	IHC - CD3 +, CD8 +, FOXP3	t-TILs	Used in a continuous scale in 10 % increments by visual grading of IHC	Anthracycline-based regimens (AC), anthracycline and taxane-based regimens (docetaxel and doxorubicin or AC followed by docetaxel). HER2-positive tumors, were treated with Herceptin-based regimens	• Higher lymphocyte infiltrates of CD8 +, CD3+ or FOXP3+ was a significant independent predictor of pCR (OR: 1.26, p = 0.024)
	Seo et al. (2013)	153	IHC -CD4+, CD8+, and FOXP3 + TILs	i-TILs	High CD4 TIL defined as ≥59.67/HPF, high CD8 as ≥16.33/HPF and high FOXP3 as ≥6.33/HPF	AC, AD or AC followed by docetaxel	• High CD4 +, CD8 +, and FOXP3 + TILs were associated with a high pCR. • Only CD8 + TILs were an independent predictive factor for pCR (OR: 9.786; 95 % CI: 2.12–45.14), irrespective of breast cancer subtype
	Aruga et al. (2009)	87	IHC - FOXP3+	s-TILs and i-TILs	High TILs defined as 6.6 c/HPF, were seen in 50.5 % patients	Anthracycline (FEC or EC) with or without Taxane (Docetaxel or Paclitaxel)	• Prognosis was better among patients with low numbers of FOXP3-positive cells in tumor. They had a better recurrence-free survival, with risk ratio of 5.81 (95 % CI: 1.09– 107.5) compared to high FOXP3-positive cells
	Liu et al. (2012)	132	IHC - FOXP3	s-TILs and i-TILs	Median was taken as the cutoff and samples above the median was considered high	Anthracycline-based regimens: FEC or CEX. Following anthracycline, docetaxel was given to 43 pts	• Decreased peritumoral Tregs were an independent predictor for pCR • High intratumoral Tregs after chemotherapy was associated with unfavorable prognosis- OS (p = 0.001) and PFS (p = 0.006)

(continued)

Table 12.3 (continued)

	Trial-Author and reference	No. of samples	Method - H&E/IHC	TILs analyzed: i-TILs, s-TILs or t-TILs	Lymphocyte predominant breast cancer	Neoadjuvant Therapy	Survival parameter in High TILs subgroup
TNBC	Dieci et al. (2014)	278	H&E	s-TILs and i-TILs	High TILs defined as >60 %, were seen in 9.7 % patients	Anthracycline with or without taxane	• High TILs versus low TILs (>60 %) – 5 yr OS—91 versus 55 % – HR: 0.19, 95 % CI: 0.06–0.6
	Ono et al. (2012)	92	H&E, IHC	s-TILs and i-TILs	High TILs (>50 %) were seen in 73 % patients	Regimens with anthracycline, taxane or both	• High TILs versus Low TILs (>50 %) – pCR = 37 versus 16 %, $p = 0.05$
	Denkert et al. (2015)	314	H&E	s-TILs and i-TILs	High TILs (>60 %) were seen in 28.3 % patients	Anthracycline and taxane, with or without carboplatin	• In the LPBC/High TILs group, the addition of carboplatin to anthracycline-plus-taxane showed a high pCR of 74 %
HER2 +	Loi et al. (2014a)	156	H&E	t-TILs	TILs used as a continuous variable, no cut-off used	Trastuzumab with chemotherapy (epirubicin/cyclophosphamide with docetaxel with or without capecitabine)	• For each 10 % increment in TILs, higher rates of pCR were seen after neoadjuvant therapy • For High versus Low TILs – Adjusted OR: 1.14, 95 %CI: 1.01–1.29
	Denkert et al. (2015)	266	H&E	s-TILs and i-TILs	High TILs (>60 %) were seen in 19.9 % patients	Anthracycline and taxane, with or without carboplatin	• In the LPBC/High TILs group, the addition of carboplatin to anthracycline-plus-taxane showed a pCR of 78 %
	Salgado et al. (2015a)	387	H&E	s-TILs	TILs used as a continuous variable, no cut-off used	Trastuzumab, lapatinib or combination ×6 weeks followed by weekly taxol ×12, followed by FEC	• Every 1 % increase in TILs was associated with a 3 % decrease in rate of event (pCR and EFS) – HR:0.97, 95 % CI: 0.95–0.99 • TILs greater than 5 % were prognostic for pCR – OR: 2.60, 95 % CI: 1.26–5.39

(continued)

Table 12.3 (continued)

	Trial-Author and reference	No. of samples	Method - H&E/IHC	TILs analyzed: i-TILs, s-TILs or t-TILs	Lymphocyte predominant breast cancer	Neoadjuvant Therapy	Survival parameter in High TILs subgroup
HER2-	Issa-Nummer et al. (2013)	313	H&E	s-TILs and i-TILs	High TILs (≥60 %) were seen in 26.2 % patients	Epirubicin, cyclophosphamide followed by Docetaxel and Bevacizumab	• Every 10 % increase in lymphocytic infiltrate was associated with an improvement in pCR • For High versus low TILs (>60 %) – pCR was 36.6 versus 14.3 %
ER-/ PR-	West et al. (2011)	113	IHC for CD3, CD8, CD4, gene expression	t-TILs	Median values of TILs markers used as cut-offs	FEC ×6 cycles or TET (docetaxel ×3 cycles followed by docetaxel plus epirubicin ×3 cycles)	• For High versus low TILs (median) – pCR = 74 % vs 31 %, OR: 6.33, 95 % CI: 2.49 - 16.08
ER +/ PR+	Chan et al. (2012)	Unable to locate article	IHC	t-TILs, CD8+/ Treg ratio	No cut-offs used	Steroidal aromatase inhibitor (AI) therapy	• Significant increase in the CD8+/ Treg ratio was detected in responders ($p = 0.028$) to neo-adjuvant endocrine therapy but not in non-responders

TILs Tumor infiltrating lymphocytes; *s-TILs* Stromal tumor infiltrating lymphocytes; *i-TILs* Intratumoral tumor infiltrating lymphocytes; *t-TILs* Total tumor infiltrating lymphocytes; H&E: Hematoxylin and eosin; *IHC* Immunohistochemistry; *CI* Confidence interval; *OR* Odds ratio; *OS* Overall survival; *HR* Hazards ratio; *pCR* Pathological complete response; *PFS* Progression free survival; *EFS* Event free survival; *LPBC* Lymphocyte predominant breast cancer; *FOXP3* Forkhead box P3; *TNBC* Triple negative breast cancer; *HER2* Human epidermal growth factor receptor 2; *AC* Doxorubicin and Cyclophosphamide; *FEC* 5-Fluorouracil, Epirubicin and Cyclophosphamide; *EC* Epirubicin and Cyclophosphamide; *CEX* Capecitabine, Epirubicin and Cyclophosphamide; *TAC* Docetaxel, Doxorubicin, and Cyclophosphamide; *AD* Doxorubicin and docetaxel

Table 12.4 Summary of key points and major conclusions

Key points
1. TIL density is a prognostic and predictive biomarker for TNBC and HER2+ breast cancer
2. Stromal TIL are a better predictor of clinical outcomes than intratumoral TIL
3. Expert-based guidelines have been developed for characterization of TIL density
4. TIL recruitment and function is influenced by various factors in the microenvironment including cytokines, regulatory cells and coinhibitory ligands expressed by the tumor

absence of platinum (46.6 vs. 33.5 % $p = 0.05$) and presence of platinum (>75 vs. 38.1 %, $p < 0.0005$). Higher TIL density has also been associated with higher pCR rates after neoadjuvant HER2-directed therapy plus chemotherapy (Salgado et al. 2015a; Denkert et al. 2014, 2015).

In a pooled meta-analysis of 13 published studies with 3555 patients, high level of TILs in pretreatment biopsy indicated higher pCR rates after neoadjuvant chemotherapy in TNBC and $HER2^+$ breast cancer. The correlation of pCR with TILs was not seen in hormone receptor positive [$HR^+/HER2^-$] disease (Mao et al. 2014). High $CD8^+$ T-lymphocytes in samples pre- (OR: 3.36; 95 % CI: 1.15–9.85) or post-neoadjuvant chemotherapy (OR: 4.71; 95 % CI: 1.29–17.27) was associated with a higher pCR. In the $HER2^+$ group, high TILs not only predict a favorable response to neoadjuvant trastuzumab, but also to chemotherapy. Study of TILs and its response to chemotherapy in 368 pretreatment tissues from two ER negative cohorts (EORTC 10994 and BIG 00-01) (West et al. 2011), showed that high level of $CD8^+$ TIL was an independent predictor of anthracycline response.

TILs and Predicting Response to Endocrine Therapy: The status of TILs following endocrine therapy is not clearly defined. In a study of patients with ER^+ breast cancer treated with neoadjuvant steroidal aromatase inhibitor (AI) therapy, changes in $CD8^+$ T cells/$Foxp3^+$ or T regulatory cells ratio before and after therapy correlated with response. A significant increase in the $CD8^+$/Treg ratio was detected after hormonal therapy in responders ($p = 0.028$) but not in nonresponders (Chan et al. 2012). Thus, the $CD8^+$/Treg ratio in surgical pathology specimens can be a potential surrogate marker for predicting responses to neoadjuvant endocrine therapy.

TILs in Residual Cancer after Neoadjuvant Chemotherapy and Prognosis: In a retrospective study of 304 TNBC patients with residual disease after primary neoadjuvant chemotherapy, the presence of TIL in residual tumor was associated with better prognosis (Dieci et al. 2014). Both sTILs and iTILs were strong prognostic factors for metastases free survival and OS. The 5-year OS rate was 91 % for high TILs and 55 % for low TILs subgroup (HR: 0.19, 95 % CI: 0.06–0.61). The prognostic impact of TILs was most significant in patients with large tumor burden (>2 cm) or lymph node metastases.

12.8 Conclusion

The key points described in this chapter are summarized in Table 12.4. First, TIL density is a prognostic biomarker, and also a predictive biomarker for response to neoadjuvant chemotherapy in TNBC and HER2 positive breast cancer. Second, characterization of sTIL density is a more practical and reproducible biomarker than iTILs, and expert-based guidelines have been developed for characterization of TIL density. Third, TIL recruitment and function is influenced by various factors in the microenvironment. Further research is needed to evaluate in detail the composition of TIL, and their subclasses in the tumor microenvironment. In case of T cells their composition, T cell receptor repertoire, neoantigens being identified by the T cells and the presence of costimulatory or coinhibitory molecules needs to be further elucidated. Additional research is also needed in order to determine whether TILs provide prognostic information in metastatic breast cancer, or predict better response to vaccines or immune checkpoint blockade.

References

Adams S, Gray RJ, Demaria S et al (2014) Prognostic value of tumor-infiltrating lymphocytes in triple-negative breast cancers from two phase III randomized adjuvant breast cancer trials: ECOG 2197 and ECOG 1199. J Clin Oncol 32(27):2959–2966

Alexandrov LB, Nik-Zainal S, Wedge DC et al (2013) Signatures of mutational processes in human cancer. Nature 500(7463):415–421

Aruga T, Suzuki E, Saji S et al (2009) A low number of tumor-infiltrating FOXP3-positive cells during primary systemic chemotherapy correlates with favorable anti-tumor response in patients with breast cancer. Oncol Rep 22(2):273–278

Bloom HJ, Richardson WW, Field JR (1970) Host resistance and survival in carcinoma of breast: a study of 104 cases of medullary carcinoma in a series of 1,411 cases of breast cancer followed for 20 years. Br Med J 3(5716):181–188

Chan MS, Wang L, Felizola SJ et al (2012) Changes of tumor infiltrating lymphocyte subtypes before and after neoadjuvant endocrine therapy in estrogen receptor-positive breast cancer patients—an immunohistochemical study of Cd8+ and Foxp3+ using double immunostaining with correlation to the pathobiological response of the patients. Int J Biol Markers 27(4):e295–e304

Chen LJ, Sun J, Wu HY et al (2011) B7-H4 expression associates with cancer progression and predicts patient's survival in human esophageal squamous cell carcinoma. Cancer Immunol Immunother 60(7):1047–1055

Cortazar P, Geyer CE Jr (2015) Pathological complete response in neoadjuvant treatment of breast cancer. Ann Surg Oncol 22(5):1441–1446

Denkert C, Loibl S, Noske A et al (2010) Tumor-associated lymphocytes as an independent predictor of response to neoadjuvant chemotherapy in breast cancer. J Clin Oncol 28(1):105–113

Denkert C, Loibl S, Salat C et al (2014) Abstract S1-06: Increased tumor-associated lymphocytes predict benefit from addition of carboplatin to neoadjuvant therapy for triple-negative and HER2-positive early breast cancer in the GeparSixto trial (GBG 66). Cancer Res 73(24 Supplement):S1-06–S01-06

Denkert C, von Minckwitz G, Brase JC et al (2015) Tumor-infiltrating lymphocytes and response to neoadjuvant chemotherapy with or without Carboplatin in human epidermal growth factor receptor 2-positive and triple-negative primary breast cancers. J Clin Oncol 33(9):983–991

Dieci MV, Criscitiello C, Goubar A et al (2014) Prognostic value of tumor-infiltrating lymphocytes on residual disease after primary chemotherapy for triple-negative breast cancer: a retrospective multicenter study. Ann Oncol 25(3):611–618

Dieci MV, Mathieu MC, Guarneri V et al (2015) Prognostic and predictive value of tumor infiltrating lymphocytes in two phase III randomized adjuvant breast cancer trials. Ann Oncol 26(8):1698–1704

Dunn GP, Old LJ, Schreiber RD (2004) The three Es of cancer immunoediting. Annu Rev Immunol 22:329–360

Fisher B, Bryant J, Wolmark N et al (1998) Effect of preoperative chemotherapy on the outcome of women with operable breast cancer. J Clin Oncol 16(8):2672–2685

Groh V, Wu J, Yee C, Spies T (2002) Tumour-derived soluble MIC ligands impair expression of NKG2D and T-cell activation. Nature 419(6908):734–738

Issa-Nummer Y, Darb-Esfahani S, Loibl S et al (2013) Prospective validation of immunological infiltrate for prediction of response to neoadjuvant chemotherapy in HER2-negative breast cancer—a substudy of the neoadjuvant GeparQuinto trial. PLoS ONE 8(12): e79775

Janakiram M, Abadi YM, Sparano JA, Zang X (2012) T cell coinhibition and immunotherapy in human breast cancer. Discov Med 14(77):229–236

Janakiram M, Chinai J, Fineberg S et al (2014) Expression, clinical significance, and receptor identification of the newest B7 family member HHLA2 protein. Clin Cancer Res 21(10):2359–2366

Jiang X, Shapiro DJ (2014) The immune system and inflammation in breast cancer. Mol Cell Endocrinol 382(1):673–682

Ladoire S, Arnould L, Apetoh L et al (2008) Pathologic complete response to neoadjuvant chemotherapy of breast carcinoma is associated with the disappearance of tumor-infiltrating foxp3+ regulatory T cells. Clin Cancer Res 14(8):2413–2420

Lakhani SR, Jacquemier J, Sloane JP et al (1998) Multifactorial analysis of differences between sporadic breast cancers and cancers involving BRCA1 and BRCA2 mutations. J Natl Cancer Inst 90(15):1138–1145

Lee HJ, Seo JY, Ahn JH, Ahn SH, Gong G (2013) Tumor-associated lymphocytes predict response to neoadjuvant chemotherapy in breast cancer patients. J Breast Cancer 16(1):32–39

Liu F, Li Y, Ren M et al (2012) Peritumoral FOXP3(+) regulatory T cell is sensitive to chemotherapy while intratumoral FOXP3(+) regulatory T cell is prognostic predictor of breast cancer patients. Breast Cancer Res Treat 135(2):459–467

Liu S, Foulkes WD, Leung S et al (2014) Prognostic significance of FOXP3 + tumor-infiltrating lymphocytes in breast cancer depends on estrogen receptor and human epidermal growth factor receptor-2 expression status and concurrent cytotoxic T-cell infiltration. Breast Cancer Res 16(5):432

Loi S, Sirtaine N, Piette F et al (2013) Prognostic and predictive value of tumor-infiltrating lymphocytes in a phase III randomized adjuvant breast cancer trial in node-positive breast cancer comparing the addition of docetaxel to doxorubicin with doxorubicin-based chemotherapy: BIG 02-98. J Clin Oncol 31(7):860–867

Loi S, Michiels S, Salgado R et al (2014a) Tumor infiltrating lymphocytes (TILs) indicate trastuzumab benefit in early-stage HER2-positive breast cancer (HER2 + BC). Cancer Res 73(24 Supplement)

Loi S, Michiels S, Salgado R et al (2014b) Tumor infiltrating lymphocytes are prognostic in triple negative breast cancer and predictive for trastuzumab benefit in early breast cancer: results from the FinHER trial. Ann Oncol 25(8):1544–1550

Mao Y, Qu Q, Zhang Y, Liu J, Chen X, Shen K (2014) The value of tumor infiltrating lymphocytes (TILs) for predicting response to neoadjuvant chemotherapy in breast cancer: a systematic review and meta-analysis. PLoS ONE 9(12):e115103

Maria Vittoria Dieci AG, Marie-Christine Mathieu, Valentina Guarneri, Pier Franco Conte, Suzette, Delaloge FA (2014) Prognostic and predictive value of tumor infiltrating lymphocytes (TIL) in two phase III randomized adjuvant breast cancer (BC) trials. J Clin Oncol 32(5s) [suppl; abstr 11087]

Miyatake T, Tringler B, Liu W et al (2007) B7-H4 (DD-O110) is overexpressed in high risk uterine endometrioid adenocarcinomas and inversely correlated with tumor T-cell infiltration. Gynecol Oncol 106(1):119–127

Moore OS Jr, Foote FW Jr (1949) The relatively favorable prognosis of medullary carcinoma of the breast. Cancer 2(4):635–642

Muenst S, Soysal SD, Gao F, Obermann EC, Oertli D, Gillanders WE (2013) The presence of programmed death 1 (PD-1)-positive tumor-infiltrating lymphocytes is associated with poor prognosis in human breast cancer. Breast Cancer Res Treat 139(3):667–676

Oda N, Shimazu K, Naoi Y et al (2012) Intratumoral regulatory T cells as an independent predictive factor for pathological complete response to neoadjuvant paclitaxel followed by 5-FU/epirubicin/cyclophosphamide in breast cancer patients. Breast Cancer Res Treat 136(1):107–116

Ohaegbulam KC, Assal A, Lazar-Molnar E, Yao Y, Zang X (2015) Human cancer immunotherapy with antibodies to the PD-1 and PD-L1 pathway. Trends Mol Med 21(1):24–33

Ono M, Tsuda H, Shimizu C et al (2012) Tumor-infiltrating lymphocytes are correlated with response to neoadjuvant chemotherapy in triple-negative breast cancer. Breast Cancer Res Treat 132(3):793–805

Perez EA BK, Anderson SK, Thompson EA, Badve SS, Bailey H, Baehner FL (2014) Stromal tumor-infiltrating lymphocytes(S-TILs). In: The alliance N9831 trial S-TILs are associated with chemotherapy benefit but not associated with trastuzumab benefit. Paper presented at the San Antonio Breast Cancer Symposium

Pickup MW, Mouw JK, Weaver VM (2014) The extracellular matrix modulates the hallmarks of cancer. EMBO Rep 15(12):1243–1253

Prowell TM, Pazdur R (2012) Pathological complete response and accelerated drug approval in early breast cancer. N Engl J Med 366(26):2438–2441

Quezada SA, Peggs KS, Simpson TR, Allison JP (2011) Shifting the equilibrium in cancer immunoediting: from tumor tolerance to eradication. Immunol Rev 241 (1):104–118

Richardson WW (1956) Medullary carcinoma of the breast; a distinctive tumour type with a relatively good prognosis following radical mastectomy. Br J Cancer 10(3):415–423

Rizvi NA, Hellmann MD, Snyder A et al (2015) Mutational landscape determines sensitivity to PD-1 blockade in non-small cell lung cancer. Science 348 (6230):124–128

Sagiv JY, Michaeli J, Assi S et al (2015) Phenotypic diversity and plasticity in circulating neutrophil subpopulations in cancer. Cell Rep 10(4):562–573

Salgado R, Denkert C, Campbell C et al (2015a) Tumor-infiltrating lymphocytes and associations with pathological complete response and event-free survival in her2-positive early-stage breast cancer treated with lapatinib and trastuzumab: a secondary analysis of the neoaltto trial. JAMA Oncology 1(4):448–454

Salgado R, Denkert C, Demaria S et al (2015b) The evaluation of tumor-infiltrating lymphocytes (TILs) in breast cancer: recommendations by an International TILs Working Group 2014. Ann Oncol 26(2):259–271

Seo AN, Lee HJ, Kim EJ et al (2013) Tumour-infiltrating CD8 + lymphocytes as an independent predictive factor for pathological complete response to primary systemic therapy in breast cancer. Br J Cancer 109 (10):2705–2713

Smith IC, Heys SD, Hutcheon AW et al (2002) Neoadjuvant chemotherapy in breast cancer: significantly enhanced response with docetaxel. J Clin Oncol 20 (6):1456–1466

Sun S, Fei X, Mao Y et al (2014) PD-1(+) immune cell infiltration inversely correlates with survival of operable breast cancer patients. Cancer Immunol Immunother 63(4):395–406

Symmans WF, Peintinger F, Hatzis C et al (2007) Measurement of residual breast cancer burden to predict survival after neoadjuvant chemotherapy. J Clin Oncol 25(28):4414–4422

Tan W, Zhang W, Strasner A et al (2011) Tumour-infiltrating regulatory T cells stimulate mammary cancer metastasis through RANKL-RANK signalling. Nature 470(7335):548–553

Telli ML, Jensen KC, Vinayak S et al (2015) Phase II study of gemcitabine, carboplatin, and iniparib as neoadjuvant therapy for triple-negative and BRCA1/2 mutation-associated breast cancer with assessment of a tumor-based measure of genomic instability: PrECOG 0105. J Clin Oncol 33(17):1895–1901

Thomas DA, Massague J (2005) TGF-beta directly targets cytotoxic T cell functions during tumor evasion of immune surveillance. Cancer Cell 8(5):369–380

Villablanca EJ, Raccosta L, Zhou D et al (2010) Tumor-mediated liver X receptor-alpha activation inhibits CC chemokine receptor-7 expression on dendritic cells and dampens antitumor responses. Nat Med 16(1):98–105

Weiss VL, Lee TH, Song H et al (2012) Trafficking of high avidity HER-2/neu-specific T cells into HER-2/neu-expressing tumors after depletion of effector/memory-like regulatory T Cells. PLoS ONE 7(2):e31962

West NR, Milne K, Truong PT, Macpherson N, Nelson BH, Watson PH (2011) Tumor-infiltrating lymphocytes predict response to anthracycline-based chemotherapy in estrogen receptor-negative breast cancer. Breast Cancer Res 13(6):R126

Yamaguchi R, Tanaka M, Yano A et al (2012) Tumor-infiltrating lymphocytes are important pathologic predictors for neoadjuvant chemotherapy in patients with breast cancer. Hum Pathol 43 (10):1688–1694

Zhang L, Wu H, Lu D et al (2013) The costimulatory molecule B7-H4 promote tumor progression and cell proliferation through translocating into nucleus. Oncogene 32(46):5347–5358

Novel Imaging Based Biomarkers in Breast Cancer

13

Christine E. Edmonds and David A. Mankoff

13.1 Introduction

Positron emission tomography (PET) plays an increasingly important role in the evaluation of breast cancer. While CT, MRI, and radiography represent the traditional imaging modalities utilized in anatomic breast cancer evaluation, molecular imaging offers the benefit of providing in vivo biochemical and metabolic information specific to the tumor. Although molecular and nuclear imaging encompasses a range of methodologies and probes, we have chosen to focus this review on PET imaging, which is, currently, the most rapidly evolving methodology used in patients.

PET employs biologically-targeted molecular probes labeled with a positron-emitting radionuclide, typically produced in a cyclotron. The emitted positron travels a short distance in the human body (less than 1–2 mm) before encountering an electron, resulting in positron-electron annihilation and giving rise to two high energy photons or gamma particles traveling in opposite directions (nearly 180° apart). PET detectors simultaneously measure these photon pairs arising from annihilations along all possible projection lines through the patient's body, allowing non-invasive reconstruction of an image of regional tracer concentration. In time-of-flight (TOF) PET, implemented in many recent scanners, the difference in the arrival times of the 2 photons at the detectors is measured with sufficient precision to help localize the emission point. Recent advances in TOF PET imaging offer reduced image noise and an improved signal to noise ratio and will likely continue to advance the field of PET imaging (Surti 2015).

PET offers the advantage of producing quantitative images of metabolic and biochemical processes at an acceptably low patient radiation dose. The administered dose of radiopharmaceutical is typically quite small (10^{-6} to 10^{-9} g) and therefore without significant pharmacological effect, thus allowing for assessment of molecular states of disease without altering the underlying biochemical or metabolic process (Fletcher et al. 2008). Among nuclear imaging techniques, PET has the advantage of a combination of high sensitivity and relatively better spatial resolution, improving the visualization and quantification of regional tracer

D.A. Mankoff (✉)
Donner 116, Division of Nuclear Medicine, Department of Radiology, Hospital of the University of Pennsylvania, 3400 Spruce Street, Philadelphia, PA 19104, USA
e-mail: david.mankoff@uphs.upenn.edu

C.E. Edmonds
Division of Breast Imaging, Department of Radiology, Massachusetts General Hospital, 55 Fruit Street, WAC 240, Boston MA 02114, USA
e-mail: cedmonds@mgh.harvard.edu

S. Badve and Y. Gökmen-Polar (eds.), *Molecular Pathology of Breast Cancer*, DOI 10.1007/978-3-319-41761-5_13

Table 13.1 Summary of the biologic pathways and their respective PET probes as described in this chapter

Biochemical/metabolic target	Radiotracer/s
Glucose metabolism	^{18}F-fluorodeoxyglucose (FDG)
Steroid receptor imagining	
Estrogen receptor	^{18}F-fluoroestradiol (FES)
Progesterone receptor	^{18}F-fluoronorpregnenedione (FFNP)
Androgen receptor	^{18}F-fluorodihydrotestosterone (FDHT)
HER2 receptor imaging	^{89}Z-trastuzumab, ^{64}Cu-DOTA-trastuzumab,
	^{18}F-fluorobenzamidoethylmaleimide (FBEM)
Cell proliferation imaging	
Thymidine analog imaging	^{18}F-fluorothymidine (FLT)
Sigma-2 receptor imaging	^{18}F-ISO-1
Other	
Membrane lipid synthesis	^{11}C-choline
Amino acid transport	^{11}C-methionine
PARP-1 activity	^{18}F-FluorThanatrace
Angiogenesis	^{18}F-galacto-RGD, ^{89}Zr-bevacizumab

concentration. The following paragraphs are a summary of the most studied and promising novel and emerging imaging biomarkers of breast cancer, organized by their biologic targeting (Table 13.1).

13.2 Glucose Metabolism Imaging

PET was developed in the mid 1970s, but it wasn't until the late 1990s that it became a widespread imaging modality in clinical oncology. The rapid rise of the application of PET was due to several factors: (1) increasing clinical experience yielded recognition of the value of PET imaging of the glucose analog, 2-[^{18}F] fluoro-2-deoxy-D-glucose (FDG), and (2) the establishment of commercial production of FDG provided more widespread access to the tracer. The development of the combination PET/CT device further accelerated clinical use of the test, as the combination of molecular and anatomic imaging improved the accuracy of the studies and the ability to interpret the images (Tagliabue and Del Sole 2014; Beyer et al. 2000). FDG-PET/CT has become an important technique in the staging and restaging of numerous malignancies, including breast cancer. The role of FDG-PET/CT in the evaluation of breast cancer continues to evolve.

FDG is formed by substituting the positron-emitting (β+) radioisotope ^{18}F, produced in a cyclotron, for the normal hydroxyl group at the 2′ position of the glucose molecule. FDG is a glucose analogue and is thus taken up via glucose transporter proteins by almost all normal tissues as well as many tumor cells. Once intracellular, FDG is phosphorylated by hexokinase and is trapped. However, because FDG lacks the 2′ hydroxyl group of normal glucose, it cannot undergo glycolysis. FDG instead undergoes intracellular decay, with a half-life of 110 min, and is a good indicator of the distribution of glucose uptake and phosphorylation. The regional retention of FDG at delayed times after injection, typically one hour (Shankar et al. 2006), largely reflects retention of phosphorylated FDG and thus the rate of glycolysis measured by the glycolytic flux through hexokinase. Increased glycolysis is a distinctive feature of many malignant tumors compared to normal tissues, with increased glucose consumption—and therefore FDG uptake and retention—compared to background. Most breast cancers overexpress molecules related to glucose consumption, including glucose transporters (GLUT1 and GLUT3), and increased hexokinase activity, leading to increased retention. In most cases, phosphorylation by hexokinase is the rate-limiting step (Bos et al. 2002; Brown and Wahl 1993; Groheux et al. 2013a).

Preclinical and human in vivo studies have elucidated factors associated with both primary tumor and metastatic disease FDG uptake (Alvarez et al. 2014; Buck et al. 2004). As glycolysis is a process downstream of many key pathways in oncogenesis, the dependence of FDG uptake on molecular features is complex and not predicted by an individual gene product or pathway activation. In general, in patients, FDG uptake varies with breast tumor histology and sub-type, and elevated uptake is associated with features that correlate with tumor aggressiveness (Humbert et al. 2015; Buck et al. 2004). Multiple studies confirm higher tumor to background uptake in invasive ductal carcinoma as compared to invasive lobular carcinoma (Buck et al. 2004; Bos et al. 2002; Humbert et al. 2015), Lobular carcinomas can often have low FDG uptake difficult to discern from background. Elevated baseline FDG SUV is strongly associated with high mitotic activity, high tumor grade, high pleomorphic score, high levels of Ki67 (a marker of cellular proliferation) and negative hormone receptor status (Berriolo- Riedinger et al. 2007; Keam et al. 2011). Of all receptor subtypes, the triple negative subtype has the highest baseline SUV (Humbert et al. 2012, 2015; Keam et al. 2011).

In the clinic, FDG-PET/CT currently serves as a valuable diagnostic tool in the evaluation of locally advanced, metastatic, and recurrent breast cancer. The National Comprehensive Cancer Network most recently recommended that FDG-PET/CT be considered in the workup of Stage III and higher breast cancer (Fletcher et al. 2008; NCCN 2016). Several recent studies suggest high sensitivity of FDG-PET/CT for the detection of both extraaxillary nodal and distant metastases (Groheux et al. 2013a; Hong et al. 2013; Lee 2013). A recent meta-analysis demonstrated that FDG-PET/CT is more sensitive and specific than bone scintigraphy for detection of breast cancer metastases to bone, especially for more lytic lesions (Rong et al. 2013). FDG-PET/CT is also among the most accurate modalities for restaging of recurrent breast cancer, particularly for disease outside of the breast, with both high sensitivity and specificity (Bourgeois et al. 2013; Aukema et al. 2010; Murakami et al. 2012) (Fig. 13.1).

In addition to serving as a primary means of detecting metastatic disease, FDG-PET/CT is also used to predict and assess response to chemotherapy. Because metabolism of glucose occurs earlier than physical changes in tumor size, the ability of FDG-PET/CT to predict treatment response is an area of ongoing investigation. FDG may be particularly valuable in the setting of neoadjuvant chemotherapy (Bourgeois et al. 2013; Humbert et al. 2015; Pahk et al. 2014; Mghanga et al. 2013) and multiple recent studies indicate that FDG offers high sensitivity as an early predictor of response following initiation of chemotherapy. A prospective study of 104 breast cancer patients on neoadjuvant chemotherapy found that a decline in tumor maximal SUV of over 45 % after the first cycle of chemotherapy predicts a pathologic response with a sensitivity of 73 % (Schwarz-Dose et al. 2009), and a second study of 52 patients with locally advanced disease found that FDG-PET/CT was able to accurately predict response after just one course of neoadjuvant chemotherapy using a 50 % decline in maximum SUV (Rousseau et al. 2011). A prospective study of stage II and III patients identified responders after one course of neoadjuvant chemotherapy with a sensitivity of 85.7 % (Keam et al. 2013). A large meta-analysis of 745 patients concluded that FDG-PET/CT predicts early response to neoadjuvant therapy with a sensitivity of 80.5 % and specificity of 78.8 %, and with a trend toward higher sensitivity after the second course compared to the first (Mghanga et al. 2013). Taken together, these studies strongly suggest that FDG-PET/CT provides an early non-invasive means of predicting chemotherapeutic response.

Recent evidence suggests that FDG-PET/CT may be utilized to predict breast cancer response to endocrine therapy as well as to demonstrate early response. Dehdashti et al. utilized a novel imaging approach to predict whether the ER may

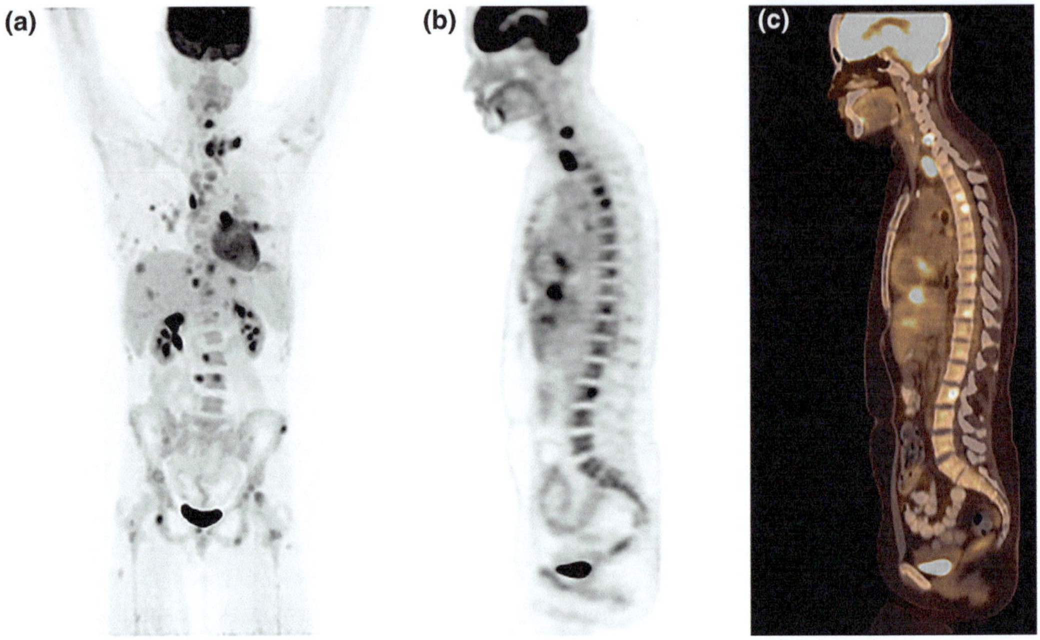

Fig. 13.1 Maximum intensity projection (**a**), sagittal (**b**), and sagittal fused PET/CT images from a restaging FDG-PET/CT in a patient with triple negative breast cancer demonstrate widespread metastatic disease, including pulmonary, hepatic, osseous, and mediastinal and supraclavicular/neck nodal metastases. Normal myocardial tracer uptake and renal tracer excretion is also demonstrated

be successfully pharmacologically blocked by administering a pre-treatment estradiol challenge to 51 women with advanced ER+ breast cancer. They found that metabolic 'flare' response on FDG-PET/CT following the challenge was predictive of response to either an aromatase inhibitor or fulvestrant. Patients underwent a baseline FDG-PET/CT and a second study following administration of 30 mg of estradiol. An increase in SUV of greater than or equal to 12 % represented metabolic flare and was correlated with a significantly longer overall survival, regardless of type of endocrine therapy (Dehdashti et al. 2009). In addition to demonstrating blockade at the level of the ER, FDG may also offer utility in demonstrating early response to upstream blockade of estrogen production. Kurland et al. found that a significant decline in FDG SUV (greater than or equal to 20 %) after two weeks of aromatase therapy was associated with low post-therapy proliferation, as measured by Ki67 in tumor biopsy specimens (Kurland et al. 2012). Preclinical experiments have elucidated the molecular basis of FDG uptake as a predictor of response to anti-estrogen therapy. The results of Ko et al. suggest that estradiol augments FDG uptake in ER+ breast cancer cells via increased glycolysis and hexokinase activity and is mediated by non-genomic membrane-initiated action (Ko et al. 2010), but further study is needed to confirm the mechanism put forth in this interesting preliminary study.

FDG-PET/CT may also play a particularly valuable role in the early assessment of HER2-targeted therapy in breast cancer. Following initial studies that suggested utility of FDG in this patient population (Groheux et al. 2013b; Humbert et al. 2014), the prospective Neo-ALTTO (Neoadjuvant Lapatinib and/or Trastuzumab Treatment Optimization) trial enrolled women with HER2 breast cancer and compared rates of pathologic complete response following anti-HER2 therapy to FDG metabolic response at 2 and 6 weeks post-treatment. Metabolic responses were evident in the primary tumors after 2 weeks of targeted therapy and were highly correlated with metabolic responses at 6 weeks. Pathologic complete responses were associated with greater declines in FDG uptake (as measured by maximum SUV) at both 2 and 6 weeks, indicating that FDG-PET/CT may identify patients with increased likelihood of complete response after neoadjuvant treatment with anti-HER2 therapy (Gebhart et al. 2013). FDG could therefore play an important role in guiding therapy decisions in this patient population.

Finally, FDG-PET/CT may be especially helpful in assessing the response of osseous breast cancer metastases to therapy, a particularly vexing clinical challenge by standard imaging. The use of FDG-PET/CT for this indication continues to grow. Clinical data have established that the initial FDG uptake within breast cancer osseous metastases is highly correlated with overall survival, after correcting for tumor phenotype, grade, and presence of visceral metastases (Morris et al. 2012). In addition, preliminary studies suggest that changes in serial FDG-PET/CT may predict time to progression in patients with bone dominant metastatic breast cancer (Specht et al. 2007). A retrospective study of 28 patients with bone dominant metastatic breast cancer who underwent serial FDG-PET found that percent decrease in SUV is predictive of time to disease progression. This study also found that a higher SUV value for an index lesion on the initial FDG-PET predicted a shorter time to a first skeletal-related event (such as pathologic fracture, spinal cord compression, or radiation to stabilize skeletal disease) (Specht et al. 2007). Evidence suggests that a decline in FDG uptake is associated with sclerosis on CT and indicates treatment response (Tateishi et al. 2008; Du et al. 2007). However, larger prospective studies are warranted to validate FDG uptake changes as a marker of treatment response.

While the clinical role of FDG-PET/CT in tumor staging and restaging continues to increase and evolve, it remains reserved as a staging modality for more advanced pathology-proven disease and plays little role in initial detection and early-stage disease (Bourgeois et al. 2013). FDG-PET/CT is not recommended to assess size of the primary tumor, nor to assess for the presence of local disease multifocality in the breast. This is primarily due to the limited spatial resolution of PET, and its variability of uptake in early-stage cancers. FDG imaging is less sensitive and less accurate than MRI for delineation of the primary tumor and assessment of multifocality (Groheux et al. 2013a; Heusner et al. 2008). Research also indicates that FDG-PET/CT cannot serve as a substitute for sentinel node biopsy due to the limited spatial resolution of PET (Groheux et al. 2013a; Cooper et al. 2011; Hindie et al. 2011; Veronesi et al. 2007; Wahl et al. 2004; Liu 2014). FDG PET/CT is not recommended for early-stage disease (stages I and IIa) in the absence of symptoms suggesting metastases (NCCN 2016), where the low incidence of disease and the imperfect specificity of FDG-PET/CT (or any systemic staging study) leads to a preponderance of false-positive studies that can lead to delays in treatment (Mankoff et al. 2012).

13.3 Steroid Receptor Imaging

13.3.1 Estrogen Receptor Imaging

Determination of the status of hormone receptors, both the estrogen receptor (ER) and progesterone receptor (PR), in breast cancer patients has become standard of care, as receptor status is an important prognostic factor and also dictates therapy (Schiavon and Smith 2014; Puhalla et al. 2012; Dunnwald et al. 2007). Approximately seventy percent of breast cancers are ER positive, and ER-directed adjuvant therapy is credited as a key factor in the decline in breast cancer mortality (Ferlay et al. 2010). Currently, the most commonly used method to assess hormonal receptor status, including the ER, is immunohistochemistry (IHC) of biopsy material. However, imaging of receptor status may offer several advantages over IHC, including noninvasiveness, potential for serial evaluation, and the ability to measure receptor expression in the entire disease burden. Biopsy of metastatic sites is often technically challenging and associated with higher morbidity than biopsy of the primary tumor. In addition, ER expression is often heterogeneous, with ER expression in the primary tumor or a metastatic site not predicting similar expression in other metastases (Spataro et al. 1992; Kuukasjarvi et al. 1996; Linden et al. 2006). Because it is not practical or feasible to biopsy every metastasis, an imaging assay to simultaneously assess ER expression at all disease sites offers the ability to both select patients who are likely to benefit from endocrine therapy and also monitor treatment response.

Current agents used to image the ER are analogs of estradiol. Estradiol, the most potent estrogen, binds with high affinity to the ER found in cell nuclei throughout the female reproductive tract and breast as well as liver, bone, pituitary, and hypothalamus. Estradiol is lipophilic and is transported in the bloodstream bound to either sex hormone-binding globulin (SHBG) or albumin, protecting it from hepatic metabolism and ensuring delivery to target tissues. Tracer binding to SHBG appears to be an important and necessary feature for a successful PET ER imaging agent (Jonson and Welch 1999).

The most successful hormonal receptor imaging agent to date is the ER imaging radiopharmaceutical 16α-[^{18}F]fluoro-17β-estradiol (FES). The binding characteristics of this positron emitting radiopharmaceutical are similar to estradiol for both the ER and SHBG (Kiesewetter et al. 1984), making it an excellent marker of ER expression. Like estradiol, the majority of FES within the blood is bound to protein, primarily SHBG and albumin, and the exact ratio depends on the concentration of SHBG (Mathias et al. 1987; Mankoff et al. 1997; Tewson et al. 1999). As with any other steroid, FES is metabolized by the liver (Mathias et al. 1987). Studies in both animal models as well as humans demonstrate that blood clearance and metabolism of FES is very rapid (Mathias et al. 1987; Mankoff et al. 1997); after two hours, most of the remaining activity in both blood and non-target tissues is due to metabolites. However, these metabolites are not selectively taken up by target tissues or tumor, and target tissue activity is primarily due to unmetabolized FES (Mathias et al. 1987). The uptake of FES by both the uterus and mammary tumors in adult rats reaches maximum levels in less than one hour (Mathias et al. 1987). Likewise, human studies demonstrate a predominance of metabolites [predominantly glucuronide and FES sulfate (Mankoff et al. 1997)] over unmetabolized FES by 20–60 min post-injection, while the radiolabeled blood metabolites persist, declining only slowly after 30 min. These metabolites do not readily bind to SHBG or penetrate the cell to bind to the nuclear receptor (Mankoff et al. 1997; Tewson et al. 1999); thus they do not contribute significantly to target tissue uptake, and delayed imaging beyond 30 min offers good visualization of ER-rich tissues (Mankoff et al. 1997).

FES measures all tumor sites, including metastases, simultaneously and thus demonstrates the tumors' ability to concentrate estrogen over the entire body (Mintun et al. 1988). The level of FES uptake in human breast tumors correlates with tumor ER expression by both radioligand binding (Mintun et al. 1988) and IHC (Peterson et al. 2008). Using a minimum standard uptake value (SUV) of 1.1 as the cutoff for determining ER-positive tumors, a concordance rate of 94 % was found between IHC results and FES uptake (Peterson et al. 2008). These early studies established FES-PET as a quantitative measure of regional ER expression. Further studies demonstrated the ability of FES-PET to assess ER expression in multiple sites of disease, including axillary lymph nodes (Mintun et al. 1988) as well as distant metastases (Mintun et al. 1988; McGuire et al. 1991) (Fig. 13.2), with good correlation between FES uptake and in vitro ER status (McGuire et al. 1991). Evidence supports the overall specificity of FES-PET for ER positive lesions, found to be 98 % (van Kruchten et al. 2013), with slightly lower sensitivity that may reflect heterogeneity in ER expression and tissue sampling error. A significant advantage of ER imaging over tissue biopsy is the ability to assess ER expression heterogeneity across multiple sites of disease (Kurland et al. 2011; Linden et al. 2006; Dehdashti et al. 1995), supported by studies that have provided new insight into the pattern of ER expression and loss of expression in recurrent disease (Linden et al. 2006; Dehdashti et al. 1995).

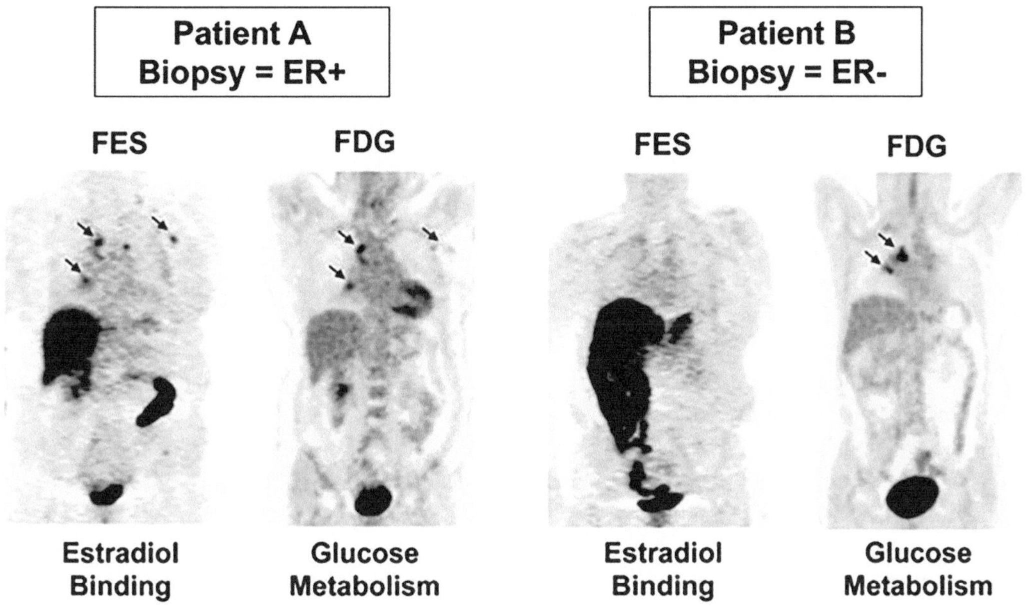

Fig. 13.2 FES- and FDG-PET images from two breast cancer patients. Patient A had mediastinal metastases appreciated by both FES as well as FDG, confirming ER expression. Patient B also had mediastinal recurrence visualized by FDG-PET. However, FES-PET demonstrated loss of the ER. Reprinted with permission from (Peterson et al. 2014)

Like measures of tissue ER expression, FES-PET can serve as a biomarker for breast cancer endocrine responsiveness. FES uptake measured by SUV predicts response to endocrine therapy with selective estrogen receptor modulators or aromatase inhibitors in both first line and salvage therapy settings (Linden et al. 2006; Mortimer et al. 2001; Dehdashti et al. 2009; Peterson et al. 2014). FES uptake, like IHC, identifies patients with tumors lacking ER expression who are unlikely to benefit from endocrine therapy. Studies to date suggest that patients with baseline tumor FES SUV values below 1.5 are unlikely to benefit from endocrine therapy (Linden et al. 2006; Humbert et al. 2015; Peterson et al. 2014) while a baseline SUV above 1.5 predicts a clinical benefit with a positive predictive value of 65 % and a negative predictive value of 88 % (Humbert et al. 2015). This is analogous to tissue assay for ER: absent ER reliably predicts a lack of endocrine responsiveness. However, only a subset of ER-expressing cancers respond to endocrine therapy.

Early evidence suggests that an early decrease in FES uptake after induction of endocrine therapy corresponds to ER blockade and is associated with disease response (Mortimer et al. 2001). In a clinical trial of forty women with ER + breast cancer treated with tamoxifen, FES successfully demonstrated early ER blockade; after 7–10 days of treatment with tamoxifen, mean tumor uptake (as measured by SUV) decreased compared to the baseline study, consistent with binding of tamoxifen to the ER. In addition, after 7–10 days of tamoxifen treatment, the percentage decrease in FES uptake was greater in patients who ultimately had a clinical response than in those patients who did not have disease response (Mortimer et al. 2001). A later study utilized FES uptake to compare regional estrogen receptor blockade in patients treated with tamoxifen versus fulvestrant. While both ER blocking therapies were effective in decreasing FES binding in both the tumor and uterus (as measured by percent SUV decrease), FES showed differences in the degree of blockade between the two agents. Tamoxifen treatment resulted in complete blockade (FES SUV of less than or equal to 1.5), while fulvestrant showed incomplete blockade (Linden et al. 2011). The lower level of blockade by fulvestrant may explain its lower clinical performance in humans compared to tamoxifen, and may be the result of inadequate dosing (Linden et al. 2011). This hypothesis is supported by a phase III trial that demonstrated increased efficacy at higher fulvestrant doses (Di Leo et al. 2010).

Studies up to this point support FES-PET in breast cancer patients as a quantitative measure of ER expression across the body and a biomarker of disease response to endocrine therapy. While clinical FES-PET/CT studies thus far are promising, multicenter studies are warranted to further evaluate sensitivity and specificity of FES and to evaluate the significance of intra- and inter-patient FES heterogeneity. Recently, multicenter trials sponsored by pharmaceutical companies have utilized FES-PET to evaluate new endocrine therapies (Wang et al. 2015), and multicenter studies validating the role of FES as a predictive biomarker for metastatic breast cancer are under development within the National Clinical Trials Network.

13.3.2 Progesterone Receptor Imaging

Approximately two thirds of the cases of breast cancer in the United States are progesterone receptor (PR) positive, and the majority of these cases also express the ER (Li et al. 2003). The PR is an estrogen-regulated gene, and its expression is indicative of a functioning ER pathway (Horwitz et al. 1978; Horwitz and McGuire 1975; Natrajan et al. 2010; Lanari et al. 2009). PR status is independently associated with disease-free and overall survival among patients on endocrine therapy, and ER+/PR+ breast cancers are more likely to respond to endocrine therapy than ER+/PR− cancers (Bardou et al. 2003). While ER+ disease responds to endocrine therapy in 55 to 60 % of patients (Dehdashti et al. 2012; Goldhirsch et al. 2002), the presence of the PR increases the likelihood of hormone responsiveness to approximately 75 % (Dehdashti et al. 2012; Keen and Davidson 2003). Thus PR status of biopsy material is routinely assessed, most often by IHC, and used to select therapy and predict prognosis.

The most promising PR radioligand to date is 21-(^{18})F-fluoro-16α,17α-[(R)-(1′-α-furylmethylidene)dioxy]-19-norpregn-4-ene-3,20-dione (FFNP), with both high affinity and selectivity for the PR (Lee et al. 2010). The first study in humans demonstrated that FFNP-PET is safe and has acceptable radiation doses. In addition, the FFNP tumor-to-normal breast uptake ratio was significantly correlated with in vitro PR status (Dehdashti et al. 2012). A preclinical study suggested that FFNP-PET may predict tumor response to endocrine therapy. Fowler et al. demonstrated an increase in FFNP uptake in the SSM3 mammary cell line implanted in mice following administration of estradiol therapy, suggesting estrogen-induced regulation of the PR gene (Fowler et al. 2012). Furthermore, FFNP uptake decreased following treatment with fulvestrant and preceded decreases in tumor size (Fowler et al. 2012). A second recent preclinical mouse study by the same group confirmed the ability of serial FFNP-PET to predict response to estrogen deprivation therapy. The group demonstrated that a significant decrease in FFNP uptake levels in ER+ tumors post-treatment compared to pretreatment levels predicted a positive response to estrogen deprivation therapy (Chan et al. 2015). Future human studies are warranted to evaluate the role of FFNP-PET as a biomarker of response to endocrine therapy following antiestrogen therapy or estradiol challenge.

13.3.3 Androgen Receptor Imaging

^{18}F-fluoro-dihydrotestosterone (FDHT) is a PET ligand targeting the androgen receptor. To date, studies have demonstrated utility of FDHT in the detection of bone metastases in androgen-sensitive prostate cancer that may remain undetected by FDG-PET or bone scan (Kircher et al. 2012). The androgen receptor (AR) has been implicated in the progression of some breast cancers (Mehta et al. 2015; Doane et al. 2006; Hickey et al. 2012). Recent evidence suggests that the AR antagonizes ER function and may oppose proliferation in ER+ breast cancers (Peters et al. 2009), while facilitating tumor growth in an androgen-dependent manner in ER −/AR+ breast cancers (Doane et al. 2006; Ni et al. 2011). These early studies suggest that FDHT may be potentially useful as a probe to evaluate AR targeting in breast cancer.

13.4 HER2 Receptor Imaging

Human epidermal growth factor receptor type 2 (HER2) is a member of the tyrosine kinase receptor family and is a strong prognostic biomarker for breast cancer (Allred et al. 1998). HER2 overexpression occurs in approximately 15–25 % of invasive breast cancers and is associated with a relatively aggressive disease and poor prognosis (Slamon et al. 1987; Slamon et al. 1989; Ross and Fletcher 1998; Sjogren et al. 1998; Ferretti et al. 2007). Overexpression, a result of DNA amplification, is associated with higher risk of relapse and death among patients with early stage breast cancer (Slamon et al. 1987). In addition, studies have demonstrated that overexpression of HER2 results in impaired response to both hormonal therapy via crosstalk with the ER (Carlomagno et al. 1996; Kurokawa and Arteaga 2003; Schiff et al. 2003; Ferretti et al. 2007) as well as certain cytotoxic chemotherapy regimens (Gusterson et al. 1992; Ferretti et al. 2007). HER2-targeted therapies have been shown to reduce development of metastatic disease and improve survival in HER2-positive breast cancer patients (Romond et al. 2005; Piccart-Gebhart et al. 2005).

Due to both prognostic and treatment implications, HER2 expression of biopsy or surgical specimens is routinely assessed, typically by IHC or fluorescence in situ hybridization (Linden and Dehdashti 2013; CAP Guidelines 2013). However, studies suggest a high error rate in laboratory testing of HER2 status, with incorrect results in approximately 20 % of HER2 tests performed by community laboratories compared to central or reference labs (Phillips et al. 2009). In addition, HER2 breast cancer is a heterogeneous disease, with intra- and intertumoral heterogeneity by IHC as high as 13 % and 30 %, respectively (Potts et al. 2012). One study found a therapeutically significant discordance of HER2 status between the primary tumor and metachronous recurrence or metastasis of 21.5 % (Santinelli et al. 2008). An imaging assay of HER2 expression may provide a useful means of noninvasively assessing the full burden of disease and both predicting and assessing response to HER2-targeted therapy.

Multiple imaging agents have been developed in recent years for noninvasive in vivo evaluation of HER2 expression, most of which are based on immune recognition. Labeled Anti-HER2 immune-based agents tested for imaging include immunoglobulins (trastuzumab and pertuzumab), immunoglobulin fragments, and novel constructs such as affibodies. Some agents are radiolabeled with single photon radionuclides (^{111}In-labeled trastuzumab and ^{99m}Tc-ICR12) while others are labeled with positron emitting radionuclides for PET (^{64}Cu-trastuzumab, ^{64}Cu-DOTA-$Z_{HER2:477}$, ^{68}Ga- trastuzumab Fab' b_2 fragments, ^{68}Ga-ABY-002, and ^{89}Zr-trastuzumab) (Linden and Dehdashti 2013; Capala and Bouchelouche 2010; Mankoff et al. 2008). One of the limitations of the clinical application of antibodies to molecular imaging is their large size, resulting in low tumor penetration and slow clearance and the need for a delay of several days to obtain images with reasonable tumor-to-blood ratios. However, one of the promising positron imaging agents is ^{89}Z-trastuzumab, with a long half-life (78.4 h), allowing antibody imaging up to 7 days after administration (Linden and Dehdashti 2013; Capala and Bouchelouche 2010). The first-in- humans study of ^{89}Z-trastuzumab-PET imaged 14 patients with HER2+ metastatic breast cancer. Delayed imaging (up to 5 days after tracer injection) demonstrated excellent tumor uptake and allowed for visualization of nearly all known metastases and several occult lesions (Dijkers et al. 2010). A similar early trial of ^{64}Cu-DOTA-trastuzumab

PET was performed in 6 patients with primary or metastatic HER2+ breast cancer. The results indicate that this agent is also safe and feasible for imaging HER2+ lesions, including brain metastases (Tamura et al. 2013).

Several research groups are now testing affibody molecules to image HER2. The small size of these proteins results in much more rapid blood clearance and better tumor penetration compared to antibodies, eliminating the need for delayed imaging. While affibodies have been radiolabeled with multiple isotopes, a group at the NIH created an ^{18}F-labeled affibody, *N*-2-(4-^{18}F-fluorobenzamido)ethyl]maleimide (^{18}F-FBEM)–*ZHER2*$_{:342}$ (Kiesewetter et al. 2008). A study of ^{18}F-FBEM-PET in mice xenografts found that tracer uptake correlated with HER2 receptor expression as assessed by IHC. In addition, mice were treated with 17-DMAG, an inhibitor of heat-shock protein 90, known to decrease HER2 expression, and the animals were scanned before and after treatment. The levels of HER2 expression estimated by PET decreased following treatment and were confirmed on pathology (Kramer-Marek et al. 2009). Additional preclinical and patient studies are warranted to further evaluate the role of HER2 as an imaging biomarker in breast cancer.

13.5 Cell Proliferation Imaging

13.5.1 Thymidine Analogs, Including Fluorothymidine (FLT)

Increased cellular proliferation is a fundamental feature of malignancy and is highly relevant to tumor growth and behavior (Tannock 2013). In breast cancer diagnosis, measurements of proliferation may be used in conjunction with tumor size, grade, nodal status, and hormone receptor status as a prognostic indicator (Beresford et al. 2006). Proliferation rates provide insight regarding prognosis and aggressiveness of tumors, and may be used to guide treatment (Beresford et al. 2006). Cell proliferation therefore provides an attractive imaging target for predicting and evaluating cancer treatment response.

While a variety of laboratory measures have been validated to evaluate and quantify cell proliferation rates in tissue specimens, including mitotic index and S-phase fraction, the most common current laboratory method of determining proliferation status is to detect Ki67 via IHC, using the antibody MIB-1 (Beresford et al. 2006). The human protein Ki67 is expressed in the nuclei of all dividing cells during G1, S, G2, and M phases, but is absent during G0 (Gerdes et al. 1991; Beresford et al. 2006), and therefore represents the total cellular proliferation regardless of DNA synthesis pathways. Studies have confirmed that higher grade cancers have higher Ki67 indices (Beresford et al. 2006; Sullivan et al. 1993), and the Ki67 index is correlated with other markers of proliferation (Beresford et al. 2006). However, IHC for Ki67 has several shortcomings, including sample variation. A study comparing Ki67 levels between core biopsies and surgical samples, without interim therapy, found significant differences between samples (Romero et al. 2011). An imaging agent targeting cell proliferation circumvents this shortcoming, and also offers a noninvasive means of evaluating proliferation.

In analogy to early studies testing the in vitro use of labeled thymidine as an indicator of breast cancer responsiveness (Thirlwell et al. 1976), the earliest studies of cellular proliferation used ^{11}C-thmyidine-PET to measure proliferation and demonstrated success in imaging tumor proliferation and changes in response to treatment (Shields et al. 1998b). However, a challenging synthesis, the short half-life of ^{11}C (approximately 20 min), and complex metabolism made ^{11}C-thmyidine impractical for routine clinical application (Mankoff et al. 2005). Subsequent investigations have largely focused on thymidine analogs as alternative PET proliferation imaging probes. The most widely used PET proliferation tracer to date is ^{18}F-fluorothymidine (FLT) (Shields et al. 1998a). The uptake of FLT is dependent on the activity of thymidine kinase-1 (TK-1), which is overexpressed during the S phase of the cell cycle (Kenny et al. 2005; Soloviev et al. 2012). TK-1 is present in cytoplasm and phosphorylates deoxythymidine during DNA synthesis. TK-1 activity is relatively high in proliferating cells, including malignant cells, but low or absent in quiescent cells (Beresford et al. 2006). FLT is transported from the extracelluar fluid into the cell via non-energy-dependent nucleoside transporters as well as Na^+-dependent carriers. Once intracellular, FLT is phosphorylated by TK-1, but due to its structure, cannot be incorporated into DNA synthesis and is instead trapped within proliferating cells; it is thus a marker of sites of proliferation (Beresford et al. 2006). FLT uptake in breast cancer patients correlates with Ki67 expression (Kenny et al. 2005; Bading and Shields 2008).

Compared to FDG-PET, FLT demonstrates lower cellular uptake and is therefore often inferior to FDG for cancer staging (Kenny et al. 2011); however, FLT was never designed or intended for use as a staging probe. In patient imaging, FLT has generally modest uptake compared to FDG (Yamamoto et al. 2007). In addition, high FLT uptake in the liver and bone marrow limits its utility for evaluation of metastatic disease in these organs (Kenny et al. 2011; Humbert et al. 2015). However, one advantage of FLT is its relative lack of accumulation at sites of inflammation, potentially reducing the false-positive results commonly encountered with FDG-PET (Humbert et al. 2015; van Waarde et al. 2004). An additional, and probably most significant, advantage of FLT is its ability to assess early response to breast cancer treatment and predict outcome (Kenny et al. 2007; Kenny et al. 2011; Pio et al. 2006) (Fig. 13.3).

Multiple recent studies have demonstrated early changes in FLT uptake after initiation of chemotherapy (Pio et al. 2006; Kenny et al. 2007; Contractor et al. 2011b; Contractor et al. 2012). An early study by Pio et al. of twelve breast cancer patients demonstrated that mean change in FLT uptake in both primary and metastatic tumors after the first course of chemotherapy significantly correlated with late changes in tumor marker levels. Change in FLT uptake was also found to be a good predictor of late changes in tumor sizes as measured by CT (Pio et al. 2006). A second small study by Kenny et al. demonstrated that FLT-PET can detect changes in proliferation at one week following chemotherapy, with a significant difference in uptake between responders and non-responders (Kenny et al. 2007). More recently, Contractor et al. have demonstrated that changes in FLT-PET uptake after 2 weeks of initiating the first or second cycle of docetaxel predict an anatomic tumor response at midtherapy (after three cycles) with high sensitivity (Contractor

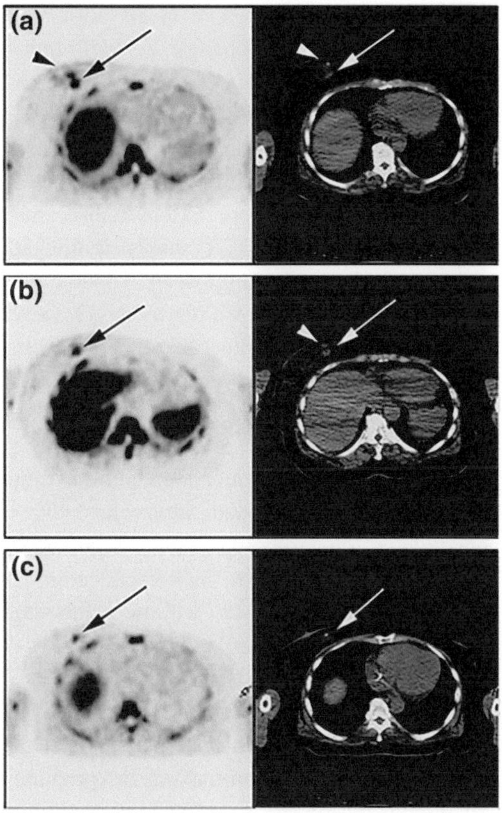

Fig. 13.3 FLT-PET/CT studies at baseline (**a**), within 1 week of completion of neoadjuvant chemotherapy (**b**), and after completion of 6 cycles of neoadjuvant therapy and before mastectomy (**c**). Baseline PET and CT images demonstrate multifocal disease in the right breast (*arrows* and *arrowheads*). Followup imaging (B&C) demonstrate progressive decline in uptake. Pathology demonstrated a residual focus of invasive carcinoma, with complete response elsewhere in the breast. Reprinted with permission from (Mankoff et al. 2014)

et al. 2011b). In addition, a small pilot study demonstrated that the change in FLT uptake within two weeks is correlated with the decrease in circulating tumor cells (Contractor et al. 2012).

The results of several more recent studies of FLT in the neoadjuvant setting are contradictory. In a study of 20 women, baseline SUV measurements of FLT-PET/CT were significantly related to Ki67, confirming that FLT uptake is, in fact, a biomarker of proliferation. However, neither the baseline uptake value nor the change in SUV after one cycle of neoadjuvant chemotherapy was predictive of response (Woolf et al. 2014). In contrast, a prospective study of 51 patients with invasive ductal carcinoma found that change in FLT uptake after one cycle of neoadjuvant chemotherapy was significantly higher for patients with pathologic complete response than for those without pathologic complete response (Kostakoglu et al. 2014).

The studies up to this point strongly indicate a significant correlation between FLT uptake and Ki67. In addition, multiple studies suggest that FLT may be an ideal biomarker for predicting and monitoring response to therapies that target proliferation. However, the results of these small patient studies need to be validated in a larger cohort or multicenter trial.

13.5.2 Alternative Approaches to Proliferation Imaging: Sigma-2 Receptor Imaging

While FLT patient studies are promising, recent studies offer alternative methods of imaging cell proliferation. Because TK-1 is expressed in the S phase of the cell cycle and is inactivated by cyclin-dependent kinase in early G2, FLT provides a snapshot of the percentage of cells in the S phase during the tracer uptake and acquisition of the PET scan. Most solid tumors are heterogeneous, containing populations of both proliferating and quiescent cells. However, FLT and other thymidine analogs cannot differentiate between proliferative cells in G1, G2, and M phases versus quiescent cells in G0, and may underestimate the proliferative status of a tumor by only detecting the fraction of cells in the S phase (Mach et al. 2009; Dehdashti et al. 2013; Shoghi et al. 2013). An alternative imaging approach targets the sigma-2 receptor.

Although the sigma-2 receptor has not yet been cloned and its endogenous ligands remain unknown, it is thought to be involved in cell survival, morphology, and differentiation (Huang et al. 2014; Guitart et al. 2004; Vilner et al. 1995a). Studies have demonstrated that the sigma-2 receptor is expressed at a 10-fold greater density in cycling tumor cells compared to quiescent tumor cells and is regulated in a manner similar to Ki67 (Mach et al. 1997; Al-Nabulsi et al. 1999; Wheeler et al. 2000). Thus sigma-2 receptor imaging offers a measure of the ratio of cycling proliferative cells to quiescent cells (P:Q ratio). Tumor cells enter quiescence during states of nutrient deprivation, such as when the tumor outgrows the blood supply, and may remain in this state for prolonged periods of time, until the tumor microenvironment again supports growth. Because many chemotherapeutics target proliferating cells and are ineffective against quiescent cells, knowledge of the P:Q ratio may have significant treatment implications (Dehdashti et al. 2013).

Early in vitro studies identified the sigma-2 receptor as a possible biomarker of breast cancer. Results demonstrated that the human breast tumor line MCF7 possesses a high density of sigma-2 receptors and a high affinity for sigma-2 radioligands (John et al. 1994; John et al. 1995; Vilner et al. 1995b). Followup in vitro and solid tumor xenograft studies in a mouse mammary adenocarcinoma model demonstrated that sigma-2 is a good biomarker of tumor proliferation in breast cancer (Mach et al. 1997; Al-Nabulsi et al. 1999; Wheeler et al. 2000).

To date, the most promising sigma-2 radioligand for PET imaging is N-(4-(6,7-dimethoxy-3,4-dihydroisoquinolin-2(1H)-yl)butyl)-2-(2-(18)F-fluoroethoxy)-5-methylbenzamide (^{18}F-ISO-1) (Dehdashti et al. 2013; Shoghi et al. 2013). In a mouse mammary tumor model, ^{18}F-ISO-1 uptake was significantly correlated with laboratory measures of proliferation status (Shoghi et al.

2013). Furthermore, ^{18}F-ISO-1 tumor uptake was significantly correlated with changes in tumor volume between consecutive MRI studies (Shoghi et al. 2013). In the first study of ^{18}F-ISO-1 in humans, there was a significant correlation between ^{18}F-ISO-1 uptake as measured by maximum SUV and Ki67 expression, including within the subset of 13 breast cancer patients (Dehdashti et al. 2013). Thus ^{18}F-ISO-1 may be useful in determining appropriate breast cancer therapy, and dedicated breast cancer clinical trials are warranted.

13.6 Other Novel Imaging Agents

13.6.1 Membrane Lipid Synthesis

Recent studies suggest that cell membrane synthesis may offer an alternative marker of cell proliferation. Proliferating tumor cells demonstrate increased lipid synthesis to form cell membranes, resulting in increased uptake of choline, a component of the membrane phospholipid phosphatidylcholine (Glunde et al. 2006). Elevated choline metabolism is considered a hallmark of tumor growth and progression, and both ^{11}C and ^{18}F-radiolabled choline have emerged as markers of tumor metabolism by PET imaging (Treglia et al. 2012). Uptake of both compounds is strongly associated with both thymidine uptake and S phase fraction (Glunde et al. 2011; Contractor et al. 2011a; Linden and Dehdashti 2013). While the primary clinical role of radiolabeled choline PET to date is in prostate cancer (Treglia et al. 2012), early studies also suggest utility in breast cancer. Contractor et al. demonstrated good visualization of ER+ breast tumors by ^{11}C-choline-PET as well as a correlation between uptake and tumor grade (Contractor et al. 2009). A recent comparison between FLT-PET and ^{11}C-choline-PET by the same group demonstrated a strong correlation between tumor uptake of ^{11}C-choline and FLT (Contractor et al. 2011a). Another recent comparison of ^{11}C-choline-PET and FDG-PET in breast cancer patients demonstrated that the degree of mitosis was independently associated with high ^{11}C-choline uptake by multiple logistic regression analysis, and of the factors analyzed (including histologic grade, nuclear grade, structural grade, and nuclear atypia), mitosis was the sole independent association (Tateishi et al. 2012). While more studies are warranted to assess the role of radiolabeled amino acids in breast cancer, these early studies support the utility of choline as a marker of proliferation.

13.6.2 Amino Acid Transport

Malignancy is associated with increased cellular utilization of nutrients, increasing the demand for and transport of amino acids. Metabolism of malignant tumors can be studied in vivo by imaging radiolabeled amino acids via PET, and the most studied radiolabeled amino acid in breast cancer imaging to date is L-methyl-^{11}C-methionine (^{11}C-methionine) (Linden and Dehdashti 2013). High uptake of ^{11}C-methionine is correlated with the S phase fraction of breast cancer tumor cells (Leskinen-Kallio et al. 1991). Several small studies of ^{11}C-methionine-PET in patients with advanced breast cancer have demonstrated that ^{11}C-methionine may provide utility in assessment of tumor response to therapy and may distinguish responders from non-responders after one or more cycles of systemic treatment (Huovinen et al. 1993; Lindholm et al. 2009).

13.6.3 PARP-1

PARP-1 is one of the most abundant members of the PARP family of nuclear enzymes and plays a central role in sensing DNA damage and facilitating repair (Hassa and Hottiger 2008). Given its role in DNA repair, PARP-1 has been actively investigated as a drug target in recent years. Because tumors with BRCA1 or BRCA2 mutations cannot undergo repair of double-strand DNA breaks via homologous recombination, they are highly dependent on PARP-1 as an alternative mechanism of DNA repair, and PARP inhibitors generate synthetic lethality in tumors with BRCA mutations, resulting in cell cycle arrest and apoptosis (Bryant et al. 2005; Farmer et al. 2005). Zhou et al. recently synthesized an ^{18}F-labeled PARP inhibitor (PARPi) known as FluorThanatrace for PET, and demonstrated high specific tracer uptake in a xenograft model of human breast cancer with innately high levels of PARP-1 activity (Zhou et al. 2014). While ^{18}F-PARPi studies are in the early phases of investigation, initial evidence suggests ^{18}F-PARPi-PET may offer utility in predicting which breast cancer patients will respond to PARP inhibitor therapy and may be particularly promising in patients with BRCA1 or BRCA2 mutations.

13.6.4 Angiogenesis

Angiogenesis is a hallmark of malignancy and is integral to the development of invasive cancer, metastasis, and progression, as well as the delivery of chemotherapy to the target tumor cells (Jain 2005). ^{15}O-water-PET permits reliable estimates of tumor blood flow in breast cancer (Wilson et al. 1992) and is predictive of response and survival in the neoadjuvant setting (Mankoff et al. 2003; Dunnwald et al. 2008). However, perfusion is not specific to tumor neovascularity. More recently, imaging probes have been developed that target integrins expressed on activated endothelial cells in neovessels. The most studied of these tracers, ^{18}F-galacto-RGD, is taken up by both primary and metastatic breast cancer (Beer et al. 2008). ^{89}Zirconium-labeled bevacizumab (^{89}Zr-bevacizumab), a radiolabeled monoclonal antibody targeting vascular endothelial growth factor (VEGF) is another promising PET tracer for in vivo analysis of tumor angiogenesis. The first clinical feasibility study of ^{89}Zr-bevacizumab-PET in breast cancer patients demonstrated uptake in the majority of primary tumors. In addition, uptake was associated with the level of VEGF-A in the tumors (Gaykema et al. 2013). These imaging agents may be particularly useful in predicting and assessing response to therapies targeting tumor angiogenesis.

13.7 Conclusion

While the role of FDG-PET in the evaluation of breast cancer continues to evolve and increase, numerous novel PET radiotracers beyond FDG also demonstrate promise in the assessment of tumor biology and prediction of treatment response. Novel tracers reviewed in this chapter, including steroid receptor, HER2 receptor, and cell proliferation imaging agents, among others, have the potential to serve as useful biomarkers in clinical medicine and may also aid in the development of targeted therapy. In the future, many of these PET tracers will likely alter and improve the approach to diagnosis and treatment of breast cancer.

Acknowledgments This work was supported in part by the following grants: Susan G. Komen, Komen SAC140060 and Department of Energy, DE-SE0012476, NIH training grant T32-EB004311, along with an institutional grant from the University of Pennsylvania Health System (Breast Cancer Translational Center of Excellence).

References

Al-Nabulsi I, Mach RH, Wang LM et al (1999) Effect of ploidy, recruitment, environmental factors, and tamoxifen treatment on the expression of sigma-2 receptors in proliferating and quiescent tumour cells. Br J Cancer 81(6):925–933

Allred DC, Harvey JM, Berardo M, Clark GM (1998) Prognostic and predictive factors in breast cancer by immunohistochemical analysis. Mod Pathol 11 (2):155–168

Alvarez JV, Belka GK, Pan TC et al (2014) Oncogene pathway activation in mammary tumors dictates FDG-PET uptake. Cancer Res 74(24):7583–7598

Aukema TS, Rutgers EJ, Vogel WV et al (2010) The role of FDG PET/CT in patients with locoregional breast cancer recurrence: a comparison to conventional imaging techniques. Eur J Surg Oncol 36(4):387–392

Bading JR, Shields AF (2008) Imaging of cell proliferation: status and prospects. J Nucl Med 49(Suppl 2):64S–80S

Bardou VJ, Arpino G, Elledge RM, Osborne CK, Clark GM (2003) Progesterone receptor status significantly improves outcome prediction over estrogen receptor status alone for adjuvant endocrine therapy in two large breast cancer databases. J Clin Oncol 21 (10):1973–1979

Beer AJ, Niemeyer M, Carlsen J et al (2008) Patterns of alphavbeta3 expression in primary and metastatic human breast cancer as shown by 18F-Galacto-RGD PET. J Nucl Med 49(2):255–259

Beresford MJ, Wilson GD, Makris A (2006) Measuring proliferation in breast cancer: practicalities and applications. Breast Cancer Res 8(6):216

Berriolo-Riedinger A, Touzery C, Riedinger JM et al (2007) [^{18}F]FDG-PET predicts complete pathological response of breast cancer to neoadjuvant chemotherapy. Eur J Nucl Med Mol Imaging 34(12):1915–1924

Beyer T, Townsend DW, Brun T et al (2000) A combined PET/CT scanner for clinical oncology. J Nucl Med 41 (8):1369–1379

Bos R, van Der Hoeven JJ, van Der Wall E et al (2002) Biologic correlates of (18)fluorodeoxyglucose uptake in human breast cancer measured by positron emission tomography. J Clin Oncol 20(2):379–387

Bourgeois AC, Warren LA, Chang TT, Embry S, Hudson K, Bradley YC (2013) Role of positron emission tomography/computed tomography in breast cancer. Radiol Clin North Am 51(5):781–798

Brown RS, Wahl RL (1993) Overexpression of Glut-1 glucose transporter in human breast cancer. An immunohistochemical study. Cancer 72(10):2979–2985

Bryant HE, Schultz N, Thomas HD et al (2005) Specific killing of BRCA2-deficient tumours with inhibitors of poly(ADP-ribose) polymerase. Nature 434 (7035):913–917

Buck AK, Schirrmeister H, Mattfeldt T, Reske SN (2004) Biological characterisation of breast cancer by means of PET. Eur J Nucl Med Mol Imaging 31(Suppl 1): S80–S87

CAP Guidelines (2013) http://www.cap.org/apps/docs/committees/immunohistochemistry/summary_of_recommendations.pdf

Capala J, Bouchelouche K (2010) Molecular imaging of HER2-positive breast cancer: a step toward an individualized 'image and treat' strategy. Curr Opin Oncol 22(6):559–566

Carlomagno C, Perrone F, Gallo C et al (1996) c-erb B2 overexpression decreases the benefit of adjuvant tamoxifen in early-stage breast cancer without axillary lymph node metastases. J Clin Oncol 14(10):2702–2708

Chan SR, Fowler AM, Allen JA et al (2015) Longitudinal noninvasive imaging of progesterone receptor as a predictive biomarker of tumor responsiveness to estrogen deprivation therapy. Clin Cancer Res 21 (5):1063–1070

Contractor KB, Kenny LM, Stebbing J et al (2009) [^{11}C]choline positron emission tomography in estrogen receptor-positive breast cancer. Clin Cancer Res 15(17):5503–5510

Contractor KB, Kenny LM, Stebbing J et al (2011a) Biological basis of [(11)C]choline-positron emission tomography in patients with breast cancer: comparison with [(18)F]fluorothymidine positron emission tomography. Nucl Med Commun 32(11):997–1004

Contractor KB, Kenny LM, Stebbing J et al (2011b) [^{18}F]-3'Deoxy-3'-fluorothymidine positron emission tomography and breast cancer response to docetaxel. Clin Cancer Res 17(24):7664–7672

Contractor K, Aboagye EO, Jacob J, Challapalli A, Coombes RC, Stebbing J (2012) Monitoring early response to taxane therapy in advanced breast cancer with circulating tumor cells and [(18)F] 3-deoxy-3-fluorothymidine PET: a pilot study. Biomark Med 6(2):231–233

Cooper KL, Harnan S, Meng Y et al (2011) Positron emission tomography (PET) for assessment of axillary lymph node status in early breast cancer: A systematic review and meta-analysis. Eur J Surg Oncol 37 (3):187–198

Dehdashti F, Mortimer JE, Siegel BA et al (1995) Positron tomographic assessment of estrogen receptors in breast cancer: comparison with FDG-PET and in vitro receptor assays. J Nucl Med 36(10):1766–1774

Dehdashti F, Mortimer JE, Trinkaus K et al (2009) PET-based estradiol challenge as a predictive biomarker of response to endocrine therapy in women with estrogen-receptor-positive breast cancer. Breast Cancer Res Treat 113(3):509–517

Dehdashti F, Laforest R, Gao F et al (2012) Assessment of progesterone receptors in breast carcinoma by PET with 21-^{18}F-fluoro-16α, 17α-[(R)-(1′-α-furylmethylidene)dioxy]-19-norpregn-4-ene-3,20-dione. J Nucl Med 53(3):363–370

Dehdashti F, Laforest R, Gao F et al (2013) Assessment of cellular proliferation in tumors by PET using ^{18}F-ISO-1. J Nucl Med 54(3):350–357

Di Leo A, Jerusalem G, Petruzelka L et al (2010) Results of the CONFIRM phase III trial comparing fulvestrant 250 mg with fulvestrant 500 mg in postmenopausal women with estrogen receptor-positive advanced breast cancer. J Clin Oncol 28(30):4594–4600

Dijkers EC, Oude Munnink TH, Kosterink JG et al (2010) Biodistribution of ^{89}Zr-trastuzumab and PET imaging of HER2-positive lesions in patients with metastatic breast cancer. Clin Pharmacol Ther 87(5):586–592

Doane AS, Danso M, Lal P et al (2006) An estrogen receptor-negative breast cancer subset characterized by a hormonally regulated transcriptional program and response to androgen. Oncogene 25(28):3994–4008

Du Y, Cullum I, Illidge TM, Ell PJ (2007) Fusion of metabolic function and morphology: sequential [^{18}F] fluorodeoxyglucose positron-emission tomography/computed tomography studies yield new insights into the natural history of bone metastases in breast cancer. J Clin Oncol 25(23):3440–3447

Dunnwald LK, Rossing MA, Li CI (2007) Hormone receptor status, tumor characteristics, and prognosis: a prospective cohort of breast cancer patients. Breast Cancer Res 9(1):R6

Dunnwald LK, Gralow JR, Ellis GK et al (2008) Tumor metabolism and blood flow changes by positron emission tomography: relation to survival in patients treated with neoadjuvant chemotherapy for locally advanced breast cancer. J Clin Oncol 26(27):4449–4457

Farmer H, McCabe N, Lord CJ et al (2005) Targeting the DNA repair defect in BRCA mutant cells as a therapeutic strategy. Nature 434(7035):917–921
Ferlay J, Shin HR, Bray F, Forman D, Mathers C, Parkin DM (2010) Estimates of worldwide burden of cancer in 2008: GLOBOCAN 2008. Int J Cancer 127 (12):2893–2917
Ferretti G, Felici A, Papaldo P, Fabi A, Cognetti F (2007) HER2/neu role in breast cancer: from a prognostic foe to a predictive friend. Curr Opin Obstet Gynecol 19 (1):56–62
Fletcher JW, Djulbegovic B, Soares HP et al (2008) Recommendations on the use of ^{18}F-FDG PET in oncology. J Nucl Med 49(3):480–508
Fowler AM, Chan SR, Sharp TL et al (2012) Small-animal PET of steroid hormone receptors predicts tumor response to endocrine therapy using a preclinical model of breast cancer. J Nucl Med 53 (7):1119–1126
Gaykema SB, Brouwers AH, Lub-de Hooge MN et al (2013) ^{89}Zr-bevacizumab PET imaging in primary breast cancer. J Nucl Med 54(7):1014–1018
Gebhart G, Gamez C, Holmes E et al (2013) ^{18}F-FDG PET/CT for early prediction of response to neoadjuvant lapatinib, trastuzumab, and their combination in HER2-positive breast cancer: results from Neo-ALTTO. J Nucl Med 54(11):1862–1868
Gerdes J, Li L, Schlueter C et al (1991) Immunobiochemical and molecular biologic characterization of the cell proliferation-associated nuclear antigen that is defined by monoclonal antibody Ki-67. Am J Pathol 138(4):867–873
Glunde K, Jacobs MA, Bhujwalla ZM (2006) Choline metabolism in cancer: implications for diagnosis and therapy. Expert Rev Mol Diagn 6(6):821–829
Glunde K, Bhujwalla ZM, Ronen SM (2011) Choline metabolism in malignant transformation. Nat Rev Cancer 11(12):835–848
Goldhirsch A, Colleoni M, Gelber RD (2002) Endocrine therapy of breast cancer. Ann Oncol 13(Suppl 4):61–68
Groheux D, Espie M, Giacchetti S, Hindie E (2013a) Performance of FDG PET/CT in the clinical management of breast cancer. Radiology 266(2):388–405
Groheux D, Giacchetti S, Hatt M et al (2013b) HER2-overexpressing breast cancer: FDG uptake after two cycles of chemotherapy predicts the outcome of neoadjuvant treatment. Br J Cancer 109(5):1157–1164
Guitart X, Codony X, Monroy X (2004) Sigma receptors: biology and therapeutic potential. Psychopharmacology 174(3):301–319
Gusterson BA, Gelber RD, Goldhirsch A et al (1992) Prognostic importance of c-erbB-2 expression in breast cancer. International (Ludwig) Breast Cancer Study Group. J Clin Oncol 10(7):1049–1056
Hassa PO, Hottiger MO (2008) The diverse biological roles of mammalian PARPS, a small but powerful family of poly-ADP-ribose polymerases. Front Biosci 13:3046–3082
Heusner TA, Kuemmel S, Umutlu L et al (2008) Breast cancer staging in a single session: whole-body PET/CT mammography. J Nucl Med 49(8):1215–1222
Hickey TE, Robinson JL, Carroll JS, Tilley WD (2012) Minireview: The androgen receptor in breast tissues: growth inhibitor, tumor suppressor, oncogene? Mol Endocrinol 26(8):1252–1267
Hindie E, Groheux D, Brenot-Rossi I, Rubello D, Moretti JL, Espie M (2011) The sentinel node procedure in breast cancer: nuclear medicine as the starting point. J Nucl Med 52(3):405–414
Hong S, Li J, Wang S (2013) ^{18}FDG PET-CT for diagnosis of distant metastases in breast cancer patients. A meta-analysis. Surg Oncol 22(2):139–143
Horwitz KB, McGuire WL (1975) Specific progesterone receptors in human breast cancer. Steroids 25(4):497–505
Horwitz KB, Koseki Y, McGuire WL (1978) Estrogen control of progesterone receptor in human breast cancer: role of estradiol and antiestrogen. Endocrinology 103(5):1742–1751
Huang YS, Lu HL, Zhang LJ, Wu Z (2014) Sigma-2 receptor ligands and their perspectives in cancer diagnosis and therapy. Med Res Rev 34(3):532–566
Humbert O, Berriolo-Riedinger A, Riedinger JM et al (2012) Changes in ^{18}F-FDG tumor metabolism after a first course of neoadjuvant chemotherapy in breast cancer: influence of tumor subtypes. Ann Oncol 23 (10):2572–2577
Humbert O, Cochet A, Riedinger JM et al (2014) HER2-positive breast cancer: (18)F-FDG PET for early prediction of response to trastuzumab plus taxane-based neoadjuvant chemotherapy. Eur J Nucl Med Mol Imaging 41(8):1525–1533
Humbert O, Cochet A, Coudert B et al (2015) Role of positron emission tomography for the monitoring of response to therapy in breast cancer. Oncologist 20 (2):94–104
Huovinen R, Leskinen-Kallio S, Nagren K, Lehikoinen P, Ruotsalainen U, Teras M (1993) Carbon-11-methionine and PET in evaluation of treatment response of breast cancer. Br J Cancer 67(4):787–791
Jain RK (2005) Antiangiogenic therapy for cancer: current and emerging concepts. Oncology (Williston Park) 19(4 Suppl 3):7–16
John CS, Vilner BJ, Bowen WD (1994) Synthesis and characterization of [^{125}I]-N-(N-benzylpiperidin-4-yl)-4- iodobenzamide, a new sigma receptor radiopharmaceutical: high-affinity binding to MCF-7 breast tumor cells. J Med Chem 37(12):1737–1739
John CS, Vilner BJ, Gulden ME et al (1995) Synthesis and pharmacological characterization of 4-[^{125}I]-N-(N-benzylpiperidin-4-yl)-4-iodobenzamide: a high affinity sigma receptor ligand for potential imaging of breast cancer. Cancer Res 55(14):3022–3027
Jonson SD, Welch MJ (1999) Synthesis, biological evaluation, and baboon PET imaging of the potential adrenal imaging agent cholesteryl-p-[^{18}F]fluorobenzoate. Nucl Med Biol 26(1):131–138

Keam B, Im SA, Koh Y et al (2011) Early metabolic response using FDG PET/CT and molecular phenotypes of breast cancer treated with neoadjuvant chemotherapy. BMC Cancer 11:452

Keam B, Im SA, Koh Y et al (2013) Predictive value of FDG PET/CT for pathologic axillary node involvement after neoadjuvant chemotherapy. Breast Cancer 20(2):167–173

Keen JC, Davidson NE (2003) The biology of breast carcinoma. Cancer 97(3 Suppl):825–833

Kenny LM, Vigushin DM, Al-Nahhas A et al (2005) Quantification of cellular proliferation in tumor and normal tissues of patients with breast cancer by [^{18}F]fluorothymidine-positron emission tomography imaging: evaluation of analytical methods. Cancer Res 65 (21):10104–10112

Kenny L, Coombes RC, Vigushin DM, Al-Nahhas A, Shousha S, Aboagye EO (2007) Imaging early changes in proliferation at 1 week post chemotherapy: a pilot study in breast cancer patients with 3′-deoxy-3′-[^{18}F]fluorothymidine positron emission tomography. Eur J Nucl Med Mol Imaging 34(9):1339–1347

Kenny LM, Al-Nahhas A, Aboagye EO (2011) Novel PET biomarkers for breast cancer imaging. Nucl Med Commun 32(5):333–335

Kiesewetter DO, Kilbourn MR, Landvatter SW, Heiman DF, Katzenellenbogen JA, Welch MJ (1984) Preparation of four fluorine- 18-labeled estrogens and their selective uptakes in target tissues of immature rats. J Nucl Med 25(11):1212–1221

Kiesewetter DO, Kramer-Marek G, Ma Y, Capala J (2008) Radiolabeling of HER2 specific Affibody(R) molecule with F-18. J Fluor Chem 129(9):799–805

Kircher MF, Hricak H, Larson SM (2012) Molecular imaging for personalized cancer care. Mol Oncol 6 (2):182–195

Ko BH, Paik JY, Jung KH, Lee KH (2010) 17beta-estradiol augments ^{18}F-FDG uptake and glycolysis of T47D breast cancer cells via membrane-initiated rapid PI3K-Akt activation. J Nucl Med 51(11):1740–1747

Kostakoglu L, Duan F, Idowu MO, Jolles PR, Bear HD, Muzi M, Cormack J, Pryma DA, Specht JM, Hovanessian Larsen L, Miliziano J, Mallett S, Shields AF, David A (2014) Mankoff phase II study of 3′-deoxy-3′-^{18}F fluorothymidine PET/CT (FLT-PET) in the assessment of early response in locally advanced breast cancer (LABC): preliminary results of ACRIN 6688. In: ASCO Annual Meeting

Kramer-Marek G, Kiesewetter DO, Capala J (2009) Changes in HER2 expression in breast cancer xenografts after therapy can be quantified using PET and (18)F-labeled affibody molecules. J Nucl Med 50 (7):1131–1139

Kurland BF, Peterson LM, Lee JH et al (2011) Between-patient and within-patient (site-to-site) variability in estrogen receptor binding, measured in vivo by ^{18}F-fluoroestradiol PET. J Nucl Med 52(10):1541–1549

Kurland BF, Gadi VK, Specht JM et al (2012) Feasibility study of FDG PET as an indicator of early response to aromatase inhibitors and trastuzumab in a heterogeneous group of breast cancer patients. EJNMMI Res 2 (1):34

Kurokawa H, Arteaga CL (2003) ErbB (HER) receptors can abrogate antiestrogen action in human breast cancer by multiple signaling mechanisms. Clin Cancer Res 9(1 Pt 2):511S–515S

Kuukasjarvi T, Kononen J, Helin H, Holli K, Isola J (1996) Loss of estrogen receptor in recurrent breast cancer is associated with poor response to endocrine therapy. J Clin Oncol 14(9):2584–2589

Lanari C, Lamb CA, Fabris VT et al (2009) The MPA mouse breast cancer model: evidence for a role of progesterone receptors in breast cancer. Endocr Relat Cancer 16(2):333–350

Lee JH (2013) Radionuclide methods for breast cancer staging. Semin Nucl Med 43(4):294–298

Lee JH, Zhou HB, Dence CS, Carlson KE, Welch MJ, Katzenellenbogen JA (2010) Development of [F-18] fluorine-substituted Tanaproget as a progesterone receptor imaging agent for positron emission tomography. Bioconjug Chem 21(6):1096–1104

Leskinen-Kallio S, Nagren K, Lehikoinen P, Ruotsalainen U, Joensuu H (1991) Uptake of ^{11}C-methionine in breast cancer studied by PET. An association with the size of S-phase fraction. Br J Cancer 64(6):1121–1124

Li CI, Daling JR, Malone KE (2003) Incidence of invasive breast cancer by hormone receptor status from 1992 to 1998. J Clin Oncol 21(1):28–34

Linden HM, Dehdashti F (2013) Novel methods and tracers for breast cancer imaging. Semin Nucl Med 43 (4):324–329

Linden HM, Stekhova SA, Link JM et al (2006) Quantitative fluoroestradiol positron emission tomography imaging predicts response to endocrine treatment in breast cancer. J Clin Oncol 24(18):2793–2799

Linden HM, Kurland BF, Peterson LM et al (2011) Fluoroestradiol positron emission tomography reveals differences in pharmacodynamics of aromatase inhibitors, tamoxifen, and fulvestrant in patients with metastatic breast cancer. Clin Cancer Res 17(14):4799–4805

Lindholm P, Lapela M, Nagren K, Lehikoinen P, Minn H, Jyrkkio S (2009) Preliminary study of carbon-11 methionine PET in the evaluation of early response to therapy in advanced breast cancer. Nucl Med Commun 30(1):30–36

Liu Y (2014) Role of FDG PET-CT in evaluation of locoregional nodal disease for initial staging of breast cancer. World J Clin Oncol 5(5):982–989

Mach RH, Smith CR, al-Nabulsi I, Whirrett BR, Childers SR, Wheeler KT (1997) Sigma 2 receptors as potential biomarkers of proliferation in breast cancer. Cancer Res 57(1):156–161

Mach RH, Dehdashti F, Wheeler KT (2009) PET radiotracers for imaging the proliferative status of solid tumors. PET Clin 4(1):1–15

Mankoff DA, Tewson TJ, Eary JF (1997) Analysis of blood clearance and labeled metabolites for the estrogen receptor tracer [F-18]-16α-fluoroestradiol (FES). Nucl Med Biol 24(4):341–348

Mankoff DA, Dunnwald LK, Gralow JR et al (2003) Changes in blood flow and metabolism in locally advanced breast cancer treated with neoadjuvant chemotherapy. J Nucl Med 44(11):1806–1814

Mankoff DA, Shields AF, Krohn KA (2005) PET imaging of cellular proliferation. Radiol Clin North Am 43 (1):153–167

Mankoff DA, Link JM, Linden HM, Sundararajan L, Krohn KA (2008) Tumor receptor imaging. J Nucl Med 49(Suppl 2):149S–163S

Mankoff DA, Specht JM, Eubank WB, Kessler L (2012) [(18)F]fluorodeoxyglucose positron emission tomography-computed tomography in breast cancer: when… and when not? J Clin Oncol 30(12):1252–1254

Mankoff DA, Pryma DA, Clark AS (2014) Molecular imaging biomarkers for oncology clinical trials. J Nucl Med 55(4):525–528

Mathias CJ, Welch MJ, Katzenellenbogen JA et al (1987) Characterization of the uptake of 16 alpha-([^{18}F] fluoro)-17 beta-estradiol in DMBA-induced mammary tumors. Int J Rad Appl Instrum B 14(1):15–25

McGuire AH, Dehdashti F, Siegel BA et al (1991) Positron tomographic assessment of 16 alpha-[^{18}F] fluoro-17 beta-estradiol uptake in metastatic breast carcinoma. J Nucl Med 32(8):1526–1531

Mehta J, Asthana S, Mandal CC, Saxena S (2015) A molecular analysis provides novel insights into androgen receptor signalling in breast cancer. PLoS ONE 10 (3):e0120622

Mghanga FP, Lan X, Bakari KH, Li C, Zhang Y (2013) Fluorine-18 fluorodeoxyglucose positron emission tomography-computed tomography in monitoring the response of breast cancer to neoadjuvant chemotherapy: a meta-analysis. Clin Breast Cancer 13(4):271–279

Mintun MA, Welch MJ, Siegel BA et al (1988) Breast cancer: PET imaging of estrogen receptors. Radiology 169(1):45–48

Morris PG, Ulaner GA, Eaton A et al (2012) Standardized uptake value by positron emission tomography/computed tomography as a prognostic variable in metastatic breast cancer. Cancer 118 (22):5454–5462

Mortimer JE, Dehdashti F, Siegel BA, Trinkaus K, Katzenellenbogen JA, Welch MJ (2001) Metabolic flare: indicator of hormone responsiveness in advanced breast cancer. J Clin Oncol 19(11):2797–2803

Murakami R, Kumita S, Yoshida T et al (2012) FDG-PET/CT in the diagnosis of recurrent breast cancer. Acta Radiol 53(1):12–16

National Comprehensive Cancer Network (NCCN). (2016) Guidelines: Invasive Breast Cancer. https://www.nccn.org/professionals/physician_gls/pdf/breast.pdf

Natrajan R, Weigelt B, Mackay A et al (2010) An integrative genomic and transcriptomic analysis reveals molecular pathways and networks regulated by copy number aberrations in basal-like, HER2 and luminal cancers. Breast Cancer Res Treat 121(3):575–589

Ni M, Chen Y, Lim E et al (2011) Targeting androgen receptor in estrogen receptor-negative breast cancer. Cancer Cell 20(1):119–131

Pahk K, Rhee S, Cho J et al (2014) The role of interim ^{18}F-FDG PET/CT in predicting early response to neoadjuvant chemotherapy in breast cancer. Anticancer Res 34(8):4447–4455

Peters AA, Buchanan G, Ricciardelli C et al (2009) Androgen receptor inhibits estrogen receptor-alpha activity and is prognostic in breast cancer. Cancer Res 69(15):6131–6140

Peterson LM, Mankoff DA, Lawton T et al (2008) Quantitative imaging of estrogen receptor expression in breast cancer with PET and ^{18}F-fluoroestradiol. J Nucl Med 49(3):367–374

Peterson LM, Kurland BF, Schubert EK et al (2014) A phase 2 study of 16alpha-[^{18}F]-fluoro-17beta-estradiol positron emission tomography (FES-PET) as a marker of hormone sensitivity in metastatic breast cancer (MBC). Mol Imaging Biol 16(3):431–440

Phillips KA, Marshall DA, Haas JS et al (2009) Clinical practice patterns and cost effectiveness of human epidermal growth receptor 2 testing strategies in breast cancer patients. Cancer 115(22):5166–5174

Piccart-Gebhart MJ, Procter M, Leyland-Jones B et al (2005) Trastuzumab after adjuvant chemotherapy in HER2-positive breast cancer. N Engl J Med 353 (16):1659–1672

Pio BS, Park CK, Pietras R et al (2006) Usefulness of 3′-[F-18]fluoro-3′-deoxythymidine with positron emission tomography in predicting breast cancer response to therapy. Mol Imaging Biol 8(1):36–42

Potts SJ, Krueger JS, Landis ND et al (2012) Evaluating tumor heterogeneity in immunohistochemistry-stained breast cancer tissue. Lab Invest 92(9):1342–1357

Puhalla S, Bhattacharya S, Davidson NE (2012) Hormonal therapy in breast cancer: a model disease for the personalization of cancer care. Mol Oncol 6(2):222–236

Romero Q, Bendahl PO, Klintman M et al (2011) Ki67 proliferation in core biopsies versus surgical samples —a model for neo-adjuvant breast cancer studies. BMC Cancer 11:341

Romond EH, Perez EA, Bryant J et al (2005) Trastuzumab plus adjuvant chemotherapy for operable HER2-positive breast cancer. N Engl J Med 353 (16):1673–1684

Rong J, Wang S, Ding Q, Yun M, Zheng Z, Ye S (2013) Comparison of ^{18}F-FDG PET-CT and bone scintigraphy for detection of bone metastases in breast cancer patients. A meta-analysis. Surg Oncol 22(2):86–91

Ross JS, Fletcher JA (1998) The HER-2/neu oncogene in breast cancer: prognostic factor, predictive factor, and target for therapy. Stem Cells 16(6):413–428

Rousseau C, Devillers A, Campone M et al (2011) FDG PET evaluation of early axillary lymph node response to neoadjuvant chemotherapy in stage II and III breast cancer patients. Eur J Nucl Med Mol Imaging 38(6):1029–1036

Santinelli A, Pisa E, Stramazzotti D, Fabris G (2008) HER-2 status discrepancy between primary breast cancer and metastatic sites. Impact on target therapy. Int J Cancer 122(5):999–1004

Schiavon G, Smith IE (2014) Status of adjuvant endocrine therapy for breast cancer. Breast Cancer Res 16(2):206

Schiff R, Massarweh S, Shou J, Osborne CK (2003) Breast cancer endocrine resistance: how growth factor signaling and estrogen receptor coregulators modulate response. Clin Cancer Res 9(1 Pt 2):447S–454S

Schwarz-Dose J, Untch M, Tiling R et al (2009) Monitoring primary systemic therapy of large and locally advanced breast cancer by using sequential positron emission tomography imaging with [^{18}F] fluorodeoxyglucose. J Clin Oncol 27(4):535–541

Shankar LK, Hoffman JM, Bacharach S et al (2006) Consensus recommendations for the use of ^{18}F-FDG PET as an indicator of therapeutic response in patients in National Cancer Institute Trials. J Nucl Med 47 (6):1059–1066

Shields AF, Grierson JR, Dohmen BM et al (1998a) Imaging proliferation in vivo with [F-18]FLT and positron emission tomography. Nat Med 4(11):1334–1336

Shields AF, Mankoff DA, Link JM et al (1998b) Carbon-11-thymidine and FDG to measure therapy response. J Nucl Med 39(10):1757–1762

Shoghi KI, Xu J, Su Y et al (2013) Quantitative receptor-based imaging of tumor proliferation with the sigma-2 ligand [(18)F]ISO-1. PLoS ONE 8(9): e74188

Sjogren S, Inganas M, Lindgren A, Holmberg L, Bergh J (1998) Prognostic and predictive value of c-erbB-2 overexpression in primary breast cancer, alone and in combination with other prognostic markers. J Clin Oncol 16(2):462–469

Slamon DJ, Clark GM, Wong SG, Levin WJ, Ullrich A, McGuire WL (1987) Human breast cancer: correlation of relapse and survival with amplification of the HER-2/neu oncogene. Science 235(4785):177–182

Slamon DJ, Godolphin W, Jones LA et al (1989) Studies of the HER-2/neu proto-oncogene in human breast and ovarian cancer. Science 244(4905):707–712

Soloviev D, Lewis D, Honess D, Aboagye E (2012) [(18) F]FLT: an imaging biomarker of tumour proliferation for assessment of tumour response to treatment. Eur J Cancer 48(4):416–424

Spataro V, Price K, Goldhirsch A et al (1992) Sequential estrogen receptor determinations from primary breast cancer and at relapse: prognostic and therapeutic relevance. The International Breast Cancer Study Group (formerly Ludwig Group). Ann Oncol 3 (9):733–740

Specht JM, Tam SL, Kurland BF et al (2007) Serial 2-[^{18}F] fluoro-2-deoxy-D-glucose positron emission tomography (FDG-PET) to monitor treatment of bone-dominant metastatic breast cancer predicts time to progression (TTP). Breast Cancer Res Treat 105 (1):87–94

Sullivan RP, Mortimer G, Muircheartaigh IO (1993) Cell proliferation in breast tumours: analysis of histological parameters Ki67 and PCNA expression. Ir J Med Sci 162(9):343–347

Surti S (2015) Update on time-of-flight PET imaging. J Nucl Med 56(1):98–105

Tagliabue L, Del Sole A (2014) Appropriate use of positron emission tomography with [(18)F] fluorodeoxyglucose for staging of oncology patients. Eur J Intern Med 25(1):6–11

Tamura K, Kurihara H, Yonemori K et al (2013) 64Cu-DOTA-trastuzumab PET imaging in patients with HER2-positive breast cancer. J Nucl Med 54 (11):1869–1875

Tannock I (2013) The basic science of oncology, 5th edn. McGraw-Hill, New York

Tateishi U, Gamez C, Dawood S, Yeung HW, Cristofanilli M, Macapinlac HA (2008) Bone metastases in patients with metastatic breast cancer: morphologic and metabolic monitoring of response to systemic therapy with integrated PET/CT. Radiology 247 (1):189–196

Tateishi U, Terauchi T, Akashi-Tanaka S et al (2012) Comparative study of the value of dual tracer PET/CT in evaluating breast cancer. Cancer Sci 103(9):1701–1707

Tewson TJ, Mankoff DA, Peterson LM, Woo I, Petra P (1999) Interactions of 16alpha-[^{18}F]-fluoroestradiol (FES) with sex steroid binding protein (SBP). Nucl Med Biol 26(8):905–913

Thirlwell MP, Livingston RB, Murphy WK, Hart JS (1976) A rapid in vitro labeling index method for predicting response of human solid tumors to chemotherapy. Cancer Res 36(9 pt.1):3279–3283

Treglia G, Giovannini E, Di Franco D et al (2012) The role of positron emission tomography using carbon-11 and fluorine-18 choline in tumors other than prostate cancer: a systematic review. Ann Nucl Med 26 (6):451–461

van Kruchten M, de Vries EG, Brown M et al (2013) PET imaging of oestrogen receptors in patients with breast cancer. Lancet Oncol 14(11):e465–e475

van Waarde A, Cobben DC, Suurmeijer AJ et al (2004) Selectivity of ^{18}F-FLT and ^{18}F-FDG for differentiating tumor from inflammation in a rodent model. J Nucl Med 45(4):695–700

Veronesi U, De Cicco C, Galimberti VE et al (2007) A comparative study on the value of FDG-PET and sentinel node biopsy to identify occult axillary metastases. Ann Oncol 18(3):473–478

Vilner BJ, de Costa BR, Bowen WD (1995a) Cytotoxic effects of sigma ligands: sigma receptor-mediated alterations in cellular morphology and viability. J Neurosci 15(1 Pt 1):117–134

Vilner BJ, John CS, Bowen WD (1995b) Sigma-1 and sigma-2 receptors are expressed in a wide variety of human and rodent tumor cell lines. Cancer Res 55 (2):408–413

Wahl RL, Siegel BA, Coleman RE, Gatsonis CG, Group PETS (2004) Prospective multicenter study of axillary nodal staging by positron emission tomography in breast cancer: a report of the staging breast cancer with PET Study Group. J Clin Oncol 22 (2):277–285

Wang Y, Ulaner G, Manning HC, Bardia A, Mayer I, Dickler M, Maneval EC, Lewis J, Baselga J, Mahmood U (2015) Validation of target engagement using ^{18}F-fluoroestradiol PET in patients undergoing therapy with selective estrogen receptor degrader, ARN-810 (GDC-0810). J Nucl Med 56:565

Wheeler KT, Wang LM, Wallen CA et al (2000) Sigma-2 receptors as a biomarker of proliferation in solid tumours. Br J Cancer 82(6):1223–1232

Wilson CB, Lammertsma AA, McKenzie CG, Sikora K, Jones T (1992) Measurements of blood flow and exchanging water space in breast tumors using positron emission tomography: a rapid and noninvasive dynamic method. Cancer Res 52(6):1592–1597

Woolf DK, Beresford M, Li SP et al (2014) Evaluation of FLT-PET-CT as an imaging biomarker of proliferation in primary breast cancer. Br J Cancer 110(12):2847–2854

Yamamoto Y, Nishiyama Y, Ishikawa S et al (2007) Correlation of ^{18}F-FLT and ^{18}F-FDG uptake on PET with Ki-67 immunohistochemistry in non-small cell lung cancer. Eur J Nucl Med Mol Imaging 34 (10):1610–1616

Zhou D, Chu W, Xu J et al (2014) Synthesis, [(18)F] radiolabeling, and evaluation of poly (ADP-ribose) polymerase-1 (PARP-1) inhibitors for in vivo imaging of PARP-1 using positron emission tomography. Bioorg Med Chem 22(5):1700–1707

Circulating Tumor Markers for Breast Cancer Management

14

Dhivya Prabhakar and Lyndsay Harris

Abstract

Many patients with early stage cancers will go on to develop metastases. Blood based tests for circulating tumor markers can provide an invaluable minimally invasive method for assessing tumor and monitoring patients. Several markers are purported to be available for this purpose. These include some newer biomarkers such as tissue polypeptide antigens and serum autoantibodies against tumor associated antigens. In this chapter, we critically evaluate the available markers and describe their advantages and more importantly their limitations. A thorough review of the data available for these biomarkers leads us to conclude that sufficient evidence exists for the use of CEA, CA15-3, CA27.29 in metastatic breast cancers. However, none of the biomarkers are suitable for routine use in patients with early stage breast cancer. Novel blood based-biomarkers are urgently required to monitor patients with early stage breast cancer and predict the long-term outcomes.

Keywords

Circulating blood biomarkers · CEA · CA15-3 · CA27.29

14.1 Introduction

Breast cancer is the most common solid tumor in women, with a lifetime risk of 1 in 8, if a woman lives to age 80. While in general, breast cancer is a very treatable disease, with 75–80 % cure rates, it accounted for an estimated 40,356 deaths in 2014 in the United States alone and approximately 400,000 deaths worldwide (Porter 2008; Kamangar et al. 2006). Improvement in survival rates have been seen over the last few decades and these are largely attributed to earlier detection and

D. Prabhakar (✉)
Division of Hematology and Oncology, Case Western Reserve University School of Medicine, Cleveland, OH, USA
e-mail: Dhivya.Prabhakar@UHhospitals.org

L. Harris
Diana Hyland Chair in Breast Cancer, Division of Hematology and Oncology, University Hospitals—Seidman Cancer Center, Case Western Reserve University School of Medicine, Cleveland, OH, USA

S. Badve and Y. Gökmen-Polar (eds.), *Molecular Pathology of Breast Cancer*, DOI 10.1007/978-3-319-41761-5_14

improvements in treatment of micro-metastases that have spread to distant organs. These achievements are the result of better screening technologies and a better understanding of the underlying molecular makeup of the disease.

Improvement in treatment of cancer is best achieved when the disease is well understood from a biological perspective. This approach has been successful in breast cancer where tumor tissue 'biomarkers' are used to classify the disease. The 'molecular classification' allows the identification of relevant targets that are most likely to eradicate micro metastatic disease in early stages of breast cancer. In addition to tissue biomarkers, the disease can be assessed by circulating markers that are typically proteins, nucleic acids and cellular fragments that are shed by the cells and represent the underlying biology of the tumor. The detection of these circulating biomarkers is a significant challenge as they are much less abundant in blood and require special techniques to measure them. While, they represent 'surrogate markers' of the tumor tissue, there are additional challenges in distinguishing these markers from those of the host, as many of them are also seen in other conditions such as inflammatory diseases and benign causes of organ dysfunction. Typically, circulating markers from cancer are more abundant than those of normal processes, although the lines become blurry when small amounts of tumor are present in the body. The applications of these markers range from early detection, to diagnosis, to treatment and the following review will focus on these areas, in the context of each marker discussed. The markers included in this chapter are serum or plasma-based markers and nucleic acid and cellular components are discussed elsewhere.

14.2 Traditional Tumor Markers

Several proteins have been classically associated with breast tumors and also detected in the circulation. Traditionally, used tumor markers include carcinoembryonic antigen (CEA), soluble mucin1 protein or MUC 1 protein (CA27.29 or CA15.3), and the ectodomain (ECD) of the human epidermal growth factor receptor (serum HER2). In addition, autoantibodies that are tumor-specific are detectable in plasma and serum and are thought to be part of the host reaction to the presence of tumor tissue. These glycoproteins are thought to be secreted by tumor cells or the cells in the tumor microenvironment and can be detected in the peripheral blood with immunoassays.

14.2.1 Carcinoembryonic Antigen (CEA)

CEA is a glycoprotein, attached to the membrane by a GPI (glycosyl phosphatidyl inositol) anchor and is involved in adhesion to the extracellular matrix and plays an important role in cancer growth, invasion and metastasis (Blumenthal et al. 2005). It is a normal constituent of mucus that is secreted into the lumen by the glandular epithelial cells. With disruption of the normal tissue architecture, CEA is released into the vascular and lymphatic system. It is thought that the release of CEA into the extracellular matrix is due to GPI anchor cleavage catalysis by GPI specific phospholipase D type enzyme in in vitro experiments, but its mechanism of release is still under study.

CEA has been evaluated as a diagnostic/screening test, a prognostic marker and to monitor breast cancer during therapy. CEA has not been found to be useful for screening at the population level, as it is not sensitive or specific enough to differentiate between benign breast disease and breast cancer (Rimsten et al. 1979).

CEA is more promising in the setting of prognosis, as it is clearly associated with important outcomes and has been found to be reflective of disease burden. In a multivariate analysis, breast cancer patients undergoing surgery with elevated pre-operative levels of CEA had worse prognosis and higher risk of relapse after therapy (Gaglia et al. 1988). In early or localized breast cancer, CEA levels were noted to be similar before and after mastectomy, however, increases in levels after mastectomy are associated with increased recurrence rate (Wang et al. 1975). In patients with metastatic disease, approximately 50–60 % of the patients have elevated CEA levels (Hogan-Ryan et al. 1980; Gray 1984; Tormey and Waalkes 1978; Veronesi et al. 1982). Furthermore, increases in CEA levels have been noted in cancer with metastasis to lymph nodes and distant organs (Laessig et al. 2007). While there is clearly a relationship between the detection and level of CEA and prognosis in early stage patients, there is no evidence that adding or changing therapy alters this prognosis. This concept, 'clinical utility', needs to be established in order for the biomarker to be recommended for clinical use. As a result, ASCO 2007 guidelines do not recommend CEA for determining prognosis among breast cancer patients, since clinical utility has not been established (Harris et al. 2007).

Perhaps the most useful setting to date for the use of CEA is in monitoring metastatic disease. Studies have shown that, among advanced breast cancer patients receiving hormonal therapy and chemotherapy, a drop in CEA levels correlates with response to therapy. Tormey et al., found that CEA levels >5 ng/ml pre therapy were associated withpoor response or early failure of chemotherapy (Tormey and Waalkes 1978). However, monitoring CEA levels does not meet the guideline requirement for clinical utility as it does not alter the prognosis when used for monitoring. Having said that, CEA and other similar markers may aid in therapy decision-making, in conjunction with other features of the clinical scenario. As a result, they are sanctioned by the ASCO Tumor Marker Guidelines Panel 2015 as reasonable adjuncts to physical examination and radiographic tests in the metastatic setting (Van Poznak et al. 2015).

14.2.2 Mucin 1 or MUC1 (CA15.3/CA27.29)

MUC1, a transmembrane glycoprotein (Fig. 14.1), is involved in oncogenesis by promotion of tyrosine kinase signaling, loss of epithelial cell polarity and constitutive activation of growth and survival pathways (Ren et al. 2006; Rajabi et al. 2014). In breast adenocarcinoma, MUC1 is overexpressed and under glycosylated resulting in loss of architectural demarcation between the apical and basolateral membrane in the cell. The most widely studied biomarkers are the soluble form of MUC1 (CA15.3), and mucin like associated antigen (MCA or CA27.29).

Similar to CEA, CA27.29 and CA15.3 have not been found to be adequately sensitive to be used for diagnosis. However, CA15.3 is found in the circulation of 10–15 % of stage I, 20–25 % and 30–45 % in stage II and stage III breast cancers, respectively (Clinical practice guidelines for the use of tumor markers in breast and colorectal cancer. Adopted on May 17, 1996 by the American Society of Clinical Oncology 1996). Its usefulness is limited as marker in early disease but can be used in advanced stages for disease monitoring.

In early stage disease, elevated levels of CA15.3 are associated with worse outcome (McLaughlin et al. 2000; Gion et al. 2002). In addition, the prognostic impact of CA15.3 is independent of the tumor size and lymph node status (Tampellini et al. 2006; Gray 1984). However, as with CEA, there is no evidence that measuring these markers at diagnosis would not influence treatment decisions in a way that affects patient outcomes.

CA15.3 has been used in follow-up of breast cancer patients after the diagnosis and treatment of early stage disease. While measurement of the marker can provide a lead-time of 5–6 months for the detection of recurrent/metastatic disease in some women (Ren et al. 2006; Rajabi et al. 2014), there is no evidence that early intervention based on this lead-time improves outcomes or quality of life (Clinical practice guidelines for the use of tumor markers in breast and colorectal cancer. Adopted on May 17, 1996 by the American Society of Clinical Oncology 1996). This is likely due to the fact that macrometastases that are detected at the time of recurrence are not curable with current treatment strategies and therefore finding these recurrences a few months earlier does not influence overall survival. This underlies the issue of sensitivity of many markers that makes them inadequate to detect micrometastases

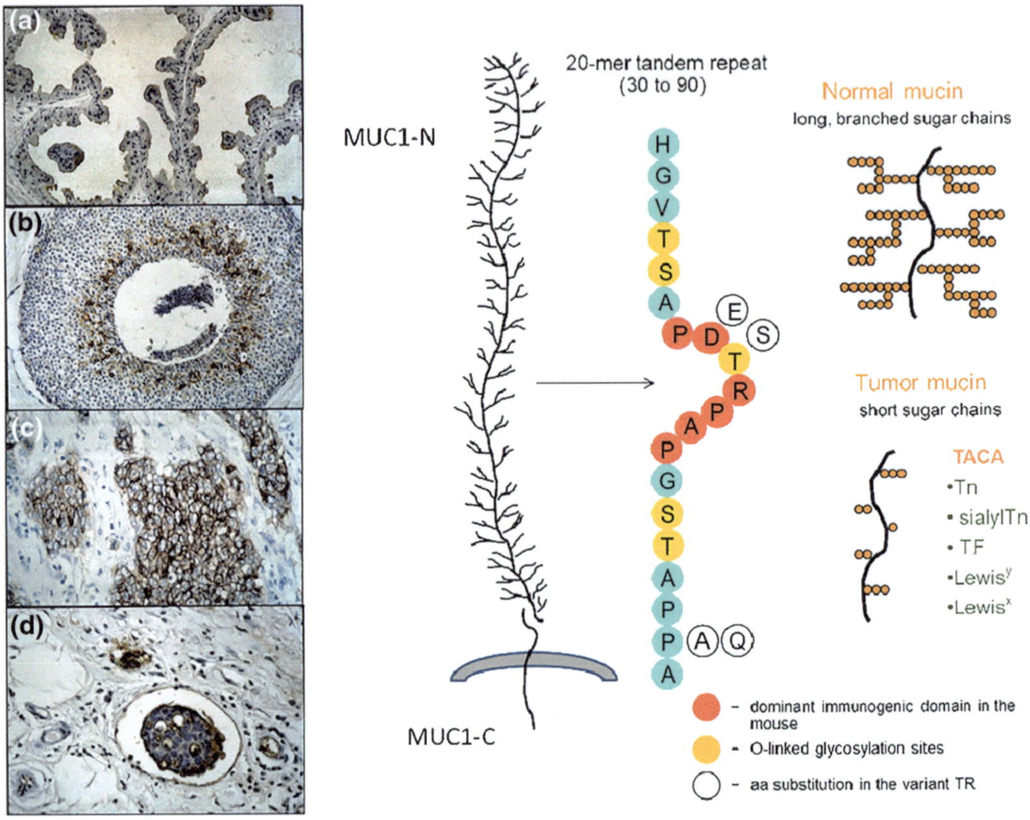

Fig. 14.1 MUC1 Molecule. To the right of the figure we have MUC1 molecule, the variant and nonvariant tandem repeat that form the major part of MUC1-N, and its glycosylation in normal and tumor associated mucin. To the left of the figure immunohistochemistry showing the expression of underglycosylated MUC1 in (**a**) apocrine metaplasia of the breast (**b**) ductal carcinoma in situ of the breast (**c**) invasive ductal adenocarcinoma of the breast (**d**) capillary with tumor embolus from an invasive ductal adenocarcinoma of the breast

at a curable stage. As with CEA, the MUC-1, CA15.3 and CA27.29 markers are not recommended for follow-up of early stage patients (Harris et al. 2007).

There have been a number of studies of CA15.3 in the metastatic setting. In an anthracycline based-phase II and III trial, median survival and clinical progression correlated with CA15.3 levels (McLaughlin et al. 2000). However, concordance with disease response was inconsistent. It has also been suggested that CA15.3 is useful for monitoring unevaluable disease such as pleural effusions, ascites, lytic and sclerotic bone disease, which are present in around one third of metastatic patients.

Studies utilizing CA15.3 and CA27.29 for monitoring patients have shown mixed results. (D'Alessandro et al. 2001; De La Lande et al. 2002; Guadagni et al. 2001; Kokko et al. 2002; Nicolini et al. 2006), and there are no randomized prospective clinical trials that determine the clinical utility of monitoring patients with metastatic disease. As a result, ASCO 2015 guidelines state that CA15.3 and CA27.29 should only be used in conjunction with other modalities like history, examination, and imaging to monitor treatment response in patients with metastatic disease (Harris et al. 2007; Van Poznak et al. 2015).

14.2.3 HER2/Neu Oncogene

The HER2 gene is located in chromosome 17q11-12 which encodes for transmembrane receptor protein with tyrosine kinase activity. The overexpression of HER2 protein is detected in 15–30 % of breast cancer patients and has traditionally correlated with poorer outcomes. The extracellular domain (ECD) of HER2 is detectable in the serum and has been proposed as a surrogate for tissue levels of HER2 to predict early relapse or response to therapy. Like the other circulating markers, HER2 also lacks sensitivity and specificity for early detection and is not recommended for use in that setting.

Circulating HER2 levels have been studied in both the early and advanced stage settings of breast cancer and are consistently associated with a worse prognosis (Lee et al. 2016; Leitzel et al. 1995; Yamauchi et al. 1997; Volas et al. 1996). Serum HER2 levels are positively correlated with tumor size, tumor grade, and worse disease free survival in early stage disease (Burstein et al. 2003). In addition, studies have shown that ECD levels are associated with response to trastuzumab and hormonal therapy. In a study done by Ali et al. (2008), data was collected from 307 metastatic breast cancer patients from seven different institutions receiving trastuzumab based therapy. The serum samples were collected at baseline and at 30–120 days after initiation of trastuzumab. Sixty two percent patients had significant decline (>20 %) in serum HER2/neu and thirty eighty percent did not. The response rate was 57 % in patients with decline in serum HER2/neu compared to 28 % who did not. Patients with decline in HER2/neu levels had significantly longer time to disease progression (320 days vs. 180 days; $p < 0.001$), longer duration of response (369 days vs. 230 days; $p < 0.0001$) and longer overall survival (898 days vs. 593 days; $p < 0.018$). Based on this study data, patients with significant decrease in the HER2/neu levels >20 % were known to have decreased benefit from trastuzumab therapy (Ali et al. 2008). Given the complexity of calculating percentage declines and the variability around this number, HER2-ECD is not felt to be a practical measure for clinical use.

HER2-ECD has also been evaluated in metastatic patients in the context of trastuzumab with hormonal therapy. In a randomized controlled trial, patients with elevated HER2-ECD had lower response to letrozole versus tamoxifen. Serial measurement of HER2-ECD levels in these two groups of patients showed that patients with elevated HER2-ECD had overall lower response rates and had no advantage of letrozole over tamoxifen (Lipton et al. 2002). This suggests that this marker might be used to determine which patients are unlikely to respond to the combination of trastuzumab and any hormonal therapy and would be better served by a chemotherapy-based HER therapy combination.

Unfortunately, associations of HER2-ECD with therapy response are confounded by the fact that HER2-ECD levels are associated with increased tumor burden and a decrease in the half-life of trastuzumab antibody due to increase in the binding sites and accelerated clearance of immune complexes. These complex interactions make the use of HER2-ECD impractical and therefore it is not recommended in either the early or advanced disease setting (Harris et al. 2007).

14.3 Tumor Markers in Development: Protein Markers

Although, no biomarker is currently approved for early detection in clinical practice, emerging research on novel biomarkers for diagnosis, prognosis and response to treatment is underway and many promising markers are under development.

14.3.1 Tissue Polypeptide Antigens (TPA)

TPA is a complex polypeptide filament made up of cytokeratin 8, 18 and 19 produced mainly during the late S and G2 phase of the cell cycle. TPA can be elevated in benign conditions like renal failure, liver failure, pregnancy, diabetes mellitus (Tramonti et al. 2000), as well as a number of cancers, limiting its utility as a biomarker for early detection or diagnosis.

In the advanced stage setting, serum TPA levels were shown to be elevated in advanced cancers (stage III and IV) patients, compared to localized breast cancer patients (Al-Youzbaki et al. 2014; Sliwowska et al. 2006). It was also shown that TPA levels are lower in breast cancer patients who received chemotherapy compared to patients who did not suggesting that it is associated with a worse prognosis as the patients who receive chemotherapy tend to have a higher disease burden and worse clinical features (Al-Youzbaki et al. 2014).

Tissue polypeptide–specific antigen (TPS) is a peptide epitope of cytokeratin 18 that can be detected in the serum (Bonfrer et al. 1994; Rydlander et al. 1996; D'Alessandro et al. 2001). As such it is thought to be a more specific serum marker than TPA and has been evaluated in several disease contexts. TPS has been found to be associated with higher tumor grade, and early stage patients with elevated tumor TPS levels have a higher risk of recurrence (O'Hanlon et al. 1996). A number of studies have suggested the utility of TPS as a prognostic marker. There are conflicting results in the literature regarding value of TPS marker in breast cancer (Given et al. 2000). On the contrary, TPS levels are known to be elevated in loco regional recurrence and significantly elevated to greater extent in metastatic diseases predicting different stages of the disease (O'Hanlon et al. 1996). Patients with elevated levels during follow up were likely to experience disease progression on further follow up. When compared to CEA or CA 15-3, TPS indicates proliferative activity, which is one of the most important phenotypic characteristics of tumor aggressiveness and is thus more beneficial as prognostic marker than serum markers as mentioned earlier (Bodenmuller et al. 1994; Weber et al. 1984; Hwa et al. 2008). Some studies have found that elevated pre-operative levels associated with poor disease free survival ($p < 0.001$) and low pre-treatment levels correlated with increased survival in advanced breast cancer patients (Ahn et al. 2013).

Several studies have suggested that TPS, particularly when combined with CA15.3, may be more specific and sensitive at predicting the likelihood of recurrence among breast cancer patients. However, larger scale studies and those aimed at clinical utility are needed to confirm these findings and support the recommendation of this marker in early stage disease. Thus, there are no recommendations as per ASCO Tumor Marker Guidelines for use of TPA or TPS in breast cancer (Harris et al. 2007).

TPS is known to be elevated in other inflammatory conditions like liver cirrhosis (van Dalen 1992) and in post-menopausal versus premenopausal women (Given et al. 2000), and is thus not specific enough to be recommended for screening or early detection.

14.3.2 Serum Autoantibodies Against Tumor Associated Antigens (TAA)

The 'Holy Grail' of serum tumor markers is to be able to use them for early detection, as this would reduce the need for non-specific radiographic screening of the entire population of women at risk for breast cancer, which currently is thought to be any woman over the age of 40 years. For many years, mammography has been the gold standard for screening that has been proven to have reduced mortality (Brooks 2009), but its sensitivity is reduced in patients with dense breasts (Brooks 2009). In addition, non-specific mammographic screening is thought to lead to over diagnosis and unnecessary treatments (Brooks 2009). Recently, there have been many serum tumor markers introduced like CEA, CA 15.3, estrogen receptor (ER) and progesterone receptor (PR), Circulating tumor cells (CTCs) which have been studied but unfortunately none of which have been approved for screening or early diagnosis of breast cancer due to lack of sensitivity and specificity of these circulating proteins. This prompted the evaluation of other serum markers that could improve these endpoints and led to intensive research on serum autoantibodies against tumor-associated antigens (Fig. 14.2).

Autoantibodies against p53 (Crawford et al. 1982), HER2 (Disis et al. 1997), MUC1 (von Mensdorff-Pouilly et al. 1996) and NY-ESO-1 (Stockert et al. 1998) were the first to be discovered in breast cancer patients. Studies have showed that serum collected prior to diagnosis, at

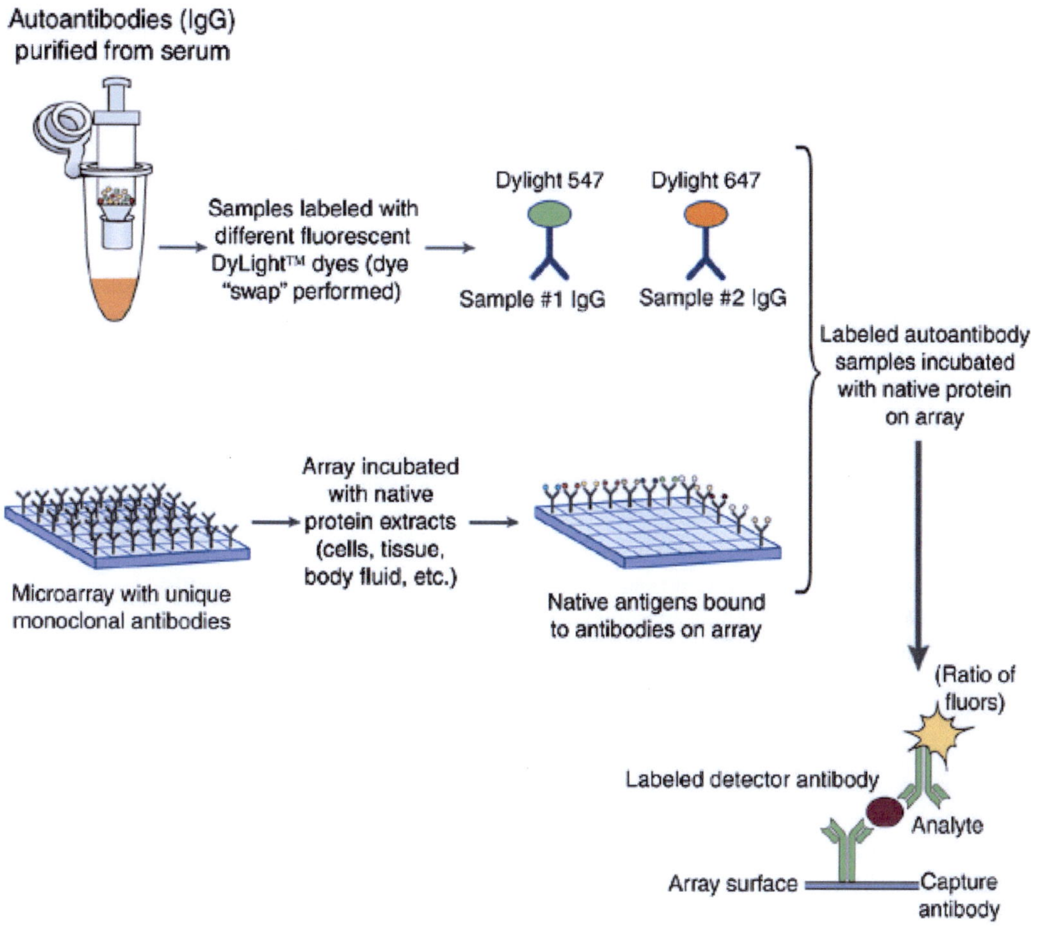

Fig. 14.2 ELISA method using antibody microarray to capture tumor associated antigens in the circulating blood. This figure depicts the use of autoantibodies purified from serum, are tagged with fluorescent dye. Native antigens in the circulating blood are bound to antibody on incubated array and result in fluorescent color from antigen antibody reaction

diagnosis, and during treatment showed that HER2 and p53 autoantibodies were significantly increased in samples from breast cancer patients. Elevated levels of HER2 and p53 autoantibodies can be detected in sera more than 150 days prior to diagnosis in breast cancer patients compared to controls (Lu et al. 2012). Recently, new autoantibodies such as SOX2 were found to be significantly elevated in patients with breast cancer (18.4 %) compared to healthy women (2.6 %) and (6.4 %) in patients with benign breast conditions. SOX2 antibodies were also associated with high tumor grade and positive nodal status. Other autoantibodies including p90/CIP2A show promising results (Sun et al. 2012) and are under investigation.

In patients with breast cancer, only 10–30 % of patients had a humoral response against a specific TAA, thought to be due to heterogeneous nature of the underlying biology (Tan et al. 2009). Looi et al. (2006) showed that p16 antibodies were relatively higher in nasopharyngeal cancer than in breast cancer. To confirm the specificity of p16 antibodies and to increase the frequency of antibody detection, a combination of TAA (p16, p53, and c-myc) was used. Antibodies to this antigen panel were found to be increased in frequency at $p < 0.01$. The combination of TAAs together increased the positive antibody detection rate to a sensitivity of 44 %. Multiple studies have looked into TAA panels and the focus later has shifted to developing TAA panels to increase the sensitivity and specificity of the test (Fernandez Madrid 2005; Lu et al. 2008). This led to developing of different TAA panels with application of SEREX (autoantibodies like XI-A, p80, S6, RPA32 (Tomkiel et al. 2002) and NY-BR-I (Fernandez-Madrid et al. 2004; Brooks 2009; Levenson 2007; Jager et al. 2001) or SERPA (autoantibodies against RNA-binding protein regulatory subunit (RS), DJ-1 oncogene, glucose 6 phosphate dehydrogenase, heat shock 70-kDa protein-1 (HS71) and dihydrolipoamide dehydrogenase (Le Naour et al. 2001; Fernandez Madrid 2005). The TAA panels also increase the sensitivity and specificity for primary breast cancer and for ductal carcinoma in situ (Chapman et al. 2007) which can help in early diagnosis and can aid along with mammography for screening breast cancer.

Mammography has been shown to decrease the breast cancer mortality rates. The relative risk reduction is only 23 % and has recall rate for additional testing is 5–10 % in whom cancer would be detected. In women undergoing screening mammography, approximately 4 to 9 % have false positive test. There is clinical need for additional tests to aid in diagnosis of breast cancer, particularly in young patients under the age of 50 years in whom mammography is less sensitive (Levenson 2007). Chapman et al. investigated the use of autoantibodies to p53, c-myc, and HER2, NY-ESO-1, BRCA2 and MUC1 antigens by using the enzyme linked immunosorbent assay (Chapman et al. 2007). It was shown that autoantibodies were elevated repeatedly for one of six antigens in 64 % of primary breast cancer patients and 45 % of patients with ductal carcinoma in situ with 85 % specificity. Individual assay specificity for each antigen varied from 91 to 98 %. Hence these autoantibody assay against panel of antigens could be used with mammography for early detection of primary breast cancer especially in young women at risk. Due to heterogeneity of breast cancer and our limited understanding about autoantibodies against TAA, we need more definitive studies before tthey can be used in clinical practice.

14.4 Challenges in Utility of Circulating Tumor Markers

Multiple studies have shown the potential for utilization of circulating biomarkers for the clinical care of breast cancer from screening and diagnosis, to prognosis and treatment monitoring. However, only a few of these markers have successfully transitioned to routine clinical use. This section addresses some of the issues surrounding these challenges.

14.4.1 Cost Effectiveness

Health care costs are continually rising and becoming an increasing concern, particularly in the United States. Adding more tests to the treatment of a patient may increase costs and offers only limited benefits. A SEER-Medicare database analysis from 2001 to 2007 of the early breast cancer survivor patients evaluated the tumor marker tests for CEA, CA 15-3, CA 27.29 and health care claims through the billing codes and found that 42 % had received these tumor marker test within 2 years of diagnosis and the utilization increased over time from 38 % in 2001 to 46 % in 2007 (Ramsey et al. 2015). They found that the total cost of care for those patients with one test performed was 29 % higher than those not tested, often due to higher rates of advanced imaging (Ramsey et al. 2015). Given the financial constraints of current medical system, it is important to consider the benefit of a test before recommending routine use.

14.4.2 Poor Specificity

Certain tumor markers are also known to be de-regulated in other benign conditions. For example, like CA15.3 is elevated in chronic hepatitis, liver cirrhosis, hypothyroidism, and sarcoidosis. Therefore, the utility of these biomarkers for early detection of breast cancer is low.

Further, paradoxically there can be increase in tumor markers concentration after commencement of chemotherapy possibly secondary to tumor cell necrosis. For example, Hayes et al. reported that there could be a spike in the CEA or CA 15-3 in 7 of 16 patients undergoing chemotherapy (Tondini et al. 1988). Therefore, many biomarkers used for monitoring ›treatment response need to be carefully defined as to when and how they are useful.

14.4.3 Lack of Reproducibility

Unfortunately, many promising new biomarkers that are reported in the literature fail to replicate in subsequent studies. For example, although circulating miRNAs were thought to hold great potential for breast cancer early detection, a review showed that the positive findings from these studies overlapped less than would be expected by chance (Tondini et al. 1988). Many studies of circulating biomarkers are not done in a rigorous manner and are done ad hoc with samples that are readily available. For example, using samples from a case-control design study to analyze a biomarker for early detection. Then, when the biomarker is tested in a sample of screening-eligible women in a prospective manner, the test does not replicate, as it is unclear how levels of these biomarkers change post-biopsy. Research networks, such as the Early Detection Research Network (EDRN) have been developed to help facilitate access to more appropriate samples.

Further, studies are often inconsistent in their protocols for collection and quantification of the biomarker. Some biomarkers, particularly many of these emerging cell-free markers, may be sensitive to time, temperature or processing. It is important for researchers from groups to collaborate and design strong biomarker studies with a number of independent replication sets.

14.5 Conclusion

Future direction towards identifying new tumor markers or new use of old tumor markers are essential. Many early stage breast cancer patients that are being treated surgically for cure, are prone to develop metastatic disease. We have insufficient data to recommend tumor markers like CEA, CA 15-3 and CA27.29 for diagnosis or monitoring of early stage disease but they can be used as adjunctive for monitoring the response to treatment in the metastatic setting. It is important that the clinicians are aware of sensitivities, specificities and limitation of each tumor marker before its use. In the recent past, investigators have focused on identifying new autoantibodies against tumor specific antigens and their role in breast cancer management. Many of these markers are still under study and have shown some promising results. It is crucial that we identify more of these tumor markers and explore their clinical applications. When new markers are identified, it is essential that we address the reliability and clinical utility of each marker. Only in this way, can we make progress in the management of breast cancer and improve outcomes for our patients.

REFERENCES:

Ahn SK, Moon HG, Ko E, Kim HS, Shin HC, Kim J, You JM, Han W, Noh DY (2013) Preoperative serum tissue polypeptide-specific antigen is a valuable prognostic marker in breast cancer. Int J Cancer 132 (4):875–881. doi:10.1002/ijc.27727

Al-Youzbaki WB, Al-Youzbaki NB, Telfah MM (2014) Tissue polypeptide antigen & interleukin-6: Are their serum levels a predictor for response to chemotherapy in breast cancer? Pak J Med Sci 30(5):1108–1112. doi:10.12669/pjms.305.5199

Ali SM, Carney WP, Esteva FJ, Fornier M, Harris L, Kostler WJ, Lotz JP, Luftner D, Pichon MF, Lipton A, Serum HERnSG (2008) Serum HER-2/neu and relative resistance to trastuzumab-based therapy in patients with metastatic breast cancer. Cancer 113 (6):1294-1301. doi:10.1002/cncr.23689

Blumenthal RD, Hansen HJ, Goldenberg DM (2005) Inhibition of adhesion, invasion, and metastasis by antibodies targeting CEACAM6 (NCA-90) and

CEACAM5 (Carcinoembryonic Antigen). Cancer Res 65(19):8809–8817. doi:10.1158/0008-5472.CAN-05-0420

Bodenmuller H, Ofenloch-Hahnle B, Lane EB, Dessauer A, Bottger V, Donie F (1994) Lung cancer-associated keratin 19 fragments: development and biochemical characterisation of the new serum assay Enzymun-Test CYFRA 21-1. Int J Biol Markers 9(2):75–81

Bonfrer JM, Groeneveld EM, Korse CM, van Dalen A, Oomen LC, Ivanyi D (1994) Monoclonal antibody M3 used in tissue polypeptide-specific antigen assay for the quantification of tissue polypeptide antigen recognizes keratin 18. Tumour Biol 15(4):210–222

Brooks M (2009) Breast cancer screening and biomarkers. Methods Mol Biol 472:307–321. doi:10.1007/978-1-60327-492-0_13

Burstein HJ, Harris LN, Gelman R, Lester SC, Nunes RA, Kaelin CM, Parker LM, Ellisen LW, Kuter I, Gadd MA, Christian RL, Kennedy PR, Borges VF, Bunnell CA, Younger J, Smith BL, Winer EP (2003) Preoperative therapy with trastuzumab and paclitaxel followed by sequential adjuvant doxorubicin/cyclophosphamide for HER2 overexpressing stage II or III breast cancer: a pilot study. J Clin Oncol 21(1):46–53

Chapman C, Murray A, Chakrabarti J, Thorpe A, Woolston C, Sahin U, Barnes A, Robertson J (2007) Autoantibodies in breast cancer: their use as an aid to early diagnosis. Ann Oncol 18(5):868–873. doi:10.1093/annonc/mdm007

Clinical practice guidelines for the use of tumor markers in breast and colorectal cancer. Adopted on May 17, 1996 by the American Society of Clinical Oncology (1996). J Clin Oncol 14 (10):2843-2877

Crawford LV, Pim DC, Bulbrook RD (1982) Detection of antibodies against the cellular protein p53 in sera from patients with breast cancer. Int J Cancer 30(4):403–408

D'Alessandro R, Roselli M, Ferroni P, Mariotti S, Spila A, Aloe S, Carone MD, Abbolito MR, Carlini S, Perri P, Ricciotti A, Botti C, Conti F, Vici P, Chiappetta NR, Cognetti F, Buonomo O, Guadagni F (2001) Serum tissue polypeptide specific antigen (TPS): a complementary tumor marker to CA 15-3 in the management of breast cancer. Breast Cancer Res Treat 68(1):9–19

De La Lande B, Hacene K, Floiras JL, Alatrakchi N, Pichon MF (2002) Prognostic value of CA 15.3 kinetics for metastatic breast cancer. Int J Biol Markers 17(4):231–238

Disis ML, Pupa SM, Gralow JR, Dittadi R, Menard S, Cheever MA (1997) High-titer HER-2/neu protein-specific antibody can be detected in patients with early-stage breast cancer. J Clin Oncol 15 (11):3363–3367

Fernandez-Madrid F, Tang N, Alansari H, Granda JL, Tait L, Amirikia KC, Moroianu M, Wang X, Karvonen RL (2004) Autoantibodies to Annexin XI-A and Other Autoantigens in the Diagnosis of Breast Cancer. Cancer Res 64(15):5089–5096. doi:10.1158/0008-5472.CAN-03-0932

Fernandez Madrid F (2005) Autoantibodies in breast cancer sera: candidate biomarkers and reporters of tumorigenesis. Cancer Lett 230(2):187–198. doi:10.1016/j.canlet.2004.12.017

Gaglia P, Caldarola B, Bussone R, Potente F, Lauro D, Jayme A, Caldarola L (1988) Prognostic value of CEA and ferritin assay in breast cancer: a multivariate analysis. Eur J Cancer Clin Oncol 24(7):1151–1155

Gion M, Boracchi P, Dittadi R, Biganzoli E, Peloso L, Mione R, Gatti C, Paccagnella A, Marubini E (2002) Prognostic role of serum CA15.3 in 362 node-negative breast cancers. An old player for a new game. Eur J Cancer 38(9):1181–1188

Given M, Scott M, Mc Grath JP, Given HF (2000) The predictive of tumour markers CA 15-3, TPS and CEA in breast cancer recurrence. Breast 9(5):277–280. doi:10.1054/brst.1999.0154

Gray BN (1984) Value of CEA in breast cancer. Aust N Z J Surg 54(1):1–2

Guadagni F, Ferroni P, Carlini S, Mariotti S, Spila A, Aloe S, D'Alessandro R, Carone MD, Cicchetti A, Ricciotti A, Venturo I, Perri P, Di Filippo F, Cognetti F, Botti C, Roselli M (2001) A re-evaluation of carcinoembryonic antigen (CEA) as a serum marker for breast cancer: a prospective longitudinal study. Clin Cancer Res 7(8):2357–2362

Harris L, Fritsche H, Mennel R, Norton L, Ravdin P, Taube S, Somerfield MR, Hayes DF, Bast RC, Jr., American Society of Clinical O (2007) American Society of Clinical Oncology 2007 update of recommendations for the use of tumor markers in breast cancer. J Clin Oncol 25(33):5287–5312. doi:10.1200/JCO.2007.14.2364

Hogan-Ryan A, Fennelly JJ, Jones M, Cantwell B, Duffy MJ (1980) Serum sialic acid and CEA concentrations in human breast cancer. Br J Cancer 41 (4):587–592

Hwa HL, Kuo WH, Chang LY, Wang MY, Tung TH, Chang KJ, Hsieh FJ (2008) Prediction of breast cancer and lymph node metastatic status with tumour markers using logistic regression models. J Eval Clin Pract 14 (2):275–280. doi:10.1111/j.1365-2753.2007.00849.x

Jager D, Stockert E, Gure AO, Scanlan MJ, Karbach J, Jager E, Knuth A, Old LJ, Chen YT (2001) Identification of a tissue-specific putative transcription factor in breast tissue by serological screening of a breast cancer library. Cancer Res 61(5):2055–2061

Kamangar F, Dores GM, Anderson WF (2006) Patterns of cancer incidence, mortality, and prevalence across five continents: defining priorities to reduce cancer disparities in different geographic regions of the world. J Clin Oncol 24(14):2137–2150. doi:10.1200/JCO.2005.05.2308

Kokko R, Holli K, Hakama M (2002) Ca 15-3 in the follow-up of localised breast cancer: a prospective study. Eur J Cancer 38(9):1189–1193

Laessig D, Nagel D, Heinemann V, Untch M, Kahlert S, Bauerfeind I, Stieber P (2007) Importance of CEA and

CA 15-3 during disease progression in metastatic breast cancer patients. Anticancer Res 27(4A):1963–1968

Le Naour F, Misek DE, Krause MC, Deneux L, Giordano TJ, Scholl S, Hanash SM (2001) Proteomics-based identification of RS/DJ-1 as a novel circulating tumor antigen in breast cancer. Clin Cancer Res 7(11):3328–3335

Lee MH, Jung SY, Kang SH, Song EJ, Park IH, Kong SY, Kwon YM, Lee KS, Kang HS, Lee ES (2016) The Significance of Serum HER2 Levels at Diagnosis on Intrinsic Subtype-Specific Outcome of Operable Breast Cancer Patients. PLoS One 11(10): e0163370. doi:10.1371/journal.pone.0163370

Leitzel K, Teramoto Y, Konrad K, Chinchilli VM, Volas G, Grossberg H, Harvey H, Demers L, Lipton A (1995) Elevated serum c-erbB-2 antigen levels and decreased response to hormone therapy of breast cancer. J Clin Oncol 13(5):1129–1135

Levenson VV (2007) Biomarkers for early detection of breast cancer: what, when, and where? Biochim Biophys Acta 1770(6):847–856. doi:10.1016/j.bbagen.2007.01.017

Lipton A, Ali SM, Leitzel K, Demers L, Chinchilli V, Engle L, Harvey HA, Brady C, Nalin CM, Dugan M, Carney W, Allard J (2002) Elevated serum Her-2/neu level predicts decreased response to hormone therapy in metastatic breast cancer. J Clin Oncol 20(6):1467–1472

Looi K, Megliorino R, Shi FD, Peng XX, Chen Y, Zhang JY (2006) Humoral immune response to p16, a cyclin-dependent kinase inhibitor in human malignancies. Oncol Rep 16(5):1105–1110

Lu H, Goodell V, Disis ML (2008) Humoral immunity directed against tumor-associated antigens as potential biomarkers for the early diagnosis of cancer. J Proteome Res 7(4):1388–1394. doi:10.1021/pr700818f

Lu H, Ladd J, Feng Z, Wu M, Goodell V, Pitteri SJ, Li CI, Prentice R, Hanash SM, Disis ML (2012) Evaluation of known oncoantibodies, HER2, p53, and cyclin B1, in prediagnostic breast cancer sera. Cancer Prev Res (Phila) 5(8):1036–1043. doi:10.1158/1940-6207.CAPR-11-0558

McLaughlin R, McGrath J, Grimes H, Given HF (2000) The prognostic value of the tumor marker CA 15-3 at initial diagnosis of patients with breast cancer. Int J Biol Markers 15(4):340–342

Nicolini A, Tartarelli G, Carpi A, Metelli MR, Ferrari P, Anselmi L, Conte M, Berti P, Miccoli P (2006) Intensive post-operative follow-up of breast cancer patients with tumour markers: CEA, TPA or CA15.3 vs MCA and MCA-CA15.3 vs CEA-TPA-CA15.3 panel in the early detection of distant metastases. BMC Cancer 6:269. doi:10.1186/1471-2407-6-269

O'Hanlon DM, Kerin MJ, O'Boyle C, Grimes H, Given HF (1996) Tissue polypeptide specific antigen (TPS) in breast cancer–an initial evaluation. Eur J Surg Oncol 22(1):38–41

Porter P (2008) "Westernizing" women's risks? Breast cancer in lower-income countries. N Engl J Med 358(3):213–216. doi:10.1056/NEJMp0708307

Rajabi H, Alam M, Takahashi H, Kharbanda A, Guha M, Ahmad R, Kufe D (2014) MUC1-C oncoprotein activates the ZEB1/miR-200c regulatory loop and epithelial-mesenchymal transition. Oncogene 33(13):1680–1689. doi:10.1038/onc.2013.114

Ramsey SD, Henry NL, Gralow JR, Mirick DK, Barlow W, Etzioni R, Mummy D, Thariani R, Veenstra DL (2015) Tumor marker usage and medical care costs among older early-stage breast cancer survivors. J Clin Oncol 33(2):149–155. doi:10.1200/JCO.2014.55.5409

Ren J, Bharti A, Raina D, Chen W, Ahmad R, Kufe D (2006) MUC1 oncoprotein is targeted to mitochondria by heregulin-induced activation of c-Src and the molecular chaperone HSP90. Oncogene 25(1):20–31. doi:10.1038/sj.onc.1209012

Rimsten A, Adami HO, Wahren B, Nordin B (1979) Carcinoembryonic antigen in serum of unselected breast-cancer patients and of non-hospitalized controls. Br J Cancer 39(2):109–115

Rydlander L, Ziegler E, Bergman T, Schoberl E, Steiner G, Bergman AC, Zetterberg A, Marberger M, Bjorklund P, Skern T, Einarsson R, Jornvall H (1996) Molecular characterization of a tissue-polypeptide-specific-antigen epitope and its relationship to human cytokeratin 18. Eur J Biochem 241(2):309–314

Sliwowska I, Kopczynski Z, Grodecka-Gazdecka S (2006) Diagnostic value of measuring serum CA 15-3, TPA, and TPS in women with breast cancer. Postepy Hig Med Dosw (Online) 60:295–299

Stockert E, Jager E, Chen YT, Scanlan MJ, Gout I, Karbach J, Arand M, Knuth A, Old LJ (1998) A survey of the humoral immune response of cancer patients to a panel of human tumor antigens. J Exp Med 187(8):1349–1354

Sun Y, Zhang R, Wang M, Zhang Y, Qi J, Li J (2012) SOX2 autoantibodies as noninvasive serum biomarker for breast carcinoma. Cancer Epidemiol Biomarkers Prev 21(11):2043–2047. doi:10.1158/1055-9965.EPI-12-0498

Tampellini M, Berruti A, Bitossi R, Gorzegno G, Alabiso I, Bottini A, Farris A, Donadio M, Sarobba MG, Manzin E, Durando A, Defabiani E, De Matteis A, Ardine M, Castiglione F, Danese S, Bertone E, Alabiso O, Massobrio M, Dogliotti L (2006) Prognostic significance of changes in CA 15-3 serum levels during chemotherapy in metastatic breast cancer patients. Breast Cancer Res Treat 98(3):241–248. doi:10.1007/s10549-005-9155-y

Tan HT, Low J, Lim SG, Chung MC (2009) Serum autoantibodies as biomarkers for early cancer detection. FEBS J 276(23):6880–6904. doi:10.1111/j.1742-4658.2009.07396.x

Tomkiel JE, Alansari H, Tang N, Virgin JB, Yang X, VandeVord P, Karvonen RL, Granda JL, Kraut MJ, Ensley JF, Fernandez-Madrid F (2002) Autoimmunity to the M(r) 32,000 subunit of replication protein A in breast cancer. Clin Cancer Res 8(3):752–758

Tondini C, Hayes DF, Gelman R, Henderson IC, Kufe DW (1988) Comparison of CA15-3 and carcinoembryonic antigen in monitoring the clinical course of patients with metastatic breast cancer. Cancer Res 48(14):4107–4112

Tormey DC, Waalkes TP (1978) Clinical correlation between CEA and breast cancer. Cancer 42(3 Suppl):1507–1511

Tramonti G, Ferdeghini M, Donadio C, Norpoth M, Annichiarico C, Bianchi R, Bianchi C (2000) Renal function and serum concentration of five tumor markers (TATI, SCC, CYFRA 21-1, TPA, and TPS) in patients without evidence of neoplasia. Cancer Detect Prev 24(1):86–90

van Dalen A (1992) TPS in breast cancer–a comparative study with carcinoembryonic antigen and CA 15–3. Tumour Biol 13(1–2):10–17

Van Poznak C, Somerfield MR, Bast RC, Cristofanilli M, Goetz MP, Gonzalez-Angulo AM, Hicks DG, Hill EG, Liu MC, Lucas W, Mayer IA, Mennel RG, Symmans WF, Hayes DF, Harris LN (2015) Use of Biomarkers to Guide Decisions on Systemic Therapy for Women With Metastatic Breast Cancer: American Society of Clinical Oncology Clinical Practice Guideline. J Clin Oncol 33(24):2695–2704. doi:10.1200/JCO.2015.61.1459

Veronesi A, Talamini R, Longhi S, Crivellari D, Galligioni E, Tirelli U, Trovo MG, Magri MD, Frustaci S, Figoli F, Zagonel V, Tumolo S, Grigoletto E (1982) Carcinoembryonic antigen (CEA) in the follow-up of disease-free breast cancer patients. Tumori 68(6):477–480

Volas GH, Leitzel K, Teramoto Y, Grossberg H, Demers L, Lipton A (1996) Serial serum c-erbB-2 levels in patients with breast carcinoma. Cancer 78 (2):267–272. doi:10.1002/(SICI)1097-0142(19960715)78:2<267:AID-CNCR12>3.0.CO;2-U

von Mensdorff-Pouilly S, Gourevitch MM, Kenemans P, Verstraeten AA, Litvinov SV, van Kamp GJ, Meijer S, Vermorken J, Hilgers J (1996) Humoral immune response to polymorphic epithelial mucin (MUC-1) in patients with benign and malignant breast tumours. Eur J Cancer 32A(8):1325–1331

Wang DY, Bulbrook RA, Hayward JL, Hendrick JC, Franchimont P (1975) Relationship between plasma carcinoembryonic antigen and prognosis in women with breast cancer. Eur J Cancer 11(9):615–618

Weber K, Osborn M, Moll R, Wiklund B, Luning B (1984) Tissue polypeptide antigen (TPA) is related to the non-epidermal keratins 8, 18 and 19 typical of simple and non-squamous epithelia: re-evaluation of a human tumor marker. EMBO J 3(11):2707–2714

Yamauchi H, O'Neill A, Gelman R, Carney W, Tenney DY, Hosch S, Hayes DF (1997) Prediction of response to antiestrogen therapy in advanced breast cancer patients by pretreatment circulating levels of extracellular domain of the HER-2/c-neu protein. J Clin Oncol 15(7):2518–2525

15 Circulating Tumor Cells

Malgorzata Banys-Paluchowski, Helen Schneck, Natalia Krawczyk and Tanja Fehm

Abstract

Breast cancer (BC) therapy has fundamentally progressed in the last 30 years with the change from radical mastectomy to recent individualized local and systemic therapy regimens. By combining the modern treatment modalities, approximately 77 % of BC patients can be cured, still leaving potential for optimization in 23 % of cases, which will develop metastatic disease due to tumor cell dissemination despite optimal treatment. It has been known since the 19th century that most of the solid cancers shed circulating tumor cells (CTCs) into the blood circulation already at a very early stage. Based on this observation, CTCs are a surrogate marker for minimal residual disease (MRD) and precursors of metastatic disease ("seed"). Current research indicates that the phenotype and genotype differ between CTCs and primary tumor, which may result in different therapeutic responses. Therefore, characterization of CTCs may be an important step for the optimization of adjuvant and metastatic systemic treatment.

Keywords

Breast cancer · Circulating tumor cell · Liquid biopsy · Molecular characterization · Biomarkers

15.1 Introduction

The presence of circulating tumor cells (CTCs) was first recognized and described by Thomas R. Ashworth in 1869 (Ashworth 1869). CTCs are cancer cells that have been released from the primary tumor into the blood stream, where they are further dispersed throughout the body (Joosse et al. 2014). In the blood circulation, CTCs may face different fates: they undergo apoptosis,

M. Banys-Paluchowski
Department of Obstetrics and Gynecology, Marienkrankenhaus Hamburg, Hamburg, Germany

H. Schneck · N. Krawczyk · T. Fehm (✉)
Department of Obstetrics and Gynecology, Henrich-Heine University Duesseldorf, Duesseldorf, Germany
e-mail: Tanja.Fehm@med.uni-duesseldorf.de

S. Badve and Y. Gökmen-Polar (eds.), *Molecular Pathology of Breast Cancer*, DOI 10.1007/978-3-319-41761-5_15

become dormant, or survive to transmigrate into secondary organs to persist and to eventually initiate metastatic disease (Banys et al. 2012; Krawczyk et al. 2014a). Recent data indicate that CTCs are shed already at an early stage and that their presence is not solely a phenomenon associated with metastatic disease (Hüsemann et al. 2008). Further, they are considered to be genotypically and phenotypically heterogeneous cells with metastatic progenitor cell characteristics. It is assumed that 1 g tumor tissue (about 10^9 cells) releases about 3×10^6 cells per day into the blood circulation. However, given that about 99 % of these cells are supposed to die in between 30 min, only 1 % of the CTCs may persist at secondary sites in distant organs, and these cells may accumulate genetic and epigenetic alterations diverging from primary tumors (Allard et al. 2004; Meng et al. 2004a; Coumans et al. 2012). Consequently, a subfraction of an estimated 0.1 % of CTCs may respond differently to treatment and develop metastatic potential indicating the inefficiency of the metastatic cascade per se (Klein 2008).

As putative founder cells of metastases, CTCs may provide significant information to better understand important features such as intrapatient genotypic and phenotypic heterogeneity, the mechanisms of tumorigenesis, invasion, metastasis and their value for treatment optimization. In support of this idea, CTC enumeration has been shown to be a clinically useful prognostic biomarker in epithelial malignancies including breast (Cristofanilli et al. 2004), colon (Cohen et al. 2008) and prostate cancer (de Bono et al. 2008). In the following review, we will discuss the current value of CTCs in the diagnosis and therapy of patients with early and metastatic breast cancer.

15.2 Isolation and Characterization of CTCs

15.2.1 CTC Enrichment

Due to the rarity of CTCs in the peripheral blood (PB) of cancer patients and the lack of a specific "tumor cell marker", CTC isolation generally requires a combination of enrichment and subsequent specific detection steps (Mostert et al. 2009). Many enrichment techniques have been developed and are currently being tested (reviewed by Barradas and Terstappen 2013). They generally follow one of two different strategies: selecting tumor cells according to morphological features (size/density) (*label-independent*), or enriching CTCs according to their immunologic profile (*label-dependent*) (Broersen et al. 2014) (Table 15.1).

Label-independent CTC enrichment based on morphologic criteria employs various filtration technologies (e.g. ISET, Parsortix, ScreenCell) or Ficoll density-gradient approaches (e.g. OncoQuick), which exploit the CTCs' differences in size and deformability (Müller et al. 2005; Lin et al. 2010; Freidin et al. 2014). Other enrichment devices based on the CTCs' physical properties such as label-free micro-fluidic approaches are promising tools since they allow isolation of viable CTCs without extensive pretreatment of blood (e.g. JETTA, DFF-chip) (Hou et al. 2013; Riahi et al. 2014). *Label-dependent* approaches, which are preferably used in the clinical and experimental setting, primarily use antibodies against the epithelial cell adhesion molecule (EpCAM) (e.g. CellSearch, CTC/HB-Chip, IsoFlux, AdnaTest) (Cristofanilli et al. 2005; Nagrath et al. 2007; Fehm et al. 2009; Harb et al. 2013). Among EpCAM-based strategies, the CellSearch assay (Janssen Diagnostics, LLC, USA) represents currently the "gold standard" for CTC detection (Riethdorf et al. 2007) and was approved by the US Food and Drug Administration in 2004. Using this approach, CTCs are isolated from PB using a ferrofluid, which is coated with EpCAM-specific antibodies, and then identified by a positive cytokeratin (CK) and DAPI staining and CD45 negativity. Other techniques such as IsoFlux, AdnaTest or MACS also use EpCAM antibody coated (micro-) beads for immunocapture of CTCs (Fehm et al. 2009; Harb et al. 2013). Within the microfluid channels of the CTC-/Herringbone-Chip, rare cells can be enriched from whole blood with the aid of EpCAM-antibody-coated microposts (Nagrath

Table 15.1 Technologies for CTC enrichment and identification

Technology	CTC enrichment (target)	CTC characterization	References
Label-independent			
Ficoll/density gradient	Density centrifugation/negative depletion	ICC, PCR, FISH	Fehm et al. (2002), Theodoropoulos et al. (2010)
EPISPOT	Density gradient centrifugation or negative depletion	Immunological detection of secreted proteins (e.g. MUC1, CK19)	Alix-Panabières (2012)
VitaAssay	Ingestion of fluorescently-labeled matrix	ICC, PCR	Lu et al. (2010)
OncoQuick	Density gradient centrifugation	ICC, PCR	Müller et al. (2005)
ISET	Size (>8 μm)	ICC, PCR, FISH	Lin et al. (2010)
Parsortix	Size (>10 μm)	ICC, PCR, FISH	ANGLE plc, UK
ScreenCell	Size	ICC, PCR	Freidin et al. (2014), Kulemann et al. (2015)
JETTA	Size	ICC, PCR, FISH	Riahi et al. (2014)
DFF-chip	Size	ICC, PCR, FISH	Hou et al. (2013)
Label-dependent			
CellSearch CTC/Profile Kit	EpCAM-ferrofluid	ICC for CK, CD45, DAPI; PCR, FISH	Cristofanilli et al. (2005), Sieuwerts et al. (2009a)
IsoFlux	EpCAM/antibody-coated beads	ICC, PCR, FISH	Harb et al. (2013)
CTC/herringbone-chip	EpCAM/EpCAM, HER2, EGFR coated microposts	ICC for CK, CD45, DAPI/EpCAM, CK5,7,8,18,19, CDH1, CDH2, PAI1, FN1; PCR	Nagrath et al. (2007), Stott et al. (2010)
Ariol system	EpCAM/CK-coated microbeads	ICC for CK8, 18, 19, CD45, DAPI	Deng et al. (2008)
GILUPI CellCollector	EpCAM-coated wire	ICC	Saucedo-Zeni et al. (2012)
AdnaTest breast cancer/EMT/stem cell	EpCAM, MUC1 ferrofluid	Multiplex RT-PCR for MUC1, GA733-2, HER2/TWIST, AKt2, PI3 K, ALDH1	Fehm et al. (2009), Kasimir-Bauer et al. (2012)
Liquid bead array	Density gradient centrifugation/EpCAM-ferrofluid	Multiplex PCR for CK19, HER2, MAGE-A3, hMAM, PBGD, TWIST1	Markou et al. (2011)
Label-independent and label-dependent			
CTC-iChip	Size and EpCAM-based selection or negative depletion	ICC, PCR, FISH	Ozkumur et al. (2013)

et al. 2007; Stott et al. 2010). Promising technologies that allow isolation of viable CTCs from larger blood volumes include leukapheresis (Fischer et al. 2013), flow chambers and the GILUPI CellCollector (Saucedo-Zeni et al. 2012).

15.2.2 CTC Detection

15.2.2.1 Antibody-Based Methods

After the enrichment step, antibody-based or molecular assays can be used for the identification of CTCs. The most extensively tested methods are antibody-based; they involve at least one antibody with specificity for antigens absent from other blood cells. These assays generally rely on affinity capture of epithelial surface antigens as no reproducible breast cancer-specific markers have been described so far. As a proof of concept, Fehm et al. provided evidence that these cells of epithelial origin are in fact malignant (Fehm et al. 2002). Table 15.2 provides an overview of possible detection markers. Antibody-based methods, such as immunocytochemistry or immunofluorescence, offer the possibility of visual evaluation, i.e. detected cells are identified both by the staining pattern and morphological properties (Fehm et al. 2005, 2006). In comparison to blood cells, CTCs display distinct biomechanical characteristics: higher nuclear-to-cytoplasmic ratio than leukocytes, larger size and different nuclear morphology (Fig. 15.1).

15.2.2.2 Molecular Methods

Molecular assays have been introduced as an alternative to antibody-based detection. Similarly, identification of CTCs rests upon capture of

Table 15.2 Markers for CTC detection and characterization

	References
Epithelial markers	
CK8, 18, 19	Cristofanilli et al. (2004), Cristofanilli et al. (2005)
E-cadherin (CDH1)	Yu et al. (2013)
EGFR	Yu et al. (2013)
EpCAM (GA733-2)	Fehm et al. (2002), Cristofanilli et al. (2004), Demel et al. (2004), Cristofanilli et al. (2005), Fehm et al. (2009), Yu et al. (2013)
HER2	Demel et al. (2004), Fehm et al. (2009), Yu et al. (2013)
MUC1	Demel et al. (2004), Fehm et al. (2009)
pan-CK	Theodoropoulos et al. (2010), Yu et al. (2013)
Mesenchymal markers	
Akt2	Aktas et al. (2009, Barriere et al. (2012), Kasimir-Bauer et al. (2012)
Fibronectin 1	Raimondi et al. (2011), Yu et al. (2013)
FoxC2	Thiery et al. (2009), Mego et al. (2012b)
N-cadherin (CDH2)	Armstrong et al. (2011), Yu et al. (2013)
PI3 K	Aktas et al. (2009), Barriere et al. (2012), Kasimir-Bauer et al. (2012)
SERPINE1/PAI1	Yu et al. (2013)
SLUG	Thiery et al. (2009, Mego et al. (2012b)
SNAIL1	Thiery et al. (2009), Mego et al. (2012a, b), Giordano et al. (2012)
TG2	Giordano et al. (2012)
TWIST1	Aktas et al. (2009), Thiery et al. (2009), Kallergi et al. (2011), Barriere et al. (2012), Kasimir-Bauer et al. (2012), Mego et al. (2012a, b), Giordano et al. (2012)

(continued)

Table 15.2 (continued)

	References
Vimentin	Raimondi et al. (2011), Kallergi et al. (2011), Armstrong et al. (2011)
ZEB1	Thiery et al. (2009), Mego et al. (2012b, Giordano et al. (2012)
ZEB2	Thiery et al. (2009)
Stem cell marker	
ALDH1	Aktas et al. (2009), Sieuwerts et al. (2009a), Theodoropoulos et al. (2010), Raimondi et al. (2011), Barriere et al. (2012), Kasimir-Bauer et al. (2012), Giordano et al. (2012), Mego et al. (2012a)
Bmi1	Barriere et al. (2012)
CD133	Giordano et al. (2012)
CD24	Theodoropoulos et al. (2010), Giordano et al. (2012), Mego et al. (2012a)
CD44	Theodoropoulos et al. (2010), Barriere et al. (2012), Giordano et al. (2012), Mego et al. (2012a). Lowes et al. (2012)

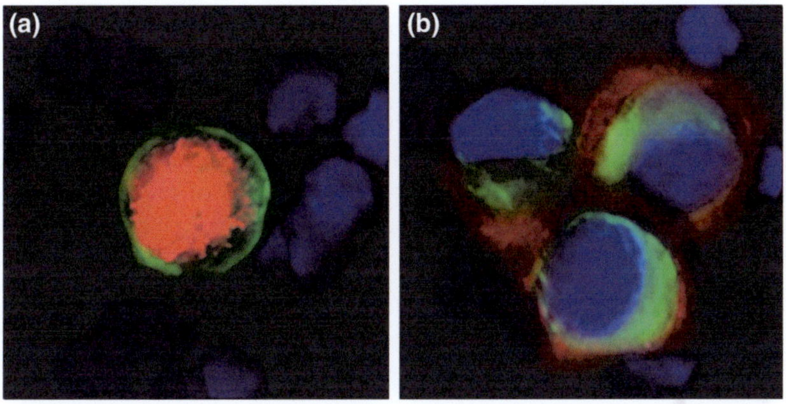

Fig. 15.1 CTC immunofluorescence staining. **a** ER alpha positive CTC: *Red*—nuclear staining for estrogen receptor alpha (ER alpha monoclonal rabbit antibody detected by a secondary with Alexa Fluor 594 labeled goat anti-rabbit antibody), *Green*—FITC cytoplasmatic staining for cytokeratin (fluorescein isothiocyanate labeled C11 antibody), *Blue*—DAPI (4′,6-Diamidin-2-phenylindol) stained nuclei. **b** HER2-positive CTC: *Red*—membranous staining for HER2 (HER2 polyclonal rabbit antibody detected by a secondary with Texas *red* labeled goat anti-rabbit antibody)

epithelial mRNA; commonly used markers include CKs, EpCAM and mammaglobin (Table 15.2). To date, the mRNA encoding CK19 has been the most widely applied in clinical trials (Stathopoulou et al. 2002; Xenidis et al. 2006; Pantel et al. 2008). The commercially available AdnaTest utilizes non-quantitative RT-PCR to identify putative transcripts of genes after immunomagnetic separation of EpCAM/MUC1-positive cells (Andreopoulou et al. 2012). Alternatively, the RNA/CTCscope assay (multiplex RNA in situ hybridization) is a promising approach to measure RNA molecules for the detection of single CTCs (Wang et al. 2012; Payne et al. 2012). RT-PCR-based detection is very sensitive; however, illegitimate gene transcription (pseudogenes) and transcription of markers present on non-malignant cells may lead to false-positive results. Molecular assays commonly involve a cutoff value to differentiate between CTC-positive and CTC-negative result. For analysis of various markers at the same time, multiplex RT-PCR can be employed.

15.2.3 CTC Characterization

Beyond the enumeration of CTCs, molecular characterization at DNA/RNA and protein levels can provide information on the presence of therapeutic targets and predict ineffective therapies. Besides the assessment of estrogen receptor (ER) and HER2, which are the most intensively investigated markers in CTCs (Fehm et al. 2009), molecular analyses provide insight into their mesenchymal, proliferative and stem cell-like features (Table 15.2) (Aktas et al. 2009; Sieuwerts et al. 2009a; Thiery et al. 2009; Barriere et al. 2012; Mego et al. 2012b).

15.2.3.1 Epithelial-Mesenchymal Transition

EMT, a process in which tumor cells undergo a series of phenotypic changes and consequently lose their epithelial features, is considered an important step in the metastatic cascade (Krawczyk et al. 2014b). Hypothetically, EMT enables single tumor cells to escape from the primary tumor into the blood circulation and eventually reach their secondary homing sites; the reverse process, i.e. mesenchymal-epithelial transition, takes place at the metastatic sites where tumor cells regain their epithelial features. Kasimir-Bauer et al. examined PB samples from 502 patients with primary BC and reported that at least one of the EMT markers (Akt2, PI3 K, TWIST) was expressed in 29 % of patients (Kasimir-Bauer et al. 2012). Since this phenomenon leads to the downregulation of EpCAM (Thiery 2002; Onder et al. 2008; Tam and Weinberg 2013), CTC detection techniques based on epithelial markers may be prone to underestimation of CTC counts; to capture all biological subsets of EpCAM-low/negative CTCs, EpCAM-independent enrichment strategies should be considered (Sieuwerts et al. 2009b).

15.2.3.2 Stem Cell Theory

It has been hypothesized that CTCs' ability to enter dormant state for very long periods may be due to their stem cell-like features. Indeed, at least a fraction of CTCs display characteristics typically attributed to cancer stem cells with self-renewal capabilities. Balic et al. observed a putative stem cell-like phenotype, defined as $CD44^{+}CD24^{-/low}$, in 65 % of detected disseminated tumor cells (DTCs) from the bone marrow of BC patients and speculated that these properties may determine their resistance to cytostatic therapy and contribute to tumor progression (Balic et al. 2006). Another "stemness" marker, ALDH1, can be identified in a significant proportion of CTCs in metastatic BC (Theodoropoulos et al. 2010). In primary BC, Aktas et al. detected ALDH1 in 69 % of CTC-positive patients (Aktas et al. 2009). Further, triple-negative (basal-like) breast cancer is composed mainly of cells resembling cancer stem cells ($CD44^{+}$, $CK5/6^{+}$); interestingly, CTCs are mostly triple-negative (Fehm et al. 2009; Krawczyk et al. 2014b).

15.2.3.3 Genotype of CTCs

Nucleic acid-based CTC detection methods are the most widely used alternative to immunocytochemical assays in order to characterize CTCs and new areas of research are directed towards high resolution molecular characterization of single cells. Assays such as those employing fluorescence in situ hybridization, whole genome amplification and array comparative genomic hybridization allow the detection of chromosomal aberrations and mutations in single cells (Fehm et al. 2002; Yu et al. 2011; Neves et al. 2014; Pantel and Alix-Panabieres 2014).

15.3 Clinical Role of CTCs

The clinical potential of CTC detection and characterization lies in three main areas: prognostication, therapy monitoring and treatment selection based on CTCs. In the following, we will review the clinical significance of CTC evaluation in both early and metastatic cancer (Table 15.3).

15.3.1 Prognostication

15.3.1.1 Early Breast Cancer

In BC, early diagnosis is crucial for successful treatment and favorable prognosis. However,

Table 15.3 Clinical role of CTCs in early and metastatic breast cancer

Potential	Early breast cancer	Metastatic breast cancer
Prognostication	Yes; CTC detection correlates significantly with DFS and OS	Yes; High CTC levels correlate with shorter PFS and OS (cut-off: 5 CTCs/7.5 ml PB)
Therapy monitoring	Unclear; changes in CTC levels correlate with response to (neo)adjuvant treatment in smaller studies; no clinical consequence so far	Possibly relevant; High CTC levels after start of first-line chemotherapy can adequately predict progression, however, patients do not benefit from a switch to another regimen (clinical trials: SWOG 0500, ongoing: CirCe01)
Treatment selection based on CTCs	Possibly relevant; evidence pending (ongoing clinical trials: TREAT CTC)	Possibly relevant; evidence pending (ongoing clinical trials: STIC CTC METABREAST, DETECT III/IVa/IVb)

DFS disease-free survival; *OS* overall survival; *PFS* progression-free survival

hematogenous spread of single tumor cells from the primary tumor may occur before the disease becomes clinically detectable; approximately one-fourth of all node-negative patients with low tumor burden will relapse despite adequate surgical and adjuvant therapy. Accordingly, CTCs can be encountered in 10–60 % of newly diagnosed non-metastatic patients (Wülfing et al. 2006; Ignatiadis et al. 2007; Slade et al. 2009; Rack et al. 2014). These CTCs may persist beyond primary treatment as minimal residual disease (MRD) and are considered to be a potential source of further metastatic spread.

Several large clinical trials investigated the impact of CTC detection on prognosis in early BC (Table 15.4). To date, the strongest evidence has been provided by the German SUCCESS trial (EUDRA-CT No. 2005-000490-21, NCT02181101). In this study, PB samples from 2026 early average-to-high risk BC patients before chemotherapy and 1492 patients after chemotherapy were analyzed by the CellSearch system. CTCs were detected in 21.5 % of the patients after surgical therapy of the primary tumor and before the start of chemotherapy (Rack et al. 2014). After a followup of 36, months a clear prognostic relevance of CTCs with respect to all clinical endpoints such as disease-free survival (DFS), distant disease-free survival (DDFS), BC-specific survival (BCSS) and overall survival (OS) was demonstrated. In an exploratory analysis, various cut-off values were evaluated (0 vs. ≥ 1; 0–1 vs. ≥ 2; 0–4 vs. ≥ 5 CTCs in 30 ml PB); a significant impact on DFS and OS was confirmed for all cut-offs, while the hazard ratios consistently increased with increasing cut-off values. Women with ≥ 5 CTCs were at highest risk for disease recurrence. After chemotherapy, 22 % of patients were CTC-positive; CTC persistence was associated with reduced DFS and OS. The SUCCESS study supports the clinical potential of CTCs to assess the individual risk of patients at the time of primary diagnosis (Rack et al. 2014). These results confirmed the findings from the neoadjuvant REMAGUS02 trial (Pierga et al. 2008; Bidard et al. 2013b), where PB samples were obtained from 115 patients with large or locally advanced tumors before and/or after neoadjuvant chemotherapy. Detection of at least one CTC in 7.5 ml blood at diagnosis was associated with reduced DDFS and OS. This effect was independent of other conventional prognostic factors, such as tumor size, nodal involvement, histological grade, receptor status etc. Interestingly, the influence of CTC detection on clinical outcome seemed to be time-dependent; i.e., CTC presence predicted reduced survival mainly during the first 36 and 48 months of followup. This is an important observation, particularly because the survival results from the largest trial on CTCs (SUCCESS) have so far been reported with a relatively short followup of 36 months (Rack et al. 2014). Whether the impact of CTCs on survival might be limited to the first 3–4 years after diagnosis remains unclear, at least until the

Table 15.4 Prognostic relevance of CTCs in early breast cancer

Author	Study collective	Number of patients	CTC pos[a] n (%)	Method	Followup (months)	Prognostic relevance
Rack et al. (2014), SUCCESS trial	Stage I–III, node-positive or high risk node-negative, all pts. received chemotherapy	2026	435 (21 %)	CellSearch	36	DFS, DDFS, BCSS, OS
Bidard et al. (2013b), REMAGUS02 trial	Neoadjuvant trial, Stage II–III, ineligible for breast conserving surgery at diagnosis or high-risk	95	22 (23 %)	CellSearch	70	DDFS, OS
Molloy et al. (2011)	Stage I–II	733	58 (8 %)	qRT-PCR (CK19, p1B, EGP-2, PS2, MmGI)	91	MFS, BCSS
Lucci et al. (2012)	Stage I–III	302	73 (24 %)	CellSearch	35	DFS, OS
Ignatiadis et al. (2007)	Stage I–III, all pts. received adjuvant chemotherapy	444 I–III	181 (41 %)	RT-PCR (CK19)	54	DFS, OS
Hwang et al. (2012)	Stage I–IIIa	166	37 (22 %)	RT-PCR (CK20)	100	MFS, OS

[a]At least one CTC per blood sample
n.s. not significant; *BCSS* BC-specific survival; *DDFS* distant disease-free survival; *DFS* disease-free survival; *OS* overall survival; *MFS* metastasis-free survival

results from the SUCCESS trial with a longer followup are published. In the REMAGUS02 trial, persistent CTCs had no significant impact on survival; however, the sample size was small (85 patients) compared to the SUCCESS trial (1493 patients).

15.3.1.2 Metastatic Breast Cancer

Twenty to thirty percent of patients, initially diagnosed with an early stage of disease, suffer from metastatic relapse several months or years later (EBCTCG Early Breast Cancer Trialists' Collaborative Group 2005). According to several studies, 40–80 % of MBC patients present with circulating tumor cells in PB, which was shown to be an independent prognostic factor associated with shorter progression-free survival (PFS) and OS by a number of groups (Table 15.5). First indications regarding the prognostic value of CTCs were provided by Cristofanilli et al. in 2004 (Cristofanilli et al. 2004). In this multicenter prospective trial, blood samples from 177 MBC patients were tested for CTC levels prior to starting a new therapy and at the first followup visit, and these levels were correlated with survival data. Patients with at least 5 CTCs/7.5 ml PB had significantly shorter PFS and OS compared to patients with less than 5 CTCs/7.5 ml (median PFS: 2.7 vs. 7.0 months; OS: 10.1 vs. 18 months) (Cristofanilli et al. 2004). Therefore, the cut-off of ≥ 5 CTCs/7.5 ml PB is generally used to distinguish between MBC patients with good and poor clinical outcome. Independent prognostic significance of CTCs for both PFS and OS in MBC patients has been confirmed with level 1 evidence by a recent pooled analysis of 20 studies including 1944 patients from 17 centres in Europe (Bidard et al. 2014).

Additionally, several studies investigated the prognostic significance of CTCs in MBC according to molecular subtypes of the primary tumor. The first trial to address this question was an analysis of 517 MBC patients by Giordano

Table 15.5 Prognostic relevance of CTCs in metastatic breast cancer

Author	Year	Number of patients	Method	CTC positivity rate	Prognostic relevance
Bidard et al. (2014) (pooled analysis)	2014	1944	CellSearch	47 %	PFS, OS
Wallwiener et al. (2013)	2013	486	CellSearch	42 %	PFS, OS
Giordano et al. (2012)	2012	517	CellSearch	40 %[a]	PFS, OS
Pierga et al. (2012)	2012	267	CellSearch	44 %[a]	PFS, OS
Müller et al. (2012)	2012	254	CellSearch AdnaTest	CSS: 50 %[a] AT: 40 %	CellSearch: OS AdnaTest: none
Giuliano et al. (2011)	2011	235	CellSearch	40 %[a]	PFS, OS
Nakamura et al. (2010)	2010	107	CellSearch	37 %[a]	PFS
Liu et al. (2009)	2009	74	CellSearch	n.s.	PFS
Tewes et al. (2009)	2009	42	AdnaTest	52 %	OS
Bidard et al. (2008)	2008	37	ICC	41 %	OS
Nolé et al. (2008)	2008	80	CellSearch	61 %	PFS
Hayes et al. (2006)	2006	177	CellSearch	54 %	PFS, OS[b]
Budd et al. (2006)	2006	138	CellSearch	43 %	OS
Benoy et al. (2006)	2006	32	RT-PCR	25–40 %	None
Cristofanilli et al. (2004)	2004	177	CellSearch	49 %	PFS, OS

[a] $\geq$5 CTC, [b] at any time during palliative treatment
n.s. not specified

et al. (2012). This retrospective trial confirmed the prognostic value of CTCs in all molecular tumor subtypes with the exception of HER2-positive BC. Since the majority of HER2-positive patients in this trial received an anti-HER2 treatment, it may be hypothesized that HER2-directed therapy effectively targets CTCs making them harmless and thus reducing their prognostic significance. Concordantly, Pierga et al. (2012) demonstrated in their prospective study a stronger CTC decrease in patients who were additionally treated with targeted therapy compared with patients who received chemotherapy alone. In contrast, prognostic significance of CTCs in MBC patients independent of the molecular subtype of the primary tumor was recently reported in a large prospective multicenter study with 468 MBC patients by Wallwiener et al. (2013). Only 6.5 % approx. one-forth of HER2-positive patients in this cohort received trastuzumab treatment. Prognostic value of CTC levels was demonstrated for HER2-positive patients untreated with targeted therapy, while no prognostic impact of CTCs was observed in patients that were pretreated with trastuzumab.

15.3.2 Therapy Monitoring

In clinical practice, imaging technologies and determination of tumor marker levels are well-established means to monitor cancer patients and estimate treatment efficacy. However, these approaches are time-intensive and waste precious time in which patients may receive non-effective treatments instead of being switched to other regimens. The half-life of

CTCs in the blood is considered to be in the range of minutes, making them an attractive candidate to monitor therapy efficacy in a minimally invasive liquid biopsy format.

15.3.2.1 Early Breast Cancer

Clinical utility of CTC assessment for monitoring of therapy efficacy in early BC has so far not been clearly demonstrated. However, recent evidence has shown that a selected group of patients benefits from extended adjuvant therapy. In the adjuvant setting, MRD monitoring is the only way to evaluate response to treatment after the primary tumor has been surgically excised. Further, PB samples are easy to obtain and do not require an invasive procedure.

Xenidis et al. (2013) reported that a significant improvement of the median DFS in a group of patients who received a taxane-based chemotherapy versus a group with a taxane-free adjuvant therapy was reflected by a change in CTC levels during chemotherapy: 50 % of patients in the taxane-based group turned CTC negative after treatment compared to 33 % in the taxane-free group. Similarly, in the SUCCESS trial, CTC persistence during adjuvant chemotherapy; i.e., failure to achieve CTC response during treatment, was associated with reduced survival (Rack et al. 2014). Pachmann et al. (2008) reported that repeated quantitative analyses of CTC levels during adjuvant chemotherapy were predictive for DFS. In the neoadjuvant setting, where therapy efficacy is monitored by changes in tumor size, contradictory results were reported. In a substudy of the Neo-ALTTO trial patients with detectable CTCs on at least one occasion (at baseline, 2 weeks and 18 weeks after start of chemotherapy) were significantly less likely to achieve pathological complete response (27 % vs. 42 %, respectively) (Azim et al. 2013), while in the REMAGUS02 trial no correlation of CTC persistence and therapy response was observed (Pierga et al. 2008).

15.3.2.2 Metastatic Breast Cancer

In metastatic setting, CTC levels after start of treatment correlate with the clinical and radiological response (Hayes and Smerage 2008; Hong and Zu 2013; Smerage et al. 2014). Hayes et al. performed a serial analysis of CTC levels in patients undergoing first-line of chemotherapy in up to 20 weeks of followup and observed dynamic changes in CTC levels in the course of the treatment. Interestingly, patients with a decrease in CTC counts showed a significantly longer PFS and OS compared to patients with persistently high CTC levels, while the prognostic power of the threshold of ≥ 5 CTCs/7.5 ml PB with regard to PFS and OS remained unchanged (Hayes et al. 2006). Detection of elevated CTC levels at any time during treatment indicates thus a subsequent rapid disease progression. Hartkopf et al. (2011) showed that changing CTC levels correlate with response to therapy measured by radiologic RECIST criteria and overall survival.

In comparison to radiological imaging, CTC enumeration is a reliable and accurate way to monitor disease progression, possibly offering an earlier and more reproducible monitoring than standard methods (Budd et al. 2006; Liu et al. 2009; De Giorgi et al. 2010). However, monitoring treatment efficacy is only reasonable when alternative—perhaps CTC-tailored—effective treatments can be offered to patients. This issue was addressed in the randomized phase III study "Circulating Tumor Cells and Response to Chemotherapy in Metastatic Breast Cancer: SWOG S0500" (NCT00382018) which revealed that in patients with MBC receiving first-line chemotherapy and displaying persistently increased CTC numbers after 21 days, early switching to an alternate cytotoxic therapy was not effective in prolonging OS. This indicates that these patients need a more effective treatment compared to standard chemotherapy (Smerage et al. 2014). Thus, persistence of CTCs might identify a collective of patients that does not respond to chemotherapy and requires alternative, possibly targeted, treatment options. The French CirCe01 (NCT01349842) trial has a similar design to SWOG 0500 and aims at clarifying whether patients with MBC whose CTC count did not decrease following first cycle of chemotherapy benefit from an early switch to another regimen.

15.3.3 Treatment Selection Based on CTCs—Liquid Biopsy

15.3.3.1 Early Breast Cancer

The clinical potential of CTCs is not limited to simple cell enumeration. Multiple assays to evaluate their phenotype and genotype have been introduced to further characterize MRD. Interestingly, expression profiles of CTCs differ from that of the primary tumor in a large proportion of patients (Fehm et al. 2008, 2010; Krawczyk et al. 2009; Aktas et al. 2011). Since the choice of adjuvant systemic treatment is currently based on the characteristics of the primary tumor, CTCs displaying different molecular features may elude adjuvant therapy and persist beyond primary treatment. Potentially, the discrepancy between CTCs and the primary tumor might be important when selecting patients who may benefit from targeted treatment.

In this context, HER2 status has been the most extensively investigated marker in CTCs. We previously reported that the concordance between CTCs and their corresponding primary tumor is low (52 %) (Fehm et al. 2009); HER2-positive CTCs may be detected in 38 % of patients with primary BC, while only 16 % of tumors are HER2-positive. Similar findings were reported regarding disseminated tumor cells (DTCs) in bone marrow; HER2-positive DTCs may be detected in patients with HER2-negative tumors at primary diagnosis and after completion of cytotoxic therapy as well (Krawczyk et al. 2009). Discordance between CTCs and the corresponding primary tumor might thus lead to undertreatment in patients with HER2-overexpressing CTCs but HER2-negative primary tumor. Rack et al. treated ten recurrence-free BC patients with persistent HER2-positive DTCs with trastuzumab; HER2-targeted treatment was able to clear HER2-positive DTCs in all patients (Rack et al. 2012). However, HER2-negative DTCs persisted in some patients; these women had a particularly poor prognosis. Whether the eradication of MRD contributes to a more favorable outcome will be addressed in the Treat CTC trial (NCT01548677). This randomized phase II trial has been initiated by the EORTC and aims at clarifying this issue: 174 CTC-positive patients with HER2-negative BC will be randomized to trastuzumab for 18 weeks versus observation. The impact of HER2-targeted therapy on CTC levels and survival will be evaluated.

Besides HER2, discrepancies regarding hormone receptor status have been reported as well (Fehm et al. 2008; Aktas et al. 2011). Loss of ER-positivity in course of the disease is considered a cause for relapse during or after endocrine treatment in patients with initially hormone receptor positive primary tumor ("nonresponders"). We examined blood samples from 431 patients with early breast cancer and evaluated the ER, PR and HER2 status in detected CTCs (Fehm et al. 2009); CTCs generally displayed a triple-negative phenotype regardless of the molecular features of the primary tumor. Older studies on isolated tumor cells in the bone marrow described a similar phenomenon: the majority of patients presented with ER-negative DTCs despite ER-positive tumor (Fehm et al. 2008). One of the factors contributing to these discrepancies on the molecular level might be the clonal heterogeneity of breast cancer: ER-negative cells have a selection advantage due to their increased invasiveness and are therefore more likely to enter blood circulation. Similarly, since HER2-positive cells possess higher extravasative capacity, they might be more likely to persist in secondary homing sites. Consequently, molecular features of CTCs do not necessarily reflect those of their corresponding tumor.

15.3.3.2 Metastatic Breast Cancer

The question whether MBC patients clinically benefit from systemic treatment targeting CTCs is being currently addressed in several trials. Since CTCs at baseline correlate with survival, high CTC levels might indicate the need for a more aggressive or longer treatment. This issue will be addressed in the ongoing STIC CTC METABREAST trial (NCT01710605); hormone receptor positive MBC patients will be randomized between the clinician choice and CTC count-driven choice. In the CTC-group, patients with high CTC levels (≥ 5 CTCs/7.5 ml PB) will receive chemotherapy; patients with low CTC levels (<5 CTCs/7.5 ml PB) will be treated with endocrine therapy only.

Hypothetically, the choice of treatment might be guided not only by CTC levels but by the molecular features of CTCs as well. Metastatic cancer is considered a dynamic heterogenous disease; its phenotype, particularly with regard to predictive markers such as HER2 and hormone receptors, may change over time. Since CTCs seem to reflect the current "status" of the disease, evaluation of these cells may provide insight into possible therapeutic targets (such as HER and hormone receptor status) and resistance mechanisms of the tumor in real time ("liquid biopsy").

Meng et al. (2004b) has shown that patients with a HER2-negative primary tumor can develop HER2-positive CTCs and HER2-positive metastases during disease progression. However, since repeated metastasis biopsies are not feasible, treatment choices are commonly based on the phenotype of the primary tumor. In this context, CTCs may become an attractive non-invasive substitute to metastasis biopsy. Whether patients in metastatic setting benefit from a systemic therapy selected on the basis of expression profiles of CTCs, remains to be seen. The ongoing DETECT III trial aims at clarifying this question (EudraCT 2010-024238-46); this prospective randomized study will analyse the effectiveness of HER2-targeted therapy with lapatinib in MBC patients with HER2-positive CTCs despite HER2-negative primary tumor (Bidard et al. 2013a). In patients with HER2-negative CTCs and HER2-negative, hormone receptor positive MBC, the impact of everolimus in combination with endocrine agents and eribulin on CTCs will be investigated in the DETECT IVa/b trial.

15.4 Conclusion/Future

In the last two decades, several promising CTC detection methods have been developed to establish and confirm enumeration of CTCs as a prognostic marker in many studies and several clinical trials. The great promise to advance CTCs' clinical relevance lies in characterizing their individual phenotype and/or genotype, so we may better understand the processes of tumor pathogenesis and metastasis, and tailor treatment decisions to the individual patient. To achieve this, we must be able to isolate single CTCs repeatedly during the course of disease and/or its treatment, to extract their molecular and functional information and finally translate this information into clinical applications. Currently, adequate and optimized integrated workflows for molecular and functional analysis of CTCs are undergoing testing, so it is still too early to implement a CTC-based therapy decision into treatment guidelines. However, recent advances in the CTC field support the ambition that CTC assessment will provide promising benefit for the patient as a non-invasive and repeatable tool for treatment individualization and monitoring. Taken together, CTC analysis will account for a more integrative predictive, preventive, and personalized medicine in the near future.

Acknowledgments We thank Dr. Anna-Sophia McKenney (Weill Cornell/Rockefeller/Sloan-Kettering Tri-Institutional MD-PhD Program, New York, NY) for critically revising the manuscript.

References

Aktas B, Müller V, Tewes M et al (2011) Comparison of estrogen and progesteronereceptor status of circulating tumor cells and the primary tumor in metastatic breast cancer patients. Gynecol Oncol 122:356–360

Aktas B, Tewes M, Fehm T et al (2009) Stem cell and epithelial-mesenchymal transition markers are frequently overexpressed in circulating tumor cells of metastatic breast cancer patients. Breast Cancer Res 11:R46

Alix-Panabières C (2012) EPISPOT assay: detection of viable DTCs/CTCs in solid tumor patients. Recent Results Cancer Res 195:69–76. doi:10.1007/978-3-642-28160-0_6

Allard WJ, Matera J, Miller MC et al (2004) Tumor cells circulate in the peripheral blood of all major carcinomas but not in healthy subjects or patients with nonmalignant diseases. Clin Cancer Res 10:6897–6904. doi:10.1158/1078-0432.CCR-04-0378

Andreopoulou E, Yang L-Y, Rangel KM et al (2012) Comparison of assay methods for detection of circulating tumor cells in metastatic breast cancer: AdnaGen AdnaTest breastcancer select/detectTM versus veridex cell searchTM system. Int J Cancer 130:1590–1597. doi:10.1002/ijc.26111

Armstrong AJ, Marengo MS, Oltean S et al (2011) Circulating tumor cells from patients with advanced prostate and breast cancer display both epithelial and mesenchymal markers. Mol Cancer Res 9:997–1007. doi:10.1158/1541-7786.MCR-10-0490

Ashworth TR (1869) A case of cancer in which cells similar to those in the tumours were seen in the blood after death. Med J 14:146–149

Azim HA, Agbor-tarh D, Bradbury I, et al (2013) Pattern of rash, diarrhea, and hepatic toxicities secondary to lapatinib and their association with age and response to neoadjuvant therapy: analysis from the NeoALTTO trial. J Clin Oncol 31:4504–4511. doi:10.1200/JCO.2013.50.9448

Balic M, Lin H, Young L, et al (2006) Most early disseminated cancer cells detected in bone marrow of breast cancer patients have a putative breast cancer stem cell phenotype. Clin Cancer Res 12:5615–5621. doi:10.1158/1078-0432.CCR-06-0169

Banys M, Hartkopf AD, Krawczyk N et al (2012) Dormancy in breast cancer. Breast Cancer (London) 4:183–191. doi:10.2147/BCTT.S26431

Barradas AMC, Terstappen LWMM (2013) Towards the biological understanding of CTC: capture technologies, definitions and potential to create metastasis. Cancers (Basel) 5:1619–1642. doi:10.3390/cancers5041619

Barriere G, Riouallon A, Renaudie J et al (2012) Mesenchymal and stemness circulating tumor cells in early breast cancer diagnosis. BMC Cancer 12:114

Benoy IH, Elst H, Philips M et al (2006) Real-time RT–PCR detection of disseminated tumour cells in bone marrow has superior prognostic significance in comparison with circulating tumour cells in patients with breast cancer. Br J Cancer 94:672–680. doi:10.1038/sj.bjc.6602985

Bidard F, Fehm T, Ignatiadis M et al (2013a) Clinical application of circulating tumor cells in breast cancer: overview of the current interventional trials. Cancer Metastasis Rev 13:179–188

Bidard F-C, Belin L, Delaloge S et al (2013b) Time-dependent prognostic impact of circulating tumor cells detection in non-metastatic breast cancer: 70-month analysis of the REMAGUS02 study. Int J Breast Cancer 2013:130470. doi:10.1155/2013/130470

Bidard F-C, Peeters DJ, Fehm T et al (2014) Clinical validity of circulating tumour cells in patients with metastatic breast cancer: a pooled analysis of individual patient data. Lancet Oncol 15:406–414. doi:10.1016/S1470-2045(14)70069-5

Bidard F-C, Vincent-Salomon A, Sigal-Zafrani B, et al (2008) Prognosis of women with stage IV breast cancer depends on detection of circulating tumor cells rather than disseminated tumor cells. Ann Oncol 19:496–500. doi:10.1093/annonc/mdm507

Broersen LA, van Pelt G, Tollenaar REM, Mesker W (2014) Clinical application of circulating tumor cells in breast cancer. Cell Oncol 37:9–15. doi:10.1007/s13402-013-0160-6

Budd GT, Cristofanilli M, Ellis MJ et al (2006) Circulating tumor cells versus imaging—predicting overall survival in metastatic breast cancer. Clin Cancer Res 12:6403–6409. doi:10.1158/1078-0432.CCR-05-1769

Cohen SJ, Punt CJA, Iannotti N, et al (2008) Relationship of circulating tumor cells to tumor response, progression-free survival, and overall survival in patients with metastatic colorectal cancer. J Clin Oncol 26:3213–3221. doi:10.1200/JCO.2007.15.8923

Coumans FAW, Ligthart ST, Uhr JW, Terstappen LWMM (2012) Challenges in the enumeration and phenotyping of CTC. Clin Cancer Res 18:5711–5718. doi:10.1158/1078-0432.CCR-12-1585

Cristofanilli M, Budd GT, Ellis MJ et al (2004) Circulating tumor cells, disease progression, and survival in metastatic breast cancer. N Engl J Med 351:781–791

Cristofanilli M, Hayes DF, Budd GT et al (2005) Circulating tumor cells: a novel prognostic factor for newly diagnosed metastatic breast cancer. J Clin Oncol 23:1420–1430

de Bono JS, Scher HI, Montgomery RB, et al (2008) Circulating tumor cells predict survival benefit from treatment in metastatic castration-resistant prostate cancer. Clin Cancer Res 14:6302–6309. doi:10.1158/1078-0432.CCR-08-0872

De Giorgi U, Valero V, Rohren E, et al (2010) Circulating tumor cells and bone metastases as detected by FDG–PET/CT in patients with metastatic breast cancer. Ann Oncol 21:33–39. doi:10.1093/annonc/mdp262

Demel U, Tilz G, Foeldes-Papp Z et al (2004) Detection of tumour cells in the peripheral blood of patients with breast cancer. Development of a new sensitive and specific immunomolecular assay. J Exp Clin Cancer Res 23:465–468

Deng G, Herrler M, Burgess D et al (2008) Enrichment with anti-cytokeratin alone or combined with anti-EpCAM antibodies significantly increases the sensitivity for circulating tumor cell detection in metastatic breast cancer patients. Breast Cancer Res 10:R69. doi:10.1186/bcr2131

EBCTCG Early Breast Cancer Trialists' Collaborative Group (2005) Effects of chemotherapy and hormonal therapy for early breast cancer on recurrence and 15-year survival: an overview of the randomised trials. Lancet 365:1687–1717. doi:10.1016/S0140-6736(05)66544-0

Fehm T, Braun S, Muller V et al (2006) A concept for the standardized detection of disseminated tumor cells in bone marrow from patients with primary breast cancer and its clinical implementation. Cancer 107:885–892. doi:10.1002/cncr.22076

Fehm T, Hoffmann O, Aktas B et al (2009) Detection and characterization of circulating tumor cells in blood of primary breast cancer patients by RT-PCR and comparison to status of bone marrow disseminated cells. Breast Cancer Res 11:R59. doi:10.1186/bcr2349

Fehm T, Krawczyk N, Solomayer E-F et al (2008) ERalpha-status of disseminated tumour cells in bone marrow of primary breast cancer patients. Breast Cancer Res 10:R76

Fehm T, Mueller V, Aktas B et al (2010) HER2 status of circulating tumor cells in patients with metastatic breast cancer: a prospective, multicenter trial. Breast Cancer Res Treat 124:403–412

Fehm T, Sagalowsky A, Clifford E et al (2002) Cytogenetic evidence that circulating epithelial cells in patients with carcinoma are malignant. Clin Cancer Res 8:2073–2084

Fehm T, Solomayer E, Meng S et al (2005) Methods for isolating circulating epithelial cells and criteria for their classification as carcinoma cells. Cytotherapy 7:171–185

Fischer JC, Niederacher D, Topp SA et al (2013) Diagnostic leukapheresis enables reliable detection of circulating tumor cells of nonmetastatic cancer patients. Proc Natl Acad Sci USA 110:16580–16585. doi:10.1073/pnas.1313594110

Freidin MB, Tay A, Freydina DV et al (2014) An assessment of diagnostic performance of a filter-based antibody-independent peripheral blood circulating tumour cell capture paired with cytomorphologic criteria for the diagnosis of cancer. Lung Cancer 85:182–185. doi:10.1016/j.lungcan.2014.05.017

Giordano A, Giuliano M, De Laurentiis M, et al (2012) Circulating tumor cells in immunohistochemical subtypes of metastatic breast cancer: lack of prediction in HER2-positive disease treated with targeted therapy. Ann Oncol 23:1144–1150. doi:10.1093/annonc/mdr434

Giuliano M, Giordano A, Jackson S et al (2011) Circulating tumor cells as prognostic and predictive markers in metastatic breast cancer patients receiving first-line systemic treatment. Breast Cancer Res 13: R67. doi:10.1186/bcr2907

Harb W, Fan A, Tran T et al (2013) Mutational analysis of circulating tumor cells using a novel microfluidic collection device and qPCR assay. Transl Oncol 6:528–538. doi:10.1593/tlo.13367

Hartkopf A, Wagner P, Wallwiener D et al (2011) Changing levels of circulating tumor cells in monitoring chemotherapy response in patients with metastatic breast cancer. Anticancer Res 31:979–984

Hayes DF, Cristofanilli M, Budd GT, et al (2006) Circulating tumor cells at each followup time point during therapy of metastatic breast cancer patients predict progression-free and overall survival. Clin Cancer Res 12:4218–4224. doi:10.1158/1078-0432.CCR-05-2821

Hayes DF, Smerage J (2008) Is there a role for circulating tumor cells in the management of breast cancer? Clin Cancer Res 14:3646–3650. doi:10.1158/1078-0432.CCR-07-4481

Hong B, Zu Y (2013) Detecting circulating tumor cells: current challenges and new trends. Theranostics 3:377–394. doi:10.7150/thno.5195

Hou HW, Warkiani ME, Khoo BL et al (2013) Isolation and retrieval of circulating tumor cells using centrifugal forces. Sci Rep 3:1259. doi:10.1038/srep01259

Hüsemann Y, Geigl JB, Schubert F et al (2008) Systemic spread is an early step in breast cancer. Cancer Cell 13:58–68. doi:10.1016/j.ccr.2007.12.003

Hwang SB, Bae JW, Lee HY, Kim HY (2012) Circulating tumor cells detected by RT-PCR for CK-20 before surgery indicate worse prognostic impact in triple-negative and HER2 subtype breast cancer. J Breast Cancer 15:34–42. doi:10.4048/jbc.2012.15.1.34

Ignatiadis M, Xenidis N, Perraki M et al (2007) Different Prognostic Value of Cytokeratin-19 mRNA positive circulating tumor cells according to estrogen receptor and HER2 status in early-stage breast cancer. J Clin Oncol 25:5194–5202

Joosse SA, Gorges TM, Pantel K (2014) Biology, detection, and clinical implications of circulating tumor cells. EMBO Mol Med 7:1–11

Kallergi G, Papadaki MA, Politaki E et al (2011) Epithelial to mesenchymal transition markers expressed in circulating tumour cells of early and metastatic breast cancer patients. Breast Cancer Res 13:R59. doi:10.1186/bcr2896

Kasimir-Bauer S, Hoffmann O, Wallwiener D et al (2012) Expression of stem cell and epithelial-mesenchymal transition markers in primary breast cancer patients with circulating tumor cells. Breast Cancer Res 14: R15. doi:10.1186/bcr3099

Klein CA (2008) The metastasis cascade. Science 321:1785–1787. doi:10.1126/science.1164853

Krawczyk N, Banys M, Neubauer H et al (2009) HER2 status on persistent disseminated tumor cells after adjuvant therapy may differ from initial HER2 status on primary tumor. Anticancer Res 29:4019–4024

Krawczyk N, Hartkopf A, Banys M et al (2014a) Prognostic relevance of induced and spontaneous apoptosis of disseminated tumor cells in primary breast cancer patients. BMC Cancer 14:394. doi:10.1186/1471-2407-14-394

Krawczyk N, Meier-Stiegen F, Banys M et al (2014b) Expression of stem cell and epithelial-mesenchymal transition markers in circulating tumor cells of breast cancer patients. Biomed Res Int 2014:415721. doi:10.1155/2014/415721

Kulemann B, Pitman MB, Liss AS et al (2015) Circulating tumor cells found in patients with localized and advanced pancreatic cancer. Pancreas 44:547–550

Lin HK, Zheng S, Williams AJ et al (2010) Portable filter-based microdevice for detection and characterization of circulating tumor cells. Clin Cancer Res 16:5011–5018. doi:10.1158/1078-0432.CCR-10-1105

Liu MC, Shields PG, Warren RD, et al (2009) Circulating tumor cells: a useful predictor of treatment efficacy in metastatic breast cancer. J Clin Oncol 27:5153–5159. doi:10.1200/JCO.2008.20.6664

Lowes LE, Hedley BD, Keeney M, Allan AL (2012) User-defined protein marker assay development for characterization of circulating tumor cells using the Cell Search system. Cytom Part A 81A:983–995. doi:10.1002/cyto.a.22158

Lu J, Fan T, Zhao Q et al (2010) Isolation of circulating epithelial and tumor progenitor cells with an invasive phenotype from breast cancer patients. Int J Cancer 126:669–683. doi:10.1002/ijc.24814

Lucci A, Hall CS, Lodhi AK et al (2012) Circulating tumour cells in non-metastatic breast cancer: a prospective study. Lancet Oncol 13:688–695. doi:10.1016/S1470-2045(12)70209-7

Markou A, Strati A, Malamos N, et al (2011) Molecular characterization of circulating tumor cells in breast cancer by a liquid bead array hybridization assay. Clin Chem 57:421–430. doi:10.1373/clinchem.2010.154328

Mego M, Gao H, Lee B-N et al (2012a) Prognostic value of EMT-circulating tumor cells in metastatic breast cancer patients undergoing high-dose chemotherapy with autologous hematopoietic stem cell transplantation. J Cancer 3:369–380. doi:10.7150/jca.5111

Mego M, Mani SA, Lee B-N et al (2012b) Expression of epithelial-mesenchymal transition-inducing transcription factors in primary breast cancer: the effect of neoadjuvant therapy. Int J Cancer 130:808–816. doi:10.1002/ijc.26037

Meng S, Tripathy D, Frenkel EP, et al (2004a) Circulating tumor cells in patients with breast cancer dormancy. Clin Cancer Res 10:8152–8162. doi:10.1158/1078-0432.CCR-04-1110

Meng S, Tripathy D, Shete S et al (2004b) HER-2 gene amplification can be acquired as breast cancer progresses. Proc Natl Acad Sci USA 101:9393–9398

Molloy TJ, Bosma AJ, Baumbusch LO et al (2011) The prognostic significance of tumour cell detection in the peripheral blood versus the bone marrow in 733 early-stage breast cancer patients. Breast Cancer Res 13:R61. doi:10.1186/bcr2898

Mostert B, Sleijfer S, Foekens JA, Gratama JW (2009) Circulating tumor cells (CTCs): detection methods and their clinical relevance in breast cancer. Cancer Treat Rev 35:463–474

Müller V, Riethdorf S, Rack B et al (2012) Prognostic impact of circulating tumor cells assessed with the cell search systemTM and AdnaTest breastTM in metastatic breast cancer patients: the DETECT study. Breast Cancer Res 14:R118. doi:10.1186/bcr3243

Müller V, Stahmann N, Riethdorf S, et al (2005) Circulating tumor cells in breast cancer: correlation to bone marrow micrometastases, heterogeneous response to systemic therapy and low proliferative activity. Clin Cancer Res 11 3678–3685. doi:10.1158/1078-0432.CCR-04-2469

Nagrath S, Sequist LV, Maheswaran S et al (2007) Isolation of rare circulating tumour cells in cancer patients by microchip technology. Nature 450:1235–1239

Nakamura S, Yagata H, Ohno S et al (2010) Multi-center study evaluating circulating tumor cells as a surrogate for response to treatment and overall survival in metastatic breast cancer. Breast Cancer 17:199–204. doi:10.1007/s12282-009-0139-3

Neves RPL, Raba K, Schmidt O et al (2014) Genomic high-resolution profiling of single CKpos/CD45neg flow-sorting purified circulating tumor cells from patients with metastatic breast cancer. Clin Chem 60:1290–1297. doi:10.1373/clinchem.2014.222331

Nolé F, Munzone E, Zorzino L, et al (2008) Variation of circulating tumor cell levels during treatment of metastatic breast cancer: prognostic and therapeutic implications. Ann Oncol 19:891–897. doi:10.1093/annonc/mdm558

Onder TT, Gupta PB, Mani SA et al (2008) Loss of E-Cadherin promotes metastasis via multiple downstream transcriptional pathways. Cancer Res 68:3645–3654. doi:10.1158/0008-5472.CAN-07-2938

Ozkumur E, Shah AM, Ciciliano JC, et al (2013) Inertial focusing for tumor antigen–dependent and –independent sorting of rare circulating tumor cells. Sci Transl Med 5:179ra47. doi:10.1126/scitranslmed.3005616

Pachmann K, Camara O, Kavallaris A, et al (2008) Monitoring the response of circulating epithelial tumor cells to adjuvant chemotherapy in breast cancer allows detection of patients at risk of early relapse. J Clin Oncol 26:1208–1215. doi:10.1200/JCO.2007.13.6523

Pantel K, Alix-Panabieres C (2014) Bone marrow as a reservoir for disseminated tumor cells: a special source for liquid biopsy in cancer patients. BoneKEy Rep 3:584

Pantel K, Brakenhoff RH, Brandt B (2008) Detection, clinical relevance and specific biological properties of disseminating tumour cells. Nat Rev Cancer 8:329–340

Payne RE, Wang F, Su N et al (2012) Viable circulating tumour cell detection using multiplex RNA in situ hybridisation predicts progression-free survival in metastatic breast cancer patients. Br J Cancer 106:1790–1797. doi:10.1038/bjc.2012.137

Pierga J-Y, Bidard F-C, Mathiot C, et al (2008) Circulating tumor cell detection predicts early metastatic relapse after neoadjuvant chemotherapy in large operable and locally advanced breast cancer in a phase II randomized trial. Clin Cancer Res 14:7004–7010. doi:10.1158/1078-0432.CCR-08-0030

Pierga J-Y, Hajage D, Bachelot T, et al (2012) High independent prognostic and predictive value of circulating tumor cells compared with serum tumor markers in a large prospective trial in first-line chemotherapy for metastatic breast cancer patients. Ann Oncol 23:618–624. doi:10.1093/annonc/mdr263

Rack B, Jückstock J, Günthner-Biller M et al (2012) Trastuzumab clears HER2/neu-positive isolated tumor cells from bone marrow in primary breast cancer patients. Arch Gynecol Obstet 285:485–492. doi:10.1007/s00404-011-1954-2

Rack B, Schindlbeck C, Jückstock J, et al (2014) Circulating tumor cells predict survival in early average-to-high risk breast cancer patients. J Natl Cancer Inst 106:dju066. doi:10.1093/jnci/dju066

Raimondi C, Gradilone A, Naso G et al (2011) Epithelial-mesenchymal transition and stemness features in circulating tumor cells from breast cancer patients. Breast Cancer Res Treat 130:449–455. doi:10.1007/s10549-011-1373-x

Riahi R, Gogoi P, Sepehri S et al (2014) A novel microchannel-based device to capture and analyze circulating tumor cells (CTCs) of breast cancer. Int J Oncol 44:1870–1878. doi:10.3892/ijo.2014.2353

Riethdorf S, Fritsche H, Müller V et al (2007) Detection of circulating tumor cells in peripheral blood of patients with metastatic breast cancer: a validation study of the cell search system. Clin Cancer Res 13:920–928. doi:10.1158/1078-0432.CCR-06-1695

Saucedo-Zeni N, Mewes S, Niestroj R et al (2012) A novel method for the in vivo isolation of circulating tumor cells from peripheral blood of cancer patients using a functionalized and structured medical wire. Int J Oncol 41:1241–1250. doi:10.3892/ijo.2012.1557

Sieuwerts A, Kraan J, Bolt-de Vries J et al (2009a) Molecular characterization of circulating tumor cells in large quantities of contaminating leukocytes by a multiplex real-time PCR. Breast Cancer Res Treat 118:455–468

Sieuwerts AM, Kraan J, Bolt J et al (2009b) Anti-epithelial cell adhesion molecule antibodies and the detection of circulating normal-like breast tumor cells. J Natl Cancer Inst 101:61–66

Slade MJ, Payne R, Riethdorf S et al (2009) Comparison of bone marrow, disseminated tumour cells and blood-circulating tumour cells in breast cancer patients after primary treatment. Br J Cancer 100:160–166. doi:10.1038/sj.bjc.6604773

Smerage JB, Barlow WE, Hortobagyi GN, et al (2014) Circulating tumor cells and response to chemotherapy in metastatic breast cancer: SWOG S0500. J Clin Oncol 32:3483–3489. doi:10.1200/JCO.2014.56.2561

Stathopoulou A, Vlachonikolis I, Mavroudis D et al (2002) Molecular Detection of cytokeratin-19-positive cells in the peripheral blood of patients with operable breast cancer: evaluation of their prognostic significance. J Clin Oncol 20:3404–3412

Stott SL, Hsu C-H, Tsukrov DI et al (2010) Isolation of circulating tumor cells using a microvortex-generating herringbone-chip. Proc Natl Acad Sci USA 107:18392–18397. doi:10.1073/pnas.1012539107

Tam WL, Weinberg RA (2013) The epigenetics of epithelial-mesenchymal plasticity in cancer. Nat Med 19:1438–1449

Tewes M, Aktas B, Welt A et al (2009) Molecular profiling and predictive value of circulating tumor cells in patients with metastatic breast cancer: an option for monitoring response to breast cancer related therapies. Breast Cancer Res Treat 115:581–590. doi:10.1007/s10549-008-0143-x

Theodoropoulos PA, Polioudaki H, Agelaki S et al (2010) Circulating tumor cells with a putative stem cell phenotype in peripheral blood of patients with breast cancer. Cancer Lett 288:99–106. doi:10.1016/j.canlet.2009.06.027

Thiery JP (2002) Epithelial-mesenchymal transitions in tumour progression. Nat Rev Cancer 2:442–454

Thiery JP, Acloque H, Huang RYJ, Nieto MA (2009) Epithelial-mesenchymal transitions in development and disease. Cell 139:871–890. doi:10.1016/j.cell.2009.11.007

Wallwiener M, Hartkopf A, Baccelli I et al (2013) The prognostic impact of circulating tumor cells in subtypes of metastatic breast cancer. Breast Cancer Res Treat 137:503–510. doi:10.1007/s10549-012-2382-0

Wang F, Flanagan J, Su N et al (2012) RNAscope: a novel in situ RNA analysis platform for formalin-fixed, paraffin-embedded tissues. J Mol Diagn 14:22–29. doi:10.1016/j.jmoldx.2011.08.002

Wülfing P, Borchard J, Buerger H, et al (2006) HER2-Positive Circulating tumor cells indicate poor clinical outcome in stage I to III breast cancer patients. Clin Cancer Res 12:1715–1720. doi:10.1158/1078-0432.CCR-05-2087

Xenidis N, Perraki M, Apostolaki S et al (2013) Differential effect of adjuvant taxane-based and taxane-free chemotherapy regimens on the CK-19 mRNA-positive circulating tumour cells in patients with early breast cancer. Br J Cancer 108:549–556. doi:10.1038/bjc.2012.597

Xenidis N, Perraki M, Kafousi M et al (2006) Predictive and prognostic value of peripheral blood cytokeratin-19 mRNA-positive cells detected by real-time polymerase chain reaction in node-negative breast cancer patients. J Clin Oncol 24:3756–3762

Yu M, Bardia A, Wittner BS, et al (2013) Circulating breast tumor cells exhibit dynamic changes in epithelial and mesenchymal composition. Science (80-) 339:580–584. doi:10.1126/science.1228522

Yu M, Stott S, Toner M et al (2011) Circulating tumor cells: approaches to isolation and characterization. J Cell Biol 192:373–382. doi:10.1083/jcb.201010021

Circulating Nucleic Acids (RNA/DNA) in Breast Cancer

16

Isabelle Gingras, Libero Santarpia and Michail Ignatiadis

Abstract

Circulating nucleic acids such as DNA and microRNA are released and circulate in the blood of cancer patients. In breast cancer, free circulating nucleic acids are being explored as potential blood biomarkers for real-time tumor monitoring. In the past decades, increasing evidence has emerged indicating potential use of circulating DNA for assessment of tumor burden and for tumor genomic and epigenetic profiling. MicroRNA profiling studies also suggest potential utility for breast cancer screening, prognosis evaluation and interrogating mechanisms of therapy resistance and tumor biology. However, a variety of preanalytical considerations must be contemplated and ultimately clinical validity and utility must be demonstrated. This book chapter will explore the main methods to detect and analyze circulating tumor DNA and circulating microRNA, and the clinical applications for circulating free nucleic acids analysis in breast cancer.

Keywords

Circulating nuclei acids · DNA · RNA · cmiRNA

I. Gingras
Hematology and Oncology Department, Hôpital du Sacré-Coeur de Montréal, Montreal, QC, Canada

L. Santarpia
Oncology Experimental Therapeutics Unit, Humanitas Clinical and Research Institute, Rozzano, Milan, Italy

M. Ignatiadis (✉)
Department of Medical Oncology and Breast Cancer Translational Research Laboratory J. C. Heuson, Institut Jules Bordet, Université libre de Bruxelles, Brussels, Belgium
e-mail: michail.ignatiadis@bordet.be

S. Badve and Y. Gökmen-Polar (eds.), *Molecular Pathology of Breast Cancer*, DOI 10.1007/978-3-319-41761-5_16

Abbrevations	
E	Endosome
EE	Early Endosome
G	Golgi
L	Lysosome
MVB	Multi-vesicular bodies
N	Nucleus
P	Protein
UP	Undigested protein

16.1 Introduction

The last two decades have witnessed a shift of treatment paradigm towards personalized medicine, with great therapeutic successes obtained with the use of drugs tailored to the genetic characteristics of the tumor. However, restricted access to tumor tissue throughout tumor evolution and lack of sensitive and specific blood biomarkers still represent major challenges to a broader use of personalized medicine in breast cancer.

The presence of circulating free nucleic acids in the human serum was first described more than 50 years ago (Mandel and Métais 1948), but it is only lately that the potential of circulating nucleic acids as tumor blood biomarkers was truly explored. Since then, researchers have investigated the possibility to interrogate the tumor biology by analyzing circulating free nucleic acids in the blood of cancer patients. This chapter will explore the main methods to detect and analyze free circulating tumor DNA (ctDNA) and circulating microRNA (cmiRNA), and the clinical applications for circulating free nucleic acids analysis in breast cancer. Analysis of "non-cell-free" nucleic acids in blood, such as analysis of RNA and DNA expression on CTCs, is beyond the scope of this chapter (Ignatiadis and Dawson 2014; Alix-Panabieres and Pantel 2014).

16.2 Circulating Tumoral DNA

16.2.1 Circulating Tumor DNA: Preanalytical Considerations and Technologies for ctDNA Detection

Circulating free DNA (cfDNA) was first discovered to be detectable in lower levels in the serum and body fluid of healthy individuals, and in higher levels in patients with various disorders, such as systemic lupus erythematous, rheumatoid arthritis, pulmonary embolism or cancer (Koffler et al. 1973; Barnett 1968; Tan et al. 1966; Leon et al. 1977). An increase in cfDNA level has also been described after trauma or following exhaustive exercise (Atamaniuk et al. 2004; Lo et al. 2000). In 1977, Leon et al. demonstrated that cfDNA was elevated in cancer patients (mean cfDNA concentration 180 ng/ml in cancer patients versus 13 ng/ml in healthy controls), and that cfDNA level was associated with tumor burden and clinical outcome (Leon et al. 1977). Other studies later confirmed that the mean cfDNA level was higher in cancer patients then in patients with benign disorders (Shapiro et al. 1983; Maebo 1990).

DNA is released into circulation following cell-death processes. Fragmentation of cfDNA is higher following apoptosis than necrosis or phagocytosis; for example, fragments longer than 10,000 bp are likely to originate from necrosis, while fragments shorter than 1000 bp are mainly observed following apoptosis (Wang et al. 2003). CtDNA fragments are typically the size of 160–180 bp, reflecting DNA degradation into nucleosomal units during the process of apoptosis (Mouliere et al. 2011).

CtDNA can represent a very small fraction of the total amount of free DNA in the plasma, especially in early-stage disease; therefore, ctDNA assays require high analytical sensitivity and specificity to overcome the bias induced by analyzing low-input material. Consideration of preanalytical factors is of critical importance to ensure the quality of the analysis (El Messaoudi et al. 2013). Plasma is favored over serum in order to reduce contamination following the lysis of white-blood cells in the samples (Umetani et al. 2006; Mouliere et al. 2011; Jung et al. 2003; Chan et al. 2005; Lui et al. 2002; El Messaoudi et al. 2013; Qin et al. 2013). EDTA coated tubes are generally preferred for blood collection; however, recently, a new collection tube (cell-free DNA BCT by Streck Inc.) was developed containing a novel chemical cocktail that can stabilize nucleated blood cells, therefore allowing for reduced changes in plasma DNA level of the samples following shaking, shipping and incubation, compared to EDTA-coated tubes (Norton et al. 2013). Further validation of these data is needed. Time delays, storage conditions and repeated freezing and thawing (more than three times) can influence the quality of the samples; prompt process and adequate storage is mandatory (El Messaoudi et al. 2013; Chan et al. 2005). Process of centrifugation must ensure adequate purification of the sample (Chiu et al. 2001). CfDNA can then be extracted using commercially available kits.

CtDNA assays have two major goals: tumor monitoring by ctDNA quantification and non-invasive tumor molecular profiling (Fig. 16.1). Different methods have been proposed to distinguish ctDNA from total cfDNA, most of them involving recognition of tumor-specific epigenetic or genomic aberrations on cfDNA (Madhavan et al. 2014; Balgkouranidou et al. 2013; Dawson et al. 2013; Chan et al. 2013a; Forshew et al. 2012; Leary et al. 2012; McBride et al. 2010; Shaw et al. 2012). One of the most sensitive and specific approaches to detect ctDNA is to identify tumor-specific genomic aberrations that are also present in primary tumor tissue samples (Leary et al. 2010; Bettegowda et al. 2014; Shaw et al. 2012).

Although the feasibility to detect genomic aberrations on ctDNA with traditional polymerase chain reaction (PCR) methods was demonstrated in the past, digital PCR using different approaches such as microfluid platforms, BEAMing (Beads, Emulsions, Amplification and Magnetics) or droplets-based system have now arisen as preferred methods for more sensitive determination of copy number variations (CNVs), for detection of rare mutant alleles and for quantification of ctDNA (Hindson et al. 2011; Wang et al. 2010b; Dressman et al. 2003; Diehl et al. 2008; Forshew et al. 2012; Taniguchi et al. 2011; Rosell et al. 2009). Moreover, next generation sequencing (NGS) technologies can be used for a more comprehensive tumor genomic analysis on cfDNA. Indeed, new methods based on NGS such as Tam-Seq, Safe-Seq, Ion AmpliSeq or CAPP-Seq have been used for the sequencing of specific regions of the genome, achieving analytical sensitivities close to PCR (Newman et al. 2014; Rothe et al. 2014; Forshew et al. 2012; Kinde et al. 2011; Carreira et al. 2014). The feasibility of performing whole-exome sequencing and whole-genome sequencing on ctDNA has also been demonstrated in few patients with high tumor burden (Murtaza et al. 2013; Chan et al. 2013b; Heidary et al. 2014).

16.2.2 Clinical Applications of CtDNA in Breast Cancer

16.2.2.1 Assessment of Tumor Burden

The feasibility to develop ctDNA detection assays by identifying tumor-specific genomic alterations such as p53 and PI3KCA mutations on cfDNA was recently demonstrated, allowing for detection

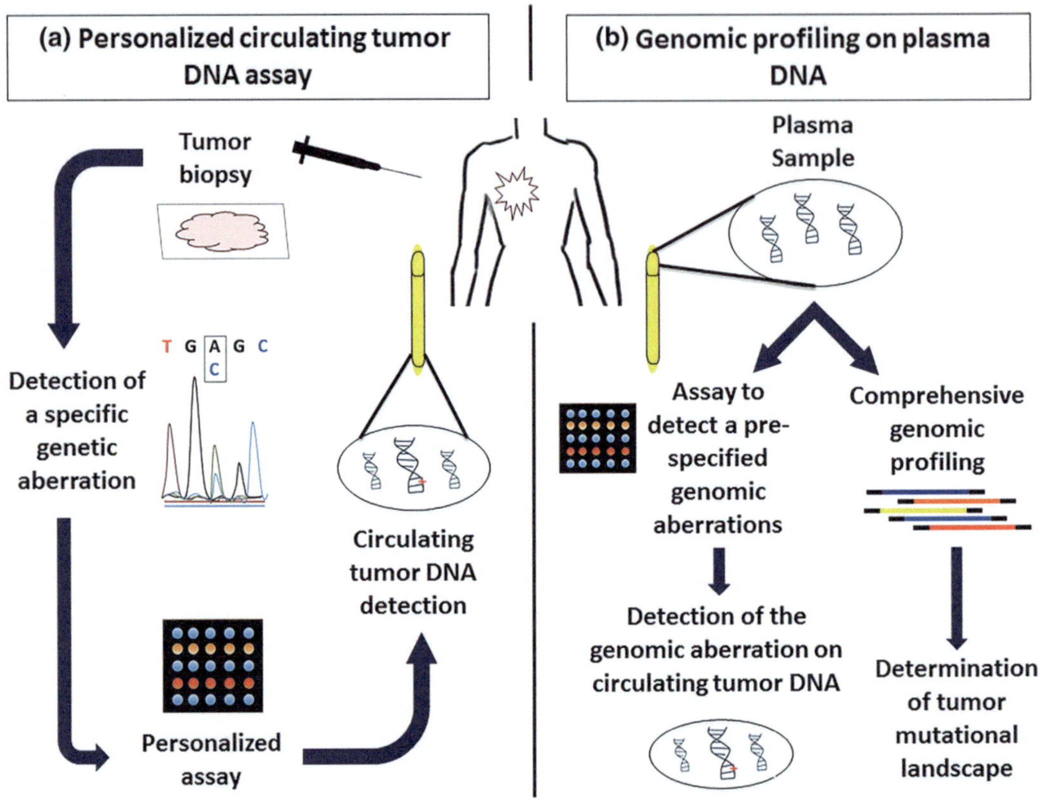

Fig. 16.1 Circulating DNA assays. **a** Development of a personalized circulating DNA assay to follow the tumor DNA level in blood. DNA is obtained from a tumor tissue sample either from a core biopsy or following tumor excision (1). Tumor genomic profiling is then performed on the tumor tissue to identify a tumor-specific genomic aberration suitable to develop a personalized circulating DNA assay (2). Upon identification of a specific tumor-genomic aberration such as genetic rearrangement, copy number alteration, point mutation, an assay is design to specifically recognize this sequence on the circulating free DNA (3). This personalized assay than allows for specific identification of circulating tumor DNA among circulating free DNA. **b** Direct interrogation of tumor genomic profile on circulating free DNA. Detection of known cancer-specific genomic aberrations in plasma is feasible with circulating DNA assay designed to detect the pre-specified genomic aberration (1). Whole-exome sequencing, whole-genome sequencing or sequencing of multiples target genes is also feasible on circulating free DNA, provided that the amount of circulating tumor DNA is sufficient (2)

of ctDNA in the metastatic and early setting (Table 16.1) (Madic et al. 2015; Beaver et al. 2014; Dawson et al. 2013; Higgins et al. 2012; Bettegowda et al. 2014). However, these assays are suitable only for the subgroup of patients whose tumor is bearing the pre-determined genomic alteration. Not unexpectedly, sensitivity of personalized ctDNA assays is usually inferior in the early than in the metastatic setting, because of lower amount of ctDNA in patients with low tumor burden (Hoque et al. 2006; Board et al. 2010; Bettegowda et al. 2014). The development of ctDNA assays with high sensitivity has also been achieved using recognition of known breast cancer DNA methylation patterns on cfDNA (Fackler et al. 2014; Hoque et al. 2006; Skvortsova et al. 2006). However, the sensitivity of this method occurs at the cost of lower specificity, and none of these assays has been validated in large dataset, retrospectively or prospectively.

Correlation between ctDNA level and tumor burden has been demonstrated in many cancers, including breast (Dawson et al. 2013; Bettegowda et al. 2014; Newman et al. 2014; Reinert

Table 16.1 Examples of assays to follow a tumor-specific genomic alteration previously identified on the primary tumor in breast cancer patients in plasma

References	Platform	Setting	Identified molecular aberration	# of patients in which a suitable mutation was identified/total # of patients screened	# of patients with ctDNA detected/total # of patients tested
Board et al. (2010)	Allele-specific PCR	EBC	PIK3CA mutations	14/30 (47 %)	0/14 (0 %)
		MBC		10/43 (23 %)	8/10 (80 %)
Leary et al. (2012)	Mate-paired sequencing	MBC	Structural variants	2/2 (100 %)	2/2 (100 %)
Higgins et al. (2012)	BEAMing	MBC	PIK3CA mutations	14/49 (29 %) (retrospective cohort) 14/51 (27 %) (prospective cohort)	14/14 (100 %) (retrospective cohort) 8/14 (57 %) (prospective cohort)[a]
Dawson et al. (2013)	Droplet-based digital PCR and Amplicon sequencing	MBC	PIK3CA mutations, TP53 mutations, structural variants	30/52 (58 %)	18/19 with dPCR 11/11 with Amplicon sequencing (total 29/30) (97 %)
Beaver et al. (2014)	Doplet-based dPCR	EBC	PIK3CA mutations	14/30 (47 %)	13/14 (92 %)
Bettegowda et al. (2014)	BEAMing, TamSeq, PCR-ligation	EBC	SNV, structural variants	19/19 (100 %)	10/19 (52 %)
		MBC		14/14 (100 %)	12/14 (86 %)
Madic et al. (2015)	Amplicon sequencing	Metastatic TNBC	TP53	26/31 (84 %)	21/26 (81 %)

[a]Blood samples and biopsy not obtained at the same time-point

BEAM Beading, emulsions, amplification and magnetics; *dPCR* digital polymerase chain reaction; *EBC* early breast cancer; *MBC* Metastatic breast cancer; *PCR* polymerase chain reaction; *SNV* single nucleotid variation; *TNBC* triple-negative breast cancer

et al. 2015). In a pivotal study by Dawson and colleagues, ctDNA level detected by personalized ctDNA assay, developed from genetic alterations identified in tumor tissue samples, proved to have better sensitivity and better correlation with tumor burden than CA 15-3 or circulating tumor cells (CTCs) in patients with metastatic breast cancer (MBC). Moreover, increase in ctDNA level often preceded by several months the establishment of progressive disease by radiological imaging. Both elevated ctDNA and CTCs were associated with poor outcomes. However, a suitable somatic genomic alteration to develop a personalized ctDNA assay was identified in only 30 of the 52 patients recruited. Hence, although highly sensitive and specific, this approach may be limited only to patients with detectable genomic aberrations in the primary tumor that can be followed in plasma (Bettegowda et al. 2014; Rothe et al. 2014).

The aforementioned study compared CTCs and ctDNA value as a biomarker; however, CTCs and ctDNA may provide complementary information. CTCs and ctDNA are of different origin (escape of a living tumor cell in circulation versus release of ctDNA in blood following apoptosis), and therefore may provide distinct knowledge on the tumor biology. CTCs and ctDNA assays each have their advantages and pitfalls, the former allowing for a more comprehensive molecular profiling and for functional analysis, but being limited by a challenging processing with the need for isolation and enrichment of the tumor cells (Ignatiadis and Dawson 2014). More studies are required to compare both assays as tumor biomarker and as tissue source for tumor molecular analysis.

Nonetheless, these studies suggest that ctDNA detected by personalized ctDNA assays has great potential to be used as a highly sensitive and specific tumor blood biomarker in breast cancer. Possible applications for ctDNA assays are cancer screening, detection of minimal residual disease or real-time tumor monitoring. However, ctDNA assays still have to demonstrate (1) sufficient sensitivity, specificity and hence analytical validity (defined as the capacity to determine accurately and reliably the measure of interest), (2) clinical validity (defined as the ability to predict a specific clinical outcome) and, ultimately, (3) clinical utility (defined as the likelihood that the test will improve clinical outcome when used in clinical practice). Standardization of the methods and validation in large prospective cohort of patients in the early and metastatic setting are needed to demonstrate such characteristics before implementation in clinical practice.

16.2.2.2 Tumor Genomic Profiling

Our knowledge on the genomic evolution of cancer has been limited by the low accessibility to tumor tissue during disease evolution. Furthermore, restricted numbers of tumor tissue samples often fail to represent all the tumor heterogeneity (Gerlinger et al. 2012). CtDNA analysis may be an alternative non-invasive method for tumor genomic profiling (Table 16.2) (Chan et al. 2013b; Murtaza et al. 2013; Board et al. 2010; Rothe et al. 2014;

Table 16.2 Studies evaluating the detection of tumor-specific genomic aberration directly in the plasma of breast cancer patient

References	Platform	Target gene(s)	Concordance between tumor tissue samples and ctDNA
Silva et al. (1999)	PCR-SSCP	TP53	58/62 patients (93 %)
Di et al. (2003)	PCR-SSCP	TP53	110/126 patients (87 %)
Board et al. (2010)	Allele-specific PCR	PIK3CA	39/41 patients (95 %)
Higgins et al. (2012)	BEAMing	PIK3CA	34/34 patients (100 %) (training cohort) 41/41 patients (100 %) (validation cohort)
Murtaza et al. (2013)	dPCR and amplicon sequencing	Whole-exome	93/151 mutations identified present in both ctDNA and synchronous biopsy—correlation coefficient 0.71 (1 patient)
Beaver et al. (2014)	Droplet-based dPCR	PIK3CA	28/29 patients (97 %)
De Mattos-Arruda et al. (2014)	Target massive parallel sequencing	Panel of 300 cancer genes	Analysis of ctDNA captured all mutations present in primary tumor and liver metastasis (1 patient)
Heidary et al. (2014)	Plasma-Seq	Whole-genome	Concordance only assessed for one patient. Unexpected low allele frequency of mutant fragments in ctDNA compared to tumor tissue and CTCs.
Rothe et al. (2014)	Amplicon sequencing	Panel of 50 cancer genes	13/17 patients (76 %)
Oshiro et al. (2015)	Chip-based PCR	PIK3CA	25/110 patients (22 %)

BEAM Beads, emulsion, amplification and magnetics; *CTCs* circulating tumor cells; *ctDNA* circulating tumor DNA; *dPCR* digital polymerase chain reaction; *PCR* polymerase chain reaction; *SSCP* single-strand conformation polymorphism

Higgins et al. 2012; De Mattos-Arruda et al. 2014; Dulaimi et al. 2004; Sharma et al. 2010b).

The ability to detect specific mutations on ctDNA has been proved in various cancers; likewise, in breast cancer, the feasibility to detect TP53 or PI3KCA mutations on ctDNA with good sensitivity and specificity has been demonstrated (Beaver et al. 2014; Board et al. 2010; Higgins et al. 2012; Page et al. 2011; Di et al. 2003). Genetic alterations that can be detected in ctDNA also include microsatellite instability and loss of heterozygosity implicating tumor suppressor genes (Fig. 16.2) (Schwarzenbach et al. 2012a; Osborne and Hamshere 2000; Chen et al. 1999; Mayall et al. 1999; Silva et al. 1999).

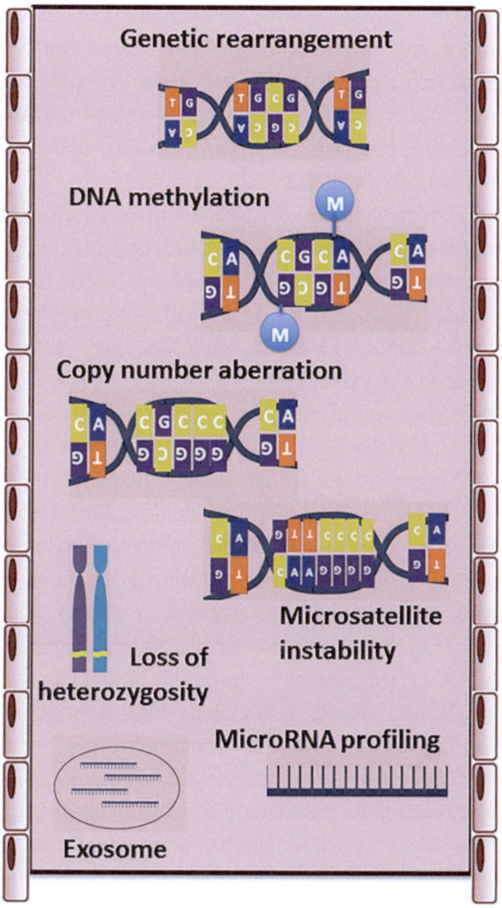

Fig. 16.2 Molecular aberration that can be detected in plasma samples from cancer patients. Circulating DNA analysis can allow for detection of tumor-specific, point mutations, genomic rearrangements, copy number variation, loss of heterozygosity or microsatellite instability in the bloodstream of cancer patients. Epigenetic modification such as DNA methylation pattern can also be analyzed on circulating DNA. Analysis of circulating microRNA allows for microRNA profiling which reflect microRNA active secretion in circulation into exosome

A more comprehensive genomic profiling is also achievable in patients with high tumor burden. In one study, massive parallel sequencing of 300 genes was performed on primary tumor, liver metastases and ctDNA of a MBC patient; ctDNA captured all mutations present in the primary tumor and liver metastases (De Mattos-Arruda et al. 2014). In another study, our group asked the question of whether plasma could be used as an alternative to metastatic biopsies for mutational analysis in breast cancer. We have used high-coverage NGS of a 50-gene panel on cfDNA to analyze plasma samples and synchronous metastatic biopsies from 17 MBC patients in a ISO-certified lab. We were able to detect genomic alterations in plasma cfDNA at allelic frequencies as low as 0.5 %, with concordance between tumor and plasma samples collected at the same time-point of 76 %; in 24 %, the results were discordant, with tumor and plasma samples providing complementary information (Rothe et al. 2014). Tumor heterogeneity may partly explain discordance between tumor tissue samples and ctDNA genomic profile. Importantly, the clinical significance of tumor-specific genomic alterations found in plasma but not in synchronous tumor tissue samples is currently unknown. Moreover, the clinical significance of genomic aberrations found in plasma at low allele frequency has not been determined. Clinical trials are needed addressing the value of ctDNA assays for treatment-related decision, independently of concordance with tumor tissue samples.

Whole-exome sequencing and whole-genome sequencing on ctDNA was also successfully performed in few MBC breast cancer patients with high tumor-burden (Murtaza et al. 2013; Chan et al. 2013b; Heidary et al. 2014). However, the applicability of comprehensive genomic profiling on ctDNA in patients with oligometastatic breast cancer has not been proven so far.

Nevertheless, ctDNA genomic assays are a unique tool for un-accessible tumor genomic profiling, with possible use for continuous monitoring of molecular evolution and detection of mutations associated with treatment resistance. These assays could be integrated in molecular screening programs as an alternative to tissue biopsies; however, clinical utility of such testing to guide treatment-related decision has yet to be demonstrated.

16.2.2.3 Epigenetic Profiling

Epigenetic alterations are now recognized as one of the most common molecular alterations in human malignancies (Esteller 2008). DNA methylation can regulate gene expression and plays major role in cancer development by silencing genes with critical function in growth or DNA repair (Baylin 2005). Pattern of DNA methylation in the bloodstream detected by methylation-specific PCR appears to correlate with that of the primary breast tumor (Shukla et al. 2006; Sharma et al. 2010b; Dulaimi et al. 2004; Chimonidou et al. 2013). Some patterns of circulating DNA methylation have been recognized to be highly specific to breast cancer patients when compared to healthy controls (Chimonidou et al. 2013; Hoque et al. 2006; Skvortsova et al. 2006). Methylation of ESR1 on cfDNA has been associated with estrogen receptor-negative status (Martinez-Galan et al. 2014). Analyses of cfDNA methylation pattern in the blood of breast cancer patients have demonstrated correlation between methylation of specific genes (BRCA1, GSTP1, RASSF1A and APC) and poor outcome in the early setting, independently of the clinicopathologic characteristics (Table 16.3) (Muller et al. 2003; Fiegl et al. 2005; Sharma et al. 2010b; Avraham et al. 2012; Gobel et al. 2011). Baseline pattern of cfDNA methylation and methylation changes with therapy may also be predictive of response to (neo)adjuvant chemotherapy (Avraham et al. 2012; Sharma et al. 2012; Fiegl et al. 2005). However, these results need to be confirmed prospectively in larger populations.

16.3 Circulating microRNA

16.3.1 Origin of microRNA and Methods for microRNA Analysis

MiRNAs are a group of fragments of single-stranded non-coding RNA that play major role in the regulation of gene expression by binding target mRNA and act as mediators of cell-cell communication (Fig. 16.3) (Pritchard et al. 2012a). Hence, miRNA are implicated in various cellular pathways that are critical for tumor genesis and biology. An altered miRNA expression pattern in tumor tissue samples has been observed in patients with various cancers including breast cancer (van Schooneveld et al. 2012; Iorio et al. 2005).

The mechanism by which miRNA enter the blood circulation is unclear; unlike DNA, RNA release in the circulation does not seem to be mostly dependent on cell death, but rather on viable cells. Cell-free miRNA are usually released in circulation in small vesicles of endocytic origin named exosomes (Cortez et al. 2011; Kosaka et al. 2010; Turchinovich et al. 2011). Exosomes are resistant to degradation by circulating RNase and can be transferred to a recipient cell by endocytic uptake. Exosomes contain miRNA that can be transferred to other cells and regulate gene expression of the target cell (Fig. 16.4) (Valadi et al. 2007). Likewise, miRNAs are present in apoptotic bodies, or they are in the blood, associated with Argonaute2 (AG02) or lipoproteins (Diederichs and Haber 2007).

Contrary to messenger RNA (mRNA), miRNAs are very stable in the serum and can be resistant to severe condition such as boiling, freezing and thawing or prolonged storage without degradation, and are therefore more interesting targets for liquid biopsy (Chen et al. 2008). Several technologies can be used for circulating microRNA (cmiRNA) expression

Table 16.3 Association between gene methylation in serum and outcomes in breast cancer

References	Gene	Setting	Prevalence (%)	Impact
Muller et al. (2003)	APC	EBC MBC	23 (EBC) 80 (MBC)	Adverse prognosis
Sharma et al. (2010b)	BRCA1	EBC	27	Adverse prognosis
Sharma et al. (2012)		EBC before NACT	53	Associated with non-response to NACT
Sharma et al. (2010b)	GSTP1	EBC	25	Adverse prognosis
Sharma et al. (2012)		EBC before NACT	43	Associated with non-response to NACT
Sharma et al. (2010a)	MDR1	EBC	100	Adverse prognosis
Sharma et al. (2012)		EBC before NACT	60	Associated with non-response to NACT
Göbel et al. (2011)	PITX2	EBC	14	Adverse prognosis
Mirza et al. (2010)	Stratifin	EBC	61	Adverse prognosis
Göbel et al. (2011)	RASSF1A	EBC	22	Adverse prognosis
Muller et al. (2003)		EBC MBC	23 (EBC) 80 (MBC)	Adverse prognosis
Fiegl et al. (2005)		EBC preoperative and 1 year after adjuvant CT	19 (before CT) 22 (1 year after CT)	Methylation status at 1 year associated with adverse outcomes
Avraham et al. (2012)		Locally advanced BC before and during NACT	40 (before NACT)	Correlation between methylation changes and response to NACT

APC Adenomatous polyposis coli; *BRCA1* breast cancer related gene-1; *CT* chemotherapy; *DAP-Kinase* death associated protein kinase; *GSTP1* glutathione-S-transferase P1; *NACT* neoadjuvant chemotherapy; *RASSF1A* RAS association domain family protein 1a

profiling, such as miRNA microarrays, quantitative real-time PCR (qRT-PCR), or NGS (Chen et al. 2008; Schrauder et al. 2012; Roth et al. 2010). A variety of preanalytical considerations need to be contemplated to ensure scientific validity (Table 16.4). Sources of variability in cmiRNA assessment are mainly related to the extraction methodology and the platform employed. This matter is further complicated by the fact that miRNAs are highly expressed in blood cells and can be released following blood cells lysis; therefore, the proportion of miRNA of hematopoietic origin (instead of tumor origin) in the sample will be influenced by the blood cell count and could be drastically affected by blood cells lysis process such as hemolysis (Pritchard et al. 2012b). Type of samples (serum or plasma) and blood sampling process can influence miRNA absolute level, but also relative miRNA levels, since all miRNA are not affected equally by the processing (Wang et al. 2012b; Cheng et al. 2013). The presence of natural polymerase

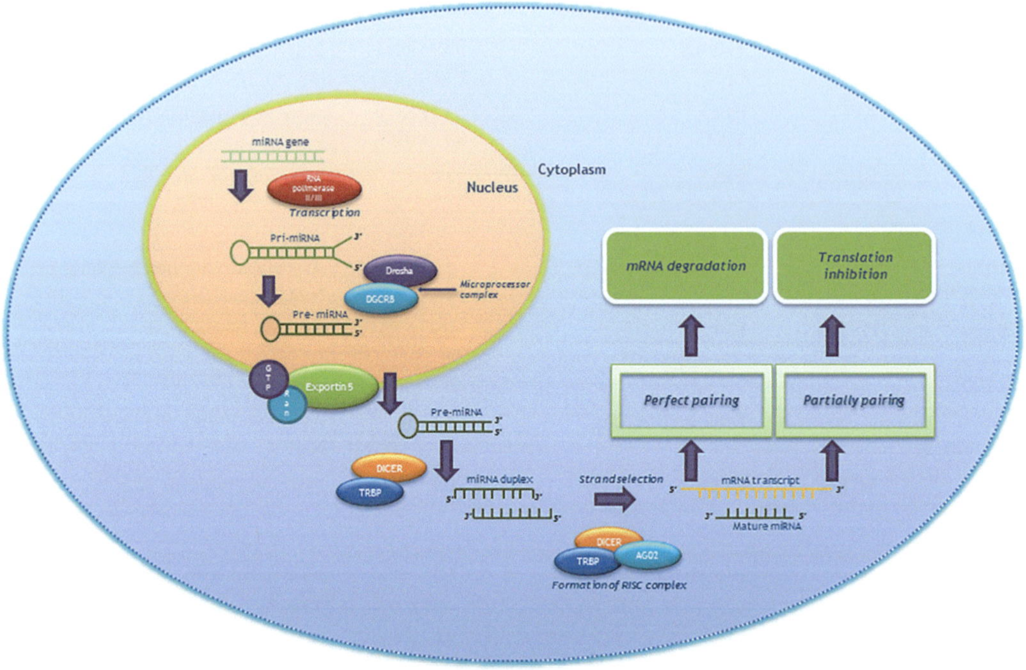

Fig. 16.3 Schematic representation of miRNA biogenesis and regulation. The miRNA biogenesis starts in the nucleus. First step is the production of the primary miRNA transcript (pri-miRNA) by RNA polymerase II or III, followed by cleavage of the pri-miRNA mediated by the microprocessor complex Drosha–DGCR8. The resulting precursor hairpin, the pre-miRNA, is exported from the nucleus by Exportin-5–Ran-GTP. In the cytoplasm, the complex DICER-TRBP (RNase and RNA-binding protein) cleaves the pre-miRNA hairpin to its mature length. The functional strand of the mature miRNA is loaded together with Argonaute (Ago2) proteins into the RNA-induced silencing complex (RISC), where it guides RISC to degrade target mRNAs or inhibit translation

inhibitors in the blood can affect detection of certain miRNA by RT-PCR (Kim et al. 2012). Additional potential confounding factors to consider should include anticoagulants (citrate and heparin should be avoided), the initial fluid volume, yield, procedural contamination and purpose of the study (profiling vs. small number of miRNAs). The centrifugation process can also significantly influence miRNA profiling (Turchinovich et al. 2011).

A crucial step is the normalization with an appropriate endogenous control, most often a reference miRNA, which is required for RT-PCR miRNA analysis. The choice of endogenous control is critical to ensure the validity of the results. To date, no universal endogenous control for miRNA in body fluids including plasma and serum, and for all experimental conditions, exist. Thus, a selection of at least 2/3 endogenous and exogenous controls with the lowest variability across all samples within a specific study should be used for normalization.

Moreover, a comprehensive survey literature review revealed that several methodological details are often overlooked, thus making the reproducibility of the data challenging or not comparable across various studies (Witwer 2015; Leidner et al. 2013).

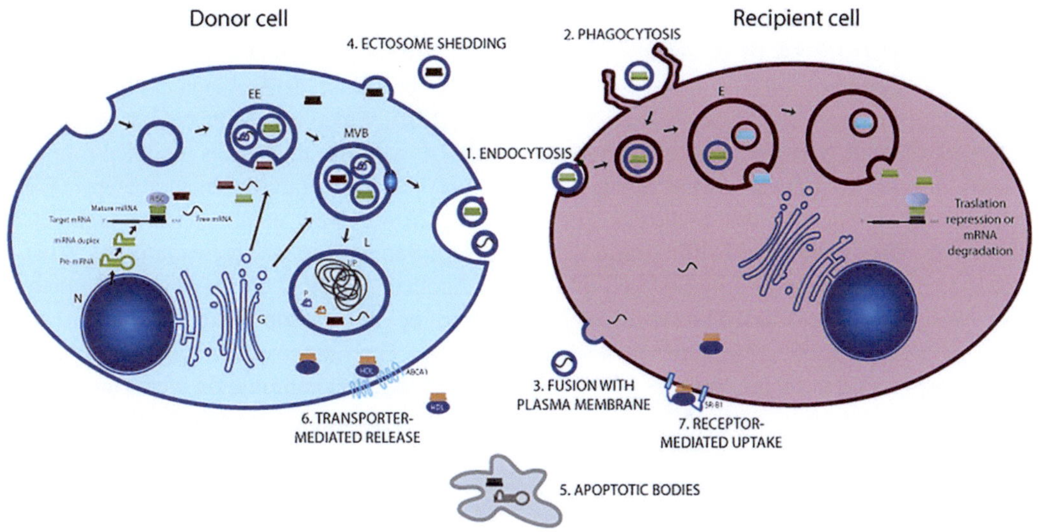

Fig. 16.4 Mechanisms of RNA transfer in cell-to-cell communication. Mechanisms underlying the transfer of RNA molecules between cells are mainly based on two systems, vesicle- and protein-mediated transport. (*1–3*) After exosome release from donor cell, RNA content is delivered into recipient cell by (*1*) the fusion of the exosome with the recipient cell membrane, by (*2*) phagocytosis- or (*3*) endocytosis-like internalization of the exosome. RNA molecules can be exported and transported out of the cells by microvesicles as (*4*) shedding ectosomes or (*5*) apoptotic bodies. (*6, 7*) Different protein complexes (*violet boxes*) including Argonaute, NPM1 and HDL proteins, bind miRNAs and are transferred out of the cell through (*6*) transporter-mediated release (ABCA1) and are translocated to target cell by (*7*) receptor-mediated uptake (SR-B1). All these pathways result in the delivery of microRNA or mRNA molecules to the cytosol of the target cell where they may contribute to post translational gene regulation

Table 16.4 Strengths and challenges of circulating nucleic acid analysis

	Circulating DNA	Circulating miRNA
Strengths	– Feasible on small sample amount – Early readout biomarker – Easy processing[a] – Potential for tumor burden monitoring – Potential to identify druggable targets – Potential to identify mutations that confer drug resistance – Potential for monitoring of clonal evolution	– Feasible on small sample amount – Early readout biomarker – Easy processing[a] – Highly stable in blood[b] – Accounts for microenvironment interaction – Potential for tumor screening – Potential to interrogate tumor biology and mechanisms of drug resistance – Potential as target for anticancer therapy
Challenges	– No standardization of preanalytical issues – Low amount in patients with low tumor burden does not allow for comprehensive genomic analysis – Unknown clinical significance of aberration found at low allele frequency – Unknown clinical significance of aberrations not find in the primary tumor or metastasis tissue sample	– No standardization of preanalytical issues – No standardization of normalization methods – Poor overlap and reproducibility of the results – Not representative of the underlying tumor

[a]Compared to circulating tumor cells
[b]Compared to messenger RNA

16.3.2 Clinical Application of cmiRNA in Breast Cancer

In 2005, Iorio et al. demonstrated deregulation of at least 29 miRNA in breast cancer tissue samples compared to normal breast tissue (Iorio et al. 2005). In that study, miR-10b, miR-125b, miR-145, miR-21 and miR-155 emerged as the most constantly deregulated. The results of this study triggered large efforts to better understand miRNA expression in breast cancer, and studies have identified a wide variety of up- or down-regulated miRNAs in early and metastatic breast cancer ever since (van Schooneveld et al. 2015). Because cmiRNAs are easily accessible and highly stable in blood, cmiRNAs are a promising source for miRNA analysis is breast cancer (Wang et al. 2010a; Ng et al. 2013).

Many studies have demonstrated the deregulation of cmiRNAs expression pattern in breast cancer patients compared to healthy controls (Wang et al. 2010a; Schrauder et al. 2012; Guo and Zhang 2012; Cuk et al. 2013; Kodahl et al. 2014a; Chan et al. 2013c). Various cmiRNA signatures including up to 240 miRNAs have been verified to be strongly associated with the presence of breast cancer in small cohorts of early breast cancer patients compared to healthy controls, highlighting the potential of cmiRNAs as a non-invasive screening tool for breast cancer (Table 16.5) (Ng et al. 2013; Roth et al. 2010; Guo and Zhang 2012; Cuk et al. 2013; Zeng et al. 2013; Heneghan et al. 2010; Asaga et al. 2011; Schrauder et al. 2012; Liu et al. 2013; Sun et al. 2012; Schwarzenbach et al. 2012b); however, none of the signatures have been validated in prospective large cohorts of patients, or compared to other screening tools such as the mammogram (Ng et al. 2013). A meta-analysis including three studies with a total of 184 breast cancer patients and 75 healthy individuals recently demonstrated the good sensitivity (79 %) and specificity (85 %) of circulating miRNA-155 expression for the diagnosis of breast cancer (AUC 0.92) (Wang et al. 2014). Small studies have demonstrated a correlation between certain cmiRNA expression pattern and advanced disease stage and tumor burden (Wang et al. 2010a; Schwarzenbach et al. 2011; Si et al. 2013; Chen et al. 2013; Asaga et al. 2011; Roth et al. 2010). Emerging evidence also suggest that miRNA expression pattern is modified following surgery or (neo)adjuvant chemotherapy (Freres et al. 2014; Gezer et al. 2014; Kodahl et al. 2014b; Sun et al. 2012; Igglezou et al. 2014).

Another potential use for cmiRNA analysis would be the determination of breast cancer subtype. Few groups have attempted to use miRNA expression profile on breast tumor tissue samples to determine the breast cancer subtype, some of them attaining high accuracy for subtype discrimination, but clinical utility has not been demonstrated yet (Mattie et al. 2006; Lowery et al. 2009). Correlation between expression of certain cmiRNA such as miRNA-17, miRNA-155 and miRNA-195 with progesterone and estrogen receptor status has been reported (Heneghan et al. 2010; Zhu et al. 2009; Wang et al. 2010a; Eichelser et al. 2013). CmiRNA-173 has been associated with HER2-negative status in another study (Eichelser et al. 2013).

Many studies have established a relation between expression of specific miRNAs in breast cancer tissue samples and prognosis (van Schooneveld et al. 2015), but the prognostic value of cmiRNA expression pattern has not been as much investigated. A four-cmiRNA signature (miRNA-18b, miRNA-103, miRNA-107, miRNA-652) was able to predict relapse and overall survival in early triple negative breast cancer (Kleivi Sahlberg et al. 2015). Correlation between cmiRNA expression and CTC-positivity has also been demonstrated (Madhavan et al. 2012). Few other cmiRNAs expression patterns have been associated with clinical outcomes in small cohort of breast cancer patients (Table 16.6) (Wu et al. 2012; Joosse et al. 2014; Madhavan et al. 2012; Kleivi Sahlberg et al. 2015).

Additionally, miRNA could possibly reveal activation of specific pathways associated with resistance to therapy. For example, an association with miRNA-125b expression level in blood and resistance to chemotherapy was demonstrated in a small study including 56 breast cancer patients;

Table 16.5 Circulating microRNA signatures for early detection of breast cancer

References	cmiRNA signature	Expression	Test performance
Heneghan et al. (2010)	Let-7a	Upregulated	Sensitivity 77.6 % Specificity 100 %
Heneghan et al. (2010)	miRNA-195	Upregulated	Sensitivity 86 % Specificity 100 %
Zhao et al. (2010)	Let-7c	Downregulated	In caucasian AUC 0.78–0.84
Zhao et al. (2010)	miRNA-589	Upregulated	In caucasian AUC 0.62–0.85
Zhao et al. (2010)	miRNA-425	Upregulated	In African American: AUC 0.79–0.83
Zhao et al. (2010)	Let-7d	Downregulated	In African American: AUC 0.73–0.99
Asaga et al. (2011)	miRNA-21	Upregulated	AUC 0.72 Sensitivity 67 % Specificity 75 % PPV 91 %
Guo and Zhang (2012)	miRNA-181a	Downregulated	AUC 0.67 Sensitivity 70 % Specificity 60 %
Liu et al. (2013)	miRNA-155	Upregulated	AUC 0.901 Sensitivity 65 %, specificity 82 %
Schrauder et al. (2012)	Signature composed of 240 different miRNAs		Sensitivity 92.5 % Specificity 78.8 %
Schwarzenbach et al. (2012b)	miRNA-214	Upregulated	AUC 0.924
Sun et al. (2012)	miRNA-155	Upregulated	AUC 0.801 Sensitivity 65 % Specificity 81.8 %
Wu et al. (2012)	miR-222	Upregulated	AUC 0.67 Sensitivity 74 % Specificity 60 %
Chan et al. (2013b)	miRNA-1 miRNA-92a miRNA-133a miRNA-133b	Upregulated Upregulated Upregulated Upregulated	AUC 0.9-0.91
Cuk et al. (2013)	miRNA-148b miRNA-409-3p miRNA-801	Upregulated Upregulated Upregulated	AUC 0.69 Sensitivity 70 % Specificity 55 %
Eichelser et al. (2013)	miRNA-34a	Upregulated	AUC 0.64 Sensitivity 60 % Specificity 76 %
Eichelser et al. (2013)	miRNA-93	Upregulated	AUC 0.70 Sensitivity 45 % Specificity 100 %
Eichelser et al. (2013)	miRNA-373	Upregulated	AUC 0.88 Sensitivity 76.6 % Specificity 100 %

(continued)

Table 16.5 (continued)

References	cmiRNA signature	Expression	Test performance
Ng et al. (2013)	miRNA-145 miRNA-451	Downregulated Upregulated	AUC 0.93-0.96 Sensitivity 83–90 % Specificity 89–92 % PPV 88–90 % NPV 92–94 %
Zeng et al. (2013)	miRNA-30a	Downregulated	Sensitivity 74 %, specificity 65.6 %
Kodahl et al. (2014a)	miRNA-15a miRNA-18a miRNA-107 miRNA-133a miRNA-139-5p miRNA-143 miRNA-145 miRNA-365 miRNA-425	Upregulated Upregulated Upregulated Downregulated Downregulated Downregulated Downregulated Downregulated Upregulated	ER-Positive only: AUC 0.67 Sensitivity 83 % Specificity 41 % PPV 62.5 % NPV 67.4 %
McDermott et al. (2014)	miRNA-29a miRNA-181a miRNA-652	Downregulated Downregulated Downregulated	For luminal A only. AUC 0.8 Sensitivity 77 % Specificity 74 %
Li et al. (2015)	Let-7c	Downregulated	AUC 0.848 87.5 % sensitivity 78.9 % specificity

AUC Area under curve; *ER* endocrine receptor; *miRNA* micro-RNA; *NPV* negative predictive value; *PPV* positive predictive value

expression of miRNA-125b was also associated with in vitro drug resistance (Wang et al. 2012a). A different study have demonstrated that cmiRNA-210 was able to predict trastuzumab sensitivity, suggesting a possible use of this miRNA to monitor the response of HER2-positive breast cancer patients to trastuzumab-based therapies (Jung et al. 2012). Another cmiRNA, *miRNA-155,* was used to monitor the sensitivity of breast cancer patients treated with taxane-containing regimens (Sun et al. 2012).

It is important to highlight that multiple-miRNA assays or miRNA signatures have a significant better diagnostic and prognostic performance than single-miRNA assays (Xin et al. 2014). Importantly, cmiRNA expression may have a complete different diagnostic and prognostic impact compared to miRNA expressed in tumor tissue samples (Zhao et al. 2010; Leidner et al. 2013).

In summary, there is evidence to support circulating extracellular miRNAs, as important players and promising biomarkers for breast cancer. However, the field still lacks consistency and standardization, therefore, the results of cmiRNA studies must be interpreted with caution. There is little overlap between the miRNA signatures identified in these studies and a partial lack of reproducibility of the results (Leidner et al. 2013). There is yet no standardized methodology to process the samples; many pre-analytical factors could affect the results and explain discordance between studies. Additionally, there is currently no established endogenous control for serum or plasma miRNA to use as control to normalize miRNA amounts (Leidner et al. 2013). As this field is continuously evolving, the analysis of cmiRNA is certainly susceptible to significant technological advancements. Meanwhile several important considerations are needed before designing studies to analyze cmiRNAs. Validation in larger cohorts of patients is needed before solid conclusion can be reached.

Table 16.6 Association between circulating microRNA expression signatures and prognosis in breast cancer

References	CmiRNA signature	Expression	N	Setting	Results
Madhavan et al. (2012)	miRNA-141 miRNA-200a miRNA-200b miRNA-200c miRNA-375 miRNA-801	Upregulated Upregulated Upregulated Upregulated Upregulated Upregulated	164	MBC	Association with lower probability of PFS ($p < 0.05$) and OS ($p < 0.008$)
Wu et al. (2012)	miRNA-122 miRNA-375	Downregulated Upregulated	Test cohort: 42 Validation cohort: 26	Stage II-III and inflammatory BC before NACT	Association with lower probability of relapse and higher probability of pCR ($p < 0.04$) Only miRNA-122 confirmed in validation cohort ($p < 0.03$)
Joosse et al. (2014)	miRNA-202	Upregulated	102	EBC	Association with poor OS ($p = 0.0001$)
Kleivi Sahlberg et al. (2015)	miRNA-18b miRNA-103 miRNA-107 miRNA-652	Upregulated Upregulated Upregulated Upregulated	Test cohort: 60 Validation cohort: 70	TNBC	Association with poor RFS and OS ($p = 0.002$ and 0.0007) Confirmed in validation cohort

BC Breast cancer; *EBC* early breast cancer; *MBC* metastatic breast cancer; *miRNA* micro-RNA; *NACT* neoadjuvant chemotherapy; *OS* overall survival; *pCR* pathological complete remission; *PFS* progression-free survival; *RFS* relapse-free survival; *TNBC* triple negative breast cancer

16.3.3 Targeting Circulating miRNAs in Breast Cancer

Exosomes-containing oncogenic miRNAs "hijack" membrane components and cytoplasmic contents of the normal (and cancer) cells thus playing an important role in intercellular communication, often inducing important biological changes in recipient cells. These tiny vesicles have been involved also in breast cancer progression and metastasis (Le et al. 2014; Melo et al. 2014). Thus, analyzing the miRNAs or RNAs harbored by exosomes could have important diagnostic and therapeutic implications. Experimental evidences show that exosomes primarily mediate interactions between cancer and normal cells, though these vesicles can also induce drug resistance of cancer cells by sequestering chemotherapeutic agent (Federici et al. 2014). Only exosomes derived from cancer cells, but not those derived from normal cells, contain key enzymes, such as Dicer, involved in miRNA biogenesis, and the membrane protein CD43 sustaining Dicer accumulation (Melo et al. 2014). Furthermore, studies have demonstrated a cancer-specific pattern of secreted miRNAs and targets (Fabbri et al. 2012). For instance, miRNAs in the cancer exosomes inhibited the expression of their respective mRNA targets, such as the phosphatase and tensin homolog (PTEN) and the transcription factor homeobox D1, in the recipient breast epithelial cells suggesting an important oncogenic effects played by these molecules on normal cells to become tumorigenic. Pre-clinical studies are now targeting these circulating molecules, for example by silencing Dicer directly in cancer cells by small interfering RNA. Alternatively, blocking CD43 expression in tumor cells with specific monoclonal antibodies could also reduce Dicer concentration within the cancer exosomes. Another way to target these oncogenic molecules will be the introduction of exosome mimetics containing antimiRs or miRNA′ sponges that either capture the incoming oncomiRs in the recipient cells or fuse with the cancer exosomes and neutralize them while still in circulation. Undoubtedly, the evaluation of such molecular mechanisms may revolutionize the development of novel cancer therapies and broaden our understanding of breast cancer progression.

16.4 Conclusion

Circulating nucleic acids are released in the circulation following tumor cells death or by active secretion; increasing evidence suggest their potential for non-invasive interrogation of tumor biology and molecular evolution. However, several preanalytical factors have to be contemplated for circulating nucleic acids analysis to ensure validity of the results. There is yet no standardized method for ctDNA or cmiRNA analysis; hence, results must be interpreted with caution.

Personalized ctDNA detection assays have been improving in sensitivity and specificity during the last few years; however, analytical validity, clinical validity and clinical utility needs to be demonstrated in prospective clinical trials. Likewise, emerging data suggest that ctDNA could be used for non-invasive analysis of the tumor genome. CfDNA genomic analysis could be integrated in molecular screening program in the research setting as an alternative to tissue biopsy to demonstrate clinical validity and utility.

cmiRNA as a valid diagnostic, prognostic and disease surveillance is still at an early stage of development. The continuous advancement of more sensitive technologies will undoubtedly help to improve the analysis applied to cmiRNA and the reproducibility of the data. Emerging data suggest the potential of cmiRNA for breast cancer screening, prognostication or to interrogate tumor biology, however, a full standardization of cmiRNA methodologies and analysis will be mandatory to develop this tool for breast cancer profiling in clinical settings.

References

Alix-Panabieres C, Pantel K (2014) Challenges in circulating tumour cell research. Nat Rev Cancer 14 (9):623–631

Asaga S, Kuo C, Nguyen T, Terpenning M, Giuliano AE, Hoon DS (2011) Direct serum assay for microRNA-21 concentrations in early and advanced breast cancer. Clin Chem 57(1):84–91

Atamaniuk J, Vidotto C, Tschan H, Bachl N, Stuhlmeier KM, Muller MM (2004) Increased concentrations of cell-free plasma DNA after exhaustive exercise. Clin Chem 50(9):1668–1670

Avraham A, Uhlmann R, Shperber A, Birnbaum M, Sandbank J, Sella A, Sukumar S, Evron E (2012) Serum DNA methylation for monitoring response to neoadjuvant chemotherapy in breast cancer patients. Int J Cancer (Journal international du cancer) 131(7): E1166–E1172

Balgkouranidou I, Karayiannakis A, Matthaios D, Bolanaki H, Tripsianis G, Tentes AA, Lianidou E, Chatzaki E, Fiska A, Lambropoulou M, Kolios G, Kakolyris S (2013) Assessment of SOX17 DNA methylation in cell free DNA from patients with operable gastric cancer. Association with prognostic variables and survival. Clin Chem Lab Med 51 (7):1505–1510

Barnett EV (1968) Detection of nuclear antigens (DNA) in normal and pathologic human fluids by quantitative complement fixation. Arthritis Rheum 11 (3):407–417

Baylin SB (2005) DNA methylation and gene silencing in cancer. Nat Clin Pract Oncol 2(Suppl 1):S4–S11

Beaver JA, Jelovac D, Balukrishna S, Cochran RL, Croessmann S, Zabransky DJ, Wong HY, Valda Toro P, Cidado J, Blair BG, Chu D, Burns T, Higgins MJ, Stearns V, Jacobs L, Habibi M, Lange J, Hurley PJ, Lauring J, VanDenBerg DA, Kessler J, Jeter S, Samuels ML, Maar D, Cope L, Cimino-Mathews A, Argani P, Wolff AC, Park BH (2014) Detection of cancer DNA in plasma of patients with early-stage breast cancer. Clin Cancer Res 20 (10):2643–2650

Bettegowda C, Sausen M, Leary RJ, Kinde I, Wang Y, Agrawal N, Bartlett BR, Wang H, Luber B, Alani RM, Antonarakis ES, Azad NS, Bardelli A, Brem H, Cameron JL, Lee CC, Fecher LA, Gallia GL, Gibbs P, Le D, Giuntoli RL, Goggins M, Hogarty MD, Holdhoff M, Hong SM, Jiao Y, Juhl HH, Kim JJ, Siravegna G, Laheru DA, Lauricella C, Lim M, Lipson EJ, Marie SK, Netto GJ, Oliner KS, Olivi A, Olsson L, Riggins GJ, Sartore-Bianchi A, Schmidt K, Shih l M, Oba-Shinjo SM, Siena S, Theodorescu D, Tie J, Harkins TT, Veronese S, Wang TL, Weingart JD, Wolfgang CL, Wood LD, Xing D, Hruban RH, Wu J, Allen PJ, Schmidt CM, Choti MA, Velculescu VE, Kinzler KW, Vogelstein B, Papadopoulos N, Diaz Jr LA (2014) Detection of circulating tumor DNA in early- and late-stage human malignancies. Sci Transl Med 6(224):224

Board RE, Wardley AM, Dixon JM, Armstrong AC, Howell S, Renshaw L, Donald E, Greystoke A, Ranson M, Hughes A, Dive C (2010) Detection of PIK3CA mutations in circulating free DNA in patients with breast cancer. Breast Cancer Res Treat 120 (2):461–467

Carreira S, Romanel A, Goodall J, Grist E, Ferraldeschi R, Miranda S, Prandi D, Lorente D, Frenel JS, Pezaro C, Omlin A, Rodrigues DN, Flohr P, Tunariu N, J SdB, Demichelis F, Attard G (2014) Tumor clone dynamics in lethal prostate cancer. Sci Transl Med 6(254):254–255

Chan KC, Yeung SW, Lui WB, Rainer TH, Lo YM (2005) Effects of preanalytical factors on the molecular size of cell-free DNA in blood. Clin Chem 51 (4):781–784

Chan KC, Jiang P, Chan CW, Sun K, Wong J, Hui EP, Chan SL, Chan WC, Hui DS, Ng SS, Chan HL, Wong CS, Ma BB, Chan AT, Lai PB, Sun H, Chiu RW, Lo YM (2013a) Noninvasive detection of cancer-associated genome-wide hypomethylation and copy number aberrations by plasma DNA bisulfite sequencing. Proc Natl Acad Sci U S A 110 (47):18761–18768

Chan KC, Jiang P, Zheng YW, Liao GJ, Sun H, Wong J, Siu SS, Chan WC, Chan SL, Chan AT, Lai PB, Chiu RW, Lo YM (2013b) Cancer genome scanning in plasma: detection of tumor-associated copy number aberrations, single-nucleotide variants, and tumoral heterogeneity by massively parallel sequencing. Clin Chem 59(1):211–224

Chan M, Liaw CS, Ji SM, Tan HH, Wong CY, Thike AA, Tan PH, Ho GH, Lee AS (2013c) Identification of circulating microRNA signatures for breast cancer detection. Clin Cancer Res 19(16):4477–4487

Chen X, Bonnefoi H, Diebold-Berger S, Lyautey J, Lederrey C, Faltin-Traub E, Stroun M, Anker P (1999) Detecting tumor-related alterations in plasma or serum DNA of patients diagnosed with breast cancer. Clin Cancer Res 5(9):2297–2303

Chen X, Ba Y, Ma L, Cai X, Yin Y, Wang K, Guo J, Zhang Y, Chen J, Guo X, Li Q, Li X, Wang W, Zhang Y, Wang J, Jiang X, Xiang Y, Xu C, Zheng P, Zhang J, Li R, Zhang H, Shang X, Gong T, Ning G, Wang J, Zen K, Zhang J, Zhang CY (2008) Characterization of microRNAs in serum: a novel class of biomarkers for diagnosis of cancer and other diseases. Cell Res 18(10):997–1006

Chen W, Cai F, Zhang B, Barekati Z, Zhong XY (2013) The level of circulating miRNA-10b and miRNA-373 in detecting lymph node metastasis of breast cancer: potential biomarkers. Tumour Biol 34 (1):455–462

Cheng HH, Yi HS, Kim Y, Kroh EM, Chien JW, Eaton KD, Goodman MT, Tait JF, Tewari M, Pritchard CC (2013) Plasma processing conditions substantially influence circulating microRNA biomarker levels. PLoS ONE 8(6):e64795

Chimonidou M, Tzitzira A, Strati A, Sotiropoulou G, Sfikas C, Malamos N, Georgoulias V, Lianidou E (2013) CST6 promoter methylation in circulating cell-free DNA of breast cancer patients. Clin Biochem 46(3):235–240

Chiu RW, Poon LL, Lau TK, Leung TN, Wong EM, Lo YM (2001) Effects of blood-processing protocols on fetal and total DNA quantification in maternal plasma. Clin Chem 47(9):1607–1613

Cortez MA, Bueso-Ramos C, Ferdin J, Lopez-Berestein G, Sood AK, Calin GA (2011) MicroRNAs in body fluids–the mix of hormones and biomarkers. Nature reviews Clinical oncology 8(8):467–477

Cuk K, Zucknick M, Heil J, Madhavan D, Schott S, Turchinovich A, Arlt D, Rath M, Sohn C, Benner A, Junkermann H, Schneeweiss A, Burwinkel B (2013) Circulating microRNAs in plasma as early detection markers for breast cancer. Int J Cancer (Journal international du cancer) 132(7):1602–1612

Dawson S-J, Tsui DWY, Murtaza M, Biggs H, Rueda OM, Chin S-F, Dunning MJ, Gale D, Forshew T, Mahler-Araujo B, Rajan S, Humphray S, Becq J, Halsall D, Wallis M, Bentley D, Caldas C, Rosenfeld N (2013) Analysis of circulating tumor dna to monitor metastatic breast cancer. N Engl J Med 368 (13):1199–1209

De Mattos-Arruda L, Weigelt B, Cortes J, Won HH, Ng CK, Nuciforo P, Bidard FC, Aura C, Saura C, Peg V, Piscuoglio S, Oliveira M, Smolders Y, Patel P, Norton L, Tabernero J, Berger MF, Seoane J, Reis-Filho JS (2014) Capturing intra-tumor genetic heterogeneity by de novo mutation profiling of circulating cell-free tumor DNA: a proof-of-principle. Ann Oncol 25(9):1729–1735

Di GH, Liu G, Wu J, Shen ZZ, Shao ZM (2003) Peripheral blood mutated p53 DNA and its clinical value in human breast cancer. Zhonghua zhong liu za zhi (Chin J Oncol) 25(2):137–140

Diederichs S, Haber DA (2007) Dual role for argonautes in microRNA processing and posttranscriptional regulation of microRNA expression. Cell 131(6):1097–1108

Diehl F, Schmidt K, Choti MA, Romans K, Goodman S, Li M, Thornton K, Agrawal N, Sokoll L, Szabo SA, Kinzler KW, Vogelstein B, Diaz LA Jr (2008) Circulating mutant DNA to assess tumor dynamics. Nat Med 14(9):985–990

Dressman D, Yan H, Traverso G, Kinzler KW, Vogelstein B (2003) Transforming single DNA molecules into fluorescent magnetic particles for detection and enumeration of genetic variations. Proc Natl Acad Sci USA 100(15):8817–8822

Dulaimi E, Hillinck J, Ibanez de Caceres I, Al-Saleem T, Cairns P (2004) Tumor suppressor gene promoter hypermethylation in serum of breast cancer patients. Clin Cancer Res 10(18 Pt 1):6189–6193

Eichelser C, Flesch-Janys D, Chang-Claude J, Pantel K, Schwarzenbach H (2013) Deregulated serum concentrations of circulating cell-free microRNAs miR-17, miR-34a, miR-155, and miR-373 in human breast cancer development and progression. Clin Chem 59 (10):1489–1496

El Messaoudi S, Rolet F, Mouliere F, Thierry AR (2013) Circulating cell free DNA: preanalytical considerations. Clin Chim Acta 424:222–230

Esteller M (2008) Epigenetics in cancer. N Engl J Med 358(11):1148–1159

Fabbri M, Paone A, Calore F, Galli R, Gaudio E, Santhanam R, Lovat F, Fadda P, Mao C, Nuovo GJ, Zanesi N, Crawford M, Ozer GH, Wernicke D, Alder H, Caligiuri MA, Nana-Sinkam P, Perrotti D, Croce CM (2012) MicroRNAs bind to toll-like receptors to induce prometastatic inflammatory response. Proc Natl Acad Sci U S A 109(31): E2110–E2116

Fackler MJ, Lopez Bujanda Z, Umbricht C, Teo WW, Cho S, Zhang Z, Visvanathan K, Jeter S, Argani P, Wang C, Lyman JP, de Brot M, Ingle JN, Boughey J, McGuire K, King TA, Carey LA, Cope L, Wolff AC, Sukumar S (2014) Novel methylated biomarkers and a robust assay to detect circulating tumor DNA in metastatic breast cancer. Cancer Res 74(8):2160–2170

Federici C, Petrucci F, Caimi S, Cesolini A, Logozzi M, Borghi M, D'Ilio S, Lugini L, Violante N, Azzarito T, Majorani C, Brambilla D, Fais S (2014) Exosome release and low pH belong to a framework of resistance of human melanoma cells to cisplatin. PLoS ONE 9(2):e88193

Fiegl H, Millinger S, Mueller-Holzner E, Marth C, Ensinger C, Berger A, Klocker H, Goebel G, Widschwendter M (2005) Circulating tumor-specific DNA: a marker for monitoring efficacy of adjuvant therapy in cancer patients. Cancer Res 65(4):1141–1145

Forshew T, Murtaza M, Parkinson C, Gale D, Tsui DW, Kaper F, Dawson SJ, Piskorz AM, Jimenez-Linan M, Bentley D, Hadfield J, May AP, Caldas C, Brenton JD, Rosenfeld N (2012) Noninvasive identification and monitoring of cancer mutations by targeted deep sequencing of plasma DNA. Sci Transl Med 4 (136):136–168

Freres P, Josse C, Bovy N, Boukerroucha M, Struman I, Bours V, Jerusalem G (2014) Neoadjuvant chemotherapy in breast cancer patients induces miR-34a and miR-122 expression. J Cell Physiol

Gerlinger M, Rowan AJ, Horswell S, Larkin J, Endesfelder D, Gronroos E, Martinez P, Matthews N, Stewart A, Tarpey P, Varela I, Phillimore B, Begum S, McDonald NQ, Butler A, Jones D, Raine K, Latimer C, Santos CR, Nohadani M, Eklund AC, Spencer-Dene B, Clark G, Pickering L, Stamp G, Gore M, Szallasi Z, Downward J, Futreal PA, Swanton C (2012) Intratumor heterogeneity and branched evolution revealed by multiregion sequencing. N Engl J Med 366(10):883–892

Gezer U, Keskin S, Igci A, Tukenmez M, Tiryakioglu D, Cetinkaya M, Disci R, Dalay N, Eralp Y (2014) Abundant circulating microRNAs in breast cancer patients fluctuate considerably during neoadjuvant chemotherapy. Oncol Lett 8(2):845–848

Gobel G, Auer D, Gaugg I, Schneitter A, Lesche R, Muller-Holzner E, Marth C, Daxenbichler G (2011) Prognostic significance of methylated RASSF1A and PITX2 genes in blood- and bone marrow plasma of breast cancer patients. Breast Cancer Res Treat 130 (1):109–117

Guo LJ, Zhang QY (2012) Decreased serum miR-181a is a potential new tool for breast cancer screening. Int J Mol Med 30(3):680–686

Heidary M, Auer M, Ulz P, Heitzer E, Petru E, Gasch C, Riethdorf S, Mauermann O, Lafer I, Pristauz G, Lax S, Pantel K, Geigl JB, Speicher MR (2014) The dynamic range of circulating tumor DNA in metastatic breast cancer. Breast Cancer Res 16(4):421

Heneghan HM, Miller N, Lowery AJ, Sweeney KJ, Newell J, Kerin MJ (2010) Circulating microRNAs as novel minimally invasive biomarkers for breast cancer. Ann Surg 251(3):499–505

Higgins MJ, Jelovac D, Barnathan E, Blair B, Slater S, Powers P, Zorzi J, Jeter SC, Oliver GR, Fetting J, Emens L, Riley C, Stearns V, Diehl F, Angenendt P, Huang P, Cope L, Argani P, Murphy KM, Bachman KE, Greshock J, Wolff AC, Park BH (2012) Detection of tumor PIK3CA status in metastatic breast cancer using peripheral blood. Clin Cancer Res 18 (12):3462–3469

Hindson BJ, Ness KD, Masquelier DA, Belgrader P, Heredia NJ, Makarewicz AJ, Bright IJ, Lucero MY, Hiddessen AL, Legler TC, Kitano TK, Hodel MR, Petersen JF, Wyatt PW, Steenblock ER, Shah PH, Bousse LJ, Troup CB, Mellen JC, Wittmann DK, Erndt NG, Cauley TH, Koehler RT, So AP, Dube S, Rose KA, Montesclaros L, Wang S, Stumbo DP, Hodges SP, Romine S, Milanovich FP, White HE, Regan JF, Karlin-Neumann GA, Hindson CM, Saxonov S, Colston BW (2011) High-throughput droplet digital PCR system for absolute quantitation of DNA copy number. Anal Chem 83(22):8604–8610

Hoque MO, Feng Q, Toure P, Dem A, Critchlow CW, Hawes SE, Wood T, Jeronimo C, Rosenbaum E, Stern J, Yu M, Trink B, Kiviat NB, Sidransky D (2006) Detection of aberrant methylation of four genes in plasma DNA for the detection of breast cancer. J Clin Oncol Off J Am Soc Clin Oncol 24(26):4262–4269

Igglezou M, Vareli K, Georgiou GK, Sainis I, Briasoulis E (2014) Kinetics of circulating levels of miR-195, miR-155 and miR-21 in patients with breast cancer undergoing mastectomy. Anticancer Res 34 (12):7443–7447

Ignatiadis M, Dawson S-J (2014) Circulating tumor cells and circulating tumor DNA for precision medicine: dream or reality? Ann Oncol

Iorio MV, Ferracin M, Liu CG, Veronese A, Spizzo R, Sabbioni S, Magri E, Pedriali M, Fabbri M, Campiglio M, Menard S, Palazzo JP, Rosenberg A, Musiani P, Volinia S, Nenci I, Calin GA, Querzoli P, Negrini M, Croce CM (2005) MicroRNA gene expression deregulation in human breast cancer. Cancer Res 65(16):7065–7070

Joosse SA, Muller V, Steinbach B, Pantel K, Schwarzenbach H (2014) Circulating cell-free cancer-testis MAGE-A RNA, BORIS RNA, let-7b and miR-202 in the blood of patients with breast cancer and benign breast diseases. Br J Cancer 111(5):909–917

Jung M, Klotzek S, Lewandowski M, Fleischhacker M, Jung K (2003) Changes in concentration of DNA in serum and plasma during storage of blood samples. Clin Chem 49(6 Pt 1):1028–1029

Jung EJ, Santarpia L, Kim J, Esteva FJ, Moretti E, Buzdar AU, Di Leo A, Le XF, Bast RC Jr, Park ST, Pusztai L, Calin GA (2012) Plasma microRNA 210 levels correlate with sensitivity to trastuzumab and tumor presence in breast cancer patients. Cancer 118 (10):2603–2614

Kim DJ, Linnstaedt S, Palma J, Park JC, Ntrivalas E, Kwak-Kim JY, Gilman-Sachs A, Beaman K, Hastings ML, Martin JN, Duelli DM (2012) Plasma components affect accuracy of circulating cancer-related microRNA quantitation. J Mol Diagn 14(1):71–80

Kinde I, Wu J, Papadopoulos N, Kinzler KW, Vogelstein B (2011) Detection and quantification of rare mutations with massively parallel sequencing. Proc Natl Acad Sci USA 108(23):9530–9535

Kleivi Sahlberg K, Bottai G, Naume B, Burwinkel B, Calin GA, Borresen-Dale AL, Santarpia L (2015) A serum microRNA signature predicts tumor relapse and survival in triple-negative breast cancer patients. Clin Cancer Res 21(5):1207–1214

Kodahl AR, Lyng MB, Binder H, Cold S, Gravgaard K, Knoop AS, Ditzel HJ (2014a) Novel circulating microRNA signature as a potential non-invasive multi-marker test in ER-positive early-stage breast cancer: a case control study. Molecular oncology 8 (5):874–883

Kodahl AR, Zeuthen P, Binder H, Knoop AS, Ditzel HJ (2014b) Alterations in circulating miRNA levels following early-stage estrogen receptor-positive breast cancer resection in post-menopausal women. PLoS ONE 9(7):e101950

Koffler D, Agnello V, Winchester R, Kunkel HG (1973) The occurrence of single-stranded DNA in the serum of patients with systemic lupus erythematosus and other diseases. J Clin Investig 52(1):198–204

Kosaka N, Iguchi H, Yoshioka Y, Takeshita F, Matsuki Y, Ochiya T (2010) Secretory mechanisms and intercellular transfer of microRNAs in living cells. J Biol Chem 285(23):17442–17452

Le MT, Hamar P, Guo C, Basar E, Perdigao-Henriques R, Balaj L, Lieberman J (2014) miR-200-containing extracellular vesicles promote breast cancer cell metastasis. J Clin Investig 124(12):5109–5128

Leary RJ, Kinde I, Diehl F, Schmidt K, Clouser C, Duncan C, Antipova A, Lee C, McKernan K, De La Vega FM, Kinzler KW, Vogelstein B, Diaz LA, Jr., Velculescu VE (2010) Development of personalized tumor biomarkers using massively parallel sequencing. Sci Transl Med 2(20):14–20

Leary RJ, Sausen M, Kinde I, Papadopoulos N, Carpten JD, Craig D, O'Shaughnessy J, Kinzler KW, Parmigiani G, Vogelstein B, Diaz LA, Jr., Velculescu VE (2012) Detection of chromosomal alterations in the circulation of cancer patients with whole-genome sequencing. Sci Transl Med 4 (162):154–162

Leidner RS, Li L, Thompson CL (2013) Dampening enthusiasm for circulating microRNA in breast cancer. PLoS ONE 8(3):e57841

Leon SA, Shapiro B, Sklaroff DM, Yaros MJ (1977) Free DNA in the serum of cancer patients and the effect of therapy. Cancer Res 37(3):646–650

Li XX, Gao SY, Wang PY, Zhou X, Li YJ, Yu Y, Yan YF, Zhang HH, Lv CJ, Zhou HH, Xie SY (2015) Reduced expression levels of let-7c in human breast cancer patients. Oncol Lett 9(3):1207–1212

Liu J, Mao Q, Liu Y, Hao X, Zhang S, Zhang J (2013) Analysis of miR-205 and miR-155 expression in the blood of breast cancer patients. Chinese journal of cancer research = Chung-kuo yen cheng yen chiu 25 (1):46-54

Lo YM, Rainer TH, Chan LY, Hjelm NM, Cocks RA (2000) Plasma DNA as a prognostic marker in trauma patients. Clin Chem 46(3):319–323

Lowery AJ, Miller N, Devaney A, McNeill RE, Davoren PA, Lemetre C, Benes V, Schmidt S, Blake J, Ball G, Kerin MJ (2009) MicroRNA signatures predict oestrogen receptor, progesterone receptor and HER2/neu receptor status in breast cancer. Breast Cancer Res 11(3):R27

Lui YY, Chik KW, Chiu RW, Ho CY, Lam CW, Lo YM (2002) Predominant hematopoietic origin of cell-free DNA in plasma and serum after sex-mismatched bone marrow transplantation. Clin Chem 48(3):421–427

Madhavan D, Zucknick M, Wallwiener M, Cuk K, Modugno C, Scharpff M, Schott S, Heil J, Turchinovich A, Yang R, Benner A, Riethdorf S, Trumpp A, Sohn C, Pantel K, Schneeweiss A, Burwinkel B (2012) Circulating miRNAs as surrogate markers for circulating tumor cells and prognostic markers in metastatic breast cancer. Clin Cancer Res 18 (21):5972–5982

Madhavan D, Wallwiener M, Bents K, Zucknick M, Nees J, Schott S, Cuk K, Riethdorf S, Trumpp A, Pantel K, Sohn C, Schneeweiss A, Surowy H, Burwinkel B (2014) Plasma DNA integrity as a biomarker for primary and metastatic breast cancer and potential marker for early diagnosis. Breast Cancer Res Treat 146(1):163–174

Madic J, Kiialainen A, Bidard FC, Birzele F, Ramey G, Leroy Q, Rio Frio T, Vaucher I, Raynal V, Bernard V, Lermine A, Clausen I, Giroud N, Schmucki R, Milder M, Horn C, Spleiss O, Lantz O, Stern MH, Pierga JY, Weisser M, Lebofsky R (2015) Circulating tumor DNA and circulating tumor cells in metastatic triple negative breast cancer patients. Int J Cancer (Journal international du cancer) 136 (9):2158–2165

Maebo A (1990) Plasma DNA level as a tumor marker in primary lung cancer. Nihon Kyobu Shikkan Gakkai zasshi 28(8):1085–1091

Mandel P, Métais P (1948) Les acides nucléiques du plasma sanguin chez l'homme. C R Acad Sci Paris 142:241–243

Martinez-Galan J, Torres-Torres B, Nunez MI, Lopez-Penalver J, Del Moral R, Ruiz De Almodovar JM, Menjon S, Concha A, Chamorro C, Rios S, Delgado JR (2014) ESR1 gene promoter region methylation in free circulating DNA and its correlation with estrogen receptor protein expression in tumor tissue in breast cancer patients. BMC Cancer 14:59

Mattie MD, Benz CC, Bowers J, Sensinger K, Wong L, Scott GK, Fedele V, Ginzinger D, Getts R, Haqq C (2006) Optimized high-throughput microRNA expression profiling provides novel biomarker assessment of clinical prostate and breast cancer biopsies. Mol Cancer 5:24

Mayall F, Fairweather S, Wilkins R, Chang B, Nicholls R (1999) Microsatellite abnormalities in plasma of patients with breast carcinoma: concordance with the primary tumour. J Clin Pathol 52(5):363–366

McBride DJ, Orpana AK, Sotiriou C, Joensuu H, Stephens PJ, Mudie LJ, Hamalainen E, Stebbings LA, Andersson LC, Flanagan AM, Durbecq V, Ignatiadis M, Kallioniemi O, Heckman CA, Alitalo K, Edgren H, Futreal PA, Stratton MR, Campbell PJ (2010) Use of cancer-specific genomic rearrangements to quantify disease burden in plasma from patients with solid tumors. Genes Chromosomes Cancer 49 (11):1062–1069

McDermott AM, Miller N, Wall D, Martyn LM, Ball G, Sweeney KJ, Kerin MJ (2014) Identification and validation of oncologic miRNA biomarkers for luminal A-like breast cancer. PLoS ONE 9(1):e87032

Melo SA, Sugimoto H, O'Connell JT, Kato N, Villanueva A, Vidal A, Qiu L, Vitkin E, Perelman LT, Melo CA, Lucci A, Ivan C, Calin GA, Kalluri R (2014) Cancer exosomes perform cell-independent microRNA biogenesis and promote tumorigenesis. Cancer Cell 26(5):707–721

Mirza S, Sharma G, Parshad R, Srivastava A, Gupta SD, Ralhan R (2010) Clinical significance of Stratifin, ERalpha and PR promoter methylation in tumor and serum DNA in Indian breast cancer patients. Clin Biochem 43(4–5):380–386

Mouliere F, Robert B, Arnau Peyrotte E, Del Rio M, Ychou M, Molina F, Gongora C, Thierry AR (2011) High fragmentation characterizes tumour-derived circulating DNA. PLoS ONE 6(9):e23418

Muller HM, Widschwendter A, Fiegl H, Ivarsson L, Goebel G, Perkmann E, Marth C, Widschwendter M (2003) DNA methylation in serum of breast cancer patients: an independent prognostic marker. Cancer Res 63(22):7641–7645

Murtaza M, Dawson SJ, Tsui DW, Gale D, Forshew T, Piskorz AM, Parkinson C, Chin SF, Kingsbury Z, Wong AS, Marass F, Humphray S, Hadfield J, Bentley D, Chin TM, Brenton JD, Caldas C, Rosenfeld N (2013) Non-invasive analysis of acquired resistance to cancer therapy by sequencing of plasma DNA. Nature 497(7447):108–112

Newman AM, Bratman SV, To J, Wynne JF, Eclov NC, Modlin LA, Liu CL, Neal JW, Wakelee HA, Merritt RE, Shrager JB, Loo BW Jr, Alizadeh AA, Diehn M (2014) An ultrasensitive method for quantitating circulating tumor DNA with broad patient coverage. Nat Med 20(5):548–554

Ng EK, Li R, Shin VY, Jin HC, Leung CP, Ma ES, Pang R, Chua D, Chu KM, Law WL, Law SY, Poon RT, Kwong A (2013) Circulating microRNAs as specific biomarkers for breast cancer detection. PLoS ONE 8(1):e53141

Norton SE, Luna KK, Lechner JM, Qin J, Fernando MR (2013) A new blood collection device minimizes cellular DNA release during sample storage and shipping when compared to a standard device. J Clin Lab Anal 27(4):305–311

Osborne RJ, Hamshere MG (2000) A genome-wide map showing common regions of loss of heterozygosity/allelic imbalance in breast cancer. Cancer Res 60(14):3706–3712

Oshiro C, Kagara N, Naoi Y, Shimoda M, Shimomura A, Maruyama N, Shimazu K, Kim SJ, Noguchi S (2015) PIK3CA mutations in serum DNA are predictive of recurrence in primary breast cancer patients. Breast Cancer Res Treat 150(2):299–307

Page K, Hava N, Ward B, Brown J, Guttery DS, Ruangpratheep C, Blighe K, Sharma A, Walker RA, Coombes RC, Shaw JA (2011) Detection of HER2 amplification in circulating free DNA in patients with breast cancer. Br J Cancer 104(8):1342–1348

Pritchard CC, Cheng HH, Tewari M (2012a) MicroRNA profiling: approaches and considerations. Nat Rev Genet 13(5):358–369

Pritchard CC, Kroh E, Wood B, Arroyo JD, Dougherty KJ, Miyaji MM, Tait JF, Tewari M (2012b) Blood cell origin of circulating microRNAs: a cautionary note for cancer biomarker studies. Cancer Prev Res (Phila) 5(3):492–497

Qin J, Williams TL, Fernando MR (2013) A novel blood collection device stabilizes cell-free RNA in blood during sample shipping and storage. BMC Res Notes 6:380

Reinert T, Scholer LV, Thomsen R, Tobiasen H, Vang S, Nordentoft I, Lamy P, Kannerup AS, Mortensen FV, Stribolt K, Hamilton-Dutoit S, Nielsen HJ, Laurberg S, Pallisgaard N, Pedersen JS, Orntoft TF, Andersen CL (2015) Analysis of circulating tumour DNA to monitor disease burden following colorectal cancer surgery. Gut

Rosell R, Moran T, Queralt C, Porta R, Cardenal F, Camps C, Majem M, Lopez-Vivanco G, Isla D, Provencio M, Insa A, Massuti B, Gonzalez-Larriba JL, Paz-Ares L, Bover I, Garcia-Campelo R, Moreno MA, Catot S, Rolfo C, Reguart N, Palmero R, Sanchez JM, Bastus R, Mayo C, Bertran-Alamillo J, Molina MA, Sanchez JJ, Taron M (2009) Screening for epidermal growth factor receptor mutations in lung cancer. New Engl J Med 361(10):958–967

Roth C, Rack B, Muller V, Janni W, Pantel K, Schwarzenbach H (2010) Circulating microRNAs as blood-based markers for patients with primary and metastatic breast cancer. Breast Cancer Res 12(6):R90

Rothe F, Laes JF, Lambrechts D, Smeets D, Vincent D, Maetens M, Fumagalli D, Michiels S, Drisis S, Moerman C, Detiffe JP, Larsimont D, Awada A, Piccart M, Sotiriou C, Ignatiadis M (2014) Plasma circulating tumor DNA as an alternative to metastatic biopsies for mutational analysis in breast cancer. Ann Oncol 25(10):1959–1965

Schrauder MG, Strick R, Schulz-Wendtland R, Strissel PL, Kahmann L, Loehberg CR, Lux MP, Jud SM, Hartmann A, Hein A, Bayer CM, Bani MR, Richter S, Adamietz BR, Wenkel E, Rauh C, Beckmann MW, Fasching PA (2012) Circulating micro-RNAs as potential blood-based markers for early stage breast cancer detection. PLoS ONE 7(1):e29770

Schwarzenbach H, Muller V, Milde-Langosch K, Steinbach B, Pantel K (2011) Evaluation of cell-free tumour DNA and RNA in patients with breast cancer and benign breast disease. Mol BioSyst 7(10):2848–2854

Schwarzenbach H, Eichelser C, Kropidlowski J, Janni W, Rack B, Pantel K (2012a) Loss of heterozygosity at tumor suppressor genes detectable on fractionated circulating cell-free tumor DNA as indicator of breast cancer progression. Clin Cancer Res 18(20):5719–5730

Schwarzenbach H, Milde-Langosch K, Steinbach B, Muller V, Pantel K (2012b) Diagnostic potential of PTEN-targeting miR-214 in the blood of breast cancer patients. Breast Cancer Res Treat 134(3):933–941

Shapiro B, Chakrabarty M, Cohn EM, Leon SA (1983) Determination of circulating DNA levels in patients with benign or malignant gastrointestinal disease. Cancer 51(11):2116–2120

Sharma G, Mirza S, Parshad R, Srivastava A, Datta Gupta S, Pandya P, Ralhan R (2010a) CpG hypomethylation of MDR1 gene in tumor and serum of invasive ductal breast carcinoma patients. Clin Biochem 43(4–5):373–379

Sharma G, Mirza S, Parshad R, Srivastava A, Gupta SD, Pandya P, Ralhan R (2010b) Clinical significance of promoter hypermethylation of DNA repair genes in tumor and serum DNA in invasive ductal breast carcinoma patients. Life Sci 87(3–4):83–91

Sharma G, Mirza S, Parshad R, Gupta SD, Ralhan R (2012) DNA methylation of circulating DNA: a marker for monitoring efficacy of neoadjuvant chemotherapy in breast cancer patients. Tumour Biol 33(6):1837–1843

Shaw JA, Page K, Blighe K, Hava N, Guttery D, Ward B, Brown J, Ruangpratheep C, Stebbing J, Payne R, Palmieri C, Cleator S, Walker RA, Coombes RC (2012) Genomic analysis of circulating cell-free DNA infers breast cancer dormancy. Genome Res 22 (2):220–231

Shukla S, Mirza S, Sharma G, Parshad R, Gupta SD, Ralhan R (2006) Detection of RASSF1A and RARbeta hypermethylation in serum DNA from breast cancer patients. Epigenetics Off J DNA Methylation Soc 1(2):88–93

Si H, Sun X, Chen Y, Cao Y, Chen S, Wang H, Hu C (2013) Circulating microRNA-92a and microRNA-21 as novel minimally invasive biomarkers for primary breast cancer. J Cancer Res Clin Oncol 139(2):223–229

Silva JM, Dominguez G, Garcia JM, Gonzalez R, Villanueva MJ, Navarro F, Provencio M, San Martin S, Espana P, Bonilla F (1999) Presence of tumor DNA in plasma of breast cancer patients: clinicopathological correlations. Cancer Res 59 (13):3251–3256

Skvortsova TE, Rykova EY, Tamkovich SN, Bryzgunova OE, Starikov AV, Kuznetsova NP, Vlassov VV, Laktionov PP (2006) Cell-free and cell-bound circulating DNA in breast tumours: DNA quantification and analysis of tumour-related gene methylation. Br J Cancer 94(10):1492–1495

Sun Y, Wang M, Lin G, Sun S, Li X, Qi J, Li J (2012) Serum microRNA-155 as a potential biomarker to track disease in breast cancer. PLoS ONE 7(10): e47003

Tan EM, Schur PH, Carr RI, Kunkel HG (1966) Deoxybonucleic acid (DNA) and antibodies to DNA in the serum of patients with systemic lupus erythematosus. J Clin Investig 45(11):1732–1740

Taniguchi K, Uchida J, Nishino K, Kumagai T, Okuyama T, Okami J, Higashiyama M, Kodama K, Imamura F, Kato K (2011) Quantitative detection of EGFR mutations in circulating tumor DNA derived from lung adenocarcinomas. Clin Cancer Res 17 (24):7808–7815

Turchinovich A, Weiz L, Langheinz A, Burwinkel B (2011) Characterization of extracellular circulating microRNA. Nucleic Acids Res 39(16):7223–7233

Umetani N, Hiramatsu S, Hoon DS (2006) Higher amount of free circulating DNA in serum than in plasma is not mainly caused by contaminated extraneous DNA during separation. Ann N Y Acad Sci 1075:299–307

Valadi H, Ekstrom K, Bossios A, Sjostrand M, Lee JJ, Lotvall JO (2007) Exosome-mediated transfer of mRNAs and microRNAs is a novel mechanism of genetic exchange between cells. Nat Cell Biol 9 (6):654–659

van Schooneveld E, Wouters MC, Van der Auwera I, Peeters DJ, Wildiers H, Van Dam PA, Vergote I, Vermeulen PB, Dirix LY, Van Laere SJ (2012) Expression profiling of cancerous and normal breast tissues identifies microRNAs that are differentially expressed in serum from patients with (metastatic) breast cancer and healthy volunteers. Breast Cancer Res 14(1):R34

van Schooneveld E, Wildiers H, Vergote I, Vermeulen PB, Dirix LY, Van Laere SJ (2015) Dysregulation of microRNAs in breast cancer and their potential role as prognostic and predictive biomarkers in patient management. Breast Cancer Res 17(1):526

Wang BG, Huang HY, Chen YC, Bristow RE, Kassauei K, Cheng CC, Roden R, Sokoll LJ, Chan DW,

Shih Ie M (2003) Increased plasma DNA integrity in cancer patients. Cancer Res 63(14):3966–3968

Wang F, Zheng Z, Guo J, Ding X (2010a) Correlation and quantitation of microRNA aberrant expression in tissues and sera from patients with breast tumor. Gynecol Oncol 119(3):586–593

Wang J, Ramakrishnan R, Tang Z, Fan W, Kluge A, Dowlati A, Jones RC, Ma PC (2010b) Quantifying EGFR alterations in the lung cancer genome with nanofluidic digital PCR arrays. Clin Chem 56(4):623–632

Wang H, Tan G, Dong L, Cheng L, Li K, Wang Z, Luo H (2012a) Circulating MiR-125b as a marker predicting chemoresistance in breast cancer. PLoS ONE 7(4): e34210

Wang K, Yuan Y, Cho JH, McClarty S, Baxter D, Galas DJ (2012b) Comparing the MicroRNA spectrum between serum and plasma. PLoS ONE 7(7): e41561

Wang F, Hou J, Jin W, Li J, Yue Y, Jin H, Wang X (2014) Increased circulating microRNA-155 as a potential biomarker for breast cancer screening: a meta-analysis. Molecules (Basel, Switzerland) 19 (5):6282–6293

Witwer KW (2015) Circulating microRNA biomarker studies: pitfalls and potential solutions. Clin Chem 61 (1):56–63

Wu X, Somlo G, Yu Y, Palomares MR, Li AX, Zhou W, Chow A, Yen Y, Rossi JJ, Gao H, Wang J, Yuan YC, Frankel P, Li S, Ashing-Giwa KT, Sun G, Wang Y, Smith R, Robinson K, Ren X, Wang SE (2012) De novo sequencing of circulating miRNAs identifies novel markers predicting clinical outcome of locally advanced breast cancer. J Transl Med 10:42

Xin H, Li X, Yang B, Zhang L, Han Z, Han C (2014) Blood-based multiple-microRNA assay displays a better diagnostic performance than single-microRNA assay in the diagnosis of breast tumor. Tumour Biol 35 (12):12635–12643

Zeng RC, Zhang W, Yan XQ, Ye ZQ, Chen ED, Huang DP, Zhang XH, Huang GL (2013) Down-regulation of miRNA-30a in human plasma is a novel marker for breast cancer. Med Oncol 30 (1):477

Zhao H, Shen J, Medico L, Wang D, Ambrosone CB, Liu S (2010) A pilot study of circulating miRNAs as potential biomarkers of early stage breast cancer. PLoS ONE 5(10):e13735

Zhu W, Qin W, Atasoy U, Sauter ER (2009) Circulating microRNAs in breast cancer and healthy subjects. BMC Res Notes 2:89

Prognostic Factors for Ductal Carcinoma in Situ of the Breast

17

Lawrence J. Solin

Abstract

Ductal carcinoma in situ of the breast is a non-obligate precursor for the development of invasive carcinoma of the breast. A number of clinical and pathologic parameters have been traditionally used to stratify cases based on the likelihood of recurrence. These include patient age, completeness of excision, method of presentation, and histologic features. Immunohistochemistry-based analysis of expression of various molecular markers have also been used to define risk of recurrence. The use of imaging studies such as magnetic resonance imaging (MRI) have not added significantly to mammography in improving local control. More recently, molecular profiling, including a gene expression-based assay, has become commercially available. Assays such as this can be successfully used to stratify patients into risk groups for clinical decision-making.

Keywords

DCIS · Risk stratification · Molecular profiling

17.1 Introduction

Ductal carcinoma in situ (DCIS; intraductal carcinoma) of the breast is a non-obligate precursor for developing invasive carcinoma of the breast. The diagnosis of DCIS poses a clinical dilemma for the patient and her physician. DCIS is typically detected as suspicious calcifications on routine screening mammography. Women with such asymptomatic mammographic findings are frequently interested in breast conservation treatment. After surgical excision (lumpectomy), adjuvant treatments (radiation and/or tamoxifen) have been shown to reduce subsequent risk (Fisher et al. 1998, 2001; Wapnir et al. 2011; Donker et al. 2013; Cuzick et al. 2011; Warnberg et al. 2014; McCormick et al. 2015; Early Breast Cancer Trialists' Collaborative Group et al. 2010; Solin 2010; Allred et al. 2012). However, adjuvant treatments are associated with a small, albeit real, risk of side effects. As a result, many patients elect to receive adjuvant treatment

L.J. Solin (✉)
Department of Radiation Oncology, Albert Einstein Healthcare Network, Philadelphia, PA, USA
e-mail: Solin@einstein.edu

S. Badve and Y. Gökmen-Polar (eds.), *Molecular Pathology of Breast Cancer*, DOI 10.1007/978-3-319-41761-5_17

(radiation and/or tamoxifen) to minimize the risk of recurrence, while other patients elect against adjuvant treatment, often because of the potential risk of side effects.

For the woman with newly diagnosed DCIS, the options for local management of the breast include surgical excision (lumpectomy) with or without radiation treatment, unilateral mastectomy, or even bilateral mastectomies (NCCN Clinical Practice Guidelines in Oncology 2015; Moran et al. 2012). As most patients with DCIS are interested in breast conservation treatment, a key management decision is whether or not to add radiation treatment after surgical excision. Excellent 10 and 15-year outcomes have been reported after lumpectomy plus radiation treatment (Solin et al. 1996, 2005). Nonetheless, population-based studies have demonstrated that a substantial fraction of patients are treated using surgical excision alone, without radiation treatment (Zujewski et al. 2011; Dodwell et al. 2007; Baxter et al. 2004; Smith et al. 2006). Although tamoxifen reduces the risk of recurrence, tamoxifen should not be considered as a substitute for radiation treatment.

17.2 Randomized Trials of Radiation Treatment and Tamoxifen

Five prospective randomized trials have demonstrated that adding radiation treatment after surgical excision for DCIS significantly reduces the risk of an ipsilateral local recurrence (also referred to as an ipsilateral breast event [IBE] or an ipsilateral breast tumor recurrence [IBTR]) (Fisher et al. 1998, 2001; Wapnir et al. 2011; Donker et al. 2013; Cuzick et al. 2011; Warnberg et al. 2014; McCormick et al. 2015; Early Breast Cancer Trialists' Collaborative Group et al. 2010). This reduction in risk is approximately 50 % for local recurrence, as well as for the subset of invasive local recurrence. Ten-year outcome data have been published from at least three of these randomized clinical trials. The risk all breast cancer events (defined as ipsilateral plus contralateral) can be further reduced by adding adjuvant tamoxifen for hormone receptor positive DCIS tumors (Fisher et al. 2001; Wapnir et al. 2011; Cuzick et al. 2011; Yi et al. 2012).

Although adding adjuvant treatment after lumpectomy reduces the rate of recurrence, randomized clinical trials have not demonstrated a benefit from adding adjuvant treatment for improving the rates of distant metastases and overall survival. The rates of freedom from distant metastases and overall survival for patients with DCIS are uniformly high in randomized clinical trials, regardless of initial treatment. In addition, prospective clinical trials have not reproducibly and reliably identified those patients for whom the risk of recurrence is sufficiently low based on conventional clinical and pathologic factors that treatment using lumpectomy alone (without radiation treatment and/or tamoxifen) is reasonable.

17.3 Risk Stratification Using Clinical and Pathologic Factors

Conventional approaches to assess and to stratify local recurrence risk typically consider various combinations of clinical and pathologic characteristics. Many studies have attempted to define prognostic factors for local control after lumpectomy, with or without radiation treatment. Those factors most consistently identified include: (a) patient age; (b) margins of resection; (c) tumor size; (d) method of presentation; and (e) pathologic features of the DCIS tumor. Although these prognostic factors are most consistently identified, other individual factors associated with local recurrence have been reported in individual studies. In addition, the specific pathologic feature(s) associated with local recurrence risk are not consistent across studies. A nomogram to determine recurrence risk after lumpectomy has been developed based on clinical, pathologic, and treatment factors, although treatment factors are heavily weighted (Rudloff et al. 2010; Yi et al. 2012). Adding breast MRI (magnetic resonance imaging) to standard mammography has not been shown to improve local control (Solin et al. 2008; Pilewskie et al. 2014).

Negative margins of resection from the lumpectomy specimen are associated with improved local control compared to close or positive margins of resection. However, after surgical excision, patients treated without radiation likely require a wider minimum negative margin width than patients treated with radiation. For the patients undergoing radiation treatment, the goal of surgical excision is to debulk the DCIS tumor burden so that adding radiation treatment has a high probability of local control. In contrast, for patients treated with lumpectomy alone (without radiation treatment), the goal of surgical excision is to completely excise the DCIS tumor.

Notwithstanding the substantial improvement in local recurrence associated with adding radiation treatment, research efforts continue to attempt to identify a subset of patients with favorable DCIS who are at sufficiently low risk of local recurrence that omitting radiation treatment after lumpectomy is reasonable (Silverstein and Lagios 2010; Hughes et al. 2009). If a group of patients could be identified with a sufficiently low risk of local recurrence after lumpectomy alone, then the risk-benefit ratio might favor not adding adjuvant treatment. Such efforts have traditionally defined "favorable" (or "low risk") DCIS using conventional clinical and pathologic factors. Although retrospective studies have suggested the possibility of omitting radiation treatment for the subset of patients with clinically "favorable" DCIS, no prospective trial has reliably and reproducibly identified such a subset of patients, especially with longer term follow-up of at least ten years.

17.4 Risk Stratification Using Molecular Profiling

Because of the inability of clinical and pathologic factors to identify consistently and reproducibly a group of patients with low risk DCIS who can be treated with lumpectomy alone, recent research efforts have focused on the potential for using molecular markers to improve the prognostic ability to separate patients into lower versus higher risk categories and to better define the risk of local recurrence for the individual patient with DCIS. By using individualized risk assessment based on molecular profiling, adding adjuvant treatment after surgical excision can be offered to higher risk patients, and omitting adjuvant treatment can be considered for lower risk patients. To be clinically useful, molecular profiling should demonstrate value beyond standard clinical and pathologic factors.

Simon et al. (2009) described the rigorous methodologic requirements for developing molecular tools for clinical practice, including the definition of levels of evidence. Molecular tools are initially developed using historical databases that include defined clinical and pathologic characteristics of the DCIS tumors as well as follow-up information for outcomes analysis. This process allows molecular tools to be developed using archived tissue specimens. Once such a molecular tool has been developed, it can then be moved into the prospective clinical trial setting. This model for developing molecular profiling has proved successful for selecting systemic therapy in the setting of invasive breast carcinoma, and thus, the groundwork has been set for developing such molecular tools for use in DCIS.

A number of studies have evaluated small numbers of genes, generally no more than three or four, using historical databases. Table 17.1 shows a literature summary of selected, recent studies of limited molecular marker panels for DCIS in the setting of breast conservation treatment. A number of these markers have been associated with local recurrence and/or the subset of invasive local recurrence. However, none of these markers have been validated in a second study. Further, many of these genes are not available in routine clinical practice. Other molecular markers have been summarized in a comprehensive literature review (Lari and Kuerer 2011).

Table 17.1 Literature summary of selected, recent studies of prognostic markers for ductal carcinoma in situ (DCIS) of the breast after breast conservation surgery (with or without radiation treatment)

Study	Number of patients	Local treatment	Molecular marker(s)	Outcome	*P* value
Toussaint et al. (2010)	154	Any[a]	CD10	Low CD10 associated with higher risk of local relapse	0.001
Kerlikowske et al. (2010)	1162	Lumpectomy alone	p16, COX-2, Ki67	Triple positive associated with higher risk of subsequent invasive cancer	<0.05
Altintas et al. (2011)	88	Any[a]	Four gene signature	VNPI-GGI associated with early relapse	<0.05
Rakovitch et al. (2012)	213	Lumpectomy ± radiation	HER2, Ki67	Both positive associated with higher DCIS local recurrence	0.001
Knudsen et al. (2012)	244	Lumpectomy alone	RB, PTEN	Loss of both associated with local recurrence and invasive local recurrence	Both < 0.001
Knudsen et al. (2013)	248	Lumpectomy alone	ALDH1, EZHZ	Both high associated with local recurrence and invasive local recurrence	0.0048 and 0.0394, respectively
Noh et al. (2013)	215	Lumpectomy plus radiation	HER2	No difference in local recurrence	0.1764
Witkiewicz et al. (2014)	226	Lumpectomy alone	ErbB2, RB	ErbB2 high and RB positive associated with higher local recurrence and invasive recurrence	0.0209 and 0.0316, respectively

VNPI-GGI Van Nuys Prognostic Index Genomic Grade Index
[a]Includes patients treated with mastectomy or breast conservation treatment

In one study, Toussaint et al. reported that low CD10 was associated with a higher risk of local relapse ($P = 0.001$) (Toussaint et al. 2010). These findings were seen in 154 patients treated with any form of local therapy, as well as for the subset of 77 patients treated with lumpectomy (with or without radiation treatment).

Kerlikowske et al. (2010) reported a case control study from a population-based cohort of 1162 women treated by lumpectomy alone. Multivariable analysis demonstrated that the combination of positive p16, COX-2, and Ki67 was associated with an increased risk of subsequent tumor events (hazard ratio = 2.2; $P < 0.05$).

Rakovitch et al. (2012) reported on using HER2 and Ki67 to evaluate the risk of local recurrence after lumpectomy, with or without radiation treatment. The combination of positive HER2 and Ki67 was associated with a higher risk of DCIS local recurrence ($P = 0.001$) and a borderline higher risk of local recurrence ($P = 0.06$).

Investigators from Thomas Jefferson University have studied a number of potential molecular markers (Knudsen et al. 2012, 2013; Witkiewicz et al. 2014). The clinical database included patients treated with lumpectomy alone, without radiation treatment. A number of potential tumor markers were identified as associated with local recurrence and the subset of invasive local recurrence.

Such retrospective studies have demonstrated the possibility of using tumor markers to predict the risks of local recurrence and the subset of invasive local recurrence. However, such studies are often limited by a number of factors, including relatively small numbers of patients as well as tumor markers that are neither routinely used nor widely available in clinical practice. Finally, these studies are all exploratory, and none has shown reproducibility in a validation study using an independent cohort of patients.

17.5 Development and Validation of the Oncotype DX DCIS Score

The 12-gene Oncotype DX DCIS Score (also referred to as the DCIS Score) was developed and validated using a multi-step strategy in accordance with the guidelines for tumor biomarker development as defined by Simon et al. (2009), (Solin et al. 2013). The need to create a molecular score for patients with DCIS was based on the observation that traditional clinical and pathologic parameters have not reproducibly and reliably identified patients at low risk after surgical excision (without radiation treatment), as well as the successful strategy for integrating molecular profiling for patients with invasive breast carcinoma. The Oncotype DX DCIS Score was therefore developed as a molecularly-based score to predict local recurrence risk after surgical excision alone (without radiation treatment), regardless of adjuvant tamoxifen.

The first step in the development process was to define which genes to include in the Oncotype DX DCIS Score and to determine the calculation algorithm. Using the 21 genes included in the Oncotype DX Recurrence Score (also referred to as the Recurrence Score) for invasive breast carcinoma, a subset of 12 genes was selected to define the Oncotype DX DCIS Score, comprised of seven cancer-related genes and five reference genes (Fig. 17.1). The proliferation group score was found to be significantly lower for DCIS tumors in comparison to invasive breast tumors. Therefore, the DCIS Score does not have a thresholding value for calculating the proliferation group score. In addition, calculation coefficients were selected to optimize the DCIS Score.

The DCIS Score was then fixed as the final step in the development process. After the development phase was completed, the ECOG-ACRIN (Eastern Cooperative Oncology Group American College of Radiology Imaging Network; formerly ECOG) E5194 specimens were used for the first validation study for the DCIS Score. Similar to the Recurrence Score (for invasive breast carcinoma), the DCIS Score was evaluated in two ways: (a) using three predefined and prespecified risk groups of low, intermediate, and high risk; and (b) as a continuous variable.

A brief description of the ECOG-ACRIN E5194 study is as follows (Hughes et al. 2009; Solin et al. 2013; Badve et al. 2012; Solin et al. 2015). In the early 1990s, ECOG-ACRIN designed the prospective clinical study E5194 for the treatment of DCIS using local excision alone (without radiation treatment) for selected patients with DCIS of the breast based on low risk clinical and pathologic features. From 1997 to 2002, patients were enrolled into one of two cohorts (not randomized): (a) Cohort 1: low or intermediate grade DCIS, tumor size 2.5 cm or less; and (b) Cohort 2: high grade DCIS, tumor size 1.0 cm or less. Cohort assignment was based on clinical and pathologic characteristics as determined by the treating institution at time of enrollment on protocol study. Adjuvant tamoxifen was allowed as optional beginning in 2000.

The results of first validation study for the DCIS Score using the ECOG-ACRIN E5194 DCIS specimens are as follows. The

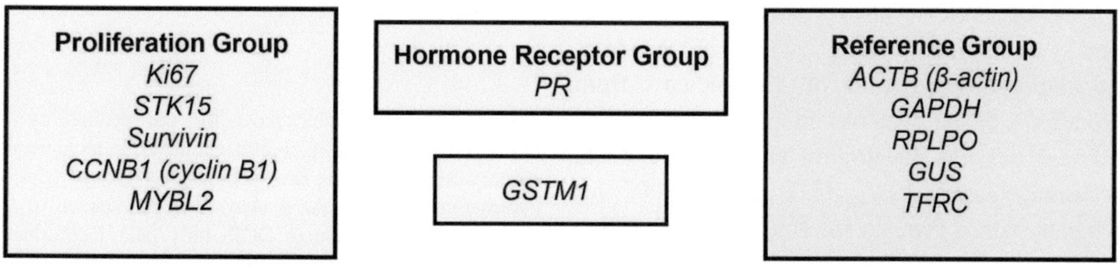

Fig. 17.1 Panel of 12 genes included in the Oncotype DX DCIS Score. There are seven cancer-related genes and five reference genes. Reproduced with permission from Oxford University Press (Solin et al. 2013)

10-year risks of developing an ipsilateral breast event (IBE; local recurrence) were 10.6 % for patients with a low DCIS Score, 26.7 % for patients with an intermediate DCIS Score, and 25.9 % for patients with a high DCIS Score ($P = 0.006$; Fig. 17.2). For the subset of invasive IBE, the 10-year risks were 3.7, 12.3, and 19.2 %, respectively ($P = 0.003$). On multivariate analysis, the DCIS Score, tumor size, and menopausal status were statistically significant for developing a local recurrence (all $P \leq 0.02$). Evaluating the DCIS Score as a continuous variable for local recurrence, the hazard ratio was 2.31 (95 % confidence interval = 1.15–4.49; $P = 0.02$). Thus, the DCIS Score quantifies the 10-year risks of local recurrence and invasive local recurrence, and provides independent information for assessing risk beyond conventional clinical and pathologic variables.

As part of the pre-specified study plan for the ECOG-ACRIN E5194 validation study, the individual 16 cancer-related genes included in the 21-gene Recurrence Score (i.e., excluding the five reference genes) were individually reviewed for the local recurrence risk and invasive local recurrence risk (Fig. 17.3). The five proliferation group genes were each individually associated with local recurrence risk and invasive local recurrence risk. However, each of these five genes (including Ki67) was less informative than the combination of these five genes. In addition, none of the nine genes included in the 21-gene Recurrence Score (but excluded from the 12-gene DCIS Score) were statistically significantly associated with local recurrence risk. These results indicate that statistical power and significant information were not lost by excluding these nine genes from the DCIS Score.

The DCIS Score has recently undergone second validation using an independent, population-based cohort of 571 patients from Ontario, Canada (Rakovitch et al. 2015). The 10-year risks of developing an ipsilateral local recurrence were 12.7, 33.0, and 27.8 % for patients with a low, an intermediate, and a high DCIS Score, respectively ($P < 0.001$; Table 17.2). For the subset of invasive local

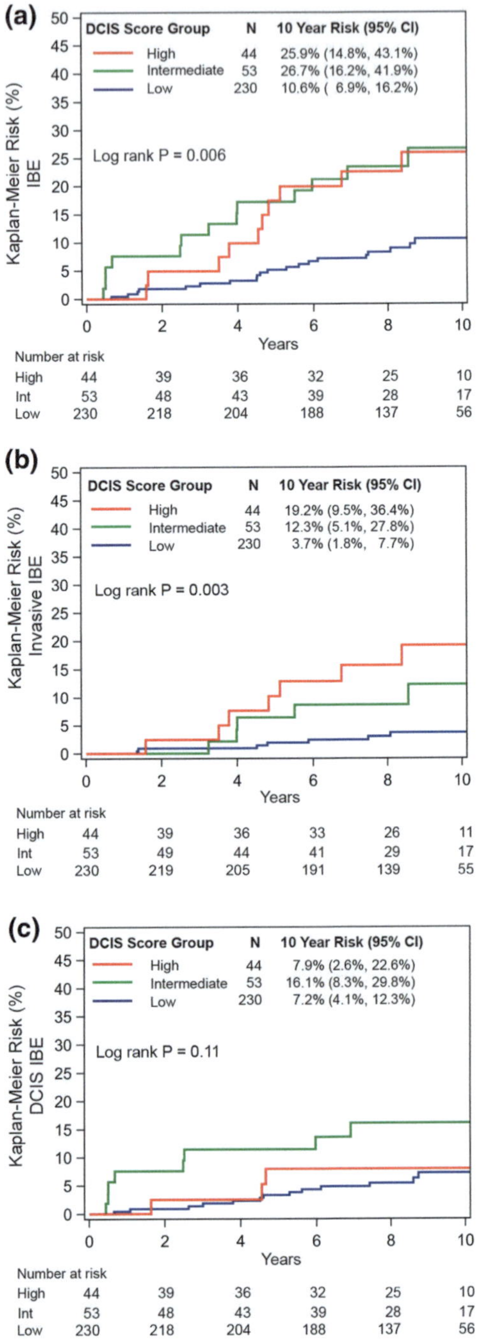

Fig. 17.2 Kaplan-Meier plots for the probability of developing an ipsilateral breast event (*IBE*; local recurrence) according to the pre-specified risk groups of low, intermediate, and high. **a** Any IBE. **b** Subset of an invasive IBE. **c** Subset of DCIS only IBE. Reproduced with permission from Oxford University Press (Solin et al. 2013)

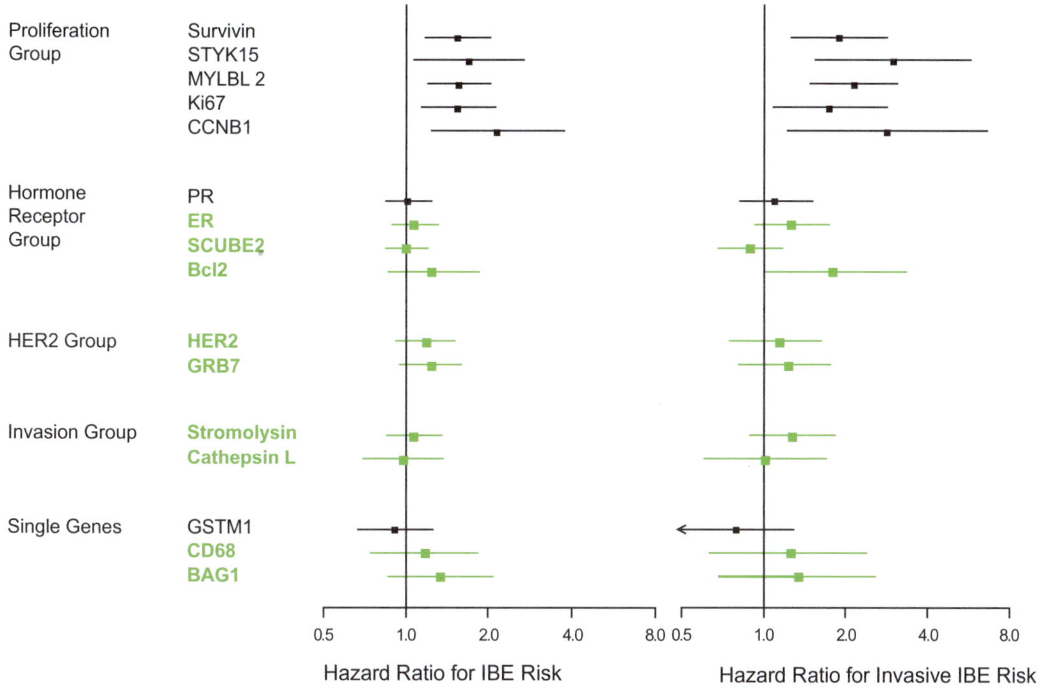

Fig. 17.3 The forest plot shows the hazard ratios for ipsilateral breast event (IBE) risk (*left side* of the figure) and invasive IBE risk (*right side* of the figure) for each of the 16 individual genes in the Oncotype DX breast cancer assay (excluding the five reference genes). The seven cancer-related genes prespecified as included in the DCIS Score are shown in *black*. The remaining nine genes (included in the Recurrence Score, but not included in the DCIS Score) are shown in *green*. The hazard ratios (with 95% confidence intervals) are calculated for a one unit difference (approximately doubling) in cycle threshold (C_T) for gene expression level. Abbreviations: Survivin = BIRC5; STK15 = aurora kinase A; MYBL2 = v-myb myeloblastosis viral oncogene homolog (avian)-like 2; Ki67 = MKI67; CCNB1 = cyclin B1; PR = progesterone receptor; ER = estrogen receptor; SCUBE2 = signal peptide, CUB domain, EGF-like 2; BCL2 = B-cell CLL/lymphoma 2; HER2 = human epidermal growth factor receptor 2; GRB7 = growth factor receptor-bound protein 7; MMP11 = stromolysin; CTSL2 = cathepsin L2; GSTM1 = glutathione S-transferase M1; CD68 = CD68 molecule; BAG1 = BCL2-associated athanogene. Reproduced with permission from Oxford University Press (Solin et al. 2013)

recurrence, the 10-year risks were 8.0, 20.9, and 15.5 %, respectively ($P = 0.03$). On multivariate analysis, the DCIS Score remained an independent, significant factor for local recurrence ($P = 0.02$), as well as age at diagnosis, tumor size, DCIS subtype, and multifocality.

Comparing the data from the ECOG-ACRIN E5194 study and the population-based cohort from Ontario, Canada demonstrates remarkably consistent results for the main study endpoints of any local recurrence, the subset of invasive local recurrence, and the subset of DCIS only local recurrence (Table 17.3). In addition, the DCIS Score is an independent and statistically significant factor for local recurrence on multivariate analysis in both studies.

Although less rigorous than 10-year clinical outcomes, comparison of the distribution of DCIS Scores also demonstrates consistent results in multiple studies (Table 17.4). In five reported studies, the distribution of DCIS Score shows a low risk DCIS Score for 62–77 % of patients.

In order to implement a tumor marker into clinical practice, both patients and physicians will want to see consistency in results between studies. As defined by Simon et al., development of molecular markers for clinical implementation requires more than one validation study (Simon et al. 2009). The high bar for clinical implementation has now been met by the DCIS Score development and validation process.

Table 17.2 Ten-year risks of local recurrence according to the Oncotype DX DCIS Score risk groups of low, intermediate, and high risk for a population-based cohort of 571 patients with DCIS from Ontario, Canada treated with breast conserving surgery alone (without radiation treatment) (Rakovitch et al. 2015)

Type of local recurrence	DCIS Score risk group	Number of patients	Local recurrence at 10 years (%)	*P* value
Any local recurrence				
	Low	121	12.7	<0.001
	Intermediate	95	33.0	
	High	355	27.8	
Subset of invasive local recurrence				
	Low	121	8.0	0.03
	Intermediate	95	20.9	
	High	355	15.5	
Subset of DCIS only local recurrence				
	Low	121	5.4	0.002
	Intermediate	95	14.1	
	High	355	13.7	

Table 17.3 Ten-year risks of local recurrence according to the Oncotype DX DCIS Score risk groups for the ECOG-ACRIN E5194 study compared to the population-based cohort from Ontario, Canada

Type of local recurrence	DCIS Score risk group	ECOG-ACRIN E5194 (Solin et al. 2013)		Ontario, Canada Cohort (Rakovitch et al. 2015)	
		Local recurrence at 10 years (%)	*P* value	Local recurrence at 10 years (%)	*P* value
Any local recurrence					
	Low	10.6	0.006	12.7	<0.001
	Intermediate	26.7		33.0	
	High	25.9		27.8	
Subset of invasive local recurrence					
	Low	3.7	0.003	8.0	0.03
	Intermediate	12.3		20.9	
	High	19.2		15.5	
Subset of DCIS only local recurrence					
	Low	7.2	0.11	5.4	0.002
	Intermediate	16.1		14.1	
	High	7.9		13.7	

Table 17.4 Distribution of the Oncotype DX DCIS Score according to risk group

Study	Number of patients	DCIS Score risk group (%)		
		Low	Intermediate	High
Solin et al. (2013)	327	70	16	13
Rakovitch et al. (2015)	571	62	17	21
Sing et al. (2014)	3947	67	17	15
Alvarado et al. (2015)	115	63	21	16
Chadha et al. (2013)	58	77	12	10

17.6 Conclusions and Future Directions

With the successful development and clinical implementation of the DCIS Score, a number of future research directions will be important. Ongoing research efforts will look at the DCIS Score as a predictive factor for the value of adding radiation treatment after lumpectomy. While current studies have evaluated molecular profiling as a prognostic factor, future studies will explore molecular profiling as a predictive factor for the benefit of adding radiation treatment after lumpectomy.

Additional research is ongoing to look at the impact of the DCIS Score on clinical decision-making, as well as an economic analysis of cost-effectiveness. Potentially extending the eligibility criteria beyond the ECOG-ACRIN E5914 study criteria will be important. For example, in the Ontario, Canada database, the definition of negative margins was no tumor on ink, rather than the 3 mm minimum negative margin width required by the ECOG-ACRIN E5194 study. Finally, future gene panels for DCIS may be refined, in particular, when full gene sequencing results become available.

In summary, prospective and retrospective studies have demonstrated that for patients with DCIS of the breast, breast conservation surgery followed by definitive radiation treatment achieves excellent long term outcomes. Adding radiation treatment after lumpectomy reduces the rates of local recurrence and invasive local recurrence by about half in randomized clinical trials. Adding adjuvant tamoxifen reduces the rate of all breast cancer events for hormone receptor positive DCIS tumors. Newer approaches using molecular profiling improve risk assessment and individualized treatment decision-making for patients with DCIS. The 12-gene Oncotype DX DCIS Score has been developed and validated in accordance with rigorous scientific principles, and is now available for use in clinical practice. The demonstrated clinical value of the Oncotype DX DCIS Score serves as proof of principle for the development and validation of molecular profiling of DCIS for clinical practice, and sets the stage for ongoing research efforts.

References

Allred DC, Anderson SJ, Paik S et al (2012) Adjuvant tamoxifen reduces subsequent breast cancer in women with estrogen receptor-positive ductal carcinoma in situ: a study based on NSABP protocol B-24. J Clin Oncol 30(12):1268–1273

Altintas S, Toussaint J, Durbecq V et al (2011) Fine tuning of the Van Nuys prognostic index (VNPI) 2003 by integrating the genomic grade index (GGI): new tools for ductal carcinoma in situ (DCIS). Breast J 17 (4):343–351

Alvarado M, Carter D, Guenther JM et al (2015) The impact of genomic testing on the recommendation for radiation therapy in patients with ductal carcinoma in situ: a prospective clinical utility assessment of the 12-gene DCIS Score result. J Surg Oncol 111(8):935–940

Badve S, Gray RJ, Baehner FL, et al (2012) Correlation between the DCIS Score and traditional clinicopathologic features in the prospectively designed E5194 clinical validation study. Presented at the 2012 American Society of Clinical Oncology (ASCO) annual meeting, Chicago, Illinois, June 1–5 (Abstract 1005)

Baxter NN, Virnig BA, Durham SB, Tuttle TM (2004) Trends in the treatment of ductal carcinoma in situ of the breast. J Natl Cancer Inst 96(6):443–448

Chadha M, Fox J, Boolbol SK et al (2013) Evaluating a role for Oncotype DX breast cancer assay in the management of ductal carcinoma in situ (Abstract 2078). Int J Radiat Oncol Biol Phys 87(Suppl):S234

Cuzick J, Sestak I, Pinder SE et al (2011) Effect of tamoxifen and radiotherapy in women with locally excised ductal carcinoma in situ: long-term results from the UK/ANZ DCIS trial. Lancet Oncol 12(1):21–29

Dodwell D, Clements K, Lawrence G et al (2007) Radiotherapy following breast-conserving surgery for screen-detected ductal carcinoma in situ: indications and utilisation in the UK. Interim findings from the Sloane Project. Br J Cancer 97(6):725–729

Donker M, Litiere S, Werutsky G et al (2013) Breast-conserving treatment with or without radiotherapy in ductal carcinoma in situ: 15-year recurrence rates and outcome after a recurrence, from the EORTC 10853 randomized phase III trial. J Clin Oncol 31 (32):4054–4059

Early Breast Cancer Trialists' Collaborative Group, Correa C, McGale P et al (2010) Overview of the randomized trials of radiotherapy in ductal carcinoma in situ of the breast. J Natl Cancer Inst Monogr 2010 (41):162–177

Fisher B, Dignam J, Wolmark N et al (1998) Lumpectomy and radiation therapy for the treatment of intraductal breast cancer: findings from National Surgical Adjuvant Breast and Bowel Project B-17. J Clin Oncol 16(2):441–452

Fisher B, Land S, Mamounas E et al (2001) Prevention of invasive breast cancer in women with ductal carcinoma in situ: an update of the National Surgical Adjuvant Breast and Bowel Project experience. Semin Oncol 28(4):400–418

Hughes LL, Wang M, Page DL et al (2009) Local excision alone without irradiation for ductal carcinoma in situ of the breast: a trial of the Eastern Cooperative Oncology Group. J Clin Oncol 27(32):5319–5324

Kerlikowske K, Molinaro AM, Gauthier ML et al (2010) Biomarker expression and risk of subsequent tumors after initial ductal carcinoma in situ diagnosis. J Natl Cancer Inst 102(9):627–637

Knudsen ES, Dervishaj O, Kleer CG et al (2013) EZH2 and ALDH1 expression in ductal carcinoma in situ: complex association with recurrence and progression to invasive breast cancer. Cell Cycle 12(13):2042–2050

Knudsen ES, Pajak TF, Qeenan M et al (2012) Retinoblastoma and phosphate and tensin homolog tumor suppressors: impact on ductal carcinoma in situ progression. J Natl Cancer Inst 104(23):1825–1836

Lari SA, Kuerer HM (2011) Biological markers in DCIS and risk of breast recurrence: a systematic review. J Cancer 2:232–261

McCormick B, Winter K, Hudis C et al (2015) RTOG 9804: a prospective randomized trial for good-risk ductal carcinoma in situ comparing radiotherapy with observation. J Clin Oncol 33(7):709–715

Moran MS, Bai HX, Harris EE et al (2012) ACR appropriateness criteria (®) ductal carcinoma in situ. Breast J 18(1):8–15

NCCN Clinical Practice Guidelines in Oncology (2015) Breast Cancer. http://www.nccn.org/professionals/physician_gls/pdf/breast.pdf. Accessed 27 Apr 2015

Noh JM, Lee J, Choi DH et al (2013) HER-2 overexpression is not associated with increased ipsilateral breast tumor recurrence in DCIS treated with breast-conserving surgery followed by radiotherapy. Breast 22(5):894–897

Pilewskie M, Olcese C, Eaton A et al (2014) Perioperative breast MRI is not associated with lower locoregional recurrence rates in DCIS patients treated with or without radiation. Ann Surg Oncol 21(5):1552–1560

Rakovitch E, Nofech-Mozes S, Hanna W et al (2015) A population-based validation study of the DCIS Score predicting recurrence risk in individuals treated by breast conserving surgery alone. Breast Cancer Res Treat 152(2):389–398

Rakovitch E, Nofech-Mozes S, Hanna W et al (2012) HER2/neu and Ki-67 expression predict non-invasive recurrence following breast-conserving therapy for ductal carcinoma in situ. Br J Cancer 106(6):1160–1165

Rudloff U, Jacks LM, Goldberg JI et al (2010) Nomogram for predicting the risk of local recurrence after breast-conserving surgery for ductal carcinoma in situ. J Clin Oncol 28(23):3762–3769

Silverstein MJ, Lagios MD (2010) Choosing treatment for patients with ductal carcinoma in situ: fine tuning the University of Southern California/Van Nuys Prognostic Index. J Natl Cancer Inst Monogr 2010(41):193–196

Simon RM, Paik S, Hayes DF (2009) Use of archived specimens in evaluation of prognostic and predictive biomarkers. J Natl Cancer Inst 101(21):1446–1452

Sing A, Tan V, Bailey H et al (2014) The 12-gene DCIS Score™ assay and quantitative gene expression for ER, PR, and HER2: experience in the first two years. Presented at the European Society for Medical Oncology congress, Madrid, Spain, 26–30 Sept 2014 (Abstract)

Smith GL, Smith BD, Haffty BG (2006) Rationalization and regionalization of treatment for ductal carcinoma in situ of the breast. Int J Radiat Oncol Biol Phys 65(5):1397–1403

Solin LJ (2010) The impact of adding radiation treatment after breast conservation surgery for ductal carcinoma in situ of the breast. J Natl Cancer Inst Monogr 2010(41):187–192

Solin LJ, Fourquet A, Vicini FA et al (2005) Long-term outcome after breast-conservation treatment with radiation for mammographically detected ductal carcinoma in situ of the breast. Cancer 103(6):1137–1146

Solin LJ, Gray R, Baehner FL et al (2013) A multigene expression assay to predict local recurrence risk for ductal carcinoma in situ of the breast. J Natl Cancer Inst 105(10):701–710

Solin LJ, Gray R, Hughes LL et al (2015) Surgical excision without radiation for ductal carcinoma in situ of the breast: 12-year results from the ECOG-ACRIN E5194 study. J Clin Oncol 33(33):3938–3944

Solin LJ, Kurtz J, Fourquet A et al (1996) Fifteen-year results of breast-conserving surgery and definitive breast irradiation for the treatment of ductal carcinoma in situ of the breast. J Clin Oncol 14(3):754–763

Solin LJ, Orel SG, Hwang WT, Harris EE, Schnall MD (2008) Relationship of breast magnetic resonance imaging to outcome after breast-conservation treatment with radiation for women with early-stage invasive breast carcinoma or ductal carcinoma in situ. J Clin Oncol 26(3):386–391

Toussaint J, Durbecq V, Altintas S et al (2010) Low CD10 mRNA expression identifies high-risk ductal carcinoma in situ (DCIS). PLoS ONE 5(8):e12100

Wapnir IL, Dignam JJ, Fisher B et al (2011) Long-term outcomes of invasive ipsilateral breast tumor

recurrences after lumpectomy in NSABP B-17 and B-24 randomized clinical trials for DCIS. J Natl Cancer Inst 103(6):478–488
Warnberg F, Garmo H, Emdin S et al (2014) Effect of radiotherapy after breast-conserving surgery for ductal carcinoma in situ: 20 years follow-up in the randomized SweDCIS Trial. J Clin Oncol 32 (32):3613–3618
Witkiewicz AK, Cox DW, Rivadeneira D et al (2014) The retinoblastoma tumor suppressor pathway modulates the invasiveness of ErbB2-positive breast cancer. Oncogene 33(30):3980–3991
Yi M, Meric-Bernstam F, Kuerer HM et al (2012) Evaluation of a breast cancer nomogram for predicting risk of ipsilateral breast tumor recurrences in patients with ductal carcinoma in situ after local excision. J Clin Oncol 30(6):600–607
Zujewski JA, Harlan LC, Morrell DM, Stevens JL (2011) Ductal carcinoma in situ: trends in treatment over time in the US. Breast Cancer Res Treat 127(1):251–257

Prognostic and Predictive Gene Expression Signatures in Breast Cancer

18

Steven Buechler and Sunil Badve

Abstract

Breast cancer patients have varying prognoses and responses to treatment due to the heterogeneity of the disease. This chapter surveys the histopathological features, molecular markers, and multigene signatures used for prognosis and prediction of treatment response. The commercially available gene expression based assays for prognostication/prediction in ER^+ breast cancer are briefly described and critically discussed. We analyze the underlying reasons for the comparable significance of these tests at the population level, while the tests are discordant for many individual patients. The current challenges to development of future assays are discussed.

Keywords

Nottingham prognostic index · Intrinsic classification · Mammaprint Oncotype DX and Prosigna

18.1 Introduction

Breast cancer is a heterogeneous disease with diverse morphologies, molecular characteristics, clinical behavior, and response to therapeutics. This complexity makes it imperative to develop tools to determine appropriate prognostic and predictive markers that can be used by physicians and patients for informed decision making. This concept is recognized in Precision Medicine wherein each patient is considered to have a *unique* tumor. The most important prognostic markers for any cancer including breast cancer, are tumor size, lymph node status, and histological features (Elston et al. 1999). Tumor size and nodal status are time dependent variables and reflect the duration for which the tumor has been present (Elston et al. 1999). Tumor size is a good prognostic marker for distant relapse in lymph node negative patients (Clark 2004; Hilsenbeck et al. 1998). However, even patients with small

S. Buechler (✉)
Department of Applied and Computational Mathematics and Statistics, University of Notre Dame, Notre Dame, IN 46556, USA
e-mail: Buechler.1@nd.edu

S. Badve
Joshua Edwards Professor of Pathology, Indiana University School of Medicine, Indianapolis, IN, USA
e-mail: sbadve@iupui.edu

S. Badve and Y. Gökmen-Polar (eds.), *Molecular Pathology of Breast Cancer*, DOI 10.1007/978-3-319-41761-5_18

tumors (<1 cm) have a 12 % chance of recurrence (Fisher et al. 2001; Rosen et al. 1989). The measurement of tumor size is confounded by several factors such as stromal desmoplastic reaction, coexisting in situ lesions and tumor multi-centricity (Fitzgibbons et al. 2000). Nodal status is predictive of both disease free and overall survival (Fisher et al. 1993; Russo et al. 1987; Smith et al. 1977). In addition, the number of positive lymph nodes directly predicts survival (Fitzgibbons et al. 2000; Clark 2004). However, 30 % of node-negative patients still develop recurrences by 10 years (Fitzgibbons et al. 2000).

18.2 Classical Prognostic Factors

Histological classification is the morphological assessment of invasive carcinomas for the degree of differentiation and the "proximity of resemblance" to normal tissue (Elston et al. 1999). There are two components to the histological classification, type and grade (Pereira et al. 1995; Elston et al. 1999). The predominant type, invasive ductal of no special type, accounts for up to 75 % of all breast cancers; this significantly limits the use of type as a prognostic factor (Elston et al. 1999; Pereira et al. 1995). Grade provides a qualitative assessment of the biological characteristics of the tumor; e.g., high grade tumors behave aggressively and have poor prognosis, while low grade tumors have better prognosis (Henson et al. 1991; Bloom and Richardson 1957; Le Doussal et al. 1989; Neville et al. 1992). However, there is only a modest interobserver agreement in the assessment of grade varying from 59 to 65 % with greater degree of agreement for poorly differentiated tumors (Paik et al. 2004). In spite of these shortcomings, grade remains a very strong prognostic factor and so far provides data comparable to molecular signatures.

The ability to perform DNA and RNA analyses in archival formalin-fixed, paraffin-embedded (FFPE) tissues has dramatically changed the tools that can be used for prognostication. Molecular classification of breast cancer broadly classifies tumors into estrogen receptor positive tumors (luminal) and those that lack these receptors. The evaluation of estrogen and progesterone receptor (ER and PR) has been part of standard of care for several decades. The original ligand binding assays have since been replaced by immunohistochemistry (IHC) (Knight et al. 1977; Pertschuk et al. 1996). One of the important shortcomings of IHC is the dependency on pre-analytical variables such as time to fixation, method(s) used for tissue processing and antigen retrieval (Rhodes et al. 2000; Hammond et al. 2010). In spite of these disadvantages, a good correlation between IHC and RT-PCR has been documented (Badve et al. 2008). ER is strongly predictive of response to anti-estrogenic therapy; however it is a weak prognostic marker (Harvey et al. 1999). It is recognized that the correlation between the molecular ER^+ (luminal) tumors and the ER^+ by clinical (IHC) assays is not perfect. The correlation in most studies is in the order of 80 %. It is currently not clear whether Luminal tumors that do not express ER will respond to endocrine therapy. However, for the purposes of the discussions below, Luminal tumors and ER^+ tumors will be considered synonyms.

The simplest (i.e., free) multi-parametric tools to aid clinical decision making include TNM staging, Nottingham prognostic index (NPI) and Adjuvant! Online. The routinely used TNM staging comprises information on tumor size, nodal status, and metastases to determine the prognosis of a patient with breast cancer (Albain et al. 2010). The NPI is a weighted index used to predict survival in patients with breast cancer based on prognostic factors such as tumor size, lymph node stage, and histological grade (D'Eredita et al. 2001; Ravdin et al. 2001). For assessment of probability of survival and benefit from specific therapies in patients with early breast cancer, the Adjuvant! Online provides a valuable tool for clinicians (Olivotto et al. 2005). The model takes into account age, menopausal status, comorbidities, ER status, tumor grade, tumor size, and number of involved axillary nodes. The prognostication capacity of these tools depends heavily on anatomical markers like size and nodal involvement and biological characteristics such as grade and ER status. In addition, they have limited utility in providing estimates for patients in subgroups such as non-Caucasian populations, younger patients, and patients with rare histological type tumors (Cufer 2008).

18.3 Molecular Prognostic Tests in ER^+ Breast Cancer

A number of gene expression based assays are commercially available for prognostication and/or prediction in ER^+ breast cancer; these are briefly described and critically discussed (Table 18.1).

18.3.1 Intrinsic Classification/ Prosigna (Nanostring, Seattle, Washington)

The PAM50 assay is based on the Intrinsic Classification of breast cancer (Sorlie et al. 2001). The original microarray based classification was initially adapted to RT-PCR and in its current form, the assay is run on the Nanostring platform. The Prosigna test computes the Risk of Recurrence score (ROR) using a form of the PAM50 classification panel (50 genes) weighted with tumor size and a proliferation indicator (Nielsen et al. 2010; Parker et al. 2009). In the Prosigna test, ROR is computed using gene expression levels measured with the Nanostring nCounter DX Analysis System from an FFPE tissue source. Prosigna is approved by the U.S. Food and Drug Administration (FDA) for use as a prognostic indicator for 10-year distant recurrence free interval (DRFI) of postmenopausal women with stage I/II lymph node-negative or stage II lymph node-positive (one to three positive nodes) ER^+ breast cancer who have undergone surgery in conjunction with locoregional treatment consistent with standard of care. Any pathology lab having the Nanostring machine can offer this approved test.

Prosigna's prognostic significance was evaluated retrospectively using samples from the transATAC clinical trial (Dowsett et al. 2013), in comparison with Oncotype DX and the IHC4 score. After computing 10-year DRFI probabilities for each value of ROR, samples were grouped into low ROR, intermediate ROR and high ROR, with risk of distant recurrence <10, 10–20, and ≥ 20 %, respectively. In the overall transATAC study group (ER^+LN^-), the percentages of samples in these risk groups are 57.9, 25.9 and 16.1 %.

The benefit to long-term recurrence-free survival due to endocrine therapy for more than 5 years (Jakesz et al. 2007; Mamounas et al. 2008; Davies et al. 2013) has increased attention on long-term risk of recurrence. ROR has been found to be prognostic 5–10 years after diagnosis as well as up to 5 years (Filipits et al. 2014; Sestak et al. 2014).

In a study (n = 180) of ER^+HER2^- patients treated with neoadjuvant chemotherapy, ROR was found to be a statistically significant predictor of pathological complete response (Prat et al. 2015). PAM50 ROR has been analyzed in the MA.21 clinical trial in which greater prognostic benefit was noted in ER-negative tumors than ER^+ tumors (Liu et al. 2015). Compared to luminal A tumors, the hazard ratio for luminal B tumors was 1.48 (95 % CI 0.92–2.37). ROR as a continuous variable was related to recurrence free survival (RFS) in chemotherapy patients.

18.3.2 Mammaprint (Agendia, Amsterdam)

The Mammaprint test measures the mRNA levels of 70 genes in a tumor sample and reports a binary classification of *low risk* or *high risk* (van de Vijver et al. 2002; van t Veer et al. 2002). Mammaprint has been approved by the FDA as an adjuvant prognostic test for breast cancer patients under 61 years of age with stage I or II disease and no more than 3 positive lymph nodes. The test originally required fresh tissue, however, it has since received FDA clearance for a version using FFPE tissue. It is offered from Agendia's central laboratory. Mammaprint classifies approximately 50 % of patients as low risk.

Table 18.1 Molecular profiling based analysis in breast cancer

Assay	Sample type	Platform	Number of genes	Target patient population	Category	Regulatory guidelines	Performance site
Mammaprint (Agendia)	FF/FFPE	Micro-array	70	Women <61 Years, T1–T2, LN	Prognostic and predictive	FDA cleared (Frozen)	Central
Oncotype DX (Genomic Health)	FFPE	qRT-PCR	21	ER+ LN-invasive cancer	Prognostic and predictive	NCCN and ASCO	Central
Blueprint (Agendia)	FFPE	Microarray	80				
Prosigna (Nanostring)	FFPE	nCounter	50 + 5	Satge I–III post-menopausal women treated with endocrine therapy		FDA cleared	Distributed kit format
EndoPredict (Sividon diagnostics)	FFPE	qRT-PCR	12	ER+/HER2-endocrine-treated pNo/pN+women	Prognostic	CE Mark	Distributed kit format
Breast cancer index (BCI) Biotheranostics	FFPE	qRT-PCR	MGI and HOXB13:IL17BR Index	ER+pNo, endocrine treated women	Prognostic	No	Central

FF fresh-frozen; *FFPE* formalin-fixed, paraffin embedded

By design, the test can be applied to both ER^+ and ER^- tumors. However, because Mammaprint classifies almost all ER^- tumors as high risk, its clinical utility is largely limited to ER^+ breast cancer. The test has been applied to multiple clinical studies and shown to predict benefit of endocrine and chemotherapy in ER^+ cancers. More recently, its utility in predicting local regional recurrences (LRR) has also been documented (Drukker et al. 2014). In a retrospective analysis of ER^+ tumors (n = 541) from multiple sites, it has been shown that systemic chemotherapy in addition to hormone therapy only improves 5-year distant relapse-free survival in the Mammaprint high risk group (Knauer et al. 2010). In an observational study (n = 427) it is also shown that patients classified as low risk by Mammaprint have 5-year (DRFI) probability 0.97 without adjuvant chemotherapy.

The MINDACT clinical trial was designed to prospectively validate Mammaprint (Piccart-Gebhart and Sotiriou 2007; Cardoso et al. 2008). This trial accrued 6600 patients by 2011. Since the primary endpoint of the study is 5-year DRFI, results are anticipated in mid-2016. In this trial, the prognostic and predictive ability of Mammaprint is tested against that of Adjuvant! Online (https://www.adjuvantonline.com/) (Ravdin 1995).

18.3.3 Oncotype DX (Genomic Health, Inc., Redwood City, California)

The Oncotype DX assay calculates a Recurrence Score (RS, 0–100) using gene expression levels of 16 of the 21 panel genes measured by qRT-PCR (Paik et al. 2004). Oncotype DX uses an FFPE tissue source and is executed in a central pathology laboratory under the regulatory category of a Laboratory Developed Test. Genomic Health, Inc., reports that Oncotype DX has been used in over 500,000 breast cancer cases, and has it undergone extensive validation to document clinical utility and economic benefit.

Oncotype DX is typically used by assigning a patient to one of three risk groups based on the RS value: low risk ($RS < 18$), intermediate risk ($18 \leq RS \leq 30$), and high risk ($RS > 30$). The National Comprehensive Cancer Network (NCCN) guidelines recommend using Oncotype DX for ER^+HER2^-, lymph-node negative (LN^-) patients to inform the decision to treat with chemotherapy. NCCN recommends treating Low Risk patients with hormone therapy alone, High Risk patients with hormone therapy plus chemotherapy, and Intermediate Risk patients with hormone therapy and perhaps chemotherapy.

Multiple studies have shown that Oncotype DX predicts the benefit of administering chemotherapy; i.e., chemotherapy significantly increases the DFRI probability in High Risk patients, but not in Low Risk patients. The benefit of chemotherapy in the Intermediate Risk group is currently unclear. The NCI sponsored clinical trial, TAILORx, is designed to clarify the relationship between RS and prognosis and survival benefit of chemotherapy. In this trial, patients with very low risk of recurrence ($RS \leq 10$) were recommended for hormone therapy alone, patients with moderately high risk ($RS \geq 26$) were recommended to receive hormone therapy and chemotherapy, and those in the TAILORx intermediate risk group ($10 < RS < 26$) were randomized to receive chemotherapy in addition to hormone therapy. The trial enrolled 10,253 patients. Preliminary results (Sparano et al. 2015) show that the set of patients with $RS \leq 10$ (15.9 %) have excellent 5-year relapse-free survival probability (0.993 for DRFI). In the TAILORx trial, 16.9 % of patients had $RS \geq 26$.

Retrospective analysis of patients from SWOG-8814 (Albain et al. 2010) suggests that $ER^+HER2^-LN^+$ patients with $RS < 18$ do not benefit from systemic chemotherapy, and patients with $RS \geq 31$ do benefit from chemotherapy. The clinical trial SWOG S1007/RxPONDER aims to validate these earlier findings.

The impact of Oncotype DX on treatment decisions population-wide depends on the number of patients in each of the risk groups. In the original study (Paik et al. 2004), the distributions of patients are Low Risk (51 %), Intermediate Risk (22 %) and High Risk (27 %). However, the cohort used in that study included $HER2^+$ patients. Since HER2 gene expression is included in the calculation of RS, we can expect different score distributions in $HER2^+$ and $HER2^-$. In one study (Kelly et al. 2010) of clinically moderate risk patients (ER^+HER2^-, stage I/II, grade I/II), the sizes of the three risk groups are 51, 40, 9 %, respectively. This suggests that when administering Oncotype DX only for $HER2^-$ patients, in accordance with NCCN guidelines, the intermediate risk group may be larger than in the original validation studies.

In the original validation study (Paik et al. 2004), it was shown that in multivariate survival analysis, Oncotype DX adds to the prognostic significance of the standard clinical variables. A refinement of Oncotype DX intermediate risk that is statistically valid is to use the RSPC score, defined by combining clinico-pathological variables (tumor size, grade and patient age) to RS to define the RSPC score (Tang et al. 2011). The dominant effect of RSPC is to reclassify some intermediate risk samples as low risk or high risk.

18.3.4 Breast Cancer Index (BioTheranostics, San Diego, California)

The Breast Cancer Index (BCI) assay predicts the risk of distant recurrence in ER^+LN^- breast cancer using the biomarkers HOXB13 and IL17BR and 5 proliferation-related genes (Ma et al. 2008; Jankowitz et al. 2011). BCI is executed with RT-PCR using FFPE tissue from a central pathology laboratory.

The BCI test is prognostic of recurrence before 5 years, hence can be used to identify patients who can forego systemic chemotherapy. BCI is also marketed to help decide whether to treat an ER^+ breast cancer patient with hormone therapy beyond 5 years. The BCI test is superior to Oncotype DX and IHC4 in prediction of distant recurrence between 5 and 10 years after diagnosis (Sgroi et al. 2013). Moreover, BCI has been shown to predict improved long-term survival following hormone therapy beyond 5 years (Sgroi et al. 2013). Patients that BCI identifies as unlikely to benefit from extended hormone therapy may decide to forego the treatment.

18.3.5 MapQuant DX (Ipsogen, Marseilles, France)

MapQuant DX is the commercial implementation of the Genomic Grade Index (GGI) (Sotiriou et al. 2006; Sotiriou and Desmedt 2006). It is executed in a central pathology laboratory using the Affymetrix hgu133plus2 microarray and a fresh tumor sample prepared with the MapQuant Pathkit (Metzger-Filho et al. 2013). GGI uses a panel of 97 genes, largely associated with proliferation. A six-gene version has also been developed that uses RT-PCR technology and can be readily applied to FFPE samples (Toussaint et al. 2009). GGI is statistically associated with pathological complete response to neoadjuvant anthracycline-taxane based chemotherapy (Liedtke et al. 2009; Ignatiadis et al. 2012), however its ability to predict improved long-term survival following chemotherapy is unclear.

18.3.6 EndoPredict (Sividon Diagnostics GmbH, Koln, Germany)

EndoPredict test calculates a risk score from the expression levels of 8 cancer-related genes and 3 control genes using RT-PCR and FFPE tissue (Filipits et al. 2011; Dubsky et al. 2013). It is sold in Europe as a diagnostic kit for execution in local pathology laboratories. EndoPredict is prognostic of distant recurrence both before 5 years and between 5 and 10 years (Dubsky et al. 2013).

18.3.7 IHC4

The IHC4 score is defined from immunohistochemical analysis of ER, PR, HER2 and Ki67. It is derived using FFPE tissue and can be executed in a local pathology laboratory using a publicly available formula (Cuzick et al. 2011). These authors also consider a score that combine standard clinical variables with IHC4. Over 50 % of $ER^{+}LN^{-}$ samples appear to have low risk of relapse under IHC4+ clinical variables; i.e., they are predicted to have 9-year relapse-free survival probability <10 %.

The prognostic significance of IHC4 is impressive considering the simplicity of methods used. However, the between-laboratory variability of quantification by IHC raises questions about the analytical validity and reproducibility of this signature. One of the methods to circumvent this issue is to perform quantitative analysis using immunofluorescence. Recent studies seem to suggest that the fears regarding interlaboratory variability may be not as significant as originally imagined (Dodson et al. 2015). In this study, a high degree of consistency was observed between four participating labs for IHC4+ C. The IHC4+ C algorithm combines data derived from immunohistochemical assessment of expression levels of four protein markers in a patient's breast cancer tissue with clinicopathological (C) parameters to identify patients with breast cancer who are at low, intermediate, or high residual risk of distant disease recurrence, therby, aiding treatment decision-making (Barton et al. 2012).

18.4 Comparisons of Tests for ER^{+} Breast Cancer

Since all of the tests described above claim to assess the risk of distant recurrence in $ER^{+}LN^{-}$ breast cancer, it is natural to ask the following questions: (1) Why are there so many tests for the same clinical problem, without significant overlap in the gene panels? (2) Do the tests identify the same group of patients as having poor prognosis? (3) Why are these tests predominantly equivalent at the population level, but assign different prognoses to many individual patients? (4) For an individual patient, do the tests report equivalent prognoses for that patient? (5) What is a sound way to resolve intermediate risk estimates or conflicting prognoses from multiple tests? (6) Are any of these tests statistically superior to others for making treatment decisions?

18.4.1 Lack of Overlap of Gene Panel

The different prognostic signatures in $ER^{+}LN^{-}$ breast cancer share one dominant feature: they all identify high proliferation rates that increases the risk of relapse. There are hundreds of genes involved in proliferation, however research in biological networks shows that these genes are tightly coexpressed (Langfelder and Horvath 2007; Venet et al. 2011). In brief, for a fixed set of tumor samples, there is a single proliferation meta-gene to which each proliferation gene is significantly correlated. Of equal importance is the fact that this meta-gene can be closely approximated as a linear combination (weighted average) of the expression vectors of *any* sufficiently large set of proliferation genes. All of the signatures described above derive a prognostic score from a set of panel genes in linear manner; i.e., by weighted averages of the component genes. Thus, all of these scores have a common "core"; i.e., the proliferation meta-gene, even if the genes used are very different (See also Wirapati et al. 2008).

It should be noted here that the proliferation meta-gene itself is not superior to the tests described above as a prognostic score. Recurrence in ER^{+} breast cancer appears to involve more processes than proliferation. For a new test to be significantly superior to the existing tests, it must identify a gene panel *and* calculate a risk score in a fundamentally different manner.

18.4.2 Discrete Classifiers Versus Continuous Predictor

Discrete risk groups have been derived from continuous scores like RS by first computing the probability of long-term recurrence-free survival for each score value, and then grouping patients by clinically relevant thresholds. For example, the Oncotype DX thresholds for defining low, intermediate and high risk groups use RS = 18 and RS = 30, at which the 10-year distant recurrence-free survival probabilities are 0.88 and 0.80, respectively (Paik et al. 2004). When a risk score is computed in a linear fashion from panel gene expression values, there will be many samples with intermediate risk values. As a result, there may be considerable variance in how different tests classify such patients. Discrete classifiers such as Mammaprint and PAM50 give the appearance of greater precision, however there are linear methods underlying their formulas that lead to some uncertainty in the classification. In short, in a quantifiable sense, there are many samples "near the boundary".

18.4.3 Concordance Between Assays

The only way to answer the sixth question is to execute the tests on the same large sample, representative of the overall population, and study the relative significance of the tests in multivariate survival models; this has been difficult. Samples from common cohorts have been analyzed with some of these same tests (Sgroi et al. 2013; Dowsett et al. 2013). The authors perform many analyses of relative significance, which we leave to the readers to interpret. Some authors have compared versions of the tests executed on a common technology platform, e.g., Affymetrix microarrays, however differences in test performance could be attributed to the alternate technology, to an unknown degree. Statistical differences in test performance may be of only academic interest unless they translate into different treatment decisions for individual patients.

Studies comparing different tests report a disturbing degree of discordance in the prognoses of individual patients. For example, in one study (Kelly et al. 2012), luminal A tumors, which comprise the majority of low risk samples under ROR, are classified by Oncotype DX as 70 % low risk and 30 % intermediate risk. Among luminal B cancers, 33 % were high risk and 48 % were intermediate risk by Oncotype DX. Ninety percent of high-risk cases by Oncotype DX were classified as luminal B and 83 % of low-risk cases were luminal A. Tumors classified as intermediate risk with Oncotype DX were divided evenly as luminal A and luminal B by PAM50. The overlap in risk classification is certainly significant, however a large group of patients receive contradictory prognoses. More recently, Bartlett et al. performed an analysis of 6 different molecular predictors of ER^+ breast cancer in the UK-OPTIMA trial. The preliminary results (Bartlett et al. 2015) seem to suggest a poor concordance in these patients. Centrally ER and HER2 status confirmed tissue samples provided for testing with Oncotype DX, Prosigna (PAM50), Mammaprint, Mammatyper, IHC4-AQUA and IHC4 using conventional biomarkers. Each test was performed at central diagnostic laboratories (OncotypeDx, Mammaprint/Blueprint, Mammatyper) or in a central laboratory (Prosigna/IHC4) strictly according to GLP practices. Oncotype DX predicted a proportion of low-risk tumors (79; 95 % CI 73–85 %) similar to that predicted as either low or intermediate risk using Prosigna ROR_P (71; 95 % CI 64–78 %) and IHC4 (69; 95 % CI 62–76 %), whilst MammaPrint identified the fewest low-risk tumors (59; 95 % CI 52–66 %). Only 71 (39 %) tumors were classified as low/intermediate risk for all four tests [Oncotype DX, MammaPrint, Prosigna ROR_P (low/int) and IHC4 (low/int)], and only 17 (9 %) tumors were high risk for all four tests. More importantly, 93 (52 %) tumors were assigned to different risk categories by different tests.

Ignoring financial limitations, suppose that a doctor could order all of the above tests for a patient. Should a treatment decision be based on the consensus prognosis under a voting scheme? More practically, if one of the tests returns an intermediate risk assessment, what is the best approach for refining the risk prediction?

No studies have shown that a consensus voting approach gives a more precise risk assessment than any single test alone. When one test reports an intermediate risk estimate for a patient, it is tempting to "ask for second opinion" by ordering an alternative test. However, no research has shown that any test is prognostically significant on the set of samples with intermediate risk under another test. For example, the OPTIMA study reported above that half of the samples in the Oncotype DX intermediate risk group are luminal A and half are luminal B under PAM50. However, it hasn't been shown that there is a different prognosis between these two subgroups.

18.5 Late Relapse

The annual rate of recurrence is at least 2 % for 15 years for patients with ER^+ breast cancer, even after 5 years of Tamoxifen treatment (Saphner et al. 1996). Long-term management of cancer survivors requires better tools for assessing the risk of recurrence continuously over both early and late time periods. The tests described above are all significantly prognostic of recurrence for at least 5 years. However, the prognostic significance of RS and PAM50 ROR decreases significantly after 8 years in ER^+LN^- breast cancer (Sestak et al. 2013, 2014). This suggests that (1) different biological processes are driving early and late relapse, and (2) the threshold between early and late relapse in ER^+LN^- breast cancer may be approximately 8 years. In the analysis of BCI (Sgroi et al. 2013), the authors describe relapse up to 5 years as "early" and relapse between 5 and 10 years as "late", but this choice of thresholds appears to be ad hoc. None of these studies explicitly consider relapse after 10 years. Many open questions remain about risk assessment over the lifetime of a breast cancer survivor.

18.6 Future Directions

Considering the full spectrum of treatment decisions across breast cancer subtypes, molecular diagnostics is in its infancy and faces many challenges. The tests described here represent a steady stream of inventions, however, they address the same clinical utility and use similar methods. Among the greatest unmet needs, are diagnostic tests that predict sensitivity and resistance to drugs for various cancer subtypes. Following are some of the obstacles that we perceive.

1. The biological processes underlying sensitivity and resistance to drugs may be highly complex and involve many different factors. Besides representing different biological processes, these factors may be represented by different molecular species. Thus, effective signatures may require measurement of mRNA, SNPs, copy number variation and miRNA. The data and methods required to derive the signature may be significantly more complex than what have been used to date.
2. Prognostic signatures have been derived using retrospective analysis of archival data. In the retrospective analysis of patients treated with a certain form of chemotherapy, it is difficult to separate the patients who would not suffer a recurrence even without treatment, from those who the drug rescues from a recurrence. There is no specific endpoint on which to train the predictive signature. Pathological complete response as a result of neoadjuvant treatment provides a useful surrogate endpoint, however, this may not imply improved long-term survival benefit, especially in ER^+ breast cancer.
3. The methods for deriving signatures used for the existing family of products may be

inadequate to address the more difficult problem of predicting drug response. Here, new methods are likely even more important than new data.

18.7 Conclusion

The decreasing cost of whole-genome analysis (RNAseq), coupled with the recognition of its value, will likely lead to a high volume of well-annotated and publicly available data concerning response to drug treatment. New methods for generating predictive signatures, developed with strict attention to clinical utility, are likely to have a significant positive impact on individual patient care and the overall cost of cancer treatment. Molecular diagnostics coupled with the expanding number of available treatments are powerful partners for improving patient care.

References

Albain KS, Barlow WE, Shak S, Hortobagyi GN, Livingston RB, Yeh IT, Ravdin P, Bugarini R, Baehner FL, Davidson NE, Sledge GW, Winer EP, Hudis C, Ingle JN, Perez EA, Pritchard KI, Shepherd L, Gralow JR, Yoshizawa C, Allred DC, Osborne CK, Hayes DF, Breast Cancer Intergroup of North America (2010) Prognostic and predictive value of the 21-gene recurrence score assay in postmenopausal women with node-positive, oestrogen-receptor-positive breast cancer on chemotherapy: a retrospective analysis of a randomised trial. Lancet Oncol 11(1):55–65. doi:10.1016/S1470-2045(09)70314-6

Badve SS, Baehner FL, Gray RP, Childs BH, Maddala T, Liu ML, Rowley SC, Shak S, Perez EA, Shulman LJ, Martino S, Davidson NE, Sledge GW, Goldstein LJ, Sparano JA (2008) Estrogen- and progesterone-receptor status in ECOG 2197: comparison of immunohistochemistry by local and central laboratories and quantitative reverse transcription polymerase chain reaction by central laboratory. J Clin Oncol 26(15):2473–2481. doi:10.1200/JCO.2007.13.6424

Bartlett JMS et al (2015) Abstract P4-11-07: comparison of multiparameter tests in the UK OPTIMA-Prelim trial. Cancer Res 57(9 Supplement):P4-11-07

Barton S, Zabaglo L, A'Hern R, Turner N, Ferguson T, O'Neill S, Hills M, Smith I, Dowsett M (2012) Assessment of the contribution of the IHC4+ C score to decision making in clinical practice in early breast cancer. Br J Cancer 106(11):1760–1765. doi:10.1038/bjc.2012.166

Bloom HJ, Richardson WW (1957) Histological grading and prognosis in breast cancer; a study of 1409 cases of which 359 have been followed for 15 years. Br J Cancer 11(3):359–377

Cardoso F et al (2008) Clinical application of the 70-gene profile: the MINDACT trial. J Clin Oncol 26(5):729–735

Clark GM (2004) Diseases of the breast. Lippincott-Raven, Philadelphia

Cufer T (2008) Which tools can I use in daily clinical practice to improve tailoring of treatment for breast cancer? The 2007 St. Gallen guidelines and/or Adjuvant! Online. Ann Oncol 19(Suppl 7):vii41–vii45. doi:10.1093/annonc/mdn439

Cuzick J et al (2011) Prognostic value of a combined estrogen receptor, progesterone receptor, Ki-67, and human epidermal growth factor receptor 2 immunohistochemical score and comparison with the Genomic Health recurrence score in early breast cancer. J Clin Oncol 29(32):4273–4278

Davies C et al (2013) Long-term effects of continuing adjuvant tamoxifen to 10 years versus stopping at 5 years after diagnosis of oestrogen receptor-positive breast cancer: ATLAS, a randomised trial. Lancet 381 (9869):805–816

D'Eredita G, Giardina C, Martellotta M, Natale T, Ferrarese F (2001) Prognostic factors in breast cancer: the predictive value of the Nottingham prognostic index in patients with a long-term follow-up that were treated in a single institution. Eur J Cancer 37(5):591–596. doi:S0959804900004354 [pii]

Dodson A et al (2015) Risk of recurrence estimates with IHC4+C are tolerant of variations in staining and scoring: an analytical validity study. J Clin Pathol. doi:10.1136/jclinpath-2015-203212

Dowsett M et al (2013) Comparison of PAM50 risk of recurrence score with oncotype DX and IHC4 for predicting risk of distant recurrence after endocrine therapy. J Clin Oncol 31(22):2783–2790

Drukker CA, Elias SG, Nijenhuis MV, Wesseling J, Bartelink H, Elkhuizen P, Fowble B, Whitworth PW, Patel RR, de Snoo FA, van 't Veer LJ, Beitsch PD, Rutgers EJ (2014) Gene expression profiling to predict the risk of locoregional recurrence in breast cancer: a pooled analysis. Breast Cancer Res Treat 148(3):599–613. doi:10.1007/s10549-014-3188-z

Dubsky P, Brase JC et al (2013) The EndoPredict score provides prognostic information on late distant metastases in ER+/HER2- breast cancer patients. Br J Cancer 109(12):2959–2964

Dubsky P, Filipits M et al (2013) EndoPredict improves the prognostic classification derived from common clinical guidelines in ER-positive, HER2-negative early breast cancer. Ann Oncol 24(3):640–647

Elston CW, Ellis IO, Pinder SE (1999) Pathological prognostic factors in breast cancer. Crit Rev Oncol

Hematol 31(3):209–223. doi:S1040842899000347 [pii]
Filipits M et al (2011) A new molecular predictor of distant recurrence in ER-positive, HER2-negative breast cancer adds independent information to conventional clinical risk factors. Clin Cancer Res 17 (18):6012–6020
Filipits M et al (2014) The PAM50 risk-of-recurrence score predicts risk for late distant recurrence after endocrine therapy in postmenopausal women with endocrine-responsive early breast cancer. Clin Cancer Res 20(5):1298–1305
Fisher ER, Anderson S, Redmond C, Fisher B (1993) Pathologic findings from the National Surgical Adjuvant Breast Project protocol B-06. 10-year pathologic and clinical prognostic discriminants. Cancer 71 (8):2507–2514
Fisher B, Dignam J, Tan-Chiu E, Anderson S, Fisher ER, Wittliff JL, Wolmark N (2001) Prognosis and treatment of patients with breast tumors of one centimeter or less and negative axillary lymph nodes. J Natl Cancer Inst 93(2):112–120
Fitzgibbons PL, Page DL, Weaver D, Thor AD, Allred DC, Clark GM, Ruby SG, O'Malley F, Simpson JF, Connolly JL, Hayes DF, Edge SB, Lichter A, Schnitt SJ (2000) Prognostic factors in breast cancer. College of American Pathologists Consensus Statement 1999. Arch Pathol Lab Med 124(7):966–978
Hammond ME, Hayes DF, Dowsett M, Allred DC, Hagerty KL, Badve S, Fitzgibbons PL, Francis G, Goldstein NS, Hayes M, Hicks DG, Lester S, Love R, Mangu PB, McShane L, Miller K, Osborne CK, Paik S, Perlmutter J, Rhodes A, Sasano H, Schwartz JN, Sweep FC, Taube S, Torlakovic EE, Valenstein P, Viale G, Visscher D, Wheeler T, Williams RB, Wittliff JL, Wolff AC (2010) American Society of Clinical Oncology/College Of American Pathologists guideline recommendations for immunohistochemical testing of estrogen and progesterone receptors in breast cancer. J Clin Oncol 28(16):2784–2795. doi:10.1200/JCO.2009.25.6529
Harvey JM, Clark GM, Osborne CK, Allred DC (1999) Estrogen receptor status by immunohistochemistry is superior to the ligand-binding assay for predicting response to adjuvant endocrine therapy in breast cancer. J Clin Oncol 17(5):1474–1481
Henson DE, Ries L, Freedman LS, Carriaga M (1991) Relationship among outcome, stage of disease, and histologic grade for 22,616 cases of breast cancer. The basis for a prognostic index. Cancer 68(10):2142–2149
Hilsenbeck SG, Ravdin PM, de Moor CA, Chamness GC, Osborne CK, Clark GM (1998) Time-dependence of hazard ratios for prognostic factors in primary breast cancer. Breast Cancer Res Treat 52(1–3):227–237
Ignatiadis M et al (2012) Gene modules and response to neoadjuvant chemotherapy in breast cancer subtypes: a pooled analysis. J Clin Oncol 30(16):1996–2004
Jakesz R et al (2007) Extended adjuvant therapy with anastrozole among postmenopausal breast cancer patients: results from the randomized Austrian Breast and Colorectal Cancer Study Group Trial 6a. J Natl Cancer Inst 99(24):1845–1853
Jankowitz RC et al (2011) Prognostic utility of the breast cancer index and comparison to Adjuvant! Online in a clinical case series of early breast cancer. Breast Cancer Res 13(5):R98
Kelly CM et al (2010) Utility of oncotype DX risk estimates in clinically intermediate risk hormone receptor-positive, HER2-normal, grade II, lymph node-negative breast cancers. Cancer 116(22):5161–5167
Kelly CM et al (2012) Agreement in risk prediction between the 21-gene recurrence score assay (Oncotype DX®) and the PAM50 breast cancer intrinsic Classifier™ in early-stage estrogen receptor-positive breast cancer. Oncologist 17(4):492–498
Knauer M et al (2010) The predictive value of the 70-gene signature for adjuvant chemotherapy in early breast cancer. Breast Cancer Res Treat 120(3):655–661
Knight WA, Livingston RB, Gregory EJ, McGuire WL (1977) Estrogen receptor as an independent prognostic factor for early recurrence in breast cancer. Cancer Res 37(12):4669–4671
Langfelder P, Horvath S (2007) Eigengene networks for studying the relationships between co-expression modules. BMC Syst Biol 1:54
Le Doussal V, Tubiana-Hulin M, Friedman S, Hacene K, Spyratos F, Brunet M (1989) Prognostic value of histologic grade nuclear components of Scarff-Bloom-Richardson (SBR). An improved score modification based on a multivariate analysis of 1262 invasive ductal breast carcinomas. Cancer 64 (9):1914–1921
Liedtke C et al (2009) Genomic grade index is associated with response to chemotherapy in patients with breast cancer. J Clin Oncol 27(19):3185–3191
Liu S, Chapman JA, Burnell MJ, Levine MN, Pritchard KI, Whelan TJ, Rugo HS, Albain KS, Perez EA, Virk S, Barry G, Gao D, O'Brien P, Shepherd LE, Nielsen TO, Gelmon KA (2015) Prognostic and predictive investigation of PAM50 intrinsic subtypes in the NCIC CTG MA.21 phase III chemotherapy trial. Breast Cancer Res Treat 149 (2):439–448. doi:10.1007/s10549-014-3259-1
Ma X-J et al (2008) A five-gene molecular grade index and HOXB13:IL17BR are complementary prognostic factors in early stage breast cancer. Clin Cancer Res 14(9):2601–2608
Mamounas EP et al (2008) Benefit from exemestane as extended adjuvant therapy after 5 years of adjuvant tamoxifen: intention-to-treat analysis of the National Surgical Adjuvant Breast and Bowel Project B-33 trial. J Clin Oncol 26(12):1965–1971
Metzger-Filho O et al (2013) Genomic Grade Index (GGI): feasibility in routine practice and impact on treatment decisions in early breast cancer. In: Glynn SA (ed) vol 8(8). PLoS ONE, pp e66848

Neville AM, Bettelheim R, Gelber RD, Save-Soderbergh J, Davis BW, Reed R, Torhorst J, Golouh R, Peterson HF, Price KN et al (1992) Factors predicting treatment responsiveness and prognosis in node-negative breast cancer. The International (Ludwig) Breast Cancer Study Group. J Clin Oncol 10 (5):696–705

Nielsen TO et al (2010) A comparison of PAM50 intrinsic subtyping with immunohistochemistry and clinical prognostic factors in tamoxifen-treated estrogen receptor-positive breast cancer. Clin Cancer Res 16 (21):5222–5232

Olivotto IA, Bajdik CD, Ravdin PM, Speers CH, Coldman AJ, Norris BD, Davis GJ, Chia SK, Gelmon KA (2005) Population-based validation of the prognostic model ADJUVANT! for early breast cancer. J Clin Oncol 23(12):2716–2725. doi:10.1200/JCO.2005.06.178 23/12/2716 [pii]

Paik S, Shak S, Tang G, Kim C, Baker J, Cronin M, Baehner FL, Walker MG, Watson D, Park T, Hiller W, Fisher ER, Wickerham DL, Bryant J, Wolmark N (2004) A multigene assay to predict recurrence of tamoxifen-treated, node-negative breast cancer. N Engl J Med 351(27):2817–2826. NEJMoa041588 [pii]. doi:10.1056/NEJMoa041588

Pereira H, Pinder SE, Sibbering DM, Galea MH, Elston CW, Blamey RW, Robertson JF, Ellis IO (1995) Pathological prognostic factors in breast cancer. IV: should you be a typer or a grader? A comparative study of two histological prognostic features in operable breast carcinoma. Histopathology 27(3):219–226

Parker JS et al (2009) Supervised risk predictor of breast cancer based on intrinsic subtypes. J Clin Oncol 27 (8):1160–1167

Pertschuk LP, Feldman JG, Kim YD, Braithwaite L, Schneider F, Braverman AS, Axiotis C (1996) Estrogen receptor immunocytochemistry in paraffin embedded tissues with ER1D5 predicts breast cancer endocrine response more accurately than H222Sp gamma in frozen sections or cytosol-based ligand-binding assays. Cancer 77(12):2514–2519. doi:10.1002/(SICI)1097-0142(19960615)77:12<2514::AID-CNCR14>3.0.CO;2-V [pii] 10.1002/(SICI)1097-0142(19960615)77:12<2514::AID-CNCR14>3.0.CO;2-V

Piccart-Gebhart MJ, Sotiriou C (2007) Adjuvant chemotherapy—yes or no? Prognostic markers in early breast cancer. Ann Oncol 18(Suppl 12):xii2–7

Prat A et al (2015) Prediction of response to neoadjuvant chemotherapy using core needle biopsy samples with the prosigna assay. Clin Cancer Res. doi:10.1158/1078-0432.CCR-15-0630

Ravdin PM (1995) A computer based program to assist in adjuvant therapy decisions for individual breast cancer patients. Bull Cancer 82(Suppl 5):561s–564s

Ravdin PM, Siminoff LA, Davis GJ, Mercer MB, Hewlett J, Gerson N, Parker HL (2001) Computer program to assist in making decisions about adjuvant therapy for women with early breast cancer. J Clin Oncol 19(4):980–991

Rhodes A, Jasani B, Balaton AJ, Miller KD (2000) Immunohistochemical demonstration of oestrogen and progesterone receptors: correlation of standards achieved on in house tumours with that achieved on external quality assessment material in over 150 laboratories from 26 countries. J Clin Pathol 53 (4):292–301

Rosen PP, Groshen S, Saigo PE, Kinne DW, Hellman S (1989) Pathological prognostic factors in stage I (T1N0M0) and stage II (T1N1M0) breast carcinoma: a study of 644 patients with median follow-up of 18 years. J Clin Oncol 7(9):1239–1251

Russo J, Frederick J, Ownby HE, Fine G, Hussain M, Krickstein HI, Robbins TO, Rosenberg B (1987) Predictors of recurrence and survival of patients with breast cancer. Am J Clin Pathol 88(2):123–131

Saphner T, Tormey DC, Gray R (1996) Annual hazard rates of recurrence for breast cancer after primary therapy. J Clin Oncol 14(10):2738–2746

Sestak I et al (2013) Factors predicting late recurrence for estrogen receptor-positive breast cancer. J Natl Cancer Inst 105(19):1504–1511

Sestak I et al (2014) Prediction of late distant recurrence after 5 years of endocrine treatment: a combined analysis of patients from the austrian breast and colorectal cancer study group 8 and arimidex, tamoxifen alone or in combination randomized trials using the PAM50 risk of recurrence score. J Clin Oncol 16 (8):916-922

Sgroi DC, Carney E et al (2013) Prediction of late disease recurrence and extended adjuvant letrozole benefit by the HOXB13/IL17BR biomarker. J Natl Cancer Inst 105(14):1036–1042

Sgroi DC, Sestak I et al (2013) Prediction of late distant recurrence in patients with oestrogen-receptor-positive breast cancer: a prospective comparison of the breast-cancer index (BCI) assay, 21-gene recurrence score, and IHC4 in the TransATAC study population. Lancet Oncol 14(11):1067–1076

Smith JA 3rd, Gamez-Araujo JJ, Gallager HS, White EC, McBride CM (1977) Carcinoma of the breast: analysis of total lymph node involvement versus level of metastasis. Cancer 39(2):527–532

Sorlie T et al (2001) Gene expression patterns of breast carcinomas distinguish tumor subclasses with clinical implications. Proc Natl Acad Sci U S A 98 (19):10869–10874

Sotiriou C, Desmedt C (2006) Gene expression profiling in breast cancer. Ann Oncol 17(Suppl 10):x259–62

Sotiriou C et al (2006) Gene expression profiling in breast cancer: understanding the molecular basis of histologic grade to improve prognosis. J Natl Cancer Inst 98(4):262–272

Sparano JA et al (2015) Prospective validation of a 21-gene expression assay in breast cancer. N Engl J Med 151015072327001

Tang G et al (2011) Risk of recurrence and chemotherapy benefit for patients with node-negative, estrogen receptor-positive breast cancer: recurrence score alone and integrated with pathologic and clinical factors. J Clin Oncol 29(33):4365–4372

Toussaint J et al (2009) Improvement of the clinical applicability of the Genomic Grade Index through a qRT-PCR test performed on frozen and formalin-fixed paraffin-embedded tissues. BMC Genomics 10(1):424

van de Vijver MJ et al (2002) A gene-expression signature as a predictor of survival in breast cancer. N Engl J Med 347(25):1999–2009

van t Veer LJ et al (2002) Gene expression profiling predicts clinical outcome of breast cancer. Nature 415 (6871):530–536

Venet D, Dumont JE, Detours V (2011) Most random gene expression signatures are significantly associated with breast cancer outcome. In: Rigoutsos I (ed) PLoS Comput Biol 7(10):e1002240

Wirapati P et al (2008) Meta-analysis of gene expression profiles in breast cancer: toward a unified understanding of breast cancer subtyping and prognosis signatures. Breast Cancer Res 10(4):R65

Genomic Markers in ER-Negative Breast Cancer

19

Thomas Karn and Christos Hatzis

Abstract

In this chapter, we will cover the role and value of genomic markers in the ER-negative subset of breast cancer. Such genomic markers encompass several different types of molecular alterations. The markers may represent proteins that can be detected by immunohistochemistry, as for example the progesterone receptor (PR), the androgen receptor (AR), or HER2. Other types of genomic markers included in this overview are markers based on gene expression data obtained from profiling breast tumor mRNA or small RNAs, as well as respective genomic tests based on such expression profiles. Furthermore, mutations in cancer genes, either hereditary or somatic, will also be covered in this chapter because of their potential prognostic and predictive value. Those mutations may represent single altered genes or mutational patterns or structural variations that have been identified through recent whole genome sequencing efforts. Regarding the value of genomic markers in ER-negative breast cancer, we distinguish between risk factors for cancer susceptibility on the one hand, and factors with prognostic or predictive value on the other. Finally, we discuss the important but complex role that immune infiltration may have in ER-negative breast cancer. What we do not cover however, are standard clinicopathologic factors, such as histopathological grading or age, which undoubtedly also have an important prognostic role in addition to the genomic markers discussed here.

T. Karn
Department of Obstetrics and Gynecology, University Hospital Frankfurt, Theodor-Stern-Kai 7, 60590 Frankfurt, Germany
e-mail: t.karn@em.uni-frankfurt.de

C. Hatzis (✉)
Yale School of Medicine, Yale Cancer Center, 333 Cedar Street, PO Box 208032, New Haven, CT 06520-8032, USA
e-mail: christos.hatzis@yale.edu

S. Badve and Y. Gökmen-Polar (eds.), *Molecular Pathology of Breast Cancer*, DOI 10.1007/978-3-319-41761-5_19

Keywords
Breast cancer · ER negative · Triple negative subtype · HER2 subtype · Genomic markers · Prognosis · Gene expression signatures · Mutation signatures · Prognosis · Tumor infiltrating lymphocytes

19.1 Breast Cancer Subtypes

Breast cancer is a heterogeneous disease consisting of different molecular subtypes, each having a distinct natural history and clinical behavior. These subtypes are recognized based on histological characteristics as well as on molecular markers (Weigelt and Reis-Filho 2009). Currently, the simplest and clinically most useful stratification of breast cancer is based on expression of the hormone receptors for both estrogen (ER) and progesterone (PgR) as well as the human epidermal growth factor receptor 2 (HER2) determined by immunohistochemistry (IHC) methods (Sotiriou and Pusztai 2009). Based on these three receptors, tumors are characterized as hormone receptor–positive, HER2-positive (i.e., amplification or overexpression of HER2), or triple-negative breast cancer (TNBC) lacking the expression of all three receptors. In addition several refined stratifications applying genomic methods or the inclusion of additional immunohistochemical markers (e.g., Ki67) allow the distinction of "Basal-like" breast cancers as well as "Luminal A" and "Luminal B" subgroups each with different prognosis and clinical behaviour (Perou et al. 2000; van't Veer et al. 2002; Prat et al. 2012; Reis-Filho and Pusztai 2011; Kaufmann et al. 2011). The basal-like and HER2-like subtypes are highly proliferative and have a poor prognosis if untreated, but exhibit an increased sensitivity to chemotherapy (Perou et al. 2000; Sorlie et al. 2001; Rouzier et al. 2005; Rody et al. 2007). Still the additional clinical value of molecular classification is limited by its close correspondence with the status of ER, PR, and HER2, along with tumor grade (Sotiriou and Pusztai 2009). Relatively high concordance (75–90 %) exists between molecular subtypes as defined by genomic methods and IHC phenotype (Reis-Filho and Pusztai 2011). Following either of these subtyping methods, the main two classes of ER-negative breast cancers are triple-negative or basal-like cancers on one hand, and HER2-positive cancers on the other. These two subtypes are fundamentally different in their biology and current clinical management and thus should be considered separately. This is of major importance given the lack of targeted therapies for TNBC and the various HER2-targeted therapeutic approaches. Consequently, HER2 amplification represents the most important genomic marker in ER-negative breast cancer to distinguish HER2-positive from triple-negative disease.

19.2 Hormone Receptor Subtypes Within ER-Negative BC

Expression of the steroid hormone receptors (HR) has long been recognized as important in the clinical management of breast cancer, having both prognostic and predictive implications for endocrine therapy. The American Society of Clinical Oncology and the College of American Pathologists recommend testing for both estrogen receptor (ER) and progesterone receptor (PR) on all newly diagnosed invasive breast cancer cases (Hammond et al. 2010). Although the importance of ER expression is well established, the clinical significance of PR expression remains controversial, especially in ER-negative breast cancer. PR expression has been hypothesized to be associated with good prognosis in certain types of HR-negative invasive carcinoma, such as adenoid cystic carcinoma and secretory carcinoma, which generally have excellent prognosis (Rakha et al. 2007b). Compared to ER−/PR−

tumors, ER−/PR+ tumors appear to have a more favorable prognosis, lower proliferation and absence of vascular invasion, but no significant difference in overall survival (Rakha et al. 2007b). In a large meta-analysis of 21,457 women with early stage breast cancer from 20 randomized trials with adjuvant tamoxifen, PR expression was not predictive of benefit from tamoxifen treatment in ER-negative breast cancer, although there was a slight early benefit from tamoxifen in ER−/PR+, but it was not statistically significant (Early Breast Cancer Trialists' Collaborative et al. 2011).

The conflicting results have raised the possibility that the ER−/PR+ classification is primarily a technical artifact caused by false-negative ER results (De Maeyer et al. 2008). In fact, with the more recent definitions of ER-positivity as minimal (1 %) ER expression, the proportion of cases reported as ER−/PR+ have decreased from about 4 % in the early 1990s to only 1 % in the recent SEER cancer registry data (Early Breast Cancer Trialists' Collaborative et al. 2011). A recent study that integrated gene expression and clinicopathologic data from 20 studies reported that PR is among the least variably expressed genes in ER-negative breast cancer and that ER−/PR+ is by far the least reproducible subtype by a secondary method (Hefti et al. 2013). Therefore, given the rarity and the questionable biological significance of the ER−/PR + phenotype, the clinical use of PR expression in ER− breast cancer is uncertain (Olivotto et al. 2004).

In addition to ER and PR, another nuclear steroid hormone receptor, the androgen receptor (AR), is widely expressed in 70–90 % of all breast cancers (Brys 2000). The role of AR as a prognostic factor or as a potential therapeutic target in breast cancer is controversial and depends on the ER status (Fioretti et al. 2014; Shah et al. 2013). In ER/PR-positive tumors expressing AR, activation of AR with the androgen dihydrotestosterone appears to decrease estrogen-dependent signaling, likely through translocation to the nucleus and competition with ER and PR for binding to the estrogen-related elements, thus reducing cell survival and promoting apoptosis. In ER-negative breast cancer, expression of AR varies widely from 9 to 50 %, and about 10–40 % of TNBC express AR (Shah et al. 2013). The effect of AR expression remains rather controversial. Molecular profiling had identified a subgroup of ER-negative/AR-positive breast tumors that had histological apocrine features and was termed the molecular apocrine subtype (Farmer et al. 2005b). This subgroup demonstrated a molecular profile consistent with increased androgen signaling and which resembled that of ER-positive tumors. Based on this, it was hypothesized that signaling though AR replaces, or at least mimics, ER-signaling and transcriptional activation through involvement of the transcription factor FOXA1 (Robinson et al. 2011) promoting cell growth. Furthermore, AR expression appears to be particularly enriched in ER-negative/HER2-positive tumors (Niemeier et al. 2010). In ER-negative/HER2-positive tumors expressing AR, androgens and AR can stimulate oncogenic Wnt and HER2 signaling pathways by FOXA1-dependent transcriptional upregulation of WNT7B and HER3 (Ni et al. 2011). These studies provided justification for targeting AR as a therapeutic strategy in patients with ER-negative or ER-negative/HER2-positive disease. A recent single-arm phase II study that evaluated the effect of the antiandrogen bicalutamide in ER-negative/PR-negative metastatic breast cancers expressing AR reported a 6-month clinical benefit rate of 19 % (Gucalp et al. 2013). TNBC tumors expressing AR also appear to be associated with a significantly higher frequency of activating PIK3CA mutations (40 vs. 4 % in AR-negative) and concurrent amplification of the PIK3CA locus, suggesting the use of AR antagonists in combination with PI3K/mTOR inhibitors as a potentially effective treatment strategy (Lehmann et al. 2014). However, these strategies have yet to be tested in the clinic.

Several studies have investigated the prognostic and predictive value of AR expression in ER-negative breast cancer, but the results appear conflicting (Shah et al. 2013; Vera-Badillo et al. 2014). In an ER-negative cohort of 303 post-menopausal women derived from the Nurses'

Health Study, 43 % of these tumors were AR-positive, but no significant association was found between AR expression and breast cancer specific mortality (Hu et al. 2011). In another cohort of 287 patients with resectable TNBC, 26 % of the cases were AR-positive and these patients had disease free survival that was significantly longer than that of patients with AR-negative breast cancer (He et al. 2012). Another single-institution study involving 282 TNBC tumors, AR expression was demonstrated in 13 % of the cases. Absence of AR expression was significantly associated with higher histologic grade, recurrence and development of distant metastases (Rakha et al. 2007a). A meta-analysis of 19 studies involving 7693 women with breast cancer reported expression of AR in 32 % of the ER-negative cases. Among ER-negative cases, there was a trend towards better 5-year overall (OS) and disease free survival (DFS) with AR expression, but the association did not reach statistical significance in either case (Vera-Badillo et al. 2014). In terms of predictive effects, results from the GeparTrio trial of early stage breast cancer women treated with neoadjuvant docetaxel/doxorubicin/cyclophosphamide, showed that among TNBC patients who achieved complete pathologic response (pCR), those with AR-positive tumors had a DFS of 100 % compared to 79 % of AR-negative tumors (Loibl et al. 2011). However, AR status was not a significant predictor of pCR rate in TNBC, as AR-positive TNBC tumors had a pCR rate of 29 % compared to 33 % in AR-negative TNBC tumors (Loibl et al. 2011). Overall, an emerging volume of evidence suggests that AR plays an important role in carcinogenesis and, as such, it could be a significant prognostic factor and may be further exploited as a novel therapeutic target in ER− disease. However, the plethora of controversial results suggests that further standardization in the estimation of AR expression, scoring systems and cut-off values would be required (Anestis et al. 2015).

19.3 Gene Expression Based Genomic Markers in Different Breast Cancer Subtypes

The clinical utility of currently available genomic tests in ER-negative breast cancer is limited since their main value is in the prognostic stratification of luminal ER-positive tumors (Prat et al. 2012; Cobain and Hayes 2015). For example, the Amsterdam 70-gene signature (Mammaprint) and the Oncotype recurrence score classify almost all ER-negative cancers as high risk. Similarly, the Genomic Grade Index, Breast Cancer Index, and EndoPredict assays are useful only in ER-positive patients (Prat et al. 2012; Gyorffy et al. 2015). While most available multigene prognostic gene signatures may provide standardized, complementary information to routine pathological variables that could assist therapeutic decision-making in ER-positive cancers, they have only very limited utility in ER-negative disease. One reason may be that these so called "first generation signatures" were developed in mixed cohorts including different subtypes, the majority of which being ER positive (Sotiriou and Pusztai 2009). It became increasingly clear that the subtype composition of a dataset can strongly influence the prognostic and predictive gene signatures derived from it (Weigelt et al. 2012). Often these "first generation" signatures represent a surrogate marker for the subtype distinction itself (Prat et al. 2012; Reis-Filho and Pusztai 2011). As a consequence subsequent guidelines have suggested to analyze subtypes of breast cancers separately and to derive subtype-specific genomic tests (Kaufmann et al. 2011; Goldhirsch et al. 2011). However, it has even been suggested that information on some problems may be lacking from the gene expression space (Hess et al. 2011), particularly for ER negative breast cancer that appears to be transcriptionally more heterogeneous than other subtypes (Jiang et al. 2014; Tofigh et al. 2014).

19.4 Gene Expression Signatures Developed in ER-Negative Breast Cancer

The realization that the different subtypes of breast cancer are fundamentally distinct in their transcriptional profiles led several groups to investigate these subgroups separately, leading to so-called second generation signatures (Reis-Filho and Pusztai 2011; Alexe et al. 2007; Teschendorff et al. 2007; Finak et al. 2008; Desmedt et al. 2008; Bianchini et al. 2010a; Lehmann et al. 2011; Hatzis et al. 2011; Rody et al. 2011; Karn et al. 2011). Some second generation prognostic signatures for TNBC could identify a subset of cases that had good prognosis when treated with standard of care chemotherapy, but since 20–25 % of these cases were predicted to relapse within 5 years, the clinical utility of these signatures was rather limited (Hatzis et al. 2011). Many of these studies identified immune cell infiltration as an important component for prognosis and prediction in ER-negative subtypes. In triple-negative breast cancer, studies also identified several subgroups besides immune cell components that can be clearly separated based on transcriptional profiles. Triple-negative disease seems to be composed of basal-like cancers, a molecular apocrine group, and the claudin-low subtype (Farmer et al. 2005b; Lehmann et al. 2011; Rody et al. 2011; Prat et al. 2010; Burstein et al. 2015). Potential therapeutic relevance of these subgroups has been suggested (Vidula and Rugo 2015; Ng et al. 2015). In contrast to these relatively stable separable groups, immune cell infiltration seems to represent a rather continuous parameter and may be detected within all three of these subgroups (Rody et al. 2011; Denkert et al. 2010; Karn et al. 2015). For ER-negative/HER2-positive disease, an important role of immune cells has also been demonstrated (Alexe et al. 2007; Ignatiadis et al. 2012; Loi et al. 2014; Denkert et al. 2015). Yet, despite refinements in the definition of ER-negative subtypes, the efforts to define clinically useful prognostic signatures in ER-negative breast cancer have had limited success (Pusztai et al. 2015).

19.5 The Role of Immune Cell Infiltration as a Marker in ER-Negative Breast Cancer

Until recently, molecular and clinical subtyping of breast cancer was solely based on the molecular features of the cancer cells without considering the importance of stromal components, such as tumor infiltrating immune cells (Perou et al. 2000; Kaufmann et al. 2011). However, an association between cancer and immune response components has long been observed (Balkwill and Mantovani 2001). Different immune cells may have either anti-tumor or tumor-promoting effects (Grivennikov et al. 2010). It is also important to recognize that the role of tumor infiltrating lymphocytes (TILs) can differ by breast cancer subtype (Karn et al. 2011; Cancer Genome Atlas Network 2012). Gene expression signal originating from immune cells is easily recognized in high throughput transcriptional profiling data, and the first microarray analyses of breast cancer tissues had already described signatures of TILs (Perou et al. 1999, 2000; Hu et al. 2006). Later on, several larger microarray studies with clinical follow up and meta-analyses revealed the strong positive prognostic value of immune signatures in ER-negative tumors (Desmedt et al. 2008; Lehmann et al. 2011; Rody et al. 2009, 2011; Schmidt et al. 2008; Bianchini et al. 2010b; Nagalla et al. 2013). The prognostic significance of immune signatures was subsequently validated with direct histological and immunohistochemical assessment of TILs and other immune components and are also in line with several earlier studies (Loi et al. 2013, 2014; Adams et al. 2014; Aaltomaa et al. 1992; Menard et al. 1997). The common theme that emerges from all these studies is a significant association of an increasing number of TILs at the tumor stroma with improved patient prognosis. It should be noted that both the presence of immune cell infiltration and its prognostic value are characteristics mainly of ER-negative cancers (Karn et al. 2015). Moreover, increased presence of TILs has been found to be predictive of improved response to neoadjuvant chemotherapy, again mainly in ER-negative tumors

(Denkert et al. 2010; Issa-Nummer et al. 2013). Finally, for HER2-positive disease, there appears to be an association of lymphocyte infiltration with benefit from trastuzumab (Loi et al. 2013; Perez et al. 2015). Thus, the "prognostic" value of TILs in ER-negative breast cancer may result from "pure prognostic" or "pure predictive" effects or a combination of both.

19.6 Complexity of Immune Cell Markers in ER-Negative Breast Cancer

Although immune gene signatures can stratify patients with ER-negative disease in terms of survival outcomes, the use of this information in clinical decision making is rather limited. Even in those patients classified as having a better prognosis, the number of relapses within 5 years remains sufficiently high to justify adjuvant chemotherapy. However, the interplay between tumor and immune system is complex because of the multiple opposing signals and feedback loops that coexist between various immune cells and cancer cells (Grivennikov et al. 2010). Therefore, subtypes of lymphocytes, macrophages, granulocytes, and antigen presenting cells may need to be considered separately when evaluating the prognostic and predictive value of the immune system. Specific metagene signatures for specialized T- and B-lymphocytes, and cells of the dendritic or macrophage/monocyte lineage have been used for this purpose (Rody et al. 2009, 2011; Schmidt et al. 2008; Bianchini et al. 2010b; Gu-Trantien et al. 2013). Similarly, large immunohistochemical studies with specific antibodies to track individual immune system components have also been performed (Karn et al. 2015). However, in most tumors co-infiltration by many different types of immune cells has been observed (Rody et al. 2009; Ruffell et al. 2012) resulting in high inter-correlation of all immune markers. Even markers linked to immunosuppressive activity, such as PD-1, PD-L1, CTLA4, show a significant positive correlation with other immune markers and with TILs (Denkert et al. 2015). These findings fit well with the intercorrelated nature of local immune biomarkers that may result from feedback loops between immune activation and suppression. Antithetical effects on prognosis have been observed for some types of immune cells, such as CD68+ and CD4+ cells, allowing their use as a combined prognostic score (Ruffell et al. 2012). Likewise, the combination of a B-cell metagene associated with good prognosis with the opposing effect of an IL-8 metagene resulted in a clinically relevant gene signature for triple-negative and basal-like breast cancer (Rody et al. 2011; Hanker et al. 2013). On the other hand, modulation of T-cell response has demonstrated clinical efficacy in solid tumors (Topalian et al. 2012). Examples include new therapeutic antibodies that unleash the antitumor properties of the immune system effectively as ipilimumab, or antibodies that block PD1 (programmed cell death 1) and PD-L1 (programmed cell death 1 ligand 1) (Herbst et al. 2014). Current results allow monitoring potential antitumor immunity in breast cancer, but we are not yet able to reliably monitor the immunosuppressive activity in the tumor immune infiltrate. Therefore, the clinical utility of immune markers in ER-negative cancer still remains marginal, but may have a greater potential in combination with the upcoming immune therapeutic approaches.

19.7 Gene Mutations as Markers in ER-Negative Breast Cancer

An additional class of genomic markers are individual mutational changes within cancer genes. In general, two types of gene mutations can contribute to cancer. Somatic mutations that occur during lifetime and generate a founder cell of a cancer or a tumor subclone (Stratton 2011), as well as germline mutations in cancer predisposition genes, that are present in all cells and increase the risk of cancer (Rahman 2014b). Examples of the latter include the BRCA1 and BRCA2 genes. The benefits of determining whether a cancer is caused by a hereditary germline mutation could be undeniable (Rahman 2014b; Narod 2010). For patients, it may provide better understanding of the genetic causes of their cancer and the higher cancer risk would justify prophylactic testing of other family members. It can also provide important information for disease management regarding surgery, radiotherapy, and chemotherapy (Narod 2010; Trainer et al. 2010). For example, platinum-based treatment is not standard for breast cancer, but can have utility in BRCA mutation carriers (Byrski et al. 2012; Turner and Tutt 2012; Foulkes and Shuen 2013). Moreover, BRCA deficiency is the basis for the synthetic lethality approach exemplified by PARP inhibitors (Foulkes and Shuen 2013; Fong et al. 2009; Farmer et al. 2005a). Testing for BRCA1 mutations in patients with breast cancer has been referred to as medical genetic testing in contrast to predictive genetic testing aimed to estimate cancer risk in unaffected people (Rahman 2014a). BRCA1 mutation frequency of 2–3 % has been reported in women with breast cancer (Malone et al. 2006) but may increase to more than 10 % among younger patients with triple-negative disease (Narod 2010; Trainer et al. 2010). This highlights the importance of BRCA1 deficiency as a genomic marker in ER negative, and especially triple-negative breast cancer. With the advent of next generation sequencing (NGS) methods (Shendure and Ji 2008) faster and more affordable testing now allows eligibility criteria to be relaxed and results to be delivered within the timeframe required to impact cancer management (Rahman 2014a). Besides the BRCA genes, a handful of rare, highly penetrant genes, including TP53, PTEN, LKB1, as well as more frequent low penetrance genes, such as CHECK2, ATM, PALB, have been described as hereditary factors associated with breast cancer (Chung and Chanock 2011). However, a clinically useful genomic marker in breast cancer would require that the respective mutation affects patient prognosis or impacts her therapeutic management. In addition to cancer predisposing genes which may also have an impact on prognosis (Fasching et al. 2012) there is additional interest in the genetic background that could result in variation in drug-response phenotypes based on metabolism, transportation elimination affecting both efficacy and toxicity of a drug (Wang et al. 2011; McLeod 2013). Such germline DNA variants may help optimize cancer drug dosing and adverse side effects to improve benefit/risk ratio of cancer treatment. This field is referred to as pharmacogenetics or pharmacogenomics. Important examples of predictive factors regarding targeted treatment have been identified in other cancers, but no validated pharmacogenomic markers for ER-negative breast cancer are yet available since those studies involve major challenges which are currently beginning to be addressed (Wang et al. 2011; McLeod 2013).

19.8 Somatically Mutated Genes in ER-Negative Breast Cancer

As already addressed, the clinically most important somatically mutated gene and genomic marker in ER-negative breast cancer is the expression of HER2, altered mainly through gene amplification, but also by activating mutations (Bose et al. 2013). Nevertheless, fueled by dramatic improvements in sequencing power and falling costs in the last decade, cancer genome sequencing projects have vastly increased our knowledge about the presence and frequency of somatic mutations in cancer. Such somatic mutations are identified by comparing tumor DNA with germline sequence obtained. e.g., from peripheral blood lymphocytes. Somatic mutations may be distinguished as either 'driver' mutations conferring a selective growth advantage to the cancer cells or 'passenger' mutations (Garraway and Lander 2013). Although this definition is simple in principle, it is more difficult to clearly identify, which somatic mutations belong into each category (Vogelstein et al. 2013). Passengers encompass all those neutral mutations that have been accumulated during normal development in the founder cell of the tumor, before the oncogenic event had occurred (Shibata 2012). These passenger mutations seem to account for roughly half of the mutations found in a typical breast cancer (Jones et al. 2008). A large part of the remaining mutations would also be passengers acquired after the tumor initiating event (Bozic et al. 2010). Individual genes can contain both driver mutations and passenger mutations. Thus the term "Mut-driver genes" has been coined to categorize genes suspected of increasing the selective growth advantage of tumor cells (Vogelstein et al. 2013). Although further cancer genome sequencing may unveil additional Mut-driver genes, the current data suggest that a plateau has being reached (Garraway and Lander 2013; Vogelstein et al. 2013). It has been estimated that for each tumor type about two thousand samples are needed to assemble the catalogue of coding mutations present in at least 2 % of tumors of a given type (Lawrence et al. 2014). For breast cancer, more than half of that number has been profiled by The Cancer Genome Atlas (TCGA). Thus, at least for the coding sequence, substantial data are available on the frequency and distribution of mutations in breast cancer subtypes (Cancer Genome Atlas Network 2012; Stephens et al. 2012). The sobering perspective on the diversity is that driver mutations are operative in many cancer genes, but only a few are commonly mutated. Many infrequently mutated genes represent the long tail of the distribution, collectively making up a substantial contribution in myriad different combinations (Stephens et al. 2012). The number of genes frequently altered in breast cancers is rather low. Only three genes (PIK3CA, TP53, GATA3) were found to be mutated in at least 10 % of breast tumors and three additional genes in at least 5 % of the patients (Cancer Genome Atlas Network 2012; Stephens et al. 2012; Shah et al. 2012). However, the majority of the 20,000 detected somatic mutations in 500 breast cancers were observed only sporadically (Cancer Genome Atlas Network 2012; Stephens et al. 2012). It appears that virtually no two tumors have a similar mutational pattern (Karn 2013). Nevertheless, different mutations may be grouped to common oncogenic pathways somewhat reducing this complexity (Cancer Genome Atlas Network 2012; Stephens et al. 2012; Garraway and Lander 2013; Vogelstein et al. 2013; Hanahan and Weinberg 2011). TP53 is the most frequently mutated gene in ER-negative breast cancer, being mutated in about 80 % of basal-like tumors and in 92 % of ER-negative, HER2-enriched breast tumors (Cancer Genome Atlas Network 2012; Stephens et al. 2012). Unfortunately, however, TP53 currently does not represent a clinically "actionable" mutation in breast cancer. Several potentially targetable mutations (MAP3K1, MAP2K4, GATA3) are seen predominantly in ER-positive tumors. In 104 triple-negative tumors, very few of the identified mutations were potentially druggable illustrating the challenges of developing new treatments and respective predictive markers for this subtype (Shah et al. 2012; Banerji et al. 2012). The frequency of PIK3CA mutations is the highest in luminal subtypes of breast cancer, but still considerable in ER-negative HER2-positive disease (Cancer Genome Atlas Network 2012). Because of the large amount of preclinical data available on activated PI3K pathway and resistance to HER2-targeted treatment, the role of this marker has been intensively studied. However, although differences in response to neoadjuvant therapy with different HER2-targeted treatments according to PIK3CA mutation status have been observed (Loibl et al. 2014; Majewski et al. 2015), these did not translate to significant clinical benefit in terms of improved overall or disease free survival (Pogue-Geile et al. 2015; Cescon and Bedard 2015). Thus, PIK3CA mutation testing is not a clinically useful test to guide treatment selection at the present time, but is should be incorporated in trials assessing the value of PI3K inhibitor combinations with HER2-targeted treatments (Cescon and Bedard 2015).

Access to next generation sequencing technology has recently spread out to basic translational research and clinical laboratories, and even if the throughput has not been adapted for high coverage genome sequencing projects, these systems are well suited for targeted sequencing of a smaller number of genes. Several cancer-specific gene panels have been introduced based on the assembled catalog of mutations from the recent cancer genome projects, and are being offered as high throughput genomic assays

(Frampton et al. 2013). The clinical utility or actionability of the respective gene mutations as genomic markers partially depends on how "actionability" is defined; e.g., either in a broad prognostic sense or narrowly regarding prediction of response to specific drugs. Several institutional, regional, and global molecular screening programs that apply such gene panels have been launched with the intent to use this information to inform clinical decision-making (Hansen and Bedard 2013). These programs may provide enrichment strategies improving the likelihood of success for testing new cancer drugs. The true merits of this approach remain to be established. But in contrast to inefficient, sequential testing of rare alterations, such comprehensive testing of multiple biomarkers early in the course of disease together with access to a broad portfolio of matched investigational or approved drugs is most likely to advance personalized cancer medicine (Hansen and Bedard 2013). Even ultra-deep sequencing of such panels can be performed to detect rare subclones coping with the problem of tumor heterogeneity. Thus personalized tumor profiling may be feasible in a clinical setting ultimately translating genome sequencing from bench to bedside (Corless 2011).

19.9 Global Genome Alterations in ER-Negative Breast Cancer

Results from TCGA revealed that on average there are 57 (range, 5–374) mutations in the coding sequence of breast cancer (Cancer Genome Atlas Network 2012). ER-negative breast cancer displays a clearly higher mutational frequency with 1.94 nonsilent coding mutations per Mb of DNA compared to 1.35 in ER-positive tumors (Ng et al. 2015). Despite this higher mutational load, TP53 represents the single most recurrently mutated gene (84.5 %) in ER-negative tumors, in contrast to PIK3CA, GATA3, and MAP3K1 that are mutated more frequently in ER-positive tumors. In addition to somatic point mutations, cancers may also be characterized by structural DNA alterations such as deletions and copy number variations. Combining genomics, transcriptomics, and epigenomics has already provided novel insights, and new genome-driven integrated classifications of breast cancer that include DNA copy number changes have been proposed (Banerji et al. 2012; Curtis et al. 2012; Dawson et al. 2013). The TCGA breast cancer study used both SNP and CGH arrays, DNA methylation analysis as well as both transcriptome, proteome, and microRNA expression analysis to obtain comprehensive portraits of the molecular subtypes through integrative analysis across platforms (Cancer Genome Atlas Network 2012). This analysis revealed that in addition to loss TP53, loss of RB1 and BRCA1 as well as high MYC activation are basal-like features. The basal-like subtype moreover displayed similarity to high grade serous ovarian cancer, which is in line with the suggested value of PARP inhibitors and platinum compounds in both diseases. Thus, it is conceivable that future genomic markers for ER-negative breast cancer may also combine several complementary molecular features. Based on the dominance of either mutational changes or copy number alterations cancers may be categorized as M or C class. While about two third of ER-positive cancers seem to belong to the M class, literally all TNBC are of the C class type as are ovarian cancers (Ciriello et al. 2013). Whole genome sequencing of some tumors has also revealed massive genomic rearrangements acquired in single catastrophic events during cancer development (Stephens et al. 2011).

Markers for deficiency in homologous DNA recombination (HRD) are of great interest since they may predict response to PARP-inhibitors and to platinum based chemotherapy, as discussed above for BRCA1. Different markers have been developed to evaluate so-called genomic scars that remained in the tumor genome (Abkevich et al. 2012; Birkbak et al. 2012; Popova et al. 2012; Vollebergh et al. 2011; Wang et al. 2012; Watkins et al. 2015). Such signatures are associated with defects in error-free repair of interstrand crosslinks (Watkins et al. 2014).

However, secondary events resulting in resistance to PARP inhibitors and DNA damaging chemotherapies limit the positive predictive value and clinical utility of these biomarkers (Watkins et al. 2014; Schouten and Linn 2015). In addition to therapies directed at HRD, other flaws in the genomic maintenance machinery that leave a detectable imprint in the genome and which may be targeted therapeutically could also become biomarkers. The large number of cancer genomes available has allowed identification of several mutational signatures giving further clues on the mutational processes shaping tumors (Alexandrov et al. 2013; Nik-Zainal et al. 2012). For example, Signature 6 of Alexandrov et al. was found to be associated with mismatch repair deficient cancers (Alexandrov et al. 2013).

Another important aspect has been observed through ultra-deep sequencing needed to establish the frequency of different subclones within the tumor. Such analyses have revealed extraordinary high intra-tumoral heterogeneity, especially in TNBC (Shah et al. 2012; Nik-Zainal et al. 2012). Those studies raised concerns that biomarker analyses from single biopsies may not cover the heterogeneous subclonality of tumors, thus ultimately leading to uncertainties in treatment decisions (McGranahan and Swanton 2015). For example tumor subclones resistant to single targeted treatments may preexist within the cancer at diagnosis. Consequently, this may suggest the need for multitarget approaches already at the start of therapy in order to eradicate the cancer (Vogelstein et al. 2013; Aparicio and Caldas 2013). On the other hand, however, the high mutational load in ER-negative breast cancer associated with this heterogeneity may be beneficial for the development of an immune response to the tumor (Rizvi et al. 2015; Le et al. 2015). In this respect, mutational derived neoantigen load may form a biomarker for potential future immunotherapy of ER-negative breast cancer and provide an incentive for the development of novel therapeutic approaches that selectively enhance T cell reactivity against this class of antigens (Schumacher and Schreiber 2015).

19.10 Current Clinical Utility of Genomic Tests for ER-Negative Breast Cancer

The clinically most useful biomarker for ER-negative breast cancer is HER2 status. Unfortunately, the clinical utility of other available genomic tests for ER-negative breast cancer is currently still limited. The Ki67 score, a proliferation marker, post chemotherapy or the reduction of the score during neoadjuvant chemotherapy was not prognostic in TNBC (Balko et al. 2014). Furthermore, gene expression based commercially available prognostic tests have value mainly in ER-positive disease (Reis-Filho and Pusztai 2011; Gyorffy et al. 2015). Substratification of TNBC by gene expression, or integrated analyses including copy number alterations, allows to further distinguish subtypes with different prognosis and potential therapeutic targets. Still those classification systems may not yet be ready for prime time (Ng et al. 2015). Immune biomarkers are established and validated prognostic and predictive factors for both triple-negative and for HER2-positive breast cancers (Karn et al. 2015). They should be used as stratification tools in future clinical trials and several biological and therapeutic hypotheses can be formulated based on these associations. However, the clinical utility of immune parameters for informing decisions about standard adjuvant therapies for TNBC or HER2-positive cancers is currently limited. A very promising research direction is to explore the potential predictive value of immune cell infiltration for future immunotherapeutic regimens; e.g., as checkpoint inhibitors. Currently, among potential analyses of mutated genes, only tests for BRCA1/2 have clinical utility regarding therapeutic decisions (Foulkes and Shuen 2013). PIK3A testing is not at present a clinically useful test to guide treatment selection in ER-negative disease (Cescon and Bedard 2015). Also, validated pharmacogenomic markers are not yet available for ER-negative breast cancer (McLeod 2013). Gene panel sequencing approaches combining comprehensive lists of genes found to be somatically mutated in tumors are currently under evaluation in several large studies. These may provide strategies for enrichment of cohorts for testing new drugs but their clinical utility has still to be established (Hansen and Bedard 2013). Several tests based on mutational scars in the genome as surrogates for DNA repair deficiencies have been developed and some of them are currently tested in clinical trials. However, final results for their use in clinical practice are not yet available (Schouten and Linn 2015).

19.11 Conclusions

One current and rapidly evolving topic in ER-negative breast cancer and in other solid tumors is the development of onco-immune therapies and the beginning understanding of the complex nature of the interface between tumor and host. It may be conceivable that a better understanding of these relationships may also provide new superior biomarkers for ER-negative breast cancers.

The recent developments in high throughput sequencing also suggest that this field may generate important novel genomic markers for cancer in general. Pilot studies have already shown that it is possible to analyze the complete genome of patients' tumors in a cost-effective and clinically relevant timeframe (Corless 2011). It is hoped that identified mutations may allow prediction of response to therapy with the ultimate aim of personalized cancer diagnostics (Corless 2011). Because of the infrequency of most alterations such methods would be germane to allow experimental "genome forward" trials or bucket trials for new therapeutics targeting such specific alterations (Bedard et al. 2013; Simon and Roychowdhury 2013). Whole genome sequencing data further suggest that each breast cancer has at least one DNA rearrangement. Thus, personalized cancer sequencing could lead to specific individual genomic markers which are suited for highly sensitive non-invasive disease monitoring by liquid biopsies (Aparicio and Caldas 2013). An important drawback for genomic markers may be the high heterogeneity and clonal diversity revealed by such methods, especially in ER-negative breast cancers (Shah et al. 2012; Nik-Zainal et al. 2012; Bedard et al. 2013). This can lead to both spatial and temporal heterogeneity within primary cancers and metastases posing questions about the value of single biopsies (McGranahan and Swanton 2015). Therefore, currently, it is also far from clear how to define a threshold for an "actionable" alteration based on its subclonal frequency in the tumor (Ng et al. 2015), while on the other hand heterogeneity itself may also represent a biomarker (McGranahan and Swanton 2015). Furthermore, it is entirely possible that what constitutes a driver mutation is not universal, but instead is cancer-specific. Inherited risk-modifying functional germline mutations could interact with somatic mutations appearing later to give rise to a founder cancer cell, whereas the same somatic mutation may be inactive in a different genetic background (Agarwal et al. 2015).

In conclusion, even when until now no new genomic markers in ER-negative breast cancers beside HER2 status have provided utility in clinical practice, their development is a constantly evolving topic. However, especially because of the poor prognosis of TNBC tremendous research efforts in this area are currently undertaken and may eventually result in the translation of clinically relevant biomarkers into the clinic.

References

Aaltomaa S, Lipponen P, Eskelinen M et al (1992) Lymphocyte infiltrates as a prognostic variable in female breast cancer. Eur J Cancer 28A(4–5):859–864

Abkevich V, Timms KM, Hennessy BT et al (2012) Patterns of genomic loss of heterozygosity predict homologous recombination repair defects in epithelial ovarian cancer. Br J Cancer 107(10):1776–1782

Adams S, Gray RJ, Demaria S et al (2014) Prognostic value of tumor-infiltrating lymphocytes in triple-negative breast cancers from two phase III

randomized adjuvant breast cancer trials: ECOG 2197 and ECOG 1199. J Clin Oncol 32(27):2959–2966
Agarwal D, Hatzis C, Pusztai L (2015) Functional polymorphisms in cancer. Oncoscience 2(2):73–74
Alexandrov LB, Nik-Zainal S, Wedge DC et al (2013) Signatures of mutational processes in human cancer. Nature 500(7463):415–421
Alexe G, Dalgin GS, Scanfeld D et al (2007) High expression of lymphocyte-associated genes in node-negative HER2+ breast cancers correlates with lower recurrence rates. Cancer Res 67(22):10669–10676
Anestis A, Karamouzis MV, Dalagiorgou G, Papavassiliou AG (2015) Is androgen receptor targeting an emerging treatment strategy for triple negative breast cancer? Cancer Treat Rev 41(6):547–553
Aparicio S, Caldas C (2013) The implications of clonal genome evolution for cancer medicine. N Engl J Med 368(9):842–851
Balko JM, Giltnane JM, Wang K et al (2014) Molecular profiling of the residual disease of triple-negative breast cancers after neoadjuvant chemotherapy identifies actionable therapeutic targets. Cancer Discov 4 (2):232–245
Balkwill F, Mantovani A (2001) Inflammation and cancer: back to Virchow? Lancet 357(9255):539–545
Banerji S, Cibulskis K, Rangel-Escareno C et al (2012) Sequence analysis of mutations and translocations across breast cancer subtypes. Nature 486(7403):405–409
Bedard PL, Hansen AR, Ratain MJ, Siu LL (2013) Tumour heterogeneity in the clinic. Nature 501 (7467):355–364
Bianchini G, Iwamoto T, Qi Y et al (2010a) Prognostic and therapeutic implications of distinct kinase expression patterns in different subtypes of breast cancer. Cancer Res 70(21):8852–8862
Bianchini G, Qi Y, Alvarez RH et al (2010b) Molecular anatomy of breast cancer stroma and its prognostic value in estrogen receptor-positive and -negative cancers. J Clin Oncol 28(28):4316–4323
Birkbak NJ, Wang ZC, Kim JY et al (2012) Telomeric allelic imbalance indicates defective DNA repair and sensitivity to DNA-damaging agents. Cancer Discov 2 (4):366–375
Bose R, Kavuri SM, Searleman AC et al (2013) Activating HER2 mutations in HER2 gene amplification negative breast cancer. Cancer Discov 3(2):224–237
Bozic I, Antal T, Ohtsuki H et al (2010) Accumulation of driver and passenger mutations during tumor progression. Proc Natl Acad Sci U S A 107(43):18545–18550
Brys M (2000) Androgens and androgen receptor: do they play a role in breast cancer? Med Sci Monit 6(2):433–438
Burstein MD, Tsimelzon A, Poage GM et al (2015) Comprehensive genomic analysis identifies novel subtypes and targets of triple-negative breast cancer. Clin Cancer Res 21(7):1688–1698
Byrski T, Dent R, Blecharz P et al (2012) Results of a phase II open-label, non-randomized trial of cisplatin chemotherapy in patients with BRCA1-positive metastatic breast cancer. Breast Cancer Res 14(4):R110
Cancer Genome Atlas Network (2012) Comprehensive molecular portraits of human breast tumours. Nature 490(7418):61–70
Cescon DW, Bedard PL (2015) PIK3CA genotype and treatment decisions in human epidermal growth factor receptor 2-positive breast cancer. J Clin Oncol 33 (12):1318–1321
Chung CC, Chanock SJ (2011) Current status of genome-wide association studies in cancer. Hum Genet 130(1):59–78
Ciriello G, Miller ML, Aksoy BA, Senbabaoglu Y, Schultz N, Sander C (2013) Emerging landscape of oncogenic signatures across human cancers. Nat Genet 45(10):1127–1133
Cobain EF, Hayes DF (2015) Indications for prognostic gene expression profiling in early breast cancer. Curr Treat Options Oncol 16(5):23
Corless CL (2011) Medicine. Personalized cancer diagnostics. Science 334(6060):1217–1218
Curtis C, Shah SP, Chin SF et al (2012) The genomic and transcriptomic architecture of 2,000 breast tumours reveals novel subgroups. Nature 486(7403):346–352
Dawson SJ, Rueda OM, Aparicio S, Caldas C (2013) A new genome-driven integrated classification of breast cancer and its implications. EMBO J 32(5):617–628
De Maeyer L, Van Limbergen E, De Nys K et al (2008) Does estrogen receptor negative/progesterone receptor positive breast carcinoma exist? J Clin Oncol 26 (2):335–336 (author reply 336–338)
Denkert C, Loibl S, Noske A et al (2010) Tumor-associated lymphocytes as an independent predictor of response to neoadjuvant chemotherapy in breast cancer. J Clin Oncol 28(1):105–113
Denkert C, von Minckwitz G, Brase JC et al (2015) Tumor-infiltrating lymphocytes and response to neoadjuvant chemotherapy with or without carboplatin in human epidermal growth factor receptor 2-positive and triple-negative primary breast cancers. J Clin Oncol 33(9):983–991
Desmedt C, Haibe-Kains B, Wirapati P et al (2008) Biological processes associated with breast cancer clinical outcome depend on the molecular subtypes. Clin Cancer Res 14(16):5158–5165
Early Breast Cancer Trialists' Collaborative Group, Davies C, Godwin J et al (2011) Relevance of breast cancer hormone receptors and other factors to the efficacy of adjuvant tamoxifen: patient-level meta-analysis of randomised trials. Lancet 378 (9793):771–784
Farmer H, McCabe N, Lord CJ et al (2005a) Targeting the DNA repair defect in BRCA mutant cells as a therapeutic strategy. Nature 434(7035):917–921

Farmer P, Bonnefoi H, Becette V et al (2005b) Identification of molecular apocrine breast tumours by microarray analysis. Oncogene 24(29):4660–4671
Fasching PA, Pharoah PD, Cox A et al (2012) The role of genetic breast cancer susceptibility variants as prognostic factors. Hum Mol Genet 21(17):3926–3939
Finak G, Bertos N, Pepin F et al (2008) Stromal gene expression predicts clinical outcome in breast cancer. Nat Med 14(5):518–527
Fioretti FM, Sita-Lumsden A, Bevan CL, Brooke GN (2014) Revising the role of the androgen receptor in breast cancer. J Mol Endocrinol 52(3):R257–R265
Fong PC, Boss DS, Yap TA et al (2009) Inhibition of poly (ADP-ribose) polymerase in tumors from BRCA mutation carriers. N Engl J Med 361(2):123–134
Foulkes WD, Shuen AY (2013) In brief: BRCA1 and BRCA2. J Pathol 230(4):347–349
Frampton GM, Fichtenholtz A, Otto GA et al (2013) Development and validation of a clinical cancer genomic profiling test based on massively parallel DNA sequencing. Nat Biotechnol 31(11):1023–1031
Garraway LA, Lander ES (2013) Lessons from the cancer genome. Cell 153(1):17–37
Goldhirsch A, Wood WC, Coates AS et al (2011) Strategies for subtypes–dealing with the diversity of breast cancer: highlights of the St. Gallen International Expert Consensus on the Primary Therapy of Early Breast Cancer 2011. Ann Oncol 22(8):1736–1747
Grivennikov SI, Greten FR, Karin M (2010) Immunity, inflammation, and cancer. Cell 140(6):883–899
Gu-Trantien C, Loi S, Garaud S et al (2013) CD4(+) follicular helper T cell infiltration predicts breast cancer survival. J Clin Invest 123(7):2873–2892
Gucalp A, Tolaney S, Isakoff SJ et al (2013) Phase II trial of bicalutamide in patients with androgen receptor-positive, estrogen receptor-negative metastatic breast cancer. Clin Cancer Res 19(19):5505–5512
Gyorffy B, Hatzis C, Sanft T, Hofstatter E, Aktas B, Pusztai L (2015) Multigene prognostic tests in breast cancer: past, present, future. Breast Cancer Res 17:11
Hammond ME, Hayes DF, Dowsett M et al (2010) American Society of Clinical Oncology/College of American Pathologists guideline recommendations for immunohistochemical testing of estrogen and progesterone receptors in breast cancer (unabridged version). Arch Pathol Lab Med 134(7):e48–e72
Hanahan D, Weinberg RA (2011) Hallmarks of cancer: the next generation. Cell 144(5):646–674
Hanker LC, Rody A, Holtrich U et al (2013) Prognostic evaluation of the B cell/IL-8 metagene in different intrinsic breast cancer subtypes. Breast Cancer Res Treat 137(2):407–416
Hansen AR, Bedard PL (2013) Clinical application of high-throughput genomic technologies for treatment selection in breast cancer. Breast Cancer Res 15(5): R97
Hatzis C, Pusztai L, Valero V et al (2011) A genomic predictor of response and survival following taxane-anthracycline chemotherapy for invasive breast cancer. JAMA 305(18):1873–1881
He J, Peng R, Yuan Z et al (2012) Prognostic value of androgen receptor expression in operable triple-negative breast cancer: a retrospective analysis based on a tissue microarray. Med Oncol 29(2):406–410
Hefti MM, Hu R, Knoblauch NW et al (2013) Estrogen receptor negative/progesterone receptor positive breast cancer is not a reproducible subtype. Breast Cancer Res 15(4):R68
Herbst RS, Soria JC, Kowanetz M et al (2014) Predictive correlates of response to the anti-PD-L1 antibody MPDL3280A in cancer patients. Nature 515 (7528):563–567
Hess KR, Wei C, Qi Y, Iwamoto T, Symmans WF, Pusztai L (2011) Lack of sufficiently strong informative features limits the potential of gene expression analysis as predictive tool for many clinical classification problems. BMC Bioinf 12:463
Hu Z, Fan C, Oh DS et al (2006) The molecular portraits of breast tumors are conserved across microarray platforms. BMC Genom 7:96
Hu R, Dawood S, Holmes MD et al (2011) Androgen receptor expression and breast cancer survival in postmenopausal women. Clin Cancer Res 17(7):1867–1874
Ignatiadis M, Singhal SK, Desmedt C et al (2012) Gene modules and response to neoadjuvant chemotherapy in breast cancer subtypes: a pooled analysis. J Clin Oncol 30(16):1996–2004
Issa-Nummer Y, Darb-Esfahani S, Loibl S et al (2013) Prospective validation of immunological infiltrate for prediction of response to neoadjuvant chemotherapy in HER2-negative breast cancer—a substudy of the neoadjuvant GeparQuinto trial. PLoS ONE 8(12): e79775
Jiang T, Shi W, Natowicz R et al (2014) Statistical measures of transcriptional diversity capture genomic heterogeneity of cancer. BMC Genom 15:876
Jones S, Chen WD, Parmigiani G et al (2008) Comparative lesion sequencing provides insights into tumor evolution. Proc Natl Acad Sci U S A 105(11):4283–4288
Karn T (2013) High-throughput gene expression and mutation profiling: current methods and future perspectives. Breast Care (Basel) 8(6):401–406
Karn T, Pusztai L, Holtrich U et al (2011) Homogeneous datasets of triple negative breast cancers enable the identification of novel prognostic and predictive signatures. PLoS ONE 6(12):e28403
Karn T, Pusztai L, Rody A, Holtrich U, Becker S (2015) The influence of host factors on the prognosis of breast cancer: stroma and immune cell components as cancer biomarkers. Curr Cancer Drug Targets 15(8):652–664
Kaufmann M, Pusztai L, Biedenkopf Expert Panel M (2011) Use of standard markers and incorporation of molecular markers into breast cancer therapy: Consensus recommendations from an International Expert Panel. Cancer 117(8):1575–1582

Lawrence MS, Stojanov P, Mermel CH et al (2014) Discovery and saturation analysis of cancer genes across 21 tumour types. Nature 505(7484):495–501

Le DT, Uram JN, Wang H et al (2015) PD-1 blockade in tumors with mismatch-repair deficiency. N Engl J Med 372(26):2509–2520

Lehmann BD, Bauer JA, Chen X et al (2011) Identification of human triple-negative breast cancer subtypes and preclinical models for selection of targeted therapies. J Clin Invest 121(7):2750–2767

Lehmann BD, Bauer JA, Schafer JM et al (2014) PIK3CA mutations in androgen receptor-positive triple negative breast cancer confer sensitivity to the combination of PI3K and androgen receptor inhibitors. Breast Cancer Res 16(4):406

Loi S, Sirtaine N, Piette F et al (2013) Prognostic and predictive value of tumor-infiltrating lymphocytes in a phase III randomized adjuvant breast cancer trial in node-positive breast cancer comparing the addition of docetaxel to doxorubicin with doxorubicin-based chemotherapy: BIG 02-98. J Clin Oncol 31(7):860–867

Loi S, Michiels S, Salgado R et al (2014) Tumor infiltrating lymphocytes are prognostic in triple negative breast cancer and predictive for trastuzumab benefit in early breast cancer: results from the FinHER trial. Ann Oncol 25(8):1544–1550

Loibl S, Muller BM, von Minckwitz G et al (2011) Androgen receptor expression in primary breast cancer and its predictive and prognostic value in patients treated with neoadjuvant chemotherapy. Breast Cancer Res Treat 130(2):477–487

Loibl S, von Minckwitz G, Schneeweiss A et al (2014) PIK3CA mutations are associated with lower rates of pathologic complete response to anti-human epidermal growth factor receptor 2 (her2) therapy in primary HER2-overexpressing breast cancer. J Clin Oncol 32 (29):3212–3220

Majewski IJ, Nuciforo P, Mittempergher L et al (2015) PIK3CA mutations are associated with decreased benefit to neoadjuvant human epidermal growth factor receptor 2-targeted therapies in breast cancer. J Clin Oncol 33(12):1334–1339

Malone KE, Daling JR, Doody DR et al (2006) Prevalence and predictors of BRCA1 and BRCA2 mutations in a population-based study of breast cancer in white and black American women ages 35 to 64 years. Cancer Res 66(16):8297–8308

McGranahan N, Swanton C (2015) Biological and therapeutic impact of intratumor heterogeneity in cancer evolution. Cancer Cell 27(1):15–26

McLeod HL (2013) Cancer pharmacogenomics: early promise, but concerted effort needed. Science 339 (6127):1563–1566

Menard S, Tomasic G, Casalini P et al (1997) Lymphoid infiltration as a prognostic variable for early-onset breast carcinomas. Clin Cancer Res 3(5):817–819

Nagalla S, Chou JW, Willingham MC et al (2013) Interactions between immunity, proliferation and molecular subtype in breast cancer prognosis. Genome Biol 14(4):R34

Narod SA (2010) BRCA mutations in the management of breast cancer: the state of the art. Nat Rev Clin Oncol 7(12):702–707

Ng CK, Schultheis AM, Bidard FC, Weigelt B, Reis-Filho JS (2015) Breast cancer genomics from microarrays to massively parallel sequencing: paradigms and new insights. J Natl Cancer Inst 107(5):[Epub ahead of print]

Ni M, Chen Y, Lim E et al (2011) Targeting androgen receptor in estrogen receptor-negative breast cancer. Cancer Cell 20(1):119–131

Niemeier LA, Dabbs DJ, Beriwal S, Striebel JM, Bhargava R (2010) Androgen receptor in breast cancer: expression in estrogen receptor-positive tumors and in estrogen receptor-negative tumors with apocrine differentiation. Mod Pathol 23(2):205–212

Nik-Zainal S, Van Loo P, Wedge DC et al (2012) The life history of 21 breast cancers. Cell 149(5):994–1007

Olivotto IA, Truong PT, Speers CH et al (2004) Time to stop progesterone receptor testing in breast cancer management. J Clin Oncol 22(9):1769–1770

Perez EA, Thompson EA, Ballman KV et al (2015) Genomic analysis reveals that immune function genes are strongly linked to clinical outcome in the North Central Cancer Treatment Group n9831 Adjuvant Trastuzumab Trial. J Clin Oncol 33(7):701–708

Perou CM, Jeffrey SS, van de Rijn M et al (1999) Distinctive gene expression patterns in human mammary epithelial cells and breast cancers. Proc Natl Acad Sci U S A 96(16):9212–9217

Perou CM, Sorlie T, Eisen MB et al (2000) Molecular portraits of human breast tumours. Nature 406 (6797):747–752

Pogue-Geile KL, Song N, Jeong JH et al (2015) Intrinsic subtypes, PIK3CA mutation, and the degree of benefit from adjuvant trastuzumab in the NSABP B-31 trial. J Clin Oncol 33(12):1340–1347

Popova T, Manie E, Rieunier G et al (2012) Ploidy and large-scale genomic instability consistently identify basal-like breast carcinomas with BRCA1/2 inactivation. Cancer Res 72(21):5454–5462

Prat A, Parker JS, Karginova O et al (2010) Phenotypic and molecular characterization of the claudin-low intrinsic subtype of breast cancer. Breast Cancer Res 12(5):R68

Prat A, Ellis MJ, Perou CM (2012) Practical implications of gene-expression-based assays for breast oncologists. Nat Rev Clin Oncol 9(1):48–57

Pusztai L, Rouzier R, Symmans WF (2015) CCR 20th anniversary commentary: divide and conquer-breast cancer subtypes and response to therapy. Clin Cancer Res 21(16):3575–3577

Rahman N (2014a) Mainstreaming genetic testing of cancer predisposition genes. Clin Med (Lond) 14 (4):436–439

Rahman N (2014b) Realizing the promise of cancer predisposition genes. Nature 505(7483):302–308

Rakha EA, El-Sayed ME, Green AR, Lee AH, Robertson JF, Ellis IO (2007a) Prognostic markers in triple-negative breast cancer. Cancer 109(1):25–32

Rakha EA, El-Sayed ME, Green AR et al (2007b) Biologic and clinical characteristics of breast cancer with single hormone receptor positive phenotype. J Clin Oncol 25(30):4772–4778

Reis-Filho JS, Pusztai L (2011) Gene expression profiling in breast cancer: classification, prognostication, and prediction. Lancet 378(9805):1812–1823

Rizvi NA, Hellmann MD, Snyder A et al (2015) Cancer immunology. Mutational landscape determines sensitivity to PD-1 blockade in non-small cell lung cancer. Science 348(6230):124–128

Robinson JL, Macarthur S, Ross-Innes CS et al (2011) Androgen receptor driven transcription in molecular apocrine breast cancer is mediated by FoxA1. EMBO J 30(15):3019–3027

Rody A, Karn T, Solbach C et al (2007) The erbB2 + cluster of the intrinsic gene set predicts tumor response of breast cancer patients receiving neoadjuvant chemotherapy with docetaxel, doxorubicin and cyclophosphamide within the GEPARTRIO trial. Breast 16(3):235–240

Rody A, Holtrich U, Pusztai L et al (2009) T-cell metagene predicts a favorable prognosis in estrogen receptor-negative and HER2-positive breast cancers. Breast Cancer Res 11(2):R15

Rody A, Karn T, Liedtke C et al (2011) A clinically relevant gene signature in triple negative and basal-like breast cancer. Breast Cancer Res 13(5):R97

Rouzier R, Perou CM, Symmans WF et al (2005) Breast cancer molecular subtypes respond differently to preoperative chemotherapy. Clin Cancer Res 11 (16):5678–5685

Ruffell B, Au A, Rugo HS, Esserman LJ, Hwang ES, Coussens LM (2012) Leukocyte composition of human breast cancer. Proc Natl Acad Sci U S A 109 (8):2796–2801

Schmidt M, Bohm D, von Torne C et al (2008) The humoral immune system has a key prognostic impact in node-negative breast cancer. Cancer Res 68 (13):5405–5413

Schouten PC, Linn SC (2015) Challenges in the use of DNA repair deficiency as a biomarker in breast cancer. J Clin Oncol 33(17):1867–1869

Schumacher TN, Schreiber RD (2015) Neoantigens in cancer immunotherapy. Science 348(6230):69–74

Shah SP, Roth A, Goya R et al (2012) The clonal and mutational evolution spectrum of primary triple-negative breast cancers. Nature 486 (7403):395–399

Shah PD, Gucalp A, Traina TA (2013) The role of the androgen receptor in triple-negative breast cancer. Womens Health (Lond Engl) 9(4):351–360

Shendure J, Ji H (2008) Next-generation DNA sequencing. Nat Biotechnol 26(10):1135–1145

Shibata D (2012) Cancer. heterogeneity and tumor history. Science 336(6079):304–305

Simon R, Roychowdhury S (2013) Implementing personalized cancer genomics in clinical trials. Nat Rev Drug Discov 12(5):358–369

Sorlie T, Perou CM, Tibshirani R et al (2001) Gene expression patterns of breast carcinomas distinguish tumor subclasses with clinical implications. Proc Natl Acad Sci U S A 98(19):10869–10874

Sotiriou C, Pusztai L (2009) Gene-expression signatures in breast cancer. N Engl J Med 360(8):790–800

Stephens PJ, Greenman CD, Fu B et al (2011) Massive genomic rearrangement acquired in a single catastrophic event during cancer development. Cell 144 (1):27–40

Stephens PJ, Tarpey PS, Davies H et al (2012) The landscape of cancer genes and mutational processes in breast cancer. Nature 486(7403):400–404

Stratton MR (2011) Exploring the genomes of cancer cells: progress and promise. Science 331(6024):1553–1558

Teschendorff AE, Miremadi A, Pinder SE, Ellis IO, Caldas C (2007) An immune response gene expression module identifies a good prognosis subtype in estrogen receptor negative breast cancer. Genome Biol 8(8):R157

Tofigh A, Suderman M, Paquet ER et al (2014) The prognostic ease and difficulty of invasive breast carcinoma. Cell Rep 9(1):129–142

Topalian SL, Hodi FS, Brahmer JR et al (2012) Safety, activity, and immune correlates of anti-PD-1 antibody in cancer. N Engl J Med 366(26):2443–2454

Trainer AH, Lewis CR, Tucker K, Meiser B, Friedlander M, Ward RL (2010) The role of BRCA mutation testing in determining breast cancer therapy. Nat Rev Clin Oncol 7(12):708–717

Turner NC, Tutt AN (2012) Platinum chemotherapy for BRCA1-related breast cancer: do we need more evidence? Breast Cancer Res 14(6):115

van't Veer LJ, Dai H, van de Vijver MJ et al (2002) Gene expression profiling predicts clinical outcome of breast cancer. Nature 415(6871):530–536

Vera-Badillo FE, Templeton AJ, de Gouveia P et al (2014) Androgen receptor expression and outcomes in early breast cancer: a systematic review and meta-analysis. J Natl Cancer Inst 106(1):djt319

Vidula N, Rugo HS (2015) Translating the molecular message of triple-negative breast cancer into targeted therapy. Clin Cancer Res 21(7):1511–1513

Vogelstein B, Papadopoulos N, Velculescu VE, Zhou S, Diaz LA Jr, Kinzler KW (2013) Cancer genome landscapes. Science 339(6127):1546–1558

Vollebergh MA, Lips EH, Nederlof PM et al (2011) An aCGH classifier derived from BRCA1-mutated breast cancer and benefit of high-dose platinum-based chemotherapy in HER2-negative breast cancer patients. Ann Oncol 22(7):1561–1570

Wang L, McLeod HL, Weinshilboum RM (2011) Genomics and drug response. N Engl J Med 364 (12):1144–1153
Wang ZC, Birkbak NJ, Culhane AC et al (2012) Profiles of genomic instability in high-grade serous ovarian cancer predict treatment outcome. Clin Cancer Res 18 (20):5806–5815
Watkins JA, Irshad S, Grigoriadis A, Tutt AN (2014) Genomic scars as biomarkers of homologous recombination deficiency and drug response in breast and ovarian cancers. Breast Cancer Res 16(3):211
Watkins J, Weekes D, Shah V et al (2015) Genomic complexity profiling reveals that HORMAD1 overexpression contributes to homologous recombination deficiency in triple-negative breast cancers. Cancer Discov 5(5):488–505
Weigelt B, Reis-Filho JS (2009) Histological and molecular types of breast cancer: is there a unifying taxonomy? Nat Rev Clin Oncol 6(12):718–730
Weigelt B, Pusztai L, Ashworth A, Reis-Filho JS (2012) Challenges translating breast cancer gene signatures into the clinic. Nat Rev Clin Oncol 9(1):58–64

Next-Generation Sequencing Based Testing for Breast Cancer

20

Shridar Ganesan and Kim M. Hirshfield

Abstract

The breast cancer can be sporadic or familial. Studies in the early 1990s lead to the recognition of the role of BRCA1 and BRCA2 genes in hereditary breast cancer. Next generation sequencing (NGS) technologies have permitted expansion of the number of genes that can be simultaneously analyzed for assessment of breast cancer risk. NGS has opened a large window into the complex biology of carcinogenesis and management of breast cancer. Mutation panels are now being commonly used in the making therapeutic decisions. In this chapter, we review the data on the gene panels being used for risk assessment and clinical management of patients and discuss the pros and cons of the approaches.

Keywords

NGS · Mutation panels · Risk assessment · Therapy

20.1 Introduction

Ever since the demonstration of germline mutations in BRCA1 and BRCA2 in high penetrance hereditary breast cancer predisposition, there has been great interest in finding other breast cancer susceptibility genes. There is now a growing set of genes for which rare germline variants may contribute to breast cancer risk (King et al. 2003; Easton et al. 2015). When compared with BRCA1 and BRCA2, in most populations, each of these genes appear to have a relatively minor contribution to breast cancer risk; however, together they may have significant impact.

Recent technical advances in the genomic sequencing technology, including targeted, massively parallel (or 'next-generation') sequencing, has allowed the development of clinical assays which can interrogate the germline sequence of multiple genes with high confidence and relatively low cost (Buermans and den Dunnen 2014; Metzker 2010; Gray et al. 2015). Multigene panels are now available for a variety of clinical uses, including pre-natal testing, These technical advances together with recent legal

S. Ganesan (✉) · K.M. Hirshfield
Rutgers Cancer Institute of New Jersey, Rutgers, The State University of New Jersey, 195 Little Albany Street, New Brunswick, NJ 08903, USA
e-mail: ganesash@cinj.rutgers.edu

S. Badve and Y. Gökmen-Polar (eds.), *Molecular Pathology of Breast Cancer*, DOI 10.1007/978-3-319-41761-5_20

rulings that have removed patent protection from assays that interrogate BRCA1 and BRCA2 (A victory for genes 2013), have led to the proliferation of commercial multigene sequencing panels for evaluation of hereditary cancer risk and for cancer therapeutics. This has led to the situation where the ability to obtain detailed genomic information on individual patients exceeds the knowledge of the actual clinical validity and utility of such information (Easton et al. 2015; Slavin et al. 2015).

In this chapter, we will review the development, clinical utility, promises and limitations of this approach in the setting of assessment of breast cancer risk and selecting therapies.

20.2 Next-Generation Sequencing

Next-generation sequencing (NGS) refers to massively parallel, short read sequencing methods based on solid substrate immobilization of templates(Buermans and den Dunnen 2014; Metzker 2010; Gray et al. 2015). This approach leads to efficient generation of a large numbers of sequence reads of limited length (75–150 bp), and requires a pre-assembled reference genome to allow mapping of individual short reads. The amount of independent sequencing reads generated and the size of the target genomic region sequenced give the relative depth (or number of independent reads that cover any given region of the target genome). For example, sequencing of the whole genome ($\sim$3.2 Gb) at 10× depth would require 32 Gb of sequencing data (or over 200 million reads of 150 bp). The key to harnessing the power of next-generation sequencing for clinical applications is specific and efficient enrichment of selected genomic regions of interest prior to sequencing (Kozarewa et al. 2015; Mamanova et al. 2010). This allows targeted sequencing of a limited region of the genome, ranging from either whole exome (32 Mb), or to just a handful of genes (<1 Mb), at very high depth.

For genomic sequencing of a limited gene panel, the target usually includes all coding exons of the genes of interest plus some region of flanking introns to cover splice sites. For some genes parts of promoter region may be included. Two main methods of genomic target enrichment are predominately used in multi-gene panels, i.e. hybrid capture and PCR-amplicon (Fig. 20.1), although other techniques including molecular inversion probe ligation (MIPL) are also available (Kozarewa et al. 2015; Mamanova et al. 2010). Hybrid capture uses sets of labeled genomic probes that correspond to genomic regions of interest. Genomic DNA is first fragmented and used for library preparation. Labeled probes are then hybridized to the genomic library, and the labels then used to purify the hybridized fragments, leaving off-target, un-hybridized genomic DNA behind. The hybridization can either be done on solid surface using immobilized probes or in solution (Hedges et al. 2011). Tiled probes covering all known exons of coding genes and some extension into flanking introns to cover conserved splice sites ($\sim$3.2 Mb) are typically used to generate "whole exome sequencing". Probe sets targeting all exons of small gene sets of interest are typically used and achieve high depth (>500×) sequencing. The enriched libraries are then subjected to NGS, and sequence reads are then mapped to the reference genome and then input into variant calling algorithms to identify genomic alterations. PCR-based enrichment uses sets of primer pairs that flank the target regions. Prepared genomic DNA is used as a template for PCR amplification. The amplified DNA can then be further modified with multiplexing tags and then subject to NGS (Kozarewa et al. 2015; Mamanova et al. 2010).

In practice, both PCR-based and hybrid-capture based target enrichment has been used to develop CLIA-certified multi-gene panels for cancer risk.

Hybrid capture approaches require more input DNA and more complex bioinformatics analysis than PCR enrichment. However they generate robust allele frequencies and can also be used to provide information on copy number variation (CNV) to identify genomic amplifications and deletions (Liu et al. 2013). PCR-based enrichment require smaller amounts of input

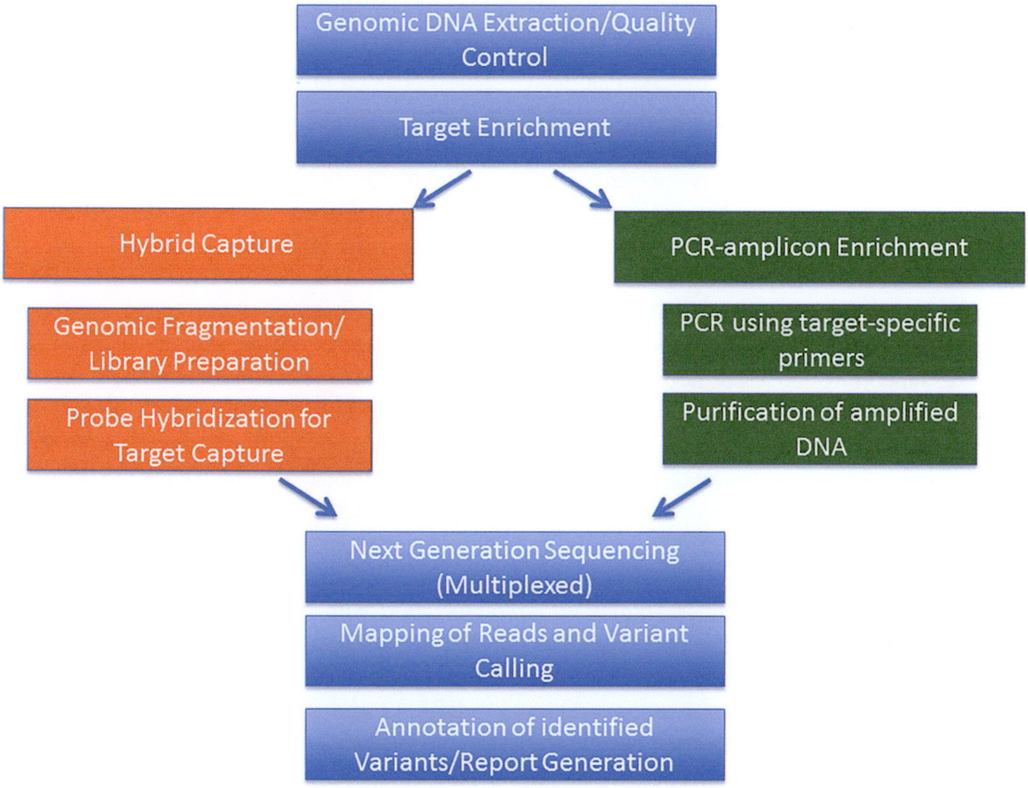

Fig. 20.1 Outline of workflow for next-generation sequencing assays using either hybrid capture or PCR-amplicon for target enrichment

DNA, require less complex bioinformatics analysis. However they may not give true sequence depth and cannot robustly identify CNVs. Both PCR-based gene panels and hybrid-capture methods may be supplemented with other assays, such as array-CGH, or multiplex ligation-dependent probe amplification (MLPA) to get information on genomic deletions, duplications or other rearrangement events (Hogervorst et al. 2003). An issue for the PCR-based approach is that rare SNPs in primer regions can dramatically affect performance of individual primer pairs. Overall, both approaches work well for analysis of germline DNA, but details of individual assays must be kept in mind to be aware of potential confounders (Samorodnitsky et al. 2015; Claes and De Leeneer 2014).

20.3 NGS Panels in Risk Assessment

In this section we will review the use of NGS approaches to identify potential germline alterations associated with breast cancer risk. The standards for clinical validity and utility will be reviewed, and then individual breast cancer risk genes will be discussed. Finally some recent clinical studies examing utility of NGS panels in risk assessment will be reviewed in detail.

20.3.1 Clinical Validity and Utility of Risk Assessment

The ACCE model, established by the CDC, defines the process for evaluating genetic tests based on four key criteria: Analytic Validity, Clinical Validity, Clinical Utility, and Ethical, legal and societal factors (Haddow and Palomaki 2003). The first of these, analytic validity, refers to the technical accuracy and reproducibility of the test used to both identify presence and absence of genomic alterations. NGS platforms have defined benchmarks for analytic validity that form the core of developing Clinical Laboratory Improvement Amendments (CLIA) certification. Clinical validity refers to the strength of evidence supporting the association of specific genomic alterations with disease risk and the magnitude of this increased risk. In other words, it answers the following question: what are the data on how a specific alteration in Gene X affects cancer risk? Clinical utility focuses on whether finding a genetic alteration has clear data to support specific clinical interventions. If a patient has an alteration in Gene X associated with increased cancer risk, what is the data showing efficacy of relevant screening or preventions strategies in reducing risk? As clinical validity and clinical utility are not part of the assessment for development of CLIA-certified laboratory tests, gene panels can be introduced for clinical use without clear data on clinical validity and/or utility (Sharfstein 2015; Hayes et al. 2013; Lander 2015).

The key questions that define Clinical Validity of a potential genetic marker of cancer risk include: What classes of gene variants contribute to increased risk, what is the magnitude of risk associated with alterations in the gene and the strength and nature of the supporting evidence? Cancer risks associated with gene variants are often presented as relative risk ratios that delineate the risk of a person with the gene variant as a multiple of the risk present in the "average" person. A relative risk (RR) >4 is usually considered "high risk", a RR of 2–4 is considered moderate risk, and a RR less than two being low risk, although different cut-offs are also used by some investigators (Easton et al. 2015; Slavin et al. 2015). Only a handful of genes are unequivocally validated as high-risk breast cancer genes (BRCA1, BRCA1, TP53, CDH1). A growing number of rare gene variants associated with moderate risk and unclear risk are now being included in gene panels. A set of genes included in most breast cancer risk panels will be considered below.

20.3.2 Genes Commonly Found in NGS Gene Panels

Intriguingly, many of these breast cancer susceptibility genes either directly interact with BRCA1 and BRCA2 or are functionally involved with DNA double strand break repair while others participate in signal transduction or cell adhesion. Mismatch repair genes are also commonly included, although their association with breast cancer risk is not certain. Some of the most common genes included, their biological role and association with breast cancer risk are summarized in Fig. 20.2. Selected individual genes are discussed in detail below.

BRCA1 and BRCA2: Both genes function in DNA repair, particularly in homologous recombination-mediated DNA double strand break repair. Germline deleterious mutations genes are clearly associated with high risk of breast cancer and other cancers and have strong data supporting both clinical validity and clinical utility (Antoniou et al. 2003; Chen and Parmigiani 2007; Mavaddat et al. 2013). Most germline mutations are truncating mutations leading to loss of protein function. Some reports suggest that protein-truncating variants (PTVs) may have different risks depending on location of truncation, although larger studies need to be done to confirm and validate these findings (Thompson and Easton 2001; Lubinski et al. 2004; Thompson and Easton 2002). Rare missense mutations and splice site mutations have also been clinically validated. Large genomic deletions/rearrangements are found in some populations, and these can be missed by PCR-amplicon based NGS assays, and may require use of complementary methods such as MLPA for their identification.

PALB2: PALB2 was initially identified as a BRCA2 interacting protein, but has since been shown to interact with both BRCA1 and BRCA2

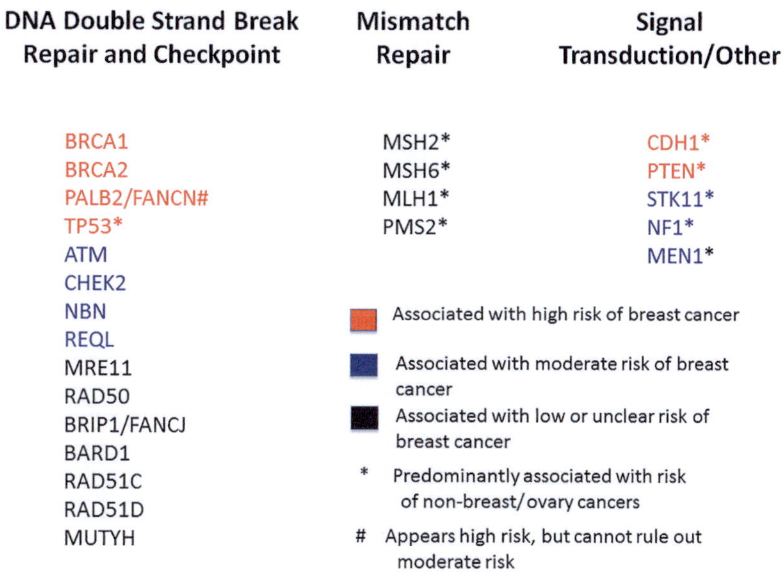

Fig. 20.2 Genes commonly found in NGS panels evaluating breast cancer risk are shown, organized by underlying function and risk category

(Xia et al. 2006; Zhang et al. 2009). Very rare bi-allelic mutations in PALB2 result in a Fanconi anemia syndrome, FANCN (Xia et al. 2007; Reid et al. 2007). Loss of function germline mutations in PALB2 also appear to be associated with a moderate to high risk of breast cancer. A meta-analysis of several studies estimated a RR of 5.3 (Easton et al. 2015; Rahman et al. 2007; Antoniou et al. 2014; Casadei et al. 2011; Erkko et al. 2007). The largest single study estimated a lifetime risk of breast cancer of 35 %, when considered independently of family history, and a lifetime risk of 58 % if there was a significant family history of breast cancer (Antoniou et al. 2014). These data suggest that PALB2 may have similar risk of breast cancer as BRCA2. However, additional data are required to justify its categorization as a high-risk breast cancer gene. Germline PALB2 mutations are also associated with a moderately increased risk of ovarian cancer, although the estimates of risk are not well defined (Antoniou et al. 2014). Germline PALB2 mutations have been identified in rare families with hereditary pancreatic cancer, although the estimate of risk also remains unclear (Jones et al. 2009). Although PALB2 mutations are much less prevalent that BRCA1/2 mutations, founder mutations in certain geographic regions may contribute more significantly to population risk (Erkko et al. 2007; Dansonka-Mieszkowska et al. 2010; Cao et al. 2009; Prokofyeva et al. 2012; Haanpaa et al. 2013).

BRIP and BARD1: Both BRIP1 and BARD1 were initially identified as BRCA1 interacting proteins. BRIP1 directly binds to the BRCT repeats of BRCA1 and bi-allelic loss of function mutations leads to a Fanconi Anemia syndrome subtype FANCJ (Cantor et al. 2001; Litman et al. 2005). Recent data show that truncating mutations in BRIP1 contributes to ovarian cancer risk, although estimates of absolute risk are much less than that seen with BRCA1 or BRCA2 (Rafnar et al. 2011). Data on breast cancer risk with BRIP1 mutations are less clear. Germline heterozygous truncating mutations have been reported to have increased risk of breast cancer with a relative risk of 2.0 (1.3–3.2) (Seal et al. 2006). However, data on associations between BRIP1 mutations and increased breast cancer risk are sparse (Aloraifi et al. 2015), and data from several other studies do not support BRIP1 mutations as having a significant contribution to breast cancer risk (Kuusisto et al. 2011). BARD1 is another key BRCA1 interacting protein that likely exists as a heterodimer with BRCA1 and contributes to the E3 ubiquitin ligase function of BRCA1 (Wu et al. 1996). Germline loss-of-function mutations in BARD1 have been implicated in breast cancer risk, however such mutations are rare and their contributions to breast cancer risk remain unclear (Thai et al. 1998; Young et al. 2016).

TP53: Germline mutations in TP53 are associated with Li-Fraumeni syndrome and with dramatically elevated risk of many cancers including sarcoma, brain cancer, adrenocortical carcinoma and rare childhood cancers (Malkin et al. 1990; Hwang et al. 2003). Germline TP53 mutations are also clearly associated with increased breast cancer risk, but well-defined estimates of relative risk are lacking given rarity of this syndrome (Malkin et al. 1990; Hwang et al. 2003; Easton et al. 2015). Most studies have estimated breast cancer risk by looking at families identified as having clinical Li-Fraumeni syndrome and thus subject to ascertainment bias. Deleterious mutations in TP53 can be both protein truncating mutations or well-characterized missense mutations. The effect of certain common polymorphisms in TP53 e.g. codon 72, has been studied extensively, but the magnitude of breast risk has varied greatly from no risk to moderate risk associations depending on population under study and breast cancer subtypes within the population (Goncalves et al. 2014; Cheng et al. 2012).

ATM: ATM is a key sensor and transducer of DNA damage signaling pathway. It is involved in both DNA double strand break repair and in response to oxidative damage (Kitagawa and Kastan 2005; Bhatti et al. 2011). Bi-allelic mutations in ATM lead to the Ataxia-Telangiectasia syndrome associated with neurologic deficits, immune deficiency and cancer predisposition (Teive et al. 2015; Chun and Gatti 2004). Heterozygous truncating mutations in ATM, are associated with moderate increased breast cancer risk in multiple studies, with an estimated relative risk of 2.8 based on a meta-analysis (van Os et al. 2015; Renwick et al. 2006; Janin et al. 1999; Thompson et al. 2005; Olsen et al. 2005; Easton et al. 2015). A rare missense mutations in ATM, V2424G, has been reported to be associated particularly high risk, greater than that associated with truncating variants, and may function as a dominant negative allele (Szabo et al. 2004; Bernstein et al. 2006; Chenevix-Trench et al. 2002). However, most missense variants of ATM found by NGS tend to be of unclear clinical significance.

CHEK2: CHEK2 is serine-threonine kinase that is phosphorylated and activated by ATM. It regulates initiation of cell-cycle checkpoints in response to DNA damage. Germline mutations in CHEK2 are associated with moderate increased risk of breast cancer in multiple studies, mostly based on case-control studies evaluating the CHEK2 c1100delC frame shift mutation. This has been reported as founder mutation in some European populations (Meijers-Heijboer et al. 2002; CHEK2*1100delC and susceptibility to breast cancer: a collaborative analysis involving 10,860 breast cancer cases and 9065 controls from 10 studies (2004; Weischer et al. 2012). A missense variant, CHEK2 I157T has also been associated with breast cancer, but is associated with lower cancer risk than the truncating mutation (Kilpivaara et al. 2004; Han et al. 2013).

NBN, MRE11 and RAD50: NBN codes for nibrin, a member of the MRN protein complex including MRE11, and RAD50. The complex plays an essential role in the recognition of DNA double strand breaks and subsequent recruitment of downstream DNA repair proteins (Williams et al. 2007). Truncating mutations of NBN, particularly c.657del5, which is present in some European populations, is associated with a RR of 2.7 (1.8–3.9) based on a meta-analysis of case-control studies (Zhang et al. 2012, 2013). Rare germline mutations in MRE11 and RAD50 have also been reported as associated with breast cancer risk, but data are too limited to develop robust risk estimates (Damiola et al. 2014; Hsu et al. 2007; Bartkova et al. 2008).

Mismatch Repair Genes: Germline loss-of-function mutations in key genes involved in mismatch repair (MSH2, MSH6, MLH1, PMS2) are associated with Lynch Syndrome and increased risk of colorectal, endometrial and other cancers (Aarnio et al. 1999; Bonadona et al. 2011). Some reports have suggested increased breast cancer risk, however the strength of evidence for increased risk based on population studies is weak (Aarnio et al. 1999; Win et al. 2013; Buerki et al. 2012; Watson et al. 2008).

MUTYH: Bi-allelic germline mutations in MUTYH are associated with a polyposis syndrome with defined, increased risk for colon cancer (Sampson and Jones 2009). A subset of initial studies suggested possible increased risk for breast cancer in heterozygous MUTYH carriers, but recent case-control studies do not support an association with increased breast cancer risk (Out et al. 2012; Win et al. 2011).

RECQL: RECQL encodes a DNA helicase that is a homolog of the prokaryotic REC Q helicase that plays critical roles in DNA repair, replication and recombination (Akbari and Cybulski 2015). Recent studies have shown that rare recurrent germline mutations were enriched in breast cancer populations in Canada and Poland, suggesting that germline mutations in RECQL are associated with increased breast cancer risk (Cybulski et al. 2015; Sun et al. 2015).

RAD51C and RAD51D: RAD51C and RAD51D encode paralogs of the key recombination protein RAD51 (Suwaki et al. 2011). Germline mutations in RAD51C and RAD51D have been associated with increased risk of ovarian cancer (Loveday et al. 2011, 2012). A screen of 1228 Danish hereditary breast or ovarian cancer families identified pathogenic RAD51C mutations in six (0.5 %) families and identified 24 variants of uncertain significance (VUS) (Pelttari et al. 2012). The role of RAD51C and RAD51D in breast cancer risk is not certain (Jonson et al. 2016).

PPM1D: PPM1D encodes a p53-inducible phosphatase (also known as WIP1) that is implicated in regulation of DNA repair checkpoint activation by ATM and ATR (Emelyanov and Bulavin 2015). A study examining protein truncating mutations in DNA repair related genes in peripheral blood lymphocytes from cohorts of patients with breast and ovarian cancer found rare protein truncating mutations of PPM1D in 25 out of 7781 cancer cases, compared with one out of 5861 controls (Ruark et al. 2013). Intriguingly, these mutations may have gain of function and were mosaic in peripheral lymphocytes, raising the question of whether these mutations were truly germline. Another study also found enrichment of PPM1D mutations in peripheral blood of 20 out of 1295 patients with ovarian cancer (Akbari et al. 2014). The authors noted that all patients who were found to have PPM1D mutations in peripheral blood had a history of treatment with platinum-based chemotherapy. Such history raised the question of whether these were acquired mutations secondary to chemotherapy exposure rather than germline mutations.

Other DNA repair genes: There is some data to suggest that germline mutations in XRCC2, FANCM, FANCC, FANCP/SLX4 are associated with increased breast cancer risk. However, these mutations are extremely rare and the significance of these associations is not certain (Park et al. 2012; Hilbers et al. 2012; Thompson et al. 2012; Kiiski et al. 2014).

CDH1: Cadherin 1 (CDH1) is a key adhesion molecule expressed in most epithelial cells. As CDH1 normally binds and sequesters β-catenin, loss of CDH1 may also lead to activation of β-catenin, loss of adhesion, and cell polarity (Priya and Yap 2015). Loss of CDH1 expression, typically through somatic mutation, is a characteristic feature of lobular breast cancers (Christgen and Derksen 2015). Germline loss-of-function mutations of CDH1 are associated with an increased risk of lobular breast cancer with a RR = 6.6 (2.2–9.9) (Pharoah et al. 2001; Masciari et al. 2007) in addition to increased risk of diffuse gastric cancer. CDH1 is considered a high-risk gastric and breast cancer susceptibility gene (Corso et al. 2014).

PTEN and STK11: These genes are related more to signal transduction pathways than DNA repair. They are associated with a multiple-cancer predisposition syndromes in which includes increase in breast cancer risk. PTEN (Phosphatase and Tensin homolog) is a lipid-phosphatase which functions as a tumor suppressor by opposing the activity of PI3K lipid kinase (Milella et al. 2015). Loss of PTEN can lead to downstream activation of PI3K/AKT pathway. Germline loss-of-function mutations in PTEN are associated with Cowden syndrome which is characterized by development of hamartomas and increased risk of breast, thyroid, endometrial and other cancers (Bubien et al. 2013; Tan et al. 2012; Ngeow and Eng 2015; Liaw et al. 1997). Some studies have reported very high relative risk of breast cancer (RR > 20) in PTEN mutation carriers (Bubien et al. 2013; Tan et al. 2012). However, these risk estimates are from analyses of families with clinical syndromes associated with PTEN loss and thus may significantly overestimate risk in the general population. Loss-of-function germline mutations in STK11 are associated with Peutz-Jeghers syndrome, which is characterized by gastrointestinal hamartomas, pigmented lesions, and increased risk of multiple cancers including breast cancer (Hearle et al. 2006; Resta et al. 2013; Lim et al. 2004). There are no clear estimates of relative risk in the setting of germline STK11 mutations. Although cumulative lifetime risks of breast cancer of up to 45 % at age 70 have been reported in families with Peutz-Jeghers, this may be an overestimate due to ascertainment bias (Hearle et al. 2006; Easton et al. 2015).

NF1 and MEN1: Loss-of-function mutations in NF1 are associated with Neurofibromatosis Type 1. Women with germline NF1 mutations have been recently shown to have a moderately elevated risk of breast cancer based on cohort studies (Madanikia et al. 2012; Seminog and Goldacre 2015). Germline mutations in MEN1 are associated with multiple-endocrine neoplasia syndrome type 1. MEN1 encodes menin, a scaffold protein involved in transcriptional regulation through interaction with chromatin regulators (Dreijerink et al. 2006). Female MEN1 mutation carriers have been reported in several independent cohorts to have a moderate risk of developing breast cancer (Dreijerink et al. 2014).

Variants of Uncertain Significance: Most of the breast cancer risk genes are thought to function as tumor suppressors with pathogenic mutations being associated with loss of function. Most pathogenic mutations are protein-truncating mutations that models clearly predict will lead to loss of protein function. However, some rare missense mutations in BRCA1 and BRCA2 and some other tumor suppressor genes, such as ATM and CHEK2, have been shown to be deleterious and associated with cancer risk. However, the majority of rare missense mutations identified by NGS have no clear data regarding effect on protein function and cancer risk, and are thus are classified as variants of unclear significance. The America College of Medical Genetics and Genomics (ACMG) has issued guidelines for classification of variants identified in clinical sequencing assays as either benign variants, pathogenic variants or variants of uncertain significance (VUS), with graded levels of supportive evidence for benign or pathogenic variants (Figs. 20.3 and 20.4) (Richards et al. 2015). These guidelines take into consideration evidence from population studies, segregation analyses, as well as biologic and in silico analysis. In many series in which multi-gene panels were employed in high-risk patient populations, VUS in non-BRCA1 and BRCA2 genes were the most common category of alterations identified (Kurian et al. 2014; Maxwell et al. 2015). The management of patients with identified VUS is challenging, and may lead to potential overtreatment. Further, both clinical data in families showing segregation of variants with cancer and/or biological data showing loss of function in cell or animal models may lead to reclassification of VUS as either benign or pathogenic with varying degrees of confidence. However, the increasing use of multi-gene panels may well lead to increasing number of patients being found to harbor VUS.

20.3.3 Clinical Use of Multi-gene Panel Sequencing for Risk Assessment

Multiple studies have looked at the clinical impact of multi-gene panel sequencing as part of genetic testing for breast cancer risk. Although data are rapidly accumulating, a subset of key published studies are summarized in Table 20.1 and is reviewed below

Kurian and colleagues evaluated blood samples from 198 women referred for genetic

	Benign		Pathogenic			
	Strong	Supporting	Supporting	Moderate	Strong	Very strong
Population data	MAF is too high for disorder BA1/BS1 **OR** observation in controls inconsistent with disease penetrance BS2			Absent in population databases PM2	Prevalence in affecteds statistically increased over controls PS4	
Computational and predictive data		Multiple lines of computational evidence suggest no impact on gene /gene product BP4 Missense in gene where only truncating cause disease BP1 Silent variant with non predicted splice impact BP7 In-frame indels in repeat w/out known function BP3	Multiple lines of computational evidence support a deleterious effect on the gene /gene product PP3	Novel missense change at an amino acid residue where a different pathogenic missense change has been seen before PM5 Protein length changing variant PM4	Same amino acid change as an established pathogenic variant PS1	Predicted null variant in a gene where LOF is a known mechanism of disease PVS1
Functional data	Well-established functional studies show no deleterious effect BS3		Missense in gene with low rate of benign missense variants and path. missenses common PP2	Mutational hot spot or well-studied functional domain without benign variation PM1	Well-established functional studies show a deleterious effect PS3	
Segregation data	Nonsegregation with disease BS4		Cosegregation with disease in multiple affected family members PP1	Increased segregation data →		
De novo data				De novo (without paternity & maternity confirmed) PM6	De novo (paternity and maternity confirmed) PS2	
Allelic data		Observed in *trans* with a dominant variant BP2 Observed in *cis* with a pathogenic variant BP2		For recessive disorders, detected in trans with a pathogenic variant PM3		
Other database		Reputable source w/out shared data = benign BP6	Reputable source = pathogenic PP5			
Other data		Found in case with an alternate cause BP5	Patient's phenotype or FH highly specific for gene PP4			

Fig. 20.3 ACMG guidelines for classification of genomic variants, from Richards et al.

BRCA1/2 testing with a 42-gene NGS panel that included BRCA1/2 and used hybrid-capture for target enrichment (Kurian et al. 2014). There was complete concordance with pathogenic BRCA1/2 mutations identified by standard clinical sequencing and results from the 42-gene panel (although one large insertion was missed by NGS analysis in a sample in which deletion/duplication analysis was not performed). In samples without pathogenic mutations in BRCA1/2, 16 pathogenic variants in 9 genes were found, 8 of which were missense mutations. The most common genes involved were MUTYH (n = 5 samples, 3 missense mutations and 2 splice acceptor mutations), SLX4/FANCP (n = 2, both truncating) and ATM (n = 2, one missense, one truncating) where overall, 15 were considered to be clinically actionable, leading to potential "actionablility" rate of 10.6 % in BRCA1/2 wild-type samples. Ten patients were successfully re-contacted, underwent genetic counseling, and interventions including increased breast cancer screening with MRI (for *ATM, BLM, CDH1, NBN,* and *SLX4/FANCP* variants) and colonoscopic screening (for *CDH1, MLH1, and MUTYH variants)* were instituted. Of note, there was an average of 2.1 VUS found per sample tested (Kurian et al. 2014).

Maxwell and colleagues used hybrid-capture based NGS to examine 22 cancer susceptibility genes in 278 women with early onset breast cancer (diagnosed age <40) who did not harbor germline mutations in BRCA1/2 (Maxwell et al. 2015). Thirty-one patients (11 %) were found to have at least one pathogenic or likely pathogenic variant. Of these, seven (2.5 %) were in genes for which there were clear clinical guidelines for management (4 cases of TP53 mutations, and one each of CKDN2A, MSH2 and a case with bi-allelic mutations in MUTYH). The other 24 were gene variants for which there exist no clear clinical guidelines including variants in ATM and CHEK2. Fifty-four patients (~19 %) had at least one VUS. Thus variants were detected overall in ~30 % of these patients, but only 2.5 % had changes which had clear clinical

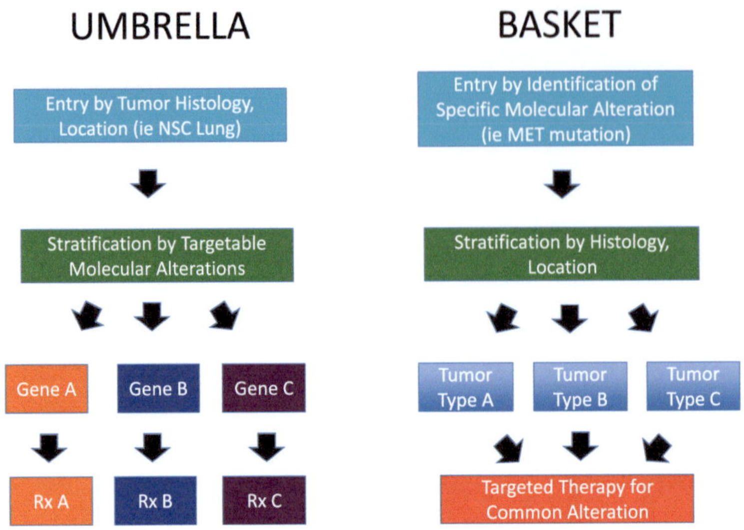

Fig. 20.4 Umbrella and basket trials

utility as determined by presence of evidence-based clinical management guidelines (Maxwell et al. 2015).

Thompson et al. (2016) performed a large, multi-center study sequencing a panel of 18 breast cancer predisposition genes (*ATM*, *ATR*, *BARD1*, *BLM*, *BRCA1*, *BRCA2*, *BRIP1*, *CDH1*, *CHEK2*, *MRE11A*, *NBN*, *NF1*, *PALB2*, *PTEN*, *RAD50*, *STK11*, *TP53*, *and XRCC2*) using NGS with HaloPlex target enrichment (Tischkowitz et al. 2007). This assay was performed on peripheral blood samples of 2000 women who tested negative for BRCA1/2 mutations and were referred to two Familial Cancer centers in Australia. Sequencing was also performed in a control set of 1994 women without a known cancer diagnosis. Six of the high-risk cases were found to harbor mutations in BRCA1/2; all 6 cases did not have full BRCA1/2 analysis at original screening and these would have been found by current BRCA1/2 testing methods. In control cases, four pathogenic mutations in BRCA1 (0.2 %) and nine pathogenic mutations in BRCA2 (0.45 %) were identified, consistent with the estimated prevalence of BRCA1/2 mutations in the general European population. In the cases without BRCA1/2 mutations, 79 pathogenic variants were detected in cases and 39 pathogenic variants were detected in controls. Only known pathogenic or novel protein truncating mutations were evaluated. The most commonly affected gene was PALB2 in which 26 pathogenic variants were identified in cases and four in controls ($p < 0.001$). There were five pathogenic TP53 mutations found in cases and none in controls ($p = 0.03$). Clear pathogenic mutations in CDH1 and PTEN were detected in one case each in the high-risk cohort and were not detected in any controls. Although potentially pathogenic mutations in ATM, CHEK2 and BRIP1 were seen in cases, these were rare and not significantly enriched above the rate seen in controls. Overall, of the 79 non-BRCA1/2 pathogenic variants found in cases, only 34 variants had evidence-based management guidelines (PALB2, TP53, CDH1, PTEN, STK11, ATM missense variant). Thus testing led to potential clinical action in 1.7 % of women referred to genetic counseling who were negative for BRCA1/2 mutations. The author concluded that frequency of validated pathogenic mutations gene panels in women with family history of breast cancer and wildtype for BRCA1/2 is low, and most results need to be interpreted with caution.

A study by Desmond et al. (2015) examined the clinical "actionability" of the results of multi-gene panel testing in a set of patients,

Table 20.1 Summary of selected studies evaluating NGS gene panels for breast cancer risk

Study	Number of patients	Number of genes sequenced	% cases with potentially deleterious mutations in non BRCA1/2 (%)	Most common non-BRCA1/2 genes	% patients with clinically actionable results (%)	Comments
Kurian et al. (2014)	198	42	10.6	MUTYH	ND	Average of 2.1 VUS/case
Maxwell et al. (2015)	278	22	11	TP53	2.5	19 % had at least 1 VUS
Thompson et al. (2016)	2000	18	4 (TR only)	PALB2	1.7	Only known/validated pathogenic variants or novel protein truncating mutations were counted 1998 control cases
Desmond et al. (2015)	1046	25 or 29	3.8	MMR genes, PALB2	<2	Actionable percentage is extrapolation of initial data set
Couch et al. (2015)	1824 (with TNBC)	17	3.7	PALB2	ND	Patients with triple negative breast cancer (TNBC) regardless of family history were analyzed
Li et al. (Li et al. 2016)	684	19	11.5	PALB2, CHEK2	<2	Analysis of other family members of cases with potentially deleterious mutations identified only 4 genes clearly associated with increased risk: PALB2, CHEK2, TP53 and CDH1

without evidence of BRCA1/2 mutations, who were referred to genetics clinics at three academic centers for hereditary breast and ovarian cancer. Patients were tested using one of two available multi-gene NGS panels covering either 25 (n = 669) or 29 (n = 377) genes. They found that 40 (3.8 %) of these BRCA1/2 negative patients harbored deleterious mutations in one potential cancer risk gene. The majority of these mutations were in moderate or low risk genes (26/40 or 65 %), while a minority were in high-risk genes including genes associated with Lynch syndrome (8/40 or 20 %), and in CDH1 (3/40 or 7.5 %), and in genes not associated with breast or ovarian cancer risk (n = 2 CDKN2A, n = 1 bi-allelic MUTYH, and n = 1 APC). To assess actionability of panel-testing results, the authors added to this an additional 23 cases with non-BRCA1/2 pathogenic mutations to give a total of 63 cases. Nearly a third of these cases (20/63) had mutations in genes that had NCCN-based guidelines for high risk cancer associated genes (CDH1, TP53, PTEN, MLH1, MSH2, MSH6, PMS2, APC, bi-allelic MUTYH) with the Lynch syndrome-associated genes being most common. An additional five had deleterious mutations in PALB2, while 28 had mutations in moderate or low risk genes, some of which had implications for increased screening. Overall, 52 % of patients identified as having deleterious mutations had findings that led to post-test recommendations for additional screening or prevention measures, above what would have been recommended based on family history alone (Desmond et al. 2015). Since in the initial screen only 3.8 % of tested patients had potential deleterious mutations, only a very small percent (<2 %) of such patients subjected to multi-gene screening would have unanticipated evidence-based clinical recommendations.

Couch and colleagues analyzed 1824 patients with triple-negative breast cancer unselected for family history (Couch et al. 2015). Germline DNA was analyzed by hybrid-capture based enrichment for a panel of 17 genes including BRCA1 and BRCA2. Deleterious mutations were found in 14.6 % of all patients, with mutations in BRCA1 (8.5 %) and BRCA2 (2.7 %) present in 11.2 %. Deleterious mutations in other genes were detected in 3.7 % of patients, with PALB2 accounting for 1.2 % and others being less frequent (0.5 % or less). These data suggest that BRCA1/2 testing should be considered for all patients with TNBC, but that the value of panel testing for other genes, with the possible exception of PALB2, is less clear (Couch et al. 2015).

Li and colleagues analyzed members from 684 families identified as having strong family history of breast and/or ovarian cancer with no known history of BRCA1/2 mutation (Li et al. 2016). Hybrid-capture based target enrichment was used to sequence coding exons of 19 genes (BRCA1, BRCA2, TP53, PALB2, ATM, CHEK2, CDH1, PTEN, STK11, BARD1, BRIP1, MRE11, NBN, RAD50, RAD51C, RAD51D, CDKN2A, CDK4 and XRCC2). Pathogenic BRCA1 and BRCA2 mutations were identified in 13 and 11 individuals, respectively, all from families without prior BRCA1/2 testing. In the remaining 660 cases, 45 were found to have deleterious mutations in other genes that may alter clinical management (14 PALB2, 14 CHEK2, 8 ATM, 6 TP53, and one each in CDH1, PTEN and STK11). Potential deleterious alterations were found in an additional 31 cases (16 BRIP1, 4 BARD1, 4 MRE11, 3 RAD51D, and one each in CDK4, RAD50, RAD51C, and NBN). From all 76 cases with deleterious or potentially deleterious alterations, DNA from an additional 558 family members was sequenced for segregation analysis. Only four genes (CDH1, CHEK2, PALB2, and TP53) were clearly associated with increased risk of breast cancer, while data for BRIP1 and ATM were equivocal. The authors conclude that panel testing results in clinically actionable findings in <2 % of cases in BRCA1/2 negative high-risk families in their cohort.

Lerner-Ellis and colleagues reviewed a set of studies reporting results of using multi-gene panel testing for hereditary breast cancer (Lerner-Ellis et al. 2015). As expected BRCA1 and BRCA2 had the highest prevalence of pathogenic mutations, found in 5.3 and 3.6 %, respectively. CHEK2 (1.3 %), PALB2 (0.9 %)

and ATM (0.8 %) were the non-BRCA1/2 genes with highest prevalence, while prevalence of PTEN (0.1 %), CDH1 (0.1 %) and STK11 (0.1 %) were quite low. ATM had the highest prevalence of VUS (9 %). The authors conclude that only PALB2 and CHEK2 were the best candidates to include in multi-gene breast cancer panels, based on the prevalence and penetrance of pathogenic mutations.

20.4 Multigene Panels for Analysis of Somatic Tumor Mutations and Therapy Selection

The basic hypothesis that mutations cause cancers and are the force that drives their progression has led to development of therapies that directly target driver mutations. The success of genomic directed therapies in diverse cancers, include targeting ABL1 translocations in CML, KIT mutations in gastro-intestinal stromal tumors and EGFR alterations in lung cancer has further strengthen this hypothesis. The recent years has seen the development of several multigene panels that uses NGS technologies to assess the somatic mutational status of the tumors. The size of the panel and the constituent genes tend to vary in the different academically developed or commercially available panels. Some panels interrogate all exons (and some introns) of a set of genes of interest (using either hybrid capture or amplicon based target enrichment), while others interrogate mutational "hotspots". The incidence of mutations identified tends to vary based on the choice of the panels. Each of these provide an output that is labeled as "actionable" mutations.

20.4.1 Advantages and Limitations of Mutation Panels: What is actionable mutation?

A minority of cancer mutations are thought to be "drivers," defined as mutations involved in the pathogenesis of the malignant state and critical for its cancer phenotype. A subset of these drivers and their component cellular pathways may be "actionable," i.e., have significant diagnostic, prognostic, or therapeutic implications in subsets of cancer patients and for specific therapies. However, the word actionable is used much more loosely in everyday practice. It is used to indicate any alteration in any gene that can be potentially targeted directly or indirectly by therapeutic agents. This definition includes genes such as Tp53 that are not directly targetable but is the most frequently mutated gene in breast cancer. In addition, the definition is agnostic to site of the mutation and whether the mutation results in a gain of function or loss of function.

It is important to clearly understand the definition since in vast majority of cases sequencing assays will identify genes and mutation sites that are distinct from the original clinical indication of the targeted therapies/drugs. To illustrate the point, vemurafenib has clear clinical activity in melanomas with the activating V600E mutations. There is some data to suggest that V600E mutations in other cancers such as thyroid cancer and hairy cell leukemia might respond to vemurafenib (Hyman et al. 2015; Tiacci et al. 2015). However, vemuranib alone does affect the progression of colon adenocarcinomas with BRAF V600E. Feedback activation of EGFR signaling present in epithelial colon cancel cells was found to limit activity of single agent vemurafenib, suggesting that a combination of EGFR-inhibitor plus BRAF-inhibitor will be required to optimally target BRAF activation in BRAF V600E mutant colon cancer (Prahallad et al. 2012). Thus the optimal way to target individual oncogenic mutations may still require consideration of the signaling networks present in the cell of origin.

Sequencing assays will also find novel BRAF alterations distinct from V600E. Some alterations have been shown to be sensitive to vemurafenib, while others, including gene fusions, have been shown to be insensitive (Sievert et al. 2013). Thus interpreting the relevance and utility of a novel BRAF alteration in a non-melanoma cancer may not be straightforward, despite such alterations being labeled "actionable".

Mutation panels provide for the simultaneous screening of multiple genes. These genes have been selected for the relevance to cancer i.e. been documented to be drivers in one or more cancer types, and may guide treatment or refine prognosis. For some genes in these panels, there are drugs with proven efficacy in certain cancer types. Therefore, identification of the target gene, at least theoretically, offers the patient a novel potentially effective treatment strategy.

The hope of targeted therapy needs to be balanced with reality. As cited above, the presence of a target mutation in one cancer does not indicate therapeutic efficacy of the same mutation in a tumor arising at a different body site. Histological parameters and tissue of origin need to be considered. More importantly, although the mutations often involve the same gene, the site of mutations may be different. In an ideal situation, one would like to characterize the nature of any novel mutations identified and its biological impact (gain or loss of function) in the tumor. At present however, there is little biological or clinical information for many novel alterations to clearly guide therapy. Another limitation of the mutation assays is that when only tumor tissue is examined, there is a potential to misidentify rare germline polymorphisms as somatic tumor-associated mutations (Jones et al. 2015).

20.4.2 Genomic Landscape of Breast Cancer Subclasses

Breast cancer comprises a very heterogeneous set of diseases. It includes multiple distinct cancer subtypes each likely with its own distinct cells of origin and molecular pathophysiology. Gene expression profiling initially identified at least 4 distinct subtypes (Luminal A, Luminal B, HER2-enriched, and basal-like), and more recent analyses on large sets of breast cancer suggest that there are at least 10 distinct subsets of breast cancer, and likely more (Perou et al. 2000; Sorlie et al. 2003; Curtis et al. 2012).

Genomic analysis is highly promising as a way to organize and categorize breast cancer. For example the presence of one genomic alteration, HER2-amplification, defines a clinically validated subclass of breast cancer. Targeted therapy aimed at the HER2 alterations has dramatically altered the natural history of this disease. This has led to great optimism that genomic characterization may both aid the proper classification of breast cancer and lead to effective targeted therapeutic approaches.

Large scale efforts to comprehensively characterize genomic alterations in breast cancer, such as The Genome Cancer Atlas have recently been completed with over 1000 breast cancer samples analyzed (Ciriello et al. 2015; Comprehensive molecular portraits of human breast tumours 2012; Gatza et al. 2014; Natrajan et al. 2010; Stephens et al. 2012). These efforts have not added immediate clarity to our classification of breast cancer. Instead these approaches have demonstrated that underlying the diversity in phenotype in breast cancer is an even greater diversity in genomic alterations. However some patterns and themes have arisen. These will be reviewed in the context of Luminal breast cancer (ER+, HER2-nonamplified, both low grade and high grade), HER2-non-amplified, high proliferation), HER2 + (HER2 amplified, can either be ER+ or ER−), and triple-negative.

20.4.2.1 Luminal Breast Cancers

In this review luminal breast cancers are characterized as having expression of the estrogen receptor and not harboring HER2-amplification. They can be further subdivided into luminal a, which have high expression of both ER and PR, and tend to have low proliferative index. Luminal B cancers are ER+, can have variable expression of pr and have higher proliferative indexes (as assayed by grade, KI67, or molecular assays such as ODx or ROS) (Ades et al. 2014; Dawood et al. 2011; Fan et al. 2006). We will review the mutations found in luminal cancers.

PIK3CA pathway alterations: Alterations in PIK3CA are the most common mutations found in luminal cancers (Comprehensive molecular portraits of human breast tumours 2012; Banerji et al. 2012). Most mutations are hotspot seen either in the helical domain or the kinase domain, and are present in ~50 % of luminal A cancers and 30 % of luminal B cancers (Dirican et al. 2016; Comprehensive molecular portraits of human breast tumours 2012; Ciriello et al. 2015). Alterations in PIK3CA are predicted to activate down stream signaling, leading to activation of AKT, and possible, downstream activation of MTOR. The PIK3CA pathway may interact with estrogen receptor (ER)-mediated signaling, suggesting that PIK3CA mutations may potentiate ER mediated signaling (Dirican et al. 2016; Fu et al. 2013). Inhibitors of PIK3CA, inhibitors of AKT and MTOR inhibitors have all been proposed as being targeted therapy for cancers harboring PIK3CA activating mutations. At present PIK3CA inhibitors and AKT inhibitors remain in early phase trials, although some data on PIK3CA pan inhibitors are promising (Ma et al. 2016; Roy-Chowdhuri et al. 2015). MTOR inhibitors are now FDA approved for metastatic ER, but several studies have failed to show that the presence of PIK3CA mutation is a marker for benefit (Loi et al. 2013; Hortobagyi et al. 2016). Other alterations in the PIK3CA pathway, including inactivating mutations in PIK3R1 (an inhibitor regulator of PIK3CA) and the PTEN phosphatase are also present in a small subset of luminal cancers (Comprehensive molecular portraits of human breast tumours 2012). At present there is no clinically validated therapy for PIK3CA mutations in breast cancer, although some are in late phase trials.

MAP3K1: MAP3K1 is part of the JNK and MAPK signaling pathway and is unusual in that it is postulated to have both ubiquitin ligase activity as well as serine-threonine kinase activity. Inactivating mutations in MAP3K1 are found in up to 14 % of Luminal cancers, with mutation being associated with high expression of estrogen receptor and low proliferation (Comprehensive molecular portraits of human breast tumours 2012; Stephens et al. 2012; Banerji et al. 2012). The exact effect of MAP3K1 loss on survival and apoptotic pathways is not clear, and at present there is no clear way to target this alteration.

GATA3. GATA3 is a master transcription factor involved in mammary epithelial development and in particular in differentiation of mammary gland into differentiated luminal epithelium. Alterations of GATA3 are found in 14 % OF Luminal A breast cancer, and associated with high expression of ER(Comprehensive molecular portraits of human breast tumours 2012; Stephens et al. 2012). At present there is no validated targeted therapy aimed at GATA alterations in breast cancer.

Estrogen receptor. The estrogen receptor is not a classic oncogene, as it is not primarily mutated, amplified in most breast cancers. However many luminal breast cancers are addicted to ER-mediated signaling for their survival and hormonal therapy with either SERMs or aromatase inhibitors is highly effective in the treatment of both early and late stage disease. In metastatic ER+ disease the development of resistance to hormonal therapy is associated with the development of specific mutations in ER (Schiavon et al. 2015; Jeselsohn et al. 2015; Robinson et al. 2013). These mutations often lead to ligand independent activation of ER (Jeselsohn et al. 2015). At present there are no validated therapies targeting the presence of ER-mutations, but these could help direct patient to non-hormonal therapies.

CDH1: Loss of function mutations (often frameshift or truncation mutations) and genomic deletion of CDH1 (E-cadherin) is seen in the majority of a specific subset of luminal cancer labeled invasive lobular breast cancer (Ciriello et al. 2015; McCart Reed et al. 2015). Loss of E-cadherin expression is thought to lead to decreased cellular cohesion, and thus contribute to the unique histologic pattern of "single-cell filing" seen in ILC. Rare gemline mutations in CHD1 are associated with herediary risk of diffuse gastric cancer and lobular brast cancer (reviewed earlier). At present there are no therapeutic interventions that specifically target loss of CDH1.

HER2: Although luminal cancer are defined in this summary as lacking HER-amplification, a small subset of ER + lobular cancers can harbor activating mutations in HER2 (Ciriello et al. 2015; Lien et al. 2015). These can include both activating mutations in the kinase domain, and mutations in the extracellular domain that are known to be activating and oncogenic. Early studies with small molecule inhibitors of HER2 such as lapatinib and neratinib suggest these agents may be active in metastatic lobular breast cancer harboring such activating mutations in HER2 (Ben-Baruch et al. 2015.

TP53. Mutations in the TP53 tumor suppressor are infrequent in low grade (~10–12 %) ER + breast cancer, with higher frequency in in the higher grade, Luminal B ER+ cancers (~30 %) (Comprehensive molecular portraits of human breast tumours 2012). Most mutations are missense mutations in the DNA binding domain. Germline mutations in TP53 are seen in Li-Fraumeni syndrome and are a rare cause of inherited breast cancer risk. There are some preclinical data showing small molecules that can "reactivate" some P53 mutations and thus potentially target a subset of p53-mutant cancers (Blanden et al. 2015). However at present there are no validated therapies that specifically target p53 mutations in breast cancer.

BRCA1/2: Cancers that arise in BRCA2 mutations carriers are mostly ER+ and fall into our luminal classification, though often have higher proliferation index and grade that standard luminal A breast cancers and may fall into luminal B category. A minority of BRCA1 associated breast cancers can be ER+; these ER+ BRCA1-associated cancers also tend to be higher grade cancers. Multiple studies have shown that BRCA1/2 mutant cancers are specifically sensitive to certain classes of DNA damaging agents such as platinum, and to the new PARP inhibitors (Kaufman et al. 2015; Livraghi and Garber 2015; Isakoff et al. 2015), and olaparib is approved for the treatment of BRCA1/2 mutant ovarian cancer. The roles of platinum and PARP inhibitors in the treatment of BRCA1/2 mutant breast cancers are now under active investigation.

8p11 amplicon: FGFR1. Amplification of FGFR1, usually as part of the larger 8p11 amplicon, is seen in ~18 % of breast cancer including luminal breast cancers (Curtis et al. 2012; Bilal et al. 2012). The 8p11 amplicon is large and includes many potential driver genes including FGFR1, so it is not clear that FGR1 is the driver gene. Presence of the 8p11 amplicon has been shown to be associated with poor outcome in ER+ breast cancers treated with hormonal therapy alone (Bilal et al. 2012; Shi et al. 2015). Initial trials with FGFR inhibitors showed little activity in breast cancers with FGFR1 amplification, other trials using newer pan-FGFR inhibitors are underway (Andre et al. 2013; Soria et al. 2014).

Cyclin D1 amplification: Amplification of the Cyclin D1 gene (CCND1) is seen in luminal cancers and is present in ~25 % of luminal A cancers and up to 60 % of luminal B cancers (Curtis et al. 2012; Burandt et al. 2016). This alteration can increase formation of an active CDK4/6-CCND1 complex, lead to increased Rb phosphorylation and drive entry into cell cycle. This alteration may render cells sensitive to CKD4/6 inhibitors such as palbociclib, which is FDA approved for the treatment of metastatic ER + breast cancers in combination with hormonal therapy (Finn et al. 2016. However at present there are no clinical data suggesting that CCND1 or CKD4 alterations in breast cancer are predictive of benefit from treatment with CKD4/6 inhibitors.

Other Amplicons: Other commonly amplified regions in luminal breast cancer include 8q24 and 17q28. These also have been shown to be associated with poor outcome in ER+ breast cancer in multiple studies (Curtis et al. 2012). Again the exact driver oncogene(s) on these regions is not characterized.

20.4.2.2 HER2 Amplified Breast Cancer

The presence of HER2 amplification is the one clinically actionable genomic alteration that is routinely assayed in clinical practice. HER2-targeted therapy, including the engineered antibodies trastuzumab and pertuzumab, now are part of the standard therapy of both early stage and advanced HER2-amplified breast cancer (Hodeib et al. 2015). HER2-amplified breast cancers are themselves diverse, with phenotypic variety in clinically prognostic features such as ER-expression and stromal lymphocytic infiltrate. They also have a wide spectrum of other genomic alterations, but very few recurrent alterations.

PIK3CA Pathway: Activating mutations in PIK3CA are seen in ~25–40 % of HER2-amplified breast cancers (Comprehensive molecular portraits of human breast tumours 2012; Curtis et al. 2012). Data from preclinical models strongly suggested that downstream activation of PIK3CA or loss of PTEN should engender primary resistance to upstream targeting of HER2 signaling (Hanker et al. 2013; Chandarlapaty et al. 2012; Nagata et al. 2004). Indeed some studies have shown that the presence of PIK3CA mutations, but not PTEN loss, is associated with a decreased path-CR rate in the setting of neo-adjuvant HER2 targeted therapy in HER2-amplified breast cancer (Loibl et al. 2014; Nuciforo et al. 2015). However large studies have shown that the presence of PIK3CA mutations not translate into decreased long-term outcome in Her2-amplified cancer treated with a trastuzumab-based regiment (Pogue-Geile et al. 2015; Nuciforo et al. 2015; Baselga et al. 2014). Interestingly, several studies strongly suggest that an important mechanism by which trastuzumab kills HER2-amplified cancer cells, especially micro-metastatic cancer cells, is through antibody-dependent cytotoxicity (Spector and Blackwell 2009; Petricevic et al. 2013). This mechanism would be independent of downstream HER2-signaling and thus be insensitive to presence of downstream activating mutations in PIK3CA or PTEN loss.

PIK3CA and PTEN mutations may lead to downstream activation of MTOR and thus provide resistance to HER2 targeted therapies, and preclinical studies suggest that MTOR inhibitors may prevent resistance to HER2 targeted therapy in HER2-amplified breast cancer. However recent data from the BOLER0-1 show little benefit to adding everolimus to trastuzumab based-therapy in first line treatment of HER2-amplified breast cancer (Hurvitz et al. 2015).

TP53: Mutation in TP53 are seen in over 50 % of HER2-amplified breast cancers with the majority of these mutations being missense mutations, mostly in the DNA binding domain (Comprehensive molecular portraits of human breast tumours 2012).

CCND1 and CDK4: Amplification of CCND1 are seen in about 38 % of HER2-amplified breast cancer and gain of CKD4 is seen in ~24 % (Comprehensive molecular portraits of human breast tumours 2012). Although CKD4/6 inhibitors could work downstream of CCND1 amplification and CKD4 gain, there are no clear data to show that presence of these alterations is associated with response to CKD4/6 inhibitors.

20.4.2.3 Triple Negative Breast Cancer

Triple negative breast cancers constitute a very heterogeneous set of cancers with at least 7 possible subclasses identified by gene expression profiling (Lehmann et al. 2011). Comprehensive analysis of genomic alterations found in these cancers show that these cancers tend to have very complex patterns of alterations characterized by a large number of genomic rearrangements (Shah et al. 2012; Banerji et al. 2012; Comprehensive Molecular Portraits of Human Breast Tumours 2012). The spectrum of point-mutations is wide and the only gene recurrently mutated at high frequency in TNBC appears to be tp53 (Comprehensive Molecular Portraits of Human Breast Tumours 2012; Holstege et al. 2010; Hirshfield and Ganesan 2014). Oncogenic driver alteration may be generated in TNBC more by genomic rearrangement and copy number alterations than by point mutations.

TP53: Over 80 % of TNBC have mutations in TP53 (Shah et al. 2012; Banerji et al. 2012; Comprehensive molecular portraits of human breast tumours 2012). Interestingly p53 mutations found in TNBC have a higher incidence of nonsense and frameshift mutations when compared to either luminal or HER2-amplified breast cancer in which missense mutations predominate (Comprehensive molecular portraits of human breast tumours 2012).

BRCA1/2: Approximately 5–10 % of TNBC have mutations in BRCA1 with most of these being associated with germline deleterious mutations (Comprehensive molecular portraits of human breast tumours 2012; Shah et al. 2012; Banerji et al. 2012). A very small subset of TNBC are associated with BRCA2 mutations.

Alterations in BRCA1 and BRCA2 are targetable by specific classes of DNA damaging agents including platinum agents and the PARP inhibitors (Kaufman et al. 2015; Livraghi and Garber 2015; Isakoff et al. 2015). PARP inhibitors are approved for the treatment of BRCA1/2 mutated ovarian cancer, but not at this time for breast cancer. Several clinical trials are underway examining the utility of both platinum and PARP inhibitors in BRCA1/2 mutant breast cancer.

PIK3CA pathway alterations: Activating mutations in PIK3CA are found in less than 10 % of TNBC (Comprehensive molecular portraits of human breast tumours 2012; Shah et al. 2012; Banerji et al. 2012). However gross genomic deletions of PTEN locus can be found in up to 30 % of these cancers (Comprehensive molecular portraits of human breast tumours 2012). Although these alterations are likely driver mutations, at present there is no validated therapeutic strategy for alterations in PIK3CA or PTEN in TNBC.

Common regions of genomic gain and loss: Amplification of MYC are found in up to 40 % of TNBC and function as a key driver in these cancers. RB1 loss is found in up to 20 % of TNBC. Although several strategies to target MYC amplification and RB loss have been developed in pre-clinical models, none have yet been validated clinically (Delmore et al. 2011).

Gene Fusions: Genomic rearrangements are a major class of genomic alterations seen in TNBC. However identifying driver oncogenic fusion genes in the setting of a larger number of rearrangement events is difficult, especially with short read sequencing used in current NGS (Banerji et al. 2012). Several new strategies that are being developed to enrich for fusions affecting known oncogenic drivers, such as Anchored Multiplex PCR may allow for more robust identification of driver fusions genes (Zheng et al. 2014).

20.4.3 Clinical Utility of Mutation Panels for Therapeutic Purposes

At present the only clinically validated genomic alteration in breast cancer is the presence of HER2-alterations, that are used to guide HER2-targeted therapy. The presence of the other mutations, discussed above, have not yet translated into any validated therapeutic strategies, although some studies, such as those examining efficacy of PARP inhibitors and other DNA damaging agents in BRCA1/2 mutant breast cancers are in progress. Despite lack of validated clinical utility, multiple CLIA-certified gene-panel assays for assessment of somatic mutations in solid tumors are currently available. Some studies assessing the use of these panels in breast cancer will be reviewed below.

Roy-Chowduri and colleagues analyzed results of a gene panel looking at hotspot mutation sites in 46 genes in 354 patients with cancer. They found a similar spectrum of mutations in their cohort as reported in The Cancer Genome Atlas, with PIK3CA mutations being most common in ER+/HER2− cancers, and TP53 mutations being most common in TNBC (Roy-Chowdhuri et al. 2015). Vasan and colleagues use a CLIA-certified hybrid-capture based targeted NGS assay that interrogated all exons of 182 cancer-related genes and select introns in 14 genes in 51 breast cancer samples (Vasan et al. 2014). They found that 84 % of cancers harbored alterations in at least one gene that had potential therapeutic implications. Again the most common "actionable" mutations were PIK3CA (9 cases), NF1 (7 cases), AKT1-3 (7 cases), BRCA1/2 (6 cases); FGFR1 (5 cases), and rare mutations in ALK, KIT (1 each). Balko and colleagues used a hybrid-capture based targeted genomic sequencing as well as digital RNA expression analysis in 74 samples of TNBC present as residual disease after neo-adjuvant chemotherapy (Balko et al. 2014). Targetable mutations were found in the majority of cases. Mutations in TP53 were present in 89 %, and MCLI amplifications in 54 % and MYC amplifications in 35 % and BRCA1/2 mutations seen in 10 %. Many individually infrequent mutations were seen, including some with potential therapeutic strategies such as TSC1 loss. These studies demonstrate that NGS sequencing can identify pathogenic mutations in clinical breast cancer samples. However the clinical utility is not yet clear, although these data can be used to enroll patients to matched early phase clinical trials.

There are only a few studies that have analyzed how data on somatic mutations affected care in metastatic breast cancer. Andre and colleagues reported the results of the multicenter SAFIR01 trial in which 423 patients with metastatic breast cancer had cancer specimens analyzed by array-CGH and Sanger sequencing for hotspot mutations in PIK3CA and AKT1 (Andre et al. 2014). CGH analysis was feasible in 283 patients (67 %) and Sanger sequencing in 297 (70 %). Potentially targetable alterations were found in 46 %, with PIK3CA being most common (25 %), followed by CCND1 amplification (19 %) and FGFR1 amplification (13 %), and AKT1 mutations found in <5 %. 55 patients (13 %) had therapy targeted to identified mutation. In 43 assessable patients, 4 had an objective response (9 %) and 9 (21 %) had stable disease. This shows that with this limited sequencing analysis, benefit was found but in only a minority of patients. Johnson and colleagues reported the results of more comprehensive genomic profiling in 103 patients, of which 26 % had breast cancer. Most of these patients (83 %) had a potentially actionable mutation, and 21 % actually received genomically-guided therapy, most often by referral to a clinical trial. These early trials are suggestive of the potential power of clinical tumor sequencing, however much more work has to be done to demonstrate true clinical utility. A key limiting feature in assessing utility is need for further clinical development of effective new targeted therapeutics, and increased access of patients to both new agents and combination therapy.

In order to assess the utility of these molecularly defined therapies, researchers have used two main approaches, umbrella and basket trials. In "Umbrella" trials, the goal is to test the impact of different drugs on different mutations in a single type of cancer. In the BATTLE umbrella trial, patients with non-small cell lung cancer were assigned to receive a particular drug, which was expected to best target the mutations identified within their tumors by molecular profiling. In contrast, within a basket trial, the goal is to examine the effect of a particular therapeutic agent on a particular genetic or molecular peculiarity regardless of the type or subtype of cancer in which it occurs. The patients with the different types of cancer can be then grouped into separate study arms, or "baskets" based on other characteristics such histology or tumor location. This trial design permits analyze the responses of patients with each type of cancer as well as to assess the impact of the drug on all of the patients with the molecular abnormality. The National Cancer Institute MATCH trial is enrolling up to 1000 people with a variety of cancers to therapies that target the specific mutations found in their tumors. The incidence of actionable mutations in metastatic cancers is still low. It was recently reported in the NCI MATCH trial that only one of the 700 patients screened matched to the molecularly defined treatment arm (https://www.genomeweb.com/molecular-diagnostics/nci-match-sees-lots-enthusiasm-initial-months-not-many-matches).

20.5 Summary

Advances in sequencing technologies have led to the development of low cost, multi-gene panels for evaluation of breast cancer risk. The methodology has outstanding technical validity, but the clinical validity and clinical utility of many genes included in these panels remain uncertain. Several recent studies suggest that use of NGS panels only leads to findings with clear clinical utility in a small percentage of patients, both in the setting of hereditary risk assessment and in somatic tumor profiling. Increasing use of these panels will also lead to more patients being found to harbor alterations of unknown significance, with potential for overtreatment. However, it is likely that multi-gene panels will become part of the care of many patients referred for genetic counseling to evaluate breast cancer risk. There is an obvious need for more data gathering and well-designed studies to establish both clinical validity and utility of most genes included in currently available multi-gene panels in order to maximize patient benefit and avoid overtreatment.

References

A victory for genes (2013). Nature medicine 19(7):792. doi:10.1038/nm.3279

Aarnio M, Sankila R, Pukkala E, Salovaara R, Aaltonen LA, de la Chapelle A, Peltomaki P, Mecklin JP, Jarvinen HJ (1999) Cancer risk in mutation carriers of DNA-mismatch-repair genes. Int J Cancer J Int Du Cancer 81(2):214–218

Ades F, Zardavas D, Bozovic-Spasojevic I, Pugliano L, Fumagalli D, de Azambuja E, Viale G, Sotiriou C, Piccart M (2014) Luminal B breast cancer: molecular characterization, clinical management, and future perspectives. J Clin Oncol: Off J Am Soc Clin Oncol 32(25):2794–2803. doi:10.1200/jco.2013.54.1870

Akbari MR, Cybulski C (2015) RECQL: a DNA helicase in breast cancer. Oncotarget 6(29):26558–26559. doi:10.18632/oncotarget.5452

Akbari MR, Lepage P, Rosen B, McLaughlin J, Risch H, Minden M, Narod SA (2014) PPM1D mutations in circulating white blood cells and the risk for ovarian cancer. J Natl Cancer Inst 106(1):djt323. doi:10.1093/jnci/djt323

Aloraifi F, McCartan D, McDevitt T, Green AJ, Bracken A, Geraghty J (2015) Protein-truncating variants in moderate-risk breast cancer susceptibility genes: a meta-analysis of high-risk case-control screening studies. Cancer genetics 208(9):455–463. doi:10.1016/j.cancergen.2015.06.001

Andre F, Bachelot T, Campone M, Dalenc F, Perez-Garcia JM, Hurvitz SA, Turner N, Rugo H, Smith JW, Deudon S, Shi M, Zhang Y, Kay A, Porta DG, Yovine A, Baselga J (2013) Targeting FGFR with dovitinib (TKI258): preclinical and clinical data in breast cancer. Clin Cancer Res: Off J Am Assoc Cancer Res 19(13):3693–3702. doi:10.1158/1078-0432.ccr-13-0190

Andre F, Bachelot T, Commo F, Campone M, Arnedos M, Dieras V, Lacroix-Triki M, Lacroix L, Cohen P, Gentien D, Adelaide J, Dalenc F, Goncalves A, Levy C, Ferrero JM, Bonneterre J, Lefeuvre C, Jimenez M, Filleron T, Bonnefoi H (2014) Comparative genomic hybridisation array and DNA sequencing to direct treatment of metastatic breast cancer: a multicentre, prospective trial (SAFIR01/UNICANCER). Lancet Oncol 15(3):267–274. doi:10.1016/s1470-2045(13)70611-9

Antoniou AC, Casadei S, Heikkinen T, Barrowdale D, Pylkas K, Roberts J, Lee A, Subramanian D, De Leeneer K, Fostira F, Tomiak E, Neuhausen SL, Teo ZL, Khan S, Aittomaki K, Moilanen JS, Turnbull C, Seal S, Mannermaa A, Kallioniemi A, Lindeman GJ, Buys SS, Andrulis IL, Radice P, Tondini C, Manoukian S, Toland AE, Miron P, Weitzel JN, Domchek SM, Poppe B, Claes KB, Yannoukakos D, Concannon P, Bernstein JL, James PA, Easton DF, Goldgar DE, Hopper JL, Rahman N, Peterlongo P, Nevanlinna H, King MC, Couch FJ, Southey MC, Winqvist R, Foulkes WD, Tischkowitz M (2014) Breast-cancer risk in families with mutations in PALB2. New Engl J Med 371(6):497–506. doi:10.1056/NEJMoa1400382

Antoniou A, Pharoah PD, Narod S, Risch HA, Eyfjord JE, Hopper JL, Loman N, Olsson H, Johannsson O, Borg A, Pasini B, Radice P, Manoukian S, Eccles DM, Tang N, Olah E, Anton-Culver H, Warner E, Lubinski J, Gronwald J, Gorski B, Tulinius H, Thorlacius S, Eerola H, Nevanlinna H, Syrjakoski K, Kallioniemi OP, Thompson D, Evans C, Peto J, Lalloo F, Evans DG, Easton DF (2003) Average risks of breast and ovarian cancer associated with BRCA1 or BRCA2 mutations detected in case Series unselected for family history: a combined analysis of 22 studies. Am J Hum Genet 72 (5):1117–1130. doi:10.1086/375033

Balko JM, Giltnane JM, Wang K, Schwarz LJ, Young CD, Cook RS, Owens P, Sanders ME, Kuba MG, Sanchez V, Kurupi R, Moore PD, Pinto JA, Doimi FD, Gomez H, Horiuchi D, Goga A, Lehmann BD, Bauer JA, Pietenpol JA, Ross JS, Palmer GA, Yelensky R, Cronin M, Miller VA, Stephens PJ, Arteaga CL (2014) Molecular profiling of the residual disease of triple-negative breast cancers after neoadjuvant chemotherapy identifies actionable therapeutic targets. Cancer Discov 4 (2):232–245. doi:10.1158/2159-8290.cd-13-0286

Banerji S, Cibulskis K, Rangel-Escareno C, Brown KK, Carter SL, Frederick AM, Lawrence MS, Sivachenko AY, Sougnez C, Zou L, Cortes ML, Fernandez-Lopez JC, Peng S, Ardlie KG, Auclair D, Bautista-Pina V, Duke F, Francis J, Jung J, Maffuz-Aziz A, Onofrio RC, Parkin M, Pho NH, Quintanar-Jurado V, Ramos AH, Rebollar-Vega R, Rodriguez-Cuevas S, Romero-Cordoba SL, Schumacher SE, Stransky N, Thompson KM, Uribe-Figueroa L, Baselga J, Beroukhim R, Polyak K, Sgroi DC, Richardson AL, Jimenez-Sanchez G, Lander ES, Gabriel SB, Garraway LA, Golub TR, Melendez-Zajgla J, Toker A, Getz G, Hidalgo-Miranda A, Meyerson M (2012) Sequence analysis of mutations and translocations across breast cancer subtypes. Nature 486(7403):405–409. doi:10.1038/nature11154

Bartkova J, Tommiska J, Oplustilova L, Aaltonen K, Tamminen A, Heikkinen T, Mistrik M, Aittomaki K, Blomqvist C, Heikkila P, Lukas J, Nevanlinna H, Bartek J (2008) Aberrations of the MRE11-RAD50-NBS1 DNA damage sensor complex in human breast cancer: MRE11 as a candidate familial cancer-predisposing gene. Mol Oncol 2 (4):296–316. doi:10.1016/j.molonc.2008.09.007

Baselga J, Cortes J, Im SA, Clark E, Ross G, Kiermaier A, Swain SM (2014) Biomarker analyses in CLEOPATRA: a phase III, placebo-controlled study of pertuzumab in human epidermal growth factor receptor

2-positive, first-line metastatic breast cancer. J Clin Oncol: Off J Am Soc Clin Oncol 32(33):3753–3761. doi:10.1200/jco.2013.54.5384

Ben-Baruch NE, Bose R, Kavuri SM, Ma CX, Ellis MJ (2015) HER2-Mutated Breast Cancer Responds to Treatment With Single-Agent Neratinib, a Second-Generation HER2/EGFR Tyrosine Kinase Inhibitor. J Natl Compr Cancer Netw: JNCCN 13 (9):1061–1064

Bernstein JL, Teraoka S, Southey MC, Jenkins MA, Andrulis IL, Knight JA, John EM, Lapinski R, Wolitzer AL, Whittemore AS, West D, Seminara D, Olson ER, Spurdle AB, Chenevix-Trench G, Giles GG, Hopper JL, Concannon P (2006) Population-based estimates of breast cancer risks associated with ATM gene variants c.7271T > G and c.1066-6T > G (IVS10-6T > G) from the breast cancer family registry. Hum Mutat 27(11):1122–1128. doi:10.1002/humu.20415

Bhatti S, Kozlov S, Farooqi AA, Naqi A, Lavin M, Khanna KK (2011) ATM protein kinase: the linchpin of cellular defenses to stress. Cell Mol Life Sci: CMLS 68(18):2977–3006. doi:10.1007/s00018-011-0683-9

Bilal E, Vassallo K, Toppmeyer D, Barnard N, Rye IH, Almendro V, Russnes H, Borresen-Dale AL, Levine AJ, Bhanot G, Ganesan S (2012) Amplified loci on chromosomes 8 and 17 predict early relapse in ER-positive breast cancers. PLoS ONE 7(6):e38575. doi:10.1371/journal.pone.0038575

Blanden AR, Yu X, Loh SN, Levine AJ, Carpizo DR (2015) Reactivating mutant p53 using small molecules as zinc metallochaperones: awakening a sleeping giant in cancer. Drug Discov Today 20(11):1391–1397. doi:10.1016/j.drudis.2015.07.006

Bonadona V, Bonaiti B, Olschwang S, Grandjouan S, Huiart L, Longy M, Guimbaud R, Buecher B, Bignon YJ, Caron O, Colas C, Nogues C, Lejeune-Dumoulin S, Olivier-Faivre L, Polycarpe-Osaer F, Nguyen TD, Desseigne F, Saurin JC, Berthet P, Leroux D, Duffour J, Manouvrier S, Frebourg T, Sobol H, Lasset C, Bonaiti-Pellie C (2011) Cancer risks associated with germline mutations in MLH1, MSH2, and MSH6 genes in Lynch syndrome. JAMA 305(22):2304–2310. doi:10.1001/jama.2011.743

Bubien V, Bonnet F, Brouste V, Hoppe S, Barouk-Simonet E, David A, Edery P, Bottani A, Layet V, Caron O, Gilbert-Dussardier B, Delnatte C, Dugast C, Fricker JP, Bonneau D, Sevenet N, Longy M, Caux F (2013) High cumulative risks of cancer in patients with PTEN hamartoma tumour syndrome. J Med Genet 50(4):255–263. doi:10.1136/jmedgenet-2012-101339

Buerki N, Gautier L, Kovac M, Marra G, Buser M, Mueller H, Heinimann K (2012) Evidence for breast cancer as an integral part of Lynch syndrome. Genes Chromosom Cancer 51(1):83–91. doi:10.1002/gcc.20935

Buermans HP, den Dunnen JT (2014) Next generation sequencing technology: advances and applications. Biochimica et biophysica acta 1842(10):1932–1941. doi:10.1016/j.bbadis.2014.06.015

Burandt E, Grunert M, Lebeau A, Choschzick M, Quaas A, Janicke F, Muller V, Scholz U, Bokemeyer C, Petersen C, Geist S, Paluchowski P, Wilke C, Heilenkotter U, Simon R, Sauter G, Wilczak W (2016) Cyclin D1 gene amplification is highly homogeneous in breast cancer. Breast cancer (Tokyo, Japan) 23(1):111–119. doi:10.1007/s12282-014-0538-y

CHEK2*1100delC and susceptibility to breast cancer: a collaborative analysis involving 10,860 breast cancer cases and 9,065 controls from 10 studies (2004). Am J Human Genet 74(6):1175–1182. doi:10.1086/421251

Cantor SB, Bell DW, Ganesan S, Kass EM, Drapkin R, Grossman S, Wahrer DC, Sgroi DC, Lane WS, Haber DA, Livingston DM (2001) BACH1, a novel helicase-like protein, interacts directly with BRCA1 and contributes to its DNA repair function. Cell 105 (1):149–160

Cao AY, Huang J, Hu Z, Li WF, Ma ZL, Tang LL, Zhang B, Su FX, Zhou J, Di GH, Shen KW, Wu J, Lu JS, Luo JM, Yuan WT, Shen ZZ, Huang W, Shao ZM (2009) The prevalence of PALB2 germline mutations in BRCA1/BRCA2 negative Chinese women with early onset breast cancer or affected relatives. Breast Cancer Res Treat 114(3):457–462. doi:10.1007/s10549-008-0036-z

Casadei S, Norquist BM, Walsh T, Stray S, Mandell JB, Lee MK, Stamatoyannopoulos JA, King MC (2011) Contribution of inherited mutations in the BRCA2-interacting protein PALB2 to familial breast cancer. Cancer Res 71(6):2222–2229. doi:10.1158/0008-5472.can-10-3958

Chandarlapaty S, Sakr RA, Giri D, Patil S, Heguy A, Morrow M, Modi S, Norton L, Rosen N, Hudis C, King TA (2012) Frequent mutational activation of the PI3 K-AKT pathway in trastuzumab-resistant breast cancer. Clin Cancer Res: Off J Am Assoc Cancer Res 18(24):6784–6791. doi:10.1158/1078-0432.ccr-12-1785

Chen S, Parmigiani G (2007) Meta-analysis of BRCA1 and BRCA2 penetrance. J Clin Oncol: Off J Am Soc Clin Oncol 25(11):1329–1333. doi:10.1200/jco.2006.09.1066

Chenevix-Trench G, Spurdle AB, Gatei M, Kelly H, Marsh A, Chen X, Donn K, Cummings M, Nyholt D, Jenkins MA, Scott C, Pupo GM, Dork T, Bendix R, Kirk J, Tucker K, McCredie MR, Hopper JL, Sambrook J, Mann GJ, Khanna KK (2002) Dominant negative ATM mutations in breast cancer families. J Natl Cancer Inst 94(3):205–215

Cheng H, Ma B, Jiang R, Wang W, Guo H, Shen N, Li D, Zhao Q, Wang R, Yi P, Zhao Y, Liu Z, Huang T (2012) Individual and combined effects of MDM2 SNP309 and TP53 Arg72Pro on breast cancer risk: an updated meta-analysis. Mol Biol Rep 39(9):9265–9274. doi:10.1007/s11033-012-1800-z

Christgen M, Derksen P (2015) Lobular breast cancer: molecular basis, mouse and cellular models. Breast

Cancer Res: BCR 17:16. doi:10.1186/s13058-015-0517-z

Chun HH, Gatti RA (2004) Ataxia-telangiectasia, an evolving phenotype. DNA Repair 3(8–9):1187–1196. doi:10.1016/j.dnarep.2004.04.010

Ciriello G, Gatza ML, Beck AH, Wilkerson MD, Rhie SK, Pastore A, Zhang H, McLellan M, Yau C, Kandoth C, Bowlby R, Shen H, Hayat S, Fieldhouse R, Lester SC, Tse GM, Factor RE, Collins LC, Allison KH, Chen YY, Jensen K, Johnson NB, Oesterreich S, Mills GB, Cherniack AD, Robertson G, Benz C, Sander C, Laird PW, Hoadley KA, King TA, Perou CM (2015) Comprehensive molecular portraits of invasive lobular breast cancer. Cell 163(2):506–519. doi:10.1016/j.cell.2015.09.033

Claes KB, De Leeneer K (2014) Dealing with pseudogenes in molecular diagnostics in the next-generation sequencing era. Meth Mol Biol (Clifton, NJ) 1167:303–315. doi:10.1007/978-1-4939-0835-6_21

Comprehensive molecular portraits of human breast tumours (2012) Nature 490(7418):61–70. doi:10.1038/nature11412

Corso G, Figueiredo J, Biffi R, Trentin C, Bonanni B, Feroce I, Serrano D, Cassano E, Annibale B, Melo S, Seruca R, De Lorenzi F, Ferrara F, Piagnerelli R, Roviello F, Galimberti V (2014) E-cadherin germline mutation carriers: clinical management and genetic implications. Cancer Metastasis Rev 33(4):1081–1094. doi:10.1007/s10555-014-9528-y

Couch FJ, Hart SN, Sharma P, Toland AE, Wang X, Miron P, Olson JE, Godwin AK, Pankratz VS, Olswold C, Slettedahl S, Hallberg E, Guidugli L, Davila JI, Beckmann MW, Janni W, Rack B, Ekici AB, Slamon DJ, Konstantopoulou I, Fostira F, Vratimos A, Fountzilas G, Pelttari LM, Tapper WJ, Durcan L, Cross SS, Pilarski R, Shapiro CL, Klemp J, Yao S, Garber J, Cox A, Brauch H, Ambrosone C, Nevanlinna H, Yannoukakos D, Slager SL, Vachon CM, Eccles DM, Fasching PA, Ramus SJ, Song H, Dicks E, Tyrer JP, Rosenthal AN, Intermaggio MP, Fraser L, Gentry-Maharaj A, Hayward J, Philpott S, Anderson C, Edlund CK, Conti D, Harrington P, Barrowdale D, Bowtell DD, Alsop K, Mitchell G, Group AS, Cicek MS, Cunningham JM, Fridley BL, Alsop J, Jimenez-Linan M, Poblete S, Lele S, Sucheston-Campbell L, Moysich KB, Sieh W, McGuire V, Lester J, Bogdanova N, Durst M, Hillemanns P, Ovarian Cancer Association C, Odunsi K, Whittemore AS, Karlan BY, Dork T, Goode EL, Menon U, Jacobs IJ, Antoniou AC, Pharoah PD, Gayther SA, Balmana J, Domchek SM, Susswein LR, Marshall ML, Nusbaum R, Vogel Postula KJ, Weissman SM, Yackowski L, Vaccari EM, Bissonnette J, Booker JK, Cremona ML, Gibellini F, Murphy PD, Pineda-Alvarez DE, Pollevick GD, Xu Z, Richard G, Bale S, Klein RT, Hruska KS, Chung WK, Ouhtit A, Gupta I, Shaikh Z (2015) Inherited mutations in 17 breast cancer susceptibility genes among a large triple-negative breast cancer cohort unselected for family history of breast cancer. J Clin Oncol: Off J Am Soc Clin Oncol 33(4):304–311. doi:10.1200/JCO.2014.57.1414, 10.1093/jnci/djv214, 10.1093/jnci/djv262, 10.1038/gim.2015.166

Curtis C, Shah SP, Chin SF, Turashvili G, Rueda OM, Dunning MJ, Speed D, Lynch AG, Samarajiwa S, Yuan Y, Graf S, Ha G, Haffari G, Bashashati A, Russell R, McKinney S, Langerod A, Green A, Provenzano E, Wishart G, Pinder S, Watson P, Markowetz F, Murphy L, Ellis I, Purushotham A, Borresen-Dale AL, Brenton JD, Tavare S, Caldas C, Aparicio S (2012) The genomic and transcriptomic architecture of 2,000 breast tumours reveals novel subgroups. Nature 486(7403):346–352. doi:10.1038/nature10983

Cybulski C, Carrot-Zhang J, Kluzniak W, Rivera B, Kashyap A, Wokolorczyk D, Giroux S, Nadaf J, Hamel N, Zhang S, Huzarski T, Gronwald J, Byrski T, Szwiec M, Jakubowska A, Rudnicka H, Lener M, Masojc B, Tonin PN, Rousseau F, Gorski B, Debniak T, Majewski J, Lubinski J, Foulkes WD, Narod SA, Akbari MR (2015) Germline RECQL mutations are associated with breast cancer susceptibility. Nat Genet 47(6):643–646. doi:10.1038/ng.3284

Damiola F, Pertesi M, Oliver J, Le Calvez-Kelm F, Voegele C, Young EL, Robinot N, Forey N, Durand G, Vallee MP, Tao K, Roane TC, Williams GJ, Hopper JL, Southey MC, Andrulis IL, John EM, Goldgar DE, Lesueur F, Tavtigian SV (2014) Rare key functional domain missense substitutions in MRE11A, RAD50, and NBN contribute to breast cancer susceptibility: results from a breast cancer family registry case-control mutation-screening study. Breast Cancer Res: BCR 16(3):R58. doi:10.1186/bcr3669

Dansonka-Mieszkowska A, Kluska A, Moes J, Dabrowska M, Nowakowska D, Niwinska A, Derlatka P, Cendrowski K, Kupryjanczyk J (2010) A novel germline PALB2 deletion in Polish breast and ovarian cancer patients. BMC Med Genet 11:20. doi:10.1186/1471-2350-11-20

Dawood S, Hu R, Homes MD, Collins LC, Schnitt SJ, Connolly J, Colditz GA, Tamimi RM (2011) Defining breast cancer prognosis based on molecular phenotypes: results from a large cohort study. Breast Cancer Res Treat 126(1):185–192. doi:10.1007/s10549-010-1113-7

Delmore JE, Issa GC, Lemieux ME, Rahl PB, Shi J, Jacobs HM, Kastritis E, Gilpatrick T, Paranal RM, Qi J, Chesi M, Schinzel AC, McKeown MR, Heffernan TP, Vakoc CR, Bergsagel PL, Ghobrial IM, Richardson PG, Young RA, Hahn WC, Anderson KC, Kung AL, Bradner JE, Mitsiades CS (2011) BET bromodomain inhibition as a therapeutic strategy to target c-Myc. Cell 146(6):904–917. doi:10.1016/j.cell.2011.08.017

Desmond A, Kurian AW, Gabree M, Mills MA, Anderson MJ, Kobayashi Y, Horick N, Yang S, Shannon KM, Tung N, Ford JM, Lincoln SE, Ellisen LW (2015) Clinical actionability of multigene panel testing for hereditary breast and ovarian cancer risk assessment. JAMA Oncol 1(7):943–951. doi:10.1001/jamaoncol.2015.2690

Dirican E, Akkiprik M, Ozer A (2016) Mutation distributions and clinical correlations of PIK3CA gene mutations in breast cancer. Tumour Biol: J Int Soc Oncodev Biol Med. doi:10.1007/s13277-016-4924-2

Dreijerink KM, Goudet P, Burgess JR, Valk GD (2014) Breast-cancer predisposition in multiple endocrine neoplasia type 1. New Engl J Med 371(6):583–584. doi:10.1056/NEJMc1406028

Dreijerink KM, Hoppener JW, Timmers HM, Lips CJ (2006) Mechanisms of disease: multiple endocrine neoplasia type 1-relation to chromatin modifications and transcription regulation. Nat Clin Pract Endocrinol Metab 2(10):562–570. doi:10.1038/ncpendmet0292

Easton DF, Pharoah PD, Antoniou AC, Tischkowitz M, Tavtigian SV, Nathanson KL, Devilee P, Meindl A, Couch FJ, Southey M, Goldgar DE, Evans DG, Chenevix-Trench G, Rahman N, Robson M, Domchek SM, Foulkes WD (2015) Gene-panel sequencing and the prediction of breast-cancer risk. New Engl J Med 372(23):2243–2257. doi:10.1056/NEJMsr1501341

Emelyanov A, Bulavin DV (2015) Wip1 phosphatase in breast cancer. Oncogene 34(34):4429–4438. doi:10.1038/onc.2014.375

Erkko H, Xia B, Nikkila J, Schleutker J, Syrjakoski K, Mannermaa A, Kallioniemi A, Pylkas K, Karppinen SM, Rapakko K, Miron A, Sheng Q, Li G, Mattila H, Bell DW, Haber DA, Grip M, Reiman M, Jukkola-Vuorinen A, Mustonen A, Kere J, Aaltonen LA, Kosma VM, Kataja V, Soini Y, Drapkin RI, Livingston DM, Winqvist R (2007) A recurrent mutation in PALB2 in Finnish cancer families. Nature 446(7133):316–319. doi:10.1038/nature05609

Fan C, Oh DS, Wessels L, Weigelt B, Nuyten DS, Nobel AB, van't Veer LJ, Perou CM (2006) Concordance among gene-expression-based predictors for breast cancer. New Engl J Med 355(6):560–569. doi:10.1056/NEJMoa052933

Finn RS, Aleshin A, Slamon DJ (2016) Targeting the cyclin-dependent kinases (CDK) 4/6 in estrogen receptor-positive breast cancers. Breast Cancer Res: BCR 18(1):17. doi:10.1186/s13058-015-0661-5

Fu X, Osborne CK, Schiff R (2013) Biology and therapeutic potential of PI3 K signaling in ER +/HER2-negative breast cancer. Breast (Edinburgh, Scotland) 22 Suppl 2:S12–18. doi:10.1016/j.breast.2013.08.001

Gatza ML, Silva GO, Parker JS, Fan C, Perou CM (2014) An integrated genomics approach identifies drivers of proliferation in luminal-subtype human breast cancer. Nat Genet 46(10):1051–1059. doi:10.1038/ng.3073

Goncalves ML, Borja SM, Cordeiro JA, Saddi VA, Ayres FM, Vilanova-Costa CA, Silva AM (2014) Association of the TP53 codon 72 polymorphism and breast cancer risk: a meta-analysis. SpringerPlus 3:749. doi:10.1186/2193-1801-3-749

Gray PN, Dunlop CL, Elliott AM (2015) Not all next generation sequencing diagnostics are created equal: understanding the nuances of solid tumor assay design for somatic mutation detection. Cancers 7(3):1313–1332. doi:10.3390/cancers7030837

Haanpaa M, Pylkas K, Moilanen JS, Winqvist R (2013) Evaluation of the need for routine clinical testing of PALB2 c.1592delT mutation in BRCA negative Northern Finnish breast cancer families. BMC Med Genet 14:82. doi:10.1186/1471-2350-14-82

Han FF, Guo CL, Liu LH (2013) The effect of CHEK2 variant I157T on cancer susceptibility: evidence from a meta-analysis. DNA Cell Biol 32(6):329–335. doi:10.1089/dna.2013.1970

Hanker AB, Pfefferle AD, Balko JM, Kuba MG, Young CD, Sanchez V, Sutton CR, Cheng H, Perou CM, Zhao JJ, Cook RS, Arteaga CL (2013) Mutant PIK3CA accelerates HER2-driven transgenic mammary tumors and induces resistance to combinations of anti-HER2 therapies. Proc Natl Acad Sci USA 110(35):14372–14377. doi:10.1073/pnas.1303204110

Hayes DF, Allen J, Compton C, Gustavsen G, Leonard DG, McCormack R, Newcomer L, Pothier K, Ransohoff D, Schilsky RL, Sigal E, Taube SE, Tunis SR (2013) Breaking a vicious cycle. Science Trans Med 5(196):196cm196. doi:10.1126/scitranslmed.3005950

Hearle N, Schumacher V, Menko FH, Olschwang S, Boardman LA, Gille JJ, Keller JJ, Westerman AM, Scott RJ, Lim W, Trimbath JD, Giardiello FM, Gruber SB, Offerhaus GJ, de Rooij FW, Wilson JH, Hansmann A, Moslein G, Royer-Pokora B, Vogel T, Phillips RK, Spigelman AD, Houlston RS (2006) Frequency and spectrum of cancers in the Peutz-Jeghers syndrome. Clinical Cancer Res: Off J Am Assoc Cancer Res 12(10):3209–3215. doi:10.1158/1078-0432.ccr-06-0083

Hedges DJ, Guettouche T, Yang S, Bademci G, Diaz A, Andersen A, Hulme WF, Linker S, Mehta A, Edwards YJ, Beecham GW, Martin ER, Pericak-Vance MA, Zuchner S, Vance JM, Gilbert JR (2011) Comparison of three targeted enrichment strategies on the SOLiD sequencing platform. PLoS ONE 6(4):e18595. doi:10.1371/journal.pone.0018595

Hilbers FS, Wijnen JT, Hoogerbrugge N, Oosterwijk JC, Collee MJ, Peterlongo P, Radice P, Manoukian S, Feroce I, Capra F, Couch FJ, Wang X, Guidugli L, Offit K, Shah S, Campbell IG, Thompson ER, James PA, Trainer AH, Gracia J, Benitez J, van Asperen CJ, Devilee P (2012) Rare variants in XRCC2 as breast cancer susceptibility alleles. J Med Genet 49(10):618–620. doi:10.1136/jmedgenet-2012-101191

Hirshfield KM, Ganesan S (2014) Triple-negative breast cancer: molecular subtypes and targeted therapy. Curr Opin Obstet Gynecol 26(1):34–40. doi:10.1097/gco.0000000000000038

Hodeib M, Serna-Gallegos T, Tewari KS (2015) A review of HER2-targeted therapy in breast and ovarian cancer: lessons from antiquity—CLEOPATRA and PENELOPE. Future Oncol (London, England) 11 (23):3113–3131. doi:10.2217/fon.15.266

Hogervorst FB, Nederlof PM, Gille JJ, McElgunn CJ, Grippeling M, Pruntel R, Regnerus R, van Welsem T, van Spaendonk R, Menko FH, Kluijt I, Dommering C, Verhoef S, Schouten JP, van't Veer LJ, Pals G (2003) Large genomic deletions and duplications in the BRCA1 gene identified by a novel quantitative method. Cancer Res 63(7):1449–1453

Holstege H, Horlings HM, Velds A, Langerod A, Borresen-Dale AL, van de Vijver MJ, Nederlof PM, Jonkers J (2010) BRCA1-mutated and basal-like breast cancers have similar aCGH profiles and a high incidence of protein truncating TP53 mutations. BMC Cancer 10:654. doi:10.1186/1471-2407-10-654

Hortobagyi GN, Chen D, Piccart M, Rugo HS, Burris HA 3rd, Pritchard KI, Campone M, Noguchi S, Perez AT, Deleu I, Shtivelband M, Masuda N, Dakhil S, Anderson I, Robinson DM, He W, Garg A, McDonald ER 3rd, Bitter H, Huang A, Taran T, Bachelot T, Lebrun F, Lebwohl D, Baselga J (2016) Correlative Analysis of Genetic Alterations and Everolimus Benefit in Hormone Receptor-Positive, Human Epidermal Growth Factor Receptor 2-Negative Advanced Breast Cancer: Results From BOLERO-2. J Clin Oncol: Off J Am Soc Clin Oncol 34(5):419–426. doi:10.1200/jco.2014.60.1971

Hsu HM, Wang HC, Chen ST, Hsu GC, Shen CY, Yu JC (2007) Breast cancer risk is associated with the genes encoding the DNA double-strand break repair Mre11/Rad50/Nbs1 complex. Cancer Epidemiol Biomarkers Prev: Publ Am Assoc Cancer Res, Cosponsored Am Soc Prev Oncol 16(10):2024–2032. doi:10.1158/1055-9965.epi-07-0116

Hurvitz SA, Andre F, Jiang Z, Shao Z, Mano MS, Neciosup SP, Tseng LM, Zhang Q, Shen K, Liu D, Dreosti LM, Burris HA, Toi M, Buyse ME, Cabaribere D, Lindsay MA, Rao S, Pacaud LB, Taran T, Slamon D (2015) Combination of everolimus with trastuzumab plus paclitaxel as first-line treatment for patients with HER2-positive advanced breast cancer (BOLERO-1): a phase 3, randomised, double-blind, multicentre trial. Lancet Oncol 16 (7):816–829. doi:10.1016/s1470-2045(15)00051-0

Hwang SJ, Lozano G, Amos CI, Strong LC (2003) Germline p53 mutations in a cohort with childhood sarcoma: sex differences in cancer risk. Am J Hum Genet 72(4):975–983. doi:10.1086/374567

Hyman DM, Puzanov I, Subbiah V, Faris JE, Chau I, Blay JY, Wolf J, Raje NS, Diamond EL, Hollebecque A, Gervais R, Elez-Fernandez ME, Italiano A, Hofheinz RD, Hidalgo M, Chan E, Schuler M, Lasserre SF, Makrutzki M, Sirzen F, Veronese ML, Tabernero J, Baselga J (2015) Vemurafenib in multiple nonmelanoma cancers with BRAF V600 mutations. New Engl J Med 373(8):726–736. doi:10.1056/NEJMoa1502309

Isakoff SJ, Mayer EL, He L, Traina TA, Carey LA, Krag KJ, Rugo HS, Liu MC, Stearns V, Come SE, Timms KM, Hartman AR, Borger DR, Finkelstein DM, Garber JE, Ryan PD, Winer EP, Goss PE, Ellisen LW (2015) TBCRC009: a multicenter phase II clinical trial of platinum monotherapy with biomarker assessment in metastatic triple-negative breast cancer. J Clin Oncol: Off J Am Soc Clin Oncol 33(17):1902–1909. doi:10.1200/jco.2014.57.6660

Haddow JE, Palomaki GE (2003) ACCE: a model process for evaluating data on emerging genetic tests. In: Khoury MJ, Little J, Burke W (eds) Human genome epidemiology: a scientific foundation for using genetic information to improve health and prevent disease. Oxford University Press, Oxford, pp 217–233

Janin N, Andrieu N, Ossian K, Lauge A, Croquette MF, Griscelli C, Debre M, Bressac-de-Paillerets B, Aurias A, Stoppa-Lyonnet D (1999) Breast cancer risk in ataxia telangiectasia (AT) heterozygotes: haplotype study in French AT families. Br J Cancer 80 (7):1042–1045. doi:10.1038/sj.bjc.6690460

Jeselsohn R, Buchwalter G, De Angelis C, Brown M, Schiff R (2015) ESR1 mutations-a mechanism for acquired endocrine resistance in breast cancer. Nat Rev Clin Oncol 12(10):573–583. doi:10.1038/nrclinonc.2015.117

Jones S, Hruban RH, Kamiyama M, Borges M, Zhang X, Parsons DW, Lin JC, Palmisano E, Brune K, Jaffee EM, Iacobuzio-Donahue CA, Maitra A, Parmigiani G, Kern SE, Velculescu VE, Kinzler KW, Vogelstein B, Eshleman JR, Goggins M, Klein AP (2009) Exomic sequencing identifies PALB2 as a pancreatic cancer susceptibility gene. Science (New York, NY) 324(5924):217. doi:10.1126/science.1171202

Jones S, Anagnostou V, Lytle K, Parpart-Li S, Nesselbush M, Riley DR, Shukla M, Chesnick B, Kadan M, Papp E, Galens KG, Murphy D, Zhang T, Kann L, Sausen M, Angiuoli SV, Diaz LA, Jr, Velculescu VE (2015) Personalized genomic analyses for cancer mutation discovery and interpretation. Sci Trans Med 7(283):283ra253. doi:10.1126/scitranslmed.aaa7161

Jonson L, Ahlborn LB, Steffensen AY, Djursby M, Ejlertsen B, Timshel S, Nielsen FC, Gerdes AM, Hansen TV (2016) Identification of six pathogenic RAD51C mutations via mutational screening of 1228 Danish individuals with increased risk of hereditary breast and/or ovarian cancer. Breast Cancer Res Treat 155(2):215–222. doi:10.1007/s10549-015-3674-y

Kaufman B, Shapira-Frommer R, Schmutzler RK, Audeh MW, Friedlander M, Balmana J, Mitchell G, Fried G, Stemmer SM, Hubert A, Rosengarten O, Steiner M, Loman N, Bowen K, Fielding A, Domchek SM (2015) Olaparib monotherapy in patients with advanced cancer and a germline BRCA1/2 mutation. J Clin Oncol: Off J Am Soc Clin Oncol 33(3):244–250. doi:10.1200/jco.2014.56.2728

Kiiski JI, Pelttari LM, Khan S, Freysteinsdottir ES, Reynisdottir I, Hart SN, Shimelis H, Vilske S,

Kallioniemi A, Schleutker J, Leminen A, Butzow R, Blomqvist C, Barkardottir RB, Couch FJ, Aittomaki K, Nevanlinna H (2014) Exome sequencing identifies FANCM as a susceptibility gene for triple-negative breast cancer. Proc Natl Acad Sci U S A 111 (42):15172–15177. doi:10.1073/pnas.1407909111

Kilpivaara O, Vahteristo P, Falck J, Syrjakoski K, Eerola H, Easton D, Bartkova J, Lukas J, Heikkila P, Aittomaki K, Holli K, Blomqvist C, Kallioniemi OP, Bartek J, Nevanlinna H (2004) CHEK2 variant I157T may be associated with increased breast cancer risk. Int J Cancer J Int du Cancer 111(4):543–547. doi:10.1002/ijc.20299

King MC, Marks JH, Mandell JB (2003) Breast and ovarian cancer risks due to inherited mutations in BRCA1 and BRCA2. Science (New York, NY) 302 (5645):643–646. doi:10.1126/science.1088759

Kitagawa R, Kastan MB (2005) The ATM-dependent DNA damage signaling pathway. Cold Spring Harb Symp Quant Biol 70:99–109. doi:10.1101/sqb.2005.70.002

Kozarewa I, Armisen J, Gardner AF, Slatko BE, Hendrickson CL (2015) Overview of target enrichment strategies. In: Frederick MA (eds) Current protocols in molecular biology. 112:7 21 21-27 21 23. doi:10.1002/0471142727.mb0721s112

Kurian AW, Hare EE, Mills MA, Kingham KE, McPherson L, Whittemore AS, McGuire V, Ladabaum U, Kobayashi Y, Lincoln SE, Cargill M, Ford JM (2014) Clinical evaluation of a multiple-gene sequencing panel for hereditary cancer risk assessment. J Clin Oncol: Off J Am Soc Clin Oncol 32(19):2001–2009. doi:10.1200/jco.2013.53.6607

Kuusisto KM, Bebel A, Vihinen M, Schleutker J, Sallinen SL (2011) Screening for BRCA1, BRCA2, CHEK2, PALB2, BRIP1, RAD50, and CDH1 mutations in high-risk Finnish BRCA1/2-founder mutation-negative breast and/or ovarian cancer individuals. Breast Cancer Res: BCR 13(1):R20. doi:10.1186/bcr2832

Lander ES (2015) Cutting the Gordian helix–regulating genomic testing in the era of precision medicine. New Engl J Med 372(13):1185–1186. doi:10.1056/NEJMp1501964

Lehmann BD, Bauer JA, Chen X, Sanders ME, Chakravarthy AB, Shyr Y, Pietenpol JA (2011) Identification of human triple-negative breast cancer subtypes and preclinical models for selection of targeted therapies. J Clin Investig 121(7):2750–2767. doi:10.1172/jci45014

Lerner-Ellis J, Khalouei S, Sopik V, Narod SA (2015) Genetic risk assessment and prevention: the role of genetic testing panels in breast cancer. Expert Rev Anticancer Ther 15(11):1315–1326. doi:10.1586/14737140.2015.1090879

Li J, Meeks H, Feng BJ, Healey S, Thorne H, Makunin I, Ellis J, Campbell I, Southey M, Mitchell G, Clouston D, Kirk J, Goldgar D, Chenevix-Trench G (2016) Targeted massively parallel sequencing of a panel of putative breast cancer susceptibility genes in a large cohort of multiple-case breast and ovarian cancer families. J Med Genet 53(1):34–42. doi:10.1136/jmedgenet-2015-103452

Liaw D, Marsh DJ, Li J, Dahia PL, Wang SI, Zheng Z, Bose S, Call KM, Tsou HC, Peacocke M, Eng C, Parsons R (1997) Germline mutations of the PTEN gene in Cowden disease, an inherited breast and thyroid cancer syndrome. Nat Genet 16(1):64–67. doi:10.1038/ng0597-64

Lien HC, Chen YL, Juang YL, Jeng YM (2015) Frequent alterations of HER2 through mutation, amplification, or overexpression in pleomorphic lobular carcinoma of the breast. Breast Cancer Res Treat 150(2):447–455. doi:10.1007/s10549-015-3336-0

Lim W, Olschwang S, Keller JJ, Westerman AM, Menko FH, Boardman LA, Scott RJ, Trimbath J, Giardiello FM, Gruber SB, Gille JJ, Offerhaus GJ, de Rooij FW, Wilson JH, Spigelman AD, Phillips RK, Houlston RS (2004) Relative frequency and morphology of cancers in STK11 mutation carriers. Gastroenterology 126(7):1788–1794

Litman R, Peng M, Jin Z, Zhang F, Zhang J, Powell S, Andreassen PR, Cantor SB (2005) BACH1 is critical for homologous recombination and appears to be the Fanconi anemia gene product FANCJ. Cancer Cell 8 (3):255–265. doi:10.1016/j.ccr.2005.08.004

Liu B, Morrison CD, Johnson CS, Trump DL, Qin M, Conroy JC, Wang J, Liu S (2013) Computational methods for detecting copy number variations in cancer genome using next generation sequencing: principles and challenges. Oncotarget 4(11):1868–1881. doi:10.18632/oncotarget.1537

Livraghi L, Garber JE (2015) PARP inhibitors in the management of breast cancer: current data and future prospects. BMC Med 13:188. doi:10.1186/s12916-015-0425-1

Loi S, Michiels S, Baselga J, Bartlett JM, Singhal SK, Sabine VS, Sims AH, Sahmoud T, Dixon JM, Piccart MJ, Sotiriou C (2013) PIK3CA genotype and a PIK3CA mutation-related gene signature and response to everolimus and letrozole in estrogen receptor positive breast cancer. PLoS ONE 8(1):e53292. doi:10.1371/journal.pone.0053292

Loibl S, von Minckwitz G, Schneeweiss A, Paepke S, Lehmann A, Rezai M, Zahm DM, Sinn P, Khandan F, Eidtmann H, Dohnal K, Heinrichs C, Huober J, Pfitzner B, Fasching PA, Andre F, Lindner JL, Sotiriou C, Dykgers A, Guo S, Gade S, Nekljudova V, Loi S, Untch M, Denkert C (2014) PIK3CA mutations are associated with lower rates of pathologic complete response to anti-human epidermal growth factor receptor 2 (her2) therapy in primary HER2-overexpressing breast cancer. J Clin Oncol: Off J Am Soc Clin Oncol 32(29):3212–3220. doi:10.1200/jco.2014.55.7876

Loveday C, Turnbull C, Ramsay E, Hughes D, Ruark E, Frankum JR, Bowden G, Kalmyrzaev B, Warren-Perry M, Snape K, Adlard JW, Barwell J, Berg J, Brady AF, Brewer C, Brice G, Chapman C, Cook J, Davidson R, Donaldson A, Douglas F,

Greenhalgh L, Henderson A, Izatt L, Kumar A, Lalloo F, Miedzybrodzka Z, Morrison PJ, Paterson J, Porteous M, Rogers MT, Shanley S, Walker L, Eccles D, Evans DG, Renwick A, Seal S, Lord CJ, Ashworth A, Reis-Filho JS, Antoniou AC, Rahman N (2011) Germline mutations in RAD51D confer susceptibility to ovarian cancer. Nat Genet 43(9):879–882. doi:10.1038/ng.893

Loveday C, Turnbull C, Ruark E, Xicola RM, Ramsay E, Hughes D, Warren-Perry M, Snape K, Eccles D, Evans DG, Gore M, Renwick A, Seal S, Antoniou AC, Rahman N (2012) Germline RAD51C mutations confer susceptibility to ovarian cancer. Nat Genet 44 (5):475–476; author reply 476. doi:10.1038/ng.2224

Lubinski J, Phelan CM, Ghadirian P, Lynch HT, Garber J, Weber B, Tung N, Horsman D, Isaacs C, Monteiro AN, Sun P, Narod SA (2004) Cancer variation associated with the position of the mutation in the BRCA2 gene. Fam Cancer 3(1):1–10. doi:10.1023/b:fame.0000026816.32400.45

Ma CX, Sanchez C, Gao F, Crowder R, Naughton M, Pluard T, Creekmore A, Guo Z, Hoog J, Lockhart AC, Doyle A, Erlichman C, Ellis MJ (2016) A Phase I Study of the AKT Inhibitor MK-2206 in combination with hormonal therapy in postmenopausal women with estrogen receptor positive metastatic breast cancer. Clin Cancer Res: Off J Am Assoc Cancer Res. doi:10.1158/1078-0432.ccr-15-2160

Madanikia SA, Bergner A, Ye X, Blakeley JO (2012) Increased risk of breast cancer in women with NF1. Am J Med Genet Part A 158A(12):3056–3060. doi:10.1002/ajmg.a.35550

Malkin D, Li FP, Strong LC, Fraumeni JF Jr, Nelson CE, Kim DH, Kassel J, Gryka MA, Bischoff FZ, Tainsky MA et al (1990) Germ line p53 mutations in a familial syndrome of breast cancer, sarcomas, and other neoplasms. Science (New York, NY) 250 (4985):1233–1238

Mamanova L, Coffey AJ, Scott CE, Kozarewa I, Turner EH, Kumar A, Howard E, Shendure J, Turner DJ (2010) Target-enrichment strategies for next-generation sequencing. Nat Methods 7(2):111–118. doi:10.1038/nmeth.1419

Masciari S, Larsson N, Senz J, Boyd N, Kaurah P, Kandel MJ, Harris LN, Pinheiro HC, Troussard A, Miron P, Tung N, Oliveira C, Collins L, Schnitt S, Garber JE, Huntsman D (2007) Germline E-cadherin mutations in familial lobular breast cancer. J Med Genet 44(11):726–731. doi:10.1136/jmg.2007.051268

Mavaddat N, Peock S, Frost D, Ellis S, Platte R, Fineberg E, Evans DG, Izatt L, Eeles RA, Adlard J, Davidson R, Eccles D, Cole T, Cook J, Brewer C, Tischkowitz M, Douglas F, Hodgson S, Walker L, Porteous ME, Morrison PJ, Side LE, Kennedy MJ, Houghton C, Donaldson A, Rogers MT, Dorkins H, Miedzybrodzka Z, Gregory H, Eason J, Barwell J, McCann E, Murray A, Antoniou AC, Easton DF (2013) Cancer risks for BRCA1 and BRCA2 mutation carriers: results from prospective analysis of EMBRACE. J Natl Cancer Inst 105(11):812–822. doi:10.1093/jnci/djt095

Maxwell KN, Wubbenhorst B, D'Andrea K, Garman B, Long JM, Powers J, Rathbun K, Stopfer JE, Zhu J, Bradbury AR, Simon MS, DeMichele A, Domchek SM, Nathanson KL (2015) Prevalence of mutations in a panel of breast cancer susceptibility genes in BRCA1/2-negative patients with early-onset breast cancer. Genet Med: Off J Am Coll Med Genet 17 (8):630–638. doi:10.1038/gim.2014.176

McCart Reed AE, Kutasovic JR, Lakhani SR, Simpson PT (2015) Invasive lobular carcinoma of the breast: morphology, biomarkers and 'omics. Breast Cancer Res: BCR 17:12. doi:10.1186/s13058-015-0519-x

Meijers-Heijboer H, van den Ouweland A, Klijn J, Wasielewski M, de Snoo A, Oldenburg R, Hollestelle A, Houben M, Crepin E, van Veghel-Plandsoen M, Elstrodt F, van Duijn C, Bartels C, Meijers C, Schutte M, McGuffog L, Thompson D, Easton D, Sodha N, Seal S, Barfoot R, Mangion J, Chang-Claude J, Eccles D, Eeles R, Evans DG, Houlston R, Murday V, Narod S, Peretz T, Peto J, Phelan C, Zhang HX, Szabo C, Devilee P, Goldgar D, Futreal PA, Nathanson KL, Weber B, Rahman N, Stratton MR (2002) Low-penetrance susceptibility to breast cancer due to CHEK2(*)1100delC in noncarriers of BRCA1 or BRCA2 mutations. Nat Genet 31 (1):55–59. doi:10.1038/ng879

Metzker ML (2010) Sequencing technologies—the next generation. Nat Rev Genet 11(1):31–46. doi:10.1038/nrg2626

Milella M, Falcone I, Conciatori F, Cesta Incani U, Del Curatolo A, Inzerilli N, Nuzzo CM, Vaccaro V, Vari S, Cognetti F, Ciuffreda L (2015) PTEN: multiple functions in human malignant tumors. Front Oncol 5:24. doi:10.3389/fonc.2015.00024

Nagata Y, Lan KH, Zhou X, Tan M, Esteva FJ, Sahin AA, Klos KS, Li P, Monia BP, Nguyen NT, Hortobagyi GN, Hung MC, Yu D (2004) PTEN activation contributes to tumor inhibition by trastuzumab, and loss of PTEN predicts trastuzumab resistance in patients. Cancer Cell 6(2):117–127. doi:10.1016/j.ccr.2004.06.022

Natrajan R, Weigelt B, Mackay A, Geyer FC, Grigoriadis A, Tan DS, Jones C, Lord CJ, Vatcheva R, Rodriguez-Pinilla SM, Palacios J, Ashworth A, Reis-Filho JS (2010) An integrative genomic and transcriptomic analysis reveals molecular pathways and networks regulated by copy number aberrations in basal-like, HER2 and luminal cancers. Breast Cancer Res Treat 121(3):575–589. doi:10.1007/s10549-009-0501-3

Ngeow J, Eng C (2015) PTEN hamartoma tumor syndrome: clinical risk assessment and management protocol. Methods (San Diego, Calif) 77–78:11–19. doi:10.1016/j.ymeth.2014.10.011

Nuciforo PG, Aura C, Holmes E, Prudkin L, Jimenez J, Martinez P, Ameels H, de la Pena L, Ellis C, Eidtmann H, Piccart-Gebhart MJ, Scaltriti M,

Baselga J (2015) Benefit to neoadjuvant anti-human epidermal growth factor receptor 2 (HER2)-targeted therapies in HER2-positive primary breast cancer is independent of phosphatase and tensin homolog deleted from chromosome 10 (PTEN) status. Ann Oncol: Off J Eur Soc Med Oncol/ESMO 26(7):1494–1500. doi:10.1093/annonc/mdv175

Olsen JH, Hahnemann JM, Borresen-Dale AL, Tretli S, Kleinerman R, Sankila R, Hammarstrom L, Robsahm TE, Kaariainen H, Bregard A, Brondum-Nielsen K, Yuen J, Tucker M (2005) Breast and other cancers in 1445 blood relatives of 75 Nordic patients with ataxia telangiectasia. Br J Cancer 93(2):260–265. doi:10.1038/sj.bjc.6602658

Out AA, Wasielewski M, Huijts PE, van Minderhout IJ, Houwing-Duistermaat JJ, Tops CM, Nielsen M, Seynaeve C, Wijnen JT, Breuning MH, van Asperen CJ, Schutte M, Hes FJ, Devilee P (2012) MUTYH gene variants and breast cancer in a Dutch case-control study. Breast Cancer Res Treat 134(1):219–227. doi:10.1007/s10549-012-1965-0

Park DJ, Lesueur F, Nguyen-Dumont T, Pertesi M, Odefrey F, Hammet F, Neuhausen SL, John EM, Andrulis IL, Terry MB, Daly M, Buys S, Le Calvez-Kelm F, Lonie A, Pope BJ, Tsimiklis H, Voegele C, Hilbers FM, Hoogerbrugge N, Barroso A, Osorio A, Giles GG, Devilee P, Benitez J, Hopper JL, Tavtigian SV, Goldgar DE, Southey MC (2012) Rare mutations in XRCC2 increase the risk of breast cancer. Am J Hum Genet 90(4):734–739. doi:10.1016/j.ajhg.2012.02.027

Pelttari LM, Kiiski J, Nurminen R, Kallioniemi A, Schleutker J, Gylfe A, Aaltonen LA, Leminen A, Heikkila P, Blomqvist C, Butzow R, Aittomaki K, Nevanlinna H (2012) A Finnish founder mutation in RAD51D: analysis in breast, ovarian, prostate, and colorectal cancer. J Med Genet 49(7):429–432. doi:10.1136/jmedgenet-2012-100852

Perou CM, Sorlie T, Eisen MB, van de Rijn M, Jeffrey SS, Rees CA, Pollack JR, Ross DT, Johnsen H, Akslen LA, Fluge O, Pergamenschikov A, Williams C, Zhu SX, Lonning PE, Borresen-Dale AL, Brown PO, Botstein D (2000) Molecular portraits of human breast tumours. Nature 406(6797):747–752. doi:10.1038/35021093

Petricevic B, Laengle J, Singer J, Sachet M, Fazekas J, Steger G, Bartsch R, Jensen-Jarolim E, Bergmann M (2013) Trastuzumab mediates antibody-dependent cell-mediated cytotoxicity and phagocytosis to the same extent in both adjuvant and metastatic HER2/neu breast cancer patients. J Trans Med 11:307. doi:10.1186/1479-5876-11-307

Pharoah PD, Guilford P, Caldas C (2001) Incidence of gastric cancer and breast cancer in CDH1 (E-cadherin) mutation carriers from hereditary diffuse gastric cancer families. Gastroenterology 121(6):1348–1353

Pogue-Geile KL, Song N, Jeong JH, Gavin PG, Kim SR, Blackmon NL, Finnigan M, Rastogi P, Fehrenbacher L, Mamounas EP, Swain SM, Wickerham DL, Geyer CE Jr, Costantino JP, Wolmark N, Paik S (2015) Intrinsic subtypes, PIK3CA mutation, and the degree of benefit from adjuvant trastuzumab in the NSABP B-31 trial. J Clin Oncol: Off J Am Soc Clin Oncol 33(12):1340–1347. doi:10.1200/jco.2014.56.2439

Prahallad A, Sun C, Huang S, Di Nicolantonio F, Salazar R, Zecchin D, Beijersbergen RL, Bardelli A, Bernards R (2012) Unresponsiveness of colon cancer to BRAF(V600E) inhibition through feedback activation of EGFR. Nature 483(7387):100–103. doi:10.1038/nature10868

Priya R, Yap AS (2015) Active tension: the role of cadherin adhesion and signaling in generating junctional contractility. Curr Top Dev Biol 112:65–102. doi:10.1016/bs.ctdb.2014.11.016

Prokofyeva D, Bogdanova N, Bermisheva M, Zinnatullina G, Hillemanns P, Khusnutdinova E, Dork T (2012) Rare occurrence of PALB2 mutations in ovarian cancer patients from the Volga-Ural region. Clin Genet 82(1):100–101. doi:10.1111/j.1399-0004.2011.01824.x

Rafnar T, Gudbjartsson DF, Sulem P, Jonasdottir A, Sigurdsson A, Jonasdottir A, Besenbacher S, Lundin P, Stacey SN, Gudmundsson J, Magnusson OT, le Roux L, Orlygsdottir G, Helgadottir HT, Johannsdottir H, Gylfason A, Tryggvadottir L, Jonasson JG, de Juan A, Ortega E, Ramon-Cajal JM, Garcia-Prats MD, Mayordomo C, Panadero A, Rivera F, Aben KK, van Altena AM, Massuger LF, Aavikko M, Kujala PM, Staff S, Aaltonen LA, Olafsdottir K, Bjornsson J, Kong A, Salvarsdottir A, Saemundsson H, Olafsson K, Benediktsdottir KR, Gulcher J, Masson G, Kiemeney LA, Mayordomo JI, Thorsteinsdottir U, Stefansson K (2011) Mutations in BRIP1 confer high risk of ovarian cancer. Nat Genet 43(11):1104–1107. doi:10.1038/ng.955

Rahman N, Seal S, Thompson D, Kelly P, Renwick A, Elliott A, Reid S, Spanova K, Barfoot R, Chagtai T, Jayatilake H, McGuffog L, Hanks S, Evans DG, Eccles D, Easton DF, Stratton MR (2007) PALB2, which encodes a BRCA2-interacting protein, is a breast cancer susceptibility gene. Nat Genet 39(2):165–167. doi:10.1038/ng1959

Reid S, Schindler D, Hanenberg H, Barker K, Hanks S, Kalb R, Neveling K, Kelly P, Seal S, Freund M, Wurm M, Batish SD, Lach FP, Yetgin S, Neitzel H, Ariffin H, Tischkowitz M, Mathew CG, Auerbach AD, Rahman N (2007) Biallelic mutations in PALB2 cause Fanconi anemia subtype FA-N and predispose to childhood cancer. Nat Genet 39(2):162–164. doi:10.1038/ng1947

Renwick A, Thompson D, Seal S, Kelly P, Chagtai T, Ahmed M, North B, Jayatilake H, Barfoot R, Spanova K, McGuffog L, Evans DG, Eccles D, Easton DF, Stratton MR, Rahman N (2006) ATM mutations that cause ataxia-telangiectasia are breast cancer susceptibility alleles. Nat Genet 38(8):873–875. doi:10.1038/ng1837

Resta N, Pierannunzio D, Lenato GM, Stella A, Capocaccia R, Bagnulo R, Lastella P, Susca FC, Bozzao C,

Loconte DC, Sabba C, Urso E, Sala P, Fornasarig M, Grammatico P, Piepoli A, Host C, Turchetti D, Viel A, Memo L, Giunti L, Stigliano V, Varesco L, Bertario L, Genuardi M, Lucci Cordisco E, Tibiletti MG, Di Gregorio C, Andriulli A, Ponz de Leon M (2013) Cancer risk associated with STK11/LKB1 germline mutations in Peutz-Jeghers syndrome patients: results of an Italian multicenter study. Dig Liver Dis: Off J Ital Soc Gastroenterol Ital Assoc Study Liver 45 (7):606–611. doi:10.1016/j.dld.2012.12.018

Richards S, Aziz N, Bale S, Bick D, Das S, Gastier-Foster J, Grody WW, Hegde M, Lyon E, Spector E, Voelkerding K, Rehm HL (2015) Standards and guidelines for the interpretation of sequence variants: a joint consensus recommendation of the American College of Medical Genetics and Genomics and the Association for Molecular Pathology. Genet Med: Off J Am Coll Med Genet 17(5):405–424. doi:10.1038/gim.2015.30

Robinson DR, Wu YM, Vats P, Su F, Lonigro RJ, Cao X, Kalyana-Sundaram S, Wang R, Ning Y, Hodges L, Gursky A, Siddiqui J, Tomlins SA, Roychowdhury S, Pienta KJ, Kim SY, Roberts JS, Rae JM, Van Poznak CH, Hayes DF, Chugh R, Kunju LP, Talpaz M, Schott AF, Chinnaiyan AM (2013) Activating ESR1 mutations in hormone-resistant metastatic breast cancer. Nat Genet 45(12):1446–1451. doi:10.1038/ng.2823

Roy-Chowdhuri S, de Melo Gagliato D, Routbort MJ, Patel KP, Singh RR, Broaddus R, Lazar AJ, Sahin A, Alvarez RH, Moulder S, Wheler JJ, Janku F, Gonzalez-Angulo AM, Chavez-MacGregor M, Valero V, Ueno NT, Mills G, Mendelsohn J, Yao H, Aldape K, Luthra R, Meric-Bernstam F (2015) Multigene clinical mutational profiling of breast carcinoma using next-generation sequencing. Am J Clin Pathol 144(5):713–721. doi:10.1309/ajcpwdeqycyc92jq

Ruark E, Snape K, Humburg P, Loveday C, Bajrami I, Brough R, Rodrigues DN, Renwick A, Seal S, Ramsay E, Duarte Sdel V, Rivas MA, Warren-Perry M, Zachariou A, Campion-Flora A, Hanks S, Murray A, Ansari Pour N, Douglas J, Gregory L, Rimmer A, Walker NM, Yang TP, Adlard JW, Barwell J, Berg J, Brady AF, Brewer C, Brice G, Chapman C, Cook J, Davidson R, Donaldson A, Douglas F, Eccles D, Evans DG, Greenhalgh L, Henderson A, Izatt L, Kumar A, Lalloo F, Miedzybrodzka Z, Morrison PJ, Paterson J, Porteous M, Rogers MT, Shanley S, Walker L, Gore M, Houlston R, Brown MA, Caufield MJ, Deloukas P, McCarthy MI, Todd JA, Turnbull C, Reis-Filho JS, Ashworth A, Antoniou AC, Lord CJ, Donnelly P, Rahman N (2013) Mosaic PPM1D mutations are associated with predisposition to breast and ovarian cancer. Nature 493(7432):406–410. doi:10.1038/nature11725

Samorodnitsky E, Jewell BM, Hagopian R, Miya J, Wing MR, Lyon E, Damodaran S, Bhatt D, Reeser JW, Datta J, Roychowdhury S (2015) Evaluation of Hybridization Capture Versus Amplicon-Based Methods for Whole-Exome Sequencing. Hum Mutat 36(9):903–914. doi:10.1002/humu.22825

Sampson JR, Jones N (2009) MUTYH-associated polyposis. Best Pract Res Clin Gastroenterol 23(2):209–218. doi:10.1016/j.bpg.2009.03.006

Schiavon G, Hrebien S, Garcia-Murillas I, Cutts RJ, Pearson A, Tarazona N, Fenwick K, Kozarewa I, Lopez-Knowles E, Ribas R, Nerurkar A, Osin P, Chandarlapaty S, Martin LA, Dowsett M, Smith IE, Turner NC (2015) Analysis of ESR1 mutation in circulating tumor DNA demonstrates evolution during therapy for metastatic breast cancer. Science Trans Med 7(313):313ra182. doi:10.1126/scitranslmed.aac7551

Seal S, Thompson D, Renwick A, Elliott A, Kelly P, Barfoot R, Chagtai T, Jayatilake H, Ahmed M, Spanova K, North B, McGuffog L, Evans DG, Eccles D, Breast Cancer Susceptibility C, Easton DF, Stratton MR, Rahman N (2006) Truncating mutations in the Fanconi anemia J gene BRIP1 are low-penetrance breast cancer susceptibility alleles. Nat Genet 38(11):1239–1241. doi:10.1038/ng1902

Seminog OO, Goldacre MJ (2015) Age-specific risk of breast cancer in women with neurofibromatosis type 1. Br J Cancer 112(9):1546–1548. doi:10.1038/bjc.2015.78

Shah SP, Roth A, Goya R, Oloumi A, Ha G, Zhao Y, Turashvili G, Ding J, Tse K, Haffari G, Bashashati A, Prentice LM, Khattra J, Burleigh A, Yap D, Bernard V, McPherson A, Shumansky K, Crisan A, Giuliany R, Heravi-Moussavi A, Rosner J, Lai D, Birol I, Varhol R, Tam A, Dhalla N, Zeng T, Ma K, Chan SK, Griffith M, Moradian A, Cheng SW, Morin GB, Watson P, Gelmon K, Chia S, Chin SF, Curtis C, Rueda OM, Pharoah PD, Damaraju S, Mackey J, Hoon K, Harkins T, Tadigotla V, Sigaroudinia M, Gascard P, Tlsty T, Costello JF, Meyer IM, Eaves CJ, Wasserman WW, Jones S, Huntsman D, Hirst M, Caldas C, Marra MA, Aparicio S (2012) The clonal and mutational evolution spectrum of primary triple-negative breast cancers. Nature 486(7403):395–399. doi:10.1038/nature10933

Sharfstein J (2015) FDA regulation of laboratory-developed diagnostic tests: protect the public, advance the science. JAMA 313(7):667–668. doi:10.1001/jama.2014.18135

Shi YJ, Tsang JY, Ni YB, Chan SK, Chan KF, Tse GM (2015) FGFR1 is an adverse outcome indicator for luminal A breast cancers. Oncotarget. doi:10.18632/oncotarget.6563

Sievert AJ, Lang SS, Boucher KL, Madsen PJ, Slaunwhite E, Choudhari N, Kellet M, Storm PB, Resnick AC (2013) Paradoxical activation and RAF inhibitor resistance of BRAF protein kinase fusions characterizing pediatric astrocytomas. Proc Natl Acad Sci U S A 110(15):5957–5962. doi:10.1073/pnas.1219232110

Slavin TP, Niell-Swiller M, Solomon I, Nehoray B, Rybak C, Blazer KR, Weitzel JN (2015) Clinical application of multigene panels: challenges of next-generation counseling and cancer risk management. Fron Oncol 5:208. doi:10.3389/fonc.2015.00208

Soria JC, DeBraud F, Bahleda R, Adamo B, Andre F, Dienstmann R, Delmonte A, Cereda R, Isaacson J, Litten J, Allen A, Dubois F, Saba C, Robert R, D'Incalci M, Zucchetti M, Camboni MG, Tabernero J (2014) Phase I/IIa study evaluating the safety, efficacy, pharmacokinetics, and pharmacodynamics of lucitanib in advanced solid tumors. Ann Oncol: Off J Eur Soc Med Oncol/ESMO 25(11):2244–2251. doi:10.1093/annonc/mdu390

Sorlie T, Tibshirani R, Parker J, Hastie T, Marron JS, Nobel A, Deng S, Johnsen H, Pesich R, Geisler S, Demeter J, Perou CM, Lonning PE, Brown PO, Borresen-Dale AL, Botstein D (2003) Repeated observation of breast tumor subtypes in independent gene expression data sets. Proc Natl Acad Sci U S A 100(14):8418–8423. doi:10.1073/pnas.0932692100

Spector NL, Blackwell KL (2009) Understanding the mechanisms behind trastuzumab therapy for human epidermal growth factor receptor 2-positive breast cancer. Journal of Clin Oncol: Off J Am Soc Clin Oncol 27(34):5838–5847. doi:10.1200/jco.2009.22.1507

Stephens PJ, Tarpey PS, Davies H, Van Loo P, Greenman C, Wedge DC, Nik-Zainal S, Martin S, Varela I, Bignell GR, Yates LR, Papaemmanuil E, Beare D, Butler A, Cheverton A, Gamble J, Hinton J, Jia M, Jayakumar A, Jones D, Latimer C, Lau KW, McLaren S, McBride DJ, Menzies A, Mudie L, Raine K, Rad R, Chapman MS, Teague J, Easton D, Langerod A, Lee MT, Shen CY, Tee BT, Huimin BW, Broeks A, Vargas AC, Turashvili G, Martens J, Fatima A, Miron P, Chin SF, Thomas G, Boyault S, Mariani O, Lakhani SR, van de Vijver M, van 't Veer L, Foekens J, Desmedt C, Sotiriou C, Tutt A, Caldas C, Reis-Filho JS, Aparicio SA, Salomon AV, Borresen-Dale AL, Richardson AL, Campbell PJ, Futreal PA, Stratton MR (2012) The landscape of cancer genes and mutational processes in breast cancer. Nature 486(7403):400–404. doi:10.1038/nature11017

Sun J, Wang Y, Xia Y, Xu Y, Ouyang T, Li J, Wang T, Fan Z, Fan T, Lin B, Lou H, Xie Y (2015) Mutations in RECQL gene are associated with predisposition to breast cancer. PLoS Genet 11(5):e1005228. doi:10.1371/journal.pgen.1005228

Suwaki N, Klare K, Tarsounas M (2011) RAD51 paralogs: roles in DNA damage signalling, recombinational repair and tumorigenesis. Semin Cell Dev Biol 22 (8):898–905. doi:10.1016/j.semcdb.2011.07.019

Szabo CI, Schutte M, Broeks A, Houwing-Duistermaat JJ, Thorstenson YR, Durocher F, Oldenburg RA, Wasielewski M, Odefrey F, Thompson D, Floore AN, Kraan J, Klijn JG, van den Ouweland AM, Wagner TM, Devilee P, Simard J, van 't Veer LJ, Goldgar DE, Meijers-Heijboer H (2004) Are ATM mutations 7271T– > G and IVS10-6T– > G really high-risk breast cancer-susceptibility alleles? Cancer Res 64(3):840–843

Tan MH, Mester JL, Ngeow J, Rybicki LA, Orloff MS, Eng C (2012) Lifetime cancer risks in individuals with germline PTEN mutations. Clin Cancer Res: Off J Am Assoc Cancer Res 18(2):400–407. doi:10.1158/1078-0432.ccr-11-2283

Teive HA, Moro A, Moscovich M, Arruda WO, Munhoz RP, Raskin S, Ashizawa T (2015) Ataxia-telangiectasia—A historical review and a proposal for a new designation: ATM syndrome. J Neurol Sci 355(1–2):3–6. doi:10.1016/j.jns.2015.05.022

Thai TH, Du F, Tsan JT, Jin Y, Phung A, Spillman MA, Massa HF, Muller CY, Ashfaq R, Mathis JM, Miller DS, Trask BJ, Baer R, Bowcock AM (1998) Mutations in the BRCA1-associated RING domain (BARD1) gene in primary breast, ovarian and uterine cancers. Hum Mol Genet 7(2):195–202

Thompson ER, Doyle MA, Ryland GL, Rowley SM, Choong DY, Tothill RW, Thorne H, Barnes DR, Li J, Ellul J, Philip GK, Antill YC, James PA, Trainer AH, Mitchell G, Campbell IG (2012) Exome sequencing identifies rare deleterious mutations in DNA repair genes FANCC and BLM as potential breast cancer susceptibility alleles. PLoS Genet 8(9):e1002894. doi:10.1371/journal.pgen.1002894

Thompson D, Duedal S, Kirner J, McGuffog L, Last J, Reiman A, Byrd P, Taylor M, Easton DF (2005) Cancer risks and mortality in heterozygous ATM mutation carriers. J Natl Cancer Inst 97(11):813–822. doi:10.1093/jnci/dji141

Thompson D, Easton D (2001) Variation in cancer risks, by mutation position, in BRCA2 mutation carriers. Am J Hum Genet 68(2):410–419. doi:10.1086/318181

Thompson D, Easton D (2002) Variation in BRCA1 cancer risks by mutation position. Cancer Epidemiol, Biomark Prev: Publ Am Assoc Cancer Res, Cosponsored Am Soc Prev Oncol 11(4):329–336

Thompson ER, Rowley SM, Li N, McInerny S, Devereux L, Wong-Brown MW, Trainer AH, Mitchell G, Scott RJ, James PA, Campbell IG (2016) Panel testing for familial breast cancer: calibrating the tension between research and clinical care. J Clin Oncol: Off J Am Soc Clin Oncol. doi:10.1200/jco.2015.63.7454

Tiacci E, Park JH, De Carolis L, Chung SS, Broccoli A, Scott S, Zaja F, Devlin S, Pulsoni A, Chung YR, Cimminiello M, Kim E, Rossi D, Stone RM, Motta G, Saven A, Varettoni M, Altman JK, Anastasia A, Grever MR, Ambrosetti A, Rai KR, Fraticelli V, Lacouture ME, Carella AM, Levine RL, Leoni P, Rambaldi A, Falzetti F, Ascani S, Capponi M, Martelli MP, Park CY, Pileri SA, Rosen N, Foa R, Berger MF, Zinzani PL, Abdel-Wahab O, Falini B, Tallman MS (2015) Targeting mutant BRAF in relapsed or refractory hairy-cell leukemia. New Engl J Med 373(18):1733–1747. doi:10.1056/NEJMoa1506583

Tischkowitz M, Xia B, Sabbaghian N, Reis-Filho JS, Hamel N, Li G, van Beers EH, Li L, Khalil T,

Quenneville LA, Omeroglu A, Poll A, Lepage P, Wong N, Nederlof PM, Ashworth A, Tonin PN, Narod SA, Livingston DM, Foulkes WD (2007) Analysis of PALB2/FANCN-associated breast cancer families. Proc Natl Acad Sci U S A 104(16):6788–6793. doi:10.1073/pnas.0701724104

van Os NJ, Roeleveld N, Weemaes CM, Jongmans MC, Janssens GO, Taylor AM, Hoogerbrugge N, Willemsen MA (2015) Health risks for ataxia-telangiectasia mutated heterozygotes: a systematic review. Clinical Genet, Meta-analysis and evidence-based guideline. doi:10.1111/cge.12710

Vasan N, Yelensky R, Wang K, Moulder S, Dzimitrowicz H, Avritscher R, Wang B, Wu Y, Cronin MT, Palmer G, Symmans WF, Miller VA, Stephens P, Pusztai L (2014) A targeted next-generation sequencing assay detects a high frequency of therapeutically targetable alterations in primary and metastatic breast cancers: implications for clinical practice. Oncologist 19(5):453–458. doi:10.1634/theoncologist.2013-0377

Watson P, Vasen HF, Mecklin JP, Bernstein I, Aarnio M, Jarvinen HJ, Myrhoj T, Sunde L, Wijnen JT, Lynch HT (2008) The risk of extra-colonic, extra-endometrial cancer in the Lynch syndrome. Int J Cancer J Int du Cancer 123(2):444–449. doi:10.1002/ijc.23508

Weischer M, Nordestgaard BG, Pharoah P, Bolla MK, Nevanlinna H, Van't Veer LJ, Garcia-Closas M, Hopper JL, Hall P, Andrulis IL, Devilee P, Fasching PA, Anton-Culver H, Lambrechts D, Hooning M, Cox A, Giles GG, Burwinkel B, Lindblom A, Couch FJ, Mannermaa A, Grenaker Alnaes G, John EM, Dork T, Flyger H, Dunning AM, Wang Q, Muranen TA, van Hien R, Figueroa J, Southey MC, Czene K, Knight JA, Tollenaar RA, Beckmann MW, Ziogas A, Christiaens MR, Collee JM, Reed MW, Severi G, Marme F, Margolin S, Olson JE, Kosma VM, Kristensen VN, Miron A, Bogdanova N, Shah M, Blomqvist C, Broeks A, Sherman M, Phillips KA, Li J, Liu J, Glendon G, Seynaeve C, Ekici AB, Leunen K, Kriege M, Cross SS, Baglietto L, Sohn C, Wang X, Kataja V, Borresen-Dale AL, Meyer A, Easton DF, Schmidt MK, Bojesen SE (2012) CHEK2*1100delC heterozygosity in women with breast cancer associated with early death, breast cancer-specific death, and increased risk of a second breast cancer. J Clin Oncol: Off J Am Soc Clin Oncol 30(35):4308–4316. doi:10.1200/jco.2012.42.7336

Williams RS, Williams JS, Tainer JA (2007) Mre11-Rad50-Nbs1 is a keystone complex connecting DNA repair machinery, double-strand break signaling, and the chromatin template. Biochemistry and cell biology. Biochimie et biologie cellulaire 85(4):509–520. doi:10.1139/o07-069

Win AK, Cleary SP, Dowty JG, Baron JA, Young JP, Buchanan DD, Southey MC, Burnett T, Parfrey PS, Green RC, Le Marchand L, Newcomb PA, Haile RW, Lindor NM, Hopper JL, Gallinger S, Jenkins MA (2011) Cancer risks for monoallelic MUTYH mutation carriers with a family history of colorectal cancer. Int J Cancer J Int du Cancer 129(9):2256–2262. doi:10.1002/ijc.25870

Win AK, Lindor NM, Jenkins MA (2013) Risk of breast cancer in Lynch syndrome: a systematic review. Breast Cancer Res: BCR 15(2):R27. doi:10.1186/bcr3405

Wu LC, Wang ZW, Tsan JT, Spillman MA, Phung A, Xu XL, Yang MC, Hwang LY, Bowcock AM, Baer R (1996) Identification of a RING protein that can interact in vivo with the BRCA1 gene product. Nat Genet 14(4):430–440. doi:10.1038/ng1296-430

Xia B, Dorsman JC, Ameziane N, de Vries Y, Rooimans MA, Sheng Q, Pals G, Errami A, Gluckman E, Llera J, Wang W, Livingston DM, Joenje H, de Winter JP (2007) Fanconi anemia is associated with a defect in the BRCA2 partner PALB2. Nat Genet 39 (2):159–161. doi:10.1038/ng1942

Xia B, Sheng Q, Nakanishi K, Ohashi A, Wu J, Christ N, Liu X, Jasin M, Couch FJ, Livingston DM (2006) Control of BRCA2 cellular and clinical functions by a nuclear partner, PALB2. Mol Cell 22(6):719–729. doi:10.1016/j.molcel.2006.05.022

Young EL, Feng BJ, Stark AW, Damiola F, Durand G, Forey N, Francy TC, Gammon A, Kohlmann WK, Kaphingst KA, McKay-Chopin S, Nguyen-Dumont T, Oliver J, Paquette AM, Pertesi M, Robinot N, Rosenthal JS, Vallee M, Voegele C, Hopper JL, Southey MC, Andrulis IL, John EM, Hashibe M, Gertz J, Le Calvez-Kelm F, Lesueur F, Goldgar DE, Tavtigian SV (2016) Multigene testing of moderate-risk genes: be mindful of the missense. J Med Genet. doi:10.1136/jmedgenet-2015-103398

Zhang F, Ma J, Wu J, Ye L, Cai H, Xia B, Yu X (2009) PALB2 links BRCA1 and BRCA2 in the DNA-damage response. Curr Biol: CB 19(6):524–529. doi:10.1016/j.cub.2009.02.018

Zhang ZH, Yang LS, Huang F, Hao JH, Su PY, Sun YH (2012) Current evidence on the relationship between two polymorphisms in the NBS1 gene and breast cancer risk: a meta-analysis. Asian Pac J Cancer Prev: APJCP 13(11):5375–5379

Zhang G, Zeng Y, Liu Z, Wei W (2013) Significant association between Nijmegen breakage syndrome 1 657del5 polymorphism and breast cancer risk. Tumour Biol: J Int Soc Oncodev Biol Med 34 (5):2753–2757. doi:10.1007/s13277-013-0830-z

Zheng Z, Liebers M, Zhelyazkova B, Cao Y, Panditi D, Lynch KD, Chen J, Robinson HE, Shim HS, Chmielecki J, Pao W, Engelman JA, Iafrate AJ, Le LP (2014) Anchored multiplex PCR for targeted next-generation sequencing. Nat Med 20(12):1479–1484. doi:10.1038/nm.3729

Epigenetic Mechanism in Breast Cancer

21

Mukesh Verma and Sunil Badve

Abstract

Breast cancer is a heterogeneous disease and markers are needed for diagnosis and prognosis of this often fatal disease. Genetic mutations and epigenetic alterations act in concert in carcinogenesis of a variety of tumors. Epigenetic alterations are being recognized as significant features in cancer development. Four major players in cancer epigenetic regulation are DNA methylation, histone modifications, noncoding RNA expression, and chromatin remodeling. Initial studies in cancer were conducted in the area of epigenetic regulation of individual genes but later on expanded systematically to larger parts of the chromosome. Hormonal induced nucleosome repositioning and its effects on transcription machinery in breast cancer development presents a better understanding on underlying mechanism. Epigenetic alterations can be used as biomarkers for diagnosis, prognosis, and follow up of treatment. Epigenetic inhibitors have been identified which reactivate tumor suppressor genes and other genes, stop cell proliferation and tumor growth in breast cancer. Among epigenetic inhibitors, histone deacetylase inhibitors are novel clinical anticancer drugs that that inhibit HDAC gene expression and induce apoptosis. The focus of this article is to understand role of epigenetics in breast cancer development. Potential therapeutic approaches of breast cancer and correlation with precision medicine have also been discussed.

M. Verma (✉)
Epidemiology and Genomics Research Program, Division of Cancer Control and Population Sciences, National Cancer Institute, National Institutes of Health, 9601 Medical Center Drive, Suite 4E102, Rockville, MD 20850, USA
e-mail: vermam@mail.nih.gov

S. Badve
Department of Pathology and Lab Medicine and Internal Medicine, Indiana University School of Medicine, Indianapolis, IN, USA

S. Badve and Y. Gökmen-Polar (eds.), *Molecular Pathology of Breast Cancer*, DOI 10.1007/978-3-319-41761-5_21

Keywords
Biomarker · Breast cancer · Epigenetics · Epidemiology · Etiology · Precision medicine · Prevention

21.1 Introduction

Breast cancer is the most frequent malignancy in female around the world. This cancer is more complex than other cancers because a number of subtypes, mainly based on different receptor expression, have been reported (Houseman and Ince 2014). Based on clinical, histopathological, and molecular characterization, following subtypes of breast cancer have been reported: luminal A–like, luminal B–like/HER2–negative, luminal B–like/HER2 positive, HER2 positive, and triple negative. Breast cancer detection, diagnosis, and prognosis is complex and needs mechanisms other than genetics, such as epigenetics. Both genetic and epigenetic mechanisms contribute to breast cancer initiation, development, and progression (Basse and Arock 2015; Xhemalce 2013). The focus of this article is to understand the epigenetic mechanism in breast cancer.

All the cells in the body have identical DNA, yet different cells have dramatically distinct morphology, and functional characteristics. It is obvious that there must be mechanisms that control these phenotypic differences; these mechanisms are often collectively referred to as epigenetic mechanisms. They contribute not only to the normal function of the cells during various stages of life such as pregnancy and aging but also play an important role in malignant transformation and resistance to therapy. More recently, these mechanisms have been also used for diagnostic purposes (as detailed below). Needless to say that these mechanisms are poorly understood. In this chapter, we will provide an overview of the basics regarding their role in breast cancer.

21.2 Basic Epigenetic Mechanisms: Four Major Components

The nucleus of the cell is composed mainly of DNA, which if were to be stretched out would measure up to 2 m in length (Kogan et al. 2006; Tessarz and Kouzarides 2014; Travers et al. 2012). It is obvious that this thread like cord needs to be packaged and stored properly to prevent entanglement and breakage. This task is assigned to a group of proteins called histones (4 pairs; H2a, H2b, H3 and H4), which form a spool around which the (147 bp) DNA is wrapped forming the nucleosome (Zhong et al. 1983). A linker segment of 20–90 bp of DNA connects the nucleosomes. The approximately 30 million nucleosomes are further packaged to form chromatin fibers, which get condensed into chromosomes during the process of cell division (Fig. 21.1).

There are at least three basic mechanisms by which access to the DNA for protein synthesis can be controlled. These act either by controlling the DNA function by DNA methylation at what are referred to as CpG islands, or by controlling the spools by histone modifications or by sequestration of chromatin by the formation of heterochromatin. In addition to these mechanisms, protein synthesis can also be controlled downstream by altering the viability and function of the mRNAs in addition to control of transfer RNA and ribosomal function. Lastly, following synthesis, there are a number of quality control mechanisms that affect protein levels. This includes unfolded protein response mechanisms whereby abnormally folded proteins can be destroyed. These latter mechanisms are beyond the scope of the current chapter.

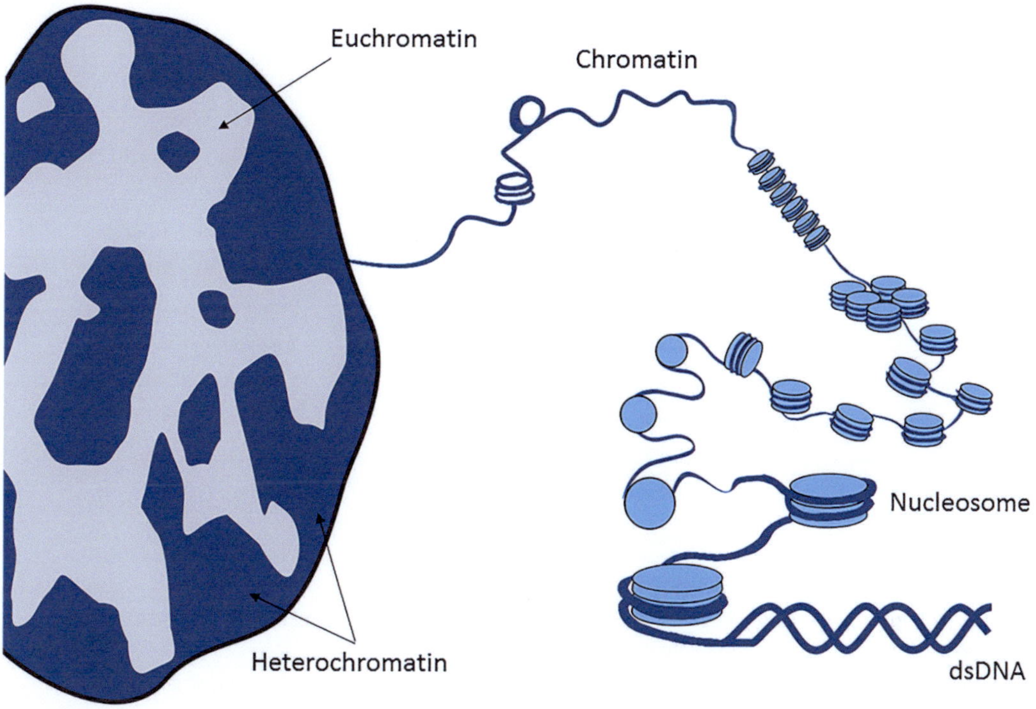

Fig. 21.1 Schematic diagram showing the coiling of double stranded DNA around nucleosomes, which are formed by histones. The nucleosomes are compacted and give rise to euchromatin composed of active elements and the more compact heterochromatin containing inactive elements. The chromatin is further compacted to form chromosomes during cell division

Epigenetics alterations do not involve nucleotide sequence change, but change in gene expression during normal development. External stimuli may influence the expression of genes by epigenetics and may contribute to cancer development. The four major players in epigenetic regulation are DNA methylation (mainly in the promoter region), histone modifications, noncoding RNA expression and chromatin modulation (Iannone et al. 2015). Enzymes involved in methylation and histone modification are well characterized. DNA (cytosine-5)-methyltransferase I (DNMT1), DNMT3a, and DNMT3b are responsible for initiation and maintenance of methylation pattern. In breast cancer, DNMTs are overexpressed. miRNAs targeting 3′ end of DNMTs have also been reported which affect the activity of DNMTs (Veeck and Esteller 2010). Advancement in technologies for detection of epigenetic changes, including dedicated platforms for measuring methylation array and miRNA profiling have made it possible to follow breast cancer progression and also response to therapy in longitudinal studies. Table 21.1 summarizes some of the genes that are regulated by epigenetics in breast cancer based on the methylation or histone modifications.

21.2.1 Methylation

DNA methylation is one of the most common molecular alterations in cancer, which refers to the covalent addition of a methyl (CH3) group from S-adenosylmethionine (SAM) onto cytosine residues of the DNA template. Cytosine molecules in the DNA are targeted by specific enzymes called DNA methyl transferases (DNMTs) and converted into 5-methyl cytosines. This typically occurs in regions of DNA where a

Table 21.1 Selected genes regulated by epigenetics in breast cancer

Gene	Mechanism/comment	References
BRCA1	Hypermethylation and breast cancer cell proliferation, biomarker of survival	Gupta et al. (2014), Zhu et al. (2015)
GSTP1		Yamamoto et al. (2012)
hMLH1	Hypermethylation, in prognosis	Alkam et al. (2013)
hMHS2	Hypermethylation, in prognosis	Alkam et al. (2013)
MGM2	Hypermethylation, in prognosis	Alkam et al. (2013)
$p16^{INK4\alpha}$	Hypermethylation, in diagnosis	Yazici et al. (2009)
RARbeta2	Hypermethylation, in detection	Yamamoto et al. (2012)
RASSF1A	Hypermethylation, in diagnosis	Yazici et al. (2009)
Sigma gene *14-3-3*	Hypermethylation, cancer detection	Gheibi et al. (2012)
T cell marker genes	Methylation, role in tumor prognosis	Dedeurwaerder and Fuks (2012)
Histone methyl transferase (HMTs)	Histone modifications at lysine 9 position	Liu et al. (2015)
histone H3K79 methylation	Histone modification at lysine 79 position with potential prediction of poor prognosis	Yokoyama et al. (2014)
Histone H3K79 methylation	Histone modification at lysine 79 position and association with survival	Zhang et al. (2014)
Histone H2A ubiquitin ligase	Histone H2A ubiquitin ligase activity was regulated by the oncoprotein TRIM37 in breast cancer	Bhatnagar et al. (2014).

cytosine nucleotide occurs next to a guanine nucleotide in the linear sequence of bases along its length are termed CpG sites (short for "-C-phosphate-G-"). CpG sites rich regions within the DNA are termed CpG islands, while regions with low density of CpG sites are termed CpG shores. The importance of this structural feature is that the methylated forms differ in how they interact with macromolecules including transcription factors and thus influence gene expression. CpG islands are typically unmethylated in normal tissues and often located at the 5′ end of genes and involved in gene regulation. This is typically the case for housekeeping genes but not for all the genes. Certain CpG islands are normally methylated; these typically are associated with the genes from inactivated X chromosome and those associated with genetic imprinting.

Methylation at the CpG islands is associated with recruitment of a number of other factors such as Methyl-CpG-binding proteins, which are involved in the translation of DNA methylation into chromatin modifications. These interact with enzymes that deacetylate histones (HDACs), methylate histones (HMT) to cause changes in chromatin.

It was believed for a long time that methylation is a permanent change. However recent studies have documented that there are several forms of modified cystosines namely 5-methyl cystosine (5mC), 5-hydroxymethylcystosine (5hmC), 5-formyl cytosine (5fC) and 5-carboxy cystosine (5caC). At least some of these forms can be converted back to cystosine by the Ten-Eleven Translocation (TET) cytosine dioxygenase family of enzymes (Song et al. 2013). Suffice to say, the exact incidence and roles of these newer forms of modified cystosines and TET enzymes are still being investigated.

21.2.1.1 DNA Methyl Transferases (DNMTs)

The pattern of DNA methylation is established by the coordinated action of DNMTs and associated factors that include polycomb proteins and S-adenosyl-methionine; the latter serves as a donor of the methyl group and is derived from folate metabolism. Mammalian DNMT family includes DNMT1, DNMT3A, DNMT3B, and DNMT3L. DNMT1 is mainly involved in maintaining the preexisting methylation pattern. More recently, expression of DNMT1 has been shown to be indispensable for mammary and cancer stem cell maintenance (Pathania et al. 2015). DNMT1 has also been shown to collaborate with EZH2 to promote the expression of miRNA200b/a/429 expression, which often lost in cancers (Ning et al. 2015). DNMT2 has weak methyltransferase activity in vitro and its depletion has little impact on global CpG methylation and no effect on developmental phenotypes (Goll et al. 2006). DNMT3A and 3B are thought to be important for de novo methylation, and have equal preference to hemimethylated and non-methylated DNA. They have nonoverlapping functions during development with distinct phenotypes and lethality stages (Okano et al. 1999). DNMT3L, although highly expressed in germ cells and embryonic cells, is catalytically inactive. It stimulates the activity of DNMT3A and DNMT3B.

The expression levels of DNMTs is increased in many cancers. In breast cancer, overexpression of the mRNA can be 14–80 fold as compared to normal breast tissues (Girault et al. 2003). Similarly, genes such as RelA/p65, component of the NFkB complex, has been shown to recruit DNMT1 and cause methylation of tumor metastases suppressor gene BRMS1 (Liu et al. 2012). Approximately 30 % of the breast cancers overexpress DNMT3A. As these tumor are typically associated high grade ER-negative status and reduced BRCA1 protein expression, an independent prognostic effect for the overexpression has not been demonstrated (Yu et al. 2015; Girault et al. 2003). Alterations in expression of DNMTs has been associated with docetaxel resistance albeit in cell line studies (Kastl et al. 2010).

Recent studies have focused on the impact of single nucleotide polymorphisms (SNP) in DNMTs and breast cancer risk. DNMT1 SNP (A201G; rs2228612) has been associated with lower risk of breast cancer in central European Caucasian population (Kullmann et al. 2013). In the Chinese Han population, rs16999593 in DNMT1 and rs2424908 in DNMT3B, have been significantly associated with breast cancer risk (Sun et al. 2012), while another study did not find any associations (Ye et al. 2010).

21.2.1.2 Methyl-CpG-Binding Proteins

There are at least 3 distinct families of proteins containing 12 members that bind the methylated DNA; these include the methyl-CpG-binding domain (MBD) family (MECP2, MBD1-6), Kaiso and Kaiso-like proteins (ZBTB4, ZBTB38) and SRA domain proteins (UHRF1, UHRF2). They have non overlapping function and can act in a sequence specific manner. All MeCPs share binding specificity for symmetrical 5meCpG, in addition, they also have other binding preferences based on the DNA sequences. MBDs mostly act as transcriptional repressors but MBD2 can also serve as an activator. The MBD domain of MBD1 has been shown to recognize 5meCpGs better within the TCGCA and TGCGCA sequences. KAISO proteins show a preference for two 5meCpGs motifs in close proximity. The SRA domain of UHRF1 recognizes and binds to hemimethylated DNA and acts in conjunction with DNMT1 to maintain DNA methylation. MBD3 is an essential subunit of the Mi-2/NuRD chromatin remodeling complex.

Analysis of the Cancer Genome Atlas (TCGA) breast cancer dataset shows that the incidence of alterations in the MBD proteins (MECP2, MBD1-6) is around 53 % while that of KAISO (ZBTB33), ZBTB4, ZBTB38 is around 24 %; and UHRF1, UHRF2 is around 16 % respectively. Collectively, alterations of these proteins amount to about 55 % in breast cancers. Most of these alterations are at the expression level and mutations within these proteins are rare (0–0.6 %).

21.2.1.3 Ten-Eleven Translocation Cytosine Dioxygenases (TETs)

TET was first described in 2003 in acute myeloid leukemia (AML). It is now recognized that there are at least 3 TET enzymes, TET1, TET2, and TET3 located on at 10q21, 4q24 and 2p13 regions respectively. They belong to the family of dioxygenases and contain three Fe(II)-and oxoglutarate-binding sites within the C-terminal catalytic domain characterized by the presence of double-stranded b-helix(DSBH) and a cysteine-rich region.TET1 and TET3 have a N-terminal CXXC zinc chelating domain through which they bind the DNA. TET2 seems to require another molecule IDAX (inhibition of Dvl1 and axin complex) to bind genomic sequences. At least 4 mechanisms of demethylation involving TET proteins have been proposed including replication-dependent passive dilution of the 5mC. The most well characterized mechanism involves removal of pyrimidine bases by thymidine-DNA glycosylase (TDG) followed by base excision repair (BER).

TET mutations have been associated with hematological malignancies including mixed lineage leukemia (MLL) and myelodysplastic syndromes (MDS). In the TGCA breast cancer dataset, TET1, TET2, and TET3 alterations have been identified in 5, 4, and 9 %, respectively. Most of these alterations are RNA upregulation, with somatic mutations in each being present in less than 1 % of cases (0.7–0.9).

21.2.2 Histone Modifications

Histone modifications are posttranslational modifications at N-terminal tails of histones that regulate chromatin structure and gene expression. These changes typically involve the lysine moiety and include acetylation, methylation, phosphorylation, sumoylation, poly (ADP) ribosylation and ubiquitination. However, modifications of the arginine, serine, threonine, tyrosine and histidine amino acids are also described. Detailed review of this topic is beyond the scope of this chapter and interested readers are directed to the recent excellent review article on this topic (see Rothbart and Strahl 2014).

Histone acetylation has been most extensively studied in cancer. Histone de-acetylating enzymes (HDACs) remove acetyl groups from the ε-amino groups of lysine residues in the N-terminal tails of the histone. This results in chromatin condensation and repression of gene expression. Histone acetyl transferases (HAT) enzymes counter this action. The readers are directed to an excellent (but older) articles by Yang and Seto (2007) for details. There are at least 3 major families of HATs: general control non-derepressible 5 (Gcn5)-related N-acetyltransferases (GNATs), p300/CBP and MYST proteins. In addition, at least another 10 proteins such as Elp3, Eco1 and CDY have been documented to have HAT activity. HATs not only affect the activity of histones but are also known to affect the activity of several transcription factors. Based on the sequence similarity and co-factor requirements, HDACs are classified into 4 classes and 2 families: the classical and silent information regulator 2 (Sir2)-related protein (Sirtuin) families. The classical family has at least 11 members (HDAC1-11) while the Sirtuin family has 7 (SIRT1-7) members.

Histone methylation is restricted to lysine (K) and arginine (R) residues but is most common in lysines. Signatures of histone (K) methylation have also been described. Briefly, Barski et al. (2007) performed high resolution methylation profiling of histones and identified a number of expression patterns. They linked mono-methylations of H3K27, H3K9, H4K20, HsK79 and H2BK5 to gene activation. In contrast, tri-methylations of H3K27, H3K9 and H3K70 were associated with gene repression. Additionally, H2A.Z histone was associated with functional regulatory elements. Similarly, Mikkelsen et al. (2007) created chromatin state maps that could distinguish pluripotent cells from lineage—committed cells.

21.2.3 Noncoding RNA Profiling

The role of noncoding RNAs such as micro RNAs (miRNAs) and long noncoding RNAs (lncRNAs) is well characterized in gene expression regulation. lncRNAs are more than 200 nt long and lack an open reading frame (Maruyama and Suzuki 2012). miRNAs are 21–25 nucleotide long small RNA molecules which are integral part of epigenetic regulatory machine in a cell (Cui et al. 2010; Kastl et al. 2012; Lee et al. 2011; Wee et al. 2012). The topic is discussed in detail in Chap. 22 of this book.

21.2.4 Chromatin Remodeling

The backbone of epigenetic regulation is chromatin structure which controls distance between nucleosomes and binding of transcription factors and other proteins involved in gene regulation. Chromatin provides stability to the genome and its functions. Understanding the complexity of interactions between the myriad proteins associated with chromatin at any given time during the development and responses to the environment is a difficult task. As stated previously, the genome of each cell is composed of approximately 30 million nucleosome. These are organized in small and large topologically associated domains (TADs) and subdomains(Ali et al. 2016). The junctions of these domains are marked by the attachment of proteins such as CTCF, which demarcate the domains from each other (Xu and Corces 2015; Corces and Corces 2016).

A number of changes can occur in the nucleosomes as they can be shifted, evicted or exchanged, and the composition of their subunits can be altered by covalent binding to different biological moieties. The relationship between chromatin modifications and gene expression is considered a hen-and-egg problem because multiple chromatin modifications can occur in the same locus and that the same modification can have different roles at different sites of a locus. One of the well characterized method for opening densely packed chromatin utilizes ATP-dependent chromatin remodeling complexes (remodelers). At least four families of these remodelers have been described namely switching defective/sucrose non-fermenting (SWI/SNF), the imitation-switch (ISWI) family, the Mi2/nucleosome remodeling and histone deacetylation (NuRD) and the inositol 80 (INO80) family (Lai and Wade 2011; Kumar et al. 2016; Dawson and Kouzarides 2012; Langst and Manelyte 2015). Each of the families are complexes composed of up to 15 subunits, which can be modified by extracellular and cytoplasmic signals. Thus the chromatin remodelers act as integrators of these signals to the nucleus for precise regulation of target gene expression (Kumar et al. 2016).

One of the first cancers to have been found to have mutations of chromatin remodelers was the Rhabdoid tumor, which harbors mutations of BAF47. This mutation is so characteristic of this tumor type that absence of the protein product (recognized by INI-1 antibody) is routinely used for diagnostic purposes. Mutations of SWI/SNF family members BRG1 and BAF250A have been identified in breast cancer (Wong et al. 2000; Jones et al. 2012; Kadoch et al. 2013). Similarly, epigenetic silencing of BRM has been described in several cancers including breast cancer(Glaros et al. 2007). In addition, members of the ISWI family (SNF2H) (Jin et al. 2015) and NuRD family (MTA-1 (metastases associated-1) and MTA-2) have also been documented to silenced in breast cancer (Jang et al. 2006; Covington et al. 2013).

Weng et al. (2015) demonstrated the oncogenic role of the high mobility group nucleosome-binding domain 5 (HMGNS5) in breast cancer. HMGNS5 affects cell proliferation, invasion and apoptosis. *CBX5* gene codes for the heterochromatin protein alpha 1 (HP1alpha) and interacts with histone H3 (in its di-methylated and tri-methylated forms) at lysine 9 position. Although this observation has been made during breast cancer development, the complete mechanism of its involvement in either development or progression of cancer is unknown (Vad-Nielsen and Nielsen 2015).

21.3 Epigenetic Biomarkers in Breast Cancer Diagnosis and Prognosis

21.3.1 DNA Methylation Biomarkers in Breast Cancer

The methylation pattern in cancer is dramatically altered. In breast cancer, like in most cancers, there is a global DNA hypomethylation, which could lead to the chromosomal instability, reactivation of transposable elements, loss of imprinting and ultimately activation of number of sequestered DNA segments/genes. This hypomethylation is, however, associated hypermethylation of a number of genes, many of which are tumor suppressors. These genes include *BRCA1*, *p16*^{INK4a}, *RASSF1A* and Cadherin superfamily genes which are required for a number of important cellular functions such as DNA repair and cell polarity. Yazici reported methylation of *RASSF1A* in plasma of breast cancer patients (Yazici et al. 2009). Hypermethylation of estrogen receptor genes *ESR1* and *ESR2* promoters results with gene silencing, which is associated with decreased expression levels of ERα and ERβ proteins in cancer cell lines. However, there are limited number of studies that demonstrated ERα and ERβ gene silencing in breast tumors. In a case control study, *BRCA1* methylation status was correlated with development of triple negative breast cancer cells (Gupta et al. 2014). Alkam et al. (2013) reported hypermethylation of genes involved in DNA repair pathway (*hMLH1*, *hMHS2*, and *MGM2*) and demonstrated their utility in basal like breast cancer prognosis. Immune components of breast tumors were also identified (T cell marker genes) and their role in tumor prognosis was proposed (Dedeurwaerder and Fuks 2012). Sigma gene 14-3-3 methylation was reported for breast cancer detection by Gheibi et al. (2012) and *GSTP1*, *RASSF1A*, and RARbeta2 were found hypermethylated in another study by Yamamoto et al. (2012). In a case control study conducted in China on tissue arrays of more than 200 triple negative cancer samples, BRCA1 biomarker was found to be associated with overall survival and disease-free survival (Zhu et al. 2015). Methylation studies on early detection of breast cancer in ductal carcinoma in situ (DCIS), a preinvasive lesion, indicated the potential of methylation markers in following progression of DCIS into breast cancer. Hypermethylation of estrogen receptor genes *ESR1* and *ESR2* promoters results with gene silencing, which is associated with decreased expression levels of ERα and ERβ proteins in cancer (Hagrass et al. 2014; Martinez-Galan et al. 2014; Wei et al. 2012). However, there are limited number of studies that demonstrated ERα and ERβ gene silencing in breast tumors. Genomewide DNA methylation analysis demonstrates that global DNA hypomethylation is highly frequent in breast cancer. In addition, hypermethylation of breast cancer specific genes such as *BRCA1, RASSF1A* and *Cadherin superfamily* genes are very often reported. In an independent genomewide methylation study of biospecimens from Melbourne Collaborative Cohort Study, a cancer risk prediction model of breast cancer was developed (Severi et al. 2014).

21.3.2 Histone Modification Biomarkers in Breast Cancer

Posttranslational histone modifications are associated with breast tumorigenesis, aggressiveness of prognosis and they are potential therapeutic targets. In one meta-analysis, lysine histone methyltransferases (HMTs) were characterized and 12 of them were found to have altered copy number (Liu et al. 2015). A role for few of the HMTs identified by these investigators in breast cancer survival and therapy was also proposed. Role of histone H3K79 methylation in self-renewal and metastatic proliferation of breast cancer was proposed by Zhang et al. (2014).

Yokoyama et al. demonstrated that loss of histone H4K20 trimethylation predicts poor prognosis of breast cancer (Yokoyama et al. 2014). Histone acetyl transferase (HAT), histone deacetyl transferase (HDAC), histone methyltransferase (HKMT

EZ2 and EHMT2) have been well characterized. HKMT EZ2 maintains repressive chromatin methylation mark H3K27me while EHMT2 maintains H3K9me methylation state (Curry et al. 2015). Curry et al. (2015) demonstrated that inhibition of both EZ2 and EHMT2 was more effective in controlling tumor growth than inhibiting single methyltransferase. Histone H2A ubiquitin ligase activity was regulated by the oncoprotein TRIM37 in breast cancer (Bhatnagar et al. 2014). This oncoprotein is overexpressed up to 40 % in breast cancer cells compared to normal breast cells.

21.3.3 Alterations in Chromosomal Conformation and Nucleosome Repositioning in Breast Cancer

Progesterone induced nucleosome positioning was observed in breast cancer (Iannone et al. 2015). Due to chromatin conformation changes, alternate splicing of specific genes was also observed. In this study, the investigators systematically demonstrated the occupancy of exon by nucleosome and alternatively by spliceosomes. In another study, the opening of chromatin as a result of hormone (estrogen) treatment was studied and proposed mechanism of histone deacetylating inhibitors was explained (Rafique et al. 2015).

21.4 Clinical Utility of Epigenetic Mechanisms

21.4.1 Epigenetic Inhibitors in Breast Cancer Treatment

Based on the receptor phenotypes, breast cancer has been divided into different subtypes. It has been observed that different subtypes become resistance to treatment at different frequencies and time durations. The most resistant one is the triple negative breast cancer, which is negative for ER, PR, and HER2 expression (Lehmann and Pietenpol 2014; Tu et al. 2012). In addition to genetic changes in breast cancer and its correlation with subgroups, response to treatment, and clinical outcome, involvement of epigenetic regulation in resistance to hormone therapy has also observed (Pathiraja et al. 2010).

21.4.1.1 DNA Methyltransferase Inhibitors

The nucleoside analogs, 5-azacytidine (AZA) and decitabine (DCA), have been the most widely used methylation inhibitors which have been approved by the Food and Drug Administration for the treatment of cancer (Connolly and Stearns 2012). Promoter methylation inhibits transcription, therefore, DNMT inhibitors (DNMTi) were used to reverse the repression of tumor suppressor genes and other genes such as estrogen receptor gene coding for *ERα*. When 5-azacytidine and 5-aza-2-deoxycytidine (nucleoside analogs) were used in combination, re-expression of *ERα* was observed. These nucleoside analogs get incorporated into DNA and replace cytosine during replication process. When DNA methylation starts, it recruits DNMTs, but the enzyme gets trapped by the analog and induces a passive DNA demethylation following DNA replication and cell division (Szyf 2009; Thakur et al. 2012). When demethylating agents are used in low doses (nanomolar range), it resulted in the development of an antitumor "memory" response which inhibited not only the growth of cancer cells but also traditionally resistant stem like cells (Tsai et al. 2012). This treatment resulted in genome-wide alteration in methylation and gene expression. Alteration in methylation levels in tumor suppressor genes, such as *ER*, *BRCA1*, *E-Cadherin*, *PTEN* and *MASPIN*, was also reported (Krawczyk and Fabianowska-Majewska 2006; Wozniak et al. 2007; Krawczyk et al. 2007). Demethylating agents have been shown to sensitize breast cancer cells by inducing tumor necrosis factor-related apoptosis-inducing ligand

(TRAIL) (Xu et al. 2007). Novel agents such as Zeburlarine, SGI-110 and NPEOC-DAC are also being developed. Apart from the nucleoside analogues, agents such as RG108, EGCG, Psammaplin, MG98 are in development. Hydralazine, an antihypertensive agent, has also been shown to affect DNMT activity.

Demethylating agents have also used in combination with other agents such as immunotherapy and chemotherapy. In one study, decitabine was used either alone or in combination with anthracycline-based chemotherapy [5 fluorouracil plus epirubicine plus cyclophosphamide, (FEC)] and results showed differential effects of decitabine and its combination on the metastatic capacity and survival of breast cancer (Ari et al. 2011).

A number of agents that have been analyzed in the chemoprevention setting also have inhibitory activity directed towards DNMT (reviewed in Cai et al. 2011; Subramaniam et al. 2014). These include the Black Raspberry derived anthocyanins with affect the methylation of the WNT pathway. Similarly, polyphenols derived from Annurca apple and coffee, acetyl-keto-β-boswellic acid (from Boswellia serrata), flavonolingnan silibinin (from thistle plant), EGCG (from Green tea), curcumin, wild thyme, genistein and number of other compounds have been shown to have DNMT modulatory activity.

21.4.1.2 Histone Deacetylase Inhibitors

In breast cancer, as suggested from different groups of investigators (Feng et al. 2007; Yarosh et al. 2008), activity of histone deacetylase has been correlated with inhibition of the expression of selected genes. Therefore, HDAC inhibitors (HDACi) have been tested to evaluate treatment response, improved survival, and reduction in tumor aggressiveness (Tu et al. 2012). Since several classes of HDACi have been identified, a number of new agents are being discovered and tested against tumor progression. This provided an opportunity for gene specific targeted therapy. Two HDAC inhibitors have been evaluated extensively: trichostatin A (TSA) and suberoylanilide hydroxamic acid (SAHA) (Komatsu et al. 2013; Min et al. 2015).

In preclinical studies, TSA induced cell death in ER^- and ER^+ cells (Chakravarty et al. 2011; Kim et al. 2010). However, the dose of the TSA was too high to be used for patients (Kim et al. 2010; Basse and Arock 2015; Reid et al. 2005; Jang et al. 2004). Also, TSA treatment sensitized TNBC cells to Tamoxifen when used in combination with Raloxifen (Tu et al. 2012). SAHA showed inhibition of tumor growth and migratory and invasive features when used in ER^+, ER + $HER2^+$, $HER2^+$, and TNBC cells (Cheng and Hung 2013; Chiu et al. 2013; Cazares Marinero Jde et al. 2013). Another HDAC inhibitor, Panobinostat, showed inhibition of aromatase (implicated in androgen metabolism) and was found to decrease estrogen levels when combined with Letrozole (Chen et al. 2010). SNDX-275 is another HDAC inhibitor which stops proliferation of HER2 cells at micromolar concentrations and was found more effective when used in combination with Trastuzumab (Huang et al. 2011; Srivastava et al. 2010). Valproic acid, either alone or in combination with Decitabine was found effective in enhancing Tamoxifen efficiency in ER^+ cells (Hodges-Gallagher et al. 2007).

HDACs interact with other nucleosomal modifier proteins, especially histone demethylating protein LSD1. In one study, combination of LSD1 inhibitor and SAHA showed tumor growth inhibition of TNBC (Huang et al. 2012; Vasilatos et al. 2013). Microarray screening of treated cells demonstrated suppression of a unique subset of genes involved in tumor development (Huang et al. 2012).

In one example, a novel HDAC inhibitor, NKHDAC-1, was identified which had antitumor proliferation properties due to inactivation of HDAC1 (Li et al. 2013). Jang et al. demonstrated that estrogen receptor alpha cells became sensitized to tamoxifen after treatment with trichostatin A, an agent with histone deacetylating properties (Jang et al. 2004). Thailandepsin A (TDP A) was recently identified as the HDAC inhibitor (Xiao et al. 2015). It inhibited apoptosis by interacting with pro-apoptotic protein Bax and inhibiting levels of anti-apoptotic protein Bcl-2, even at nanomolar concentrations.

Although epigenetic inhibitors have been used for the treatment of breast cancer, they are not specific and there is a potential of harmful effects of using these inhibitors. Combination therapy may work better for the treatment of breast cancer (Basse and Arock 2015; Thakur et al. 2012). Six new hybrid compounds that combined Tamoxifen structural motifs with SAHA were found more effective agents and less toxic than Tamoxifen and SAHA alone (Cazares Marinero Jde et al. 2013). When Decitabine was used before TSA or Tamoxifen treatment, the ER levels were higher than TSA or Tamoxifen alone (Fan et al. 2008). In combination epigenetics therapy, it is important to know the sequence in which these therapies are administrered.

One important approach for prevention of breast cancer is the use of phytochemicals which are biologically active food components with epigenetic inhibiting properties. In this direction, use of isothiocynates from cruciferous vegetables or genistein from soybean in a population study has been proposed for the prevention of breast cancer (Basse and Arock 2015). Histone deacetylases (HDACs) are overexpressed in breast cancer (and other cancers) and they are considered attractive targets for cancer therapy. Targeted delivery of epigenetic inhibitors is also a matter of concern but recent development in using disulfide cross-linked micelles (DCMs) has been successful where TDP-A was used to inhibit breast cancer cell growth (Xiao et al. 2015). Epigenetic therapy will represent further opportunity to treat breast cancer tumors by reversing the resistance to hormonal therapy.

21.4.1.3 Chromatin Remodeling Based Therapies

Chromatin remodelers are multi-protein complex that were thought to be difficult to target for therapeutics. Alterations in these proteins have been documented to led/contribute to resistance to chemo- targeted therapies as well as radiation (Kumar et al. 2016). Recent work has therefore focused on developing inhibitors. A number of agents that are directed at the chromo- and bromo-domains are in development (Gallenkamp et al. 2014; Kumar et al. 2016).

A recent study identified Bromodomain Containing 4 (BRD4) as a potential target in luminal/HER2 breast cancer and in a subset of triple negative breast cancer cells using a high-throughput shRNA screens on 77 breast cancer cell lines (Marcotte et al. 2016). BRD4 is a member of Bromodomain and extra terminal domain (BET) family. Furthermore, the study indicated the potential use of BET inhibitors which are currently in clinical trials for leukemia. The same study also reported that the presence of PIK3CA mutations may confer resistance to BET-inhibitors. Taken together, these data supports the potential use of BET inhibitors in the clinical setting. In addition, these inhibitors have the potential for combination studies with Everolimus or other Rapalogs/Torkinibs to overcome resistance in tumors harboring PIK3CA mutations.

21.5 Concluding Remarks

Breast cancer is a significantly heterogeneous disease in histology, genetics and prognosis. Many biomarkers have been identified for breast cancer detection; however, in the absence of a unique biomarker with sufficient specificity and sensitivity, a panel of multiple biomarkers should be used. Epigenetic approaches may be useful in personalized medicine in breast cancer (longitudinal prospective studies, follow up with epigenetic profiling at different times). Because of the heterogeneity and complexity of breast cancer, therapies should be tailored for individuals so that proper followup of response to therapy can be followed. Targeting distinct epigenetic pathways can be more effective in breast cancer treatment. Similarly, targeting one epigenetic pathway with multiple agents could also be effective in synergizing the effects of more than one therapeutic agent.

References

Ali T, Renkawitz R, Bartkuhn M (2016) Insulators and domains of gene expression. Curr Opin Genet Dev 37:17–26. doi:10.1016/j.gde.2015.11.009

Alkam Y, Mitomi H, Nakai K, Himuro T, Saito T, Takahashi M, Arakawa A, Yao T, Saito M (2013) Protein expression and methylation of DNA repair genes hMLH1, hMSH2, MGMT and BRCA1 and their correlation with clinicopathological parameters and prognosis in basal-like breast cancer. Histopathology 63(5):713–725. doi:10.1111/his.12220

Ari F, Napieralski R, Ulukaya E, Dere E, Colling C, Honert K, Kruger A, Kiechle M, Schmitt M (2011) Modulation of protein expression levels and DNA methylation status of breast cancer metastasis genes by anthracycline-based chemotherapy and the demethylating agent decitabine. Cell Biochem Funct 29 (8):651–659. doi:10.1002/cbf.1801

Barski A, Cuddapah S, Cui K, Roh TY, Schones DE, Wang Z, Wei G, Chepelev I, Zhao K (2007) High-resolution profiling of histone methylations in the human genome. Cell 129(4):823–837. doi:10.1016/j.cell.2007.05.009

Basse C, Arock M (2015) The increasing roles of epigenetics in breast cancer: Implications for pathogenicity, biomarkers, prevention and treatment. Int J Cancer 137(12):2785–2794. doi:10.1002/ijc.29347

Bhatnagar S, Gazin C, Chamberlain L, Ou J, Zhu X, Tushir JS, Virbasius CM, Lin L, Zhu LJ, Wajapeyee N, Green MR (2014) TRIM37 is a new histone H2A ubiquitin ligase and breast cancer oncoprotein. Nature 516(7529):116–120. doi:10.1038/nature13955

Cai FF, Kohler C, Zhang B, Wang MH, Chen WJ, Zhong XY (2011) Epigenetic therapy for breast cancer. Int J Mol Sci 12(7):4465–4487. doi:10.3390/ijms12074465

Cazares Marinero Jde J, Lapierre M, Cavailles V, Saint-Fort R, Vessieres A, Top S, Jaouen G (2013) Efficient new constructs against triple negative breast cancer cells: synthesis and preliminary biological study of ferrocifen-SAHA hybrids and related species. Dalton Trans 42(43):15489–15501. doi:10.1039/c3dt51917a

Chakravarty G, Rider B, Mondal D (2011) Cytoplasmic compartmentalization of SOX9 abrogates the growth arrest response of breast cancer cells that can be rescued by trichostatin A treatment. Cancer Biol Ther 11(1):71–83

Chen S, Ye J, Kijima I, Evans D (2010) The HDAC inhibitor LBH589 (panobinostat) is an inhibitory modulator of aromatase gene expression. Proc Natl Acad Sci USA 107(24):11032–11037. doi:10.1073/pnas.1000917107

Cheng HT, Hung WC (2013) Inhibition of lymphangiogenic factor VEGF-C expression and production by the histone deacetylase inhibitor suberoylanilide hydroxamic acid in breast cancer cells. Oncol Rep 29(3):1238–1244. doi:10.3892/or.2012.2188

Chiu HW, Yeh YL, Wang YC, Huang WJ, Chen YA, Chiou YS, Ho SY, Lin P, Wang YJ (2013) Suberoylanilide hydroxamic acid, an inhibitor of histone deacetylase, enhances radiosensitivity and suppresses lung metastasis in breast cancer in vitro and in vivo. PLoS ONE 8(10):e76340. doi:10.1371/journal.pone.0076340

Connolly R, Stearns V (2012) Epigenetics as a therapeutic target in breast cancer. J Mammary Gland Biol Neoplasia 17(3–4):191–204. doi:10.1007/s10911-012-9263-3

Corces MR, Corces VG (2016) The three-dimensional cancer genome. Curr Opin Genet Dev 36:1–7. doi:10.1016/j.gde.2016.01.002

Covington KR, Brusco L, Barone I, Tsimelzon A, Selever J, Corona-Rodriguez A, Brown P, Kumar R, Hilsenbeck SG, Fuqua SA (2013) Metastasis tumor-associated protein 2 enhances metastatic behavior and is associated with poor outcomes in estrogen receptor-negative breast cancer. Breast Cancer Res Treat. doi:10.1007/s10549-013-2709-5

Cui W, Zhang Y, Hu N, Shan C, Zhang S, Zhang W, Zhang X, Ye L (2010) miRNA-520b and miR-520e sensitize breast cancer cells to complement attack via directly targeting 3'UTR of CD46. Cancer Biol Ther 10(3):232–241

Curry E, Green I, Chapman-Rothe N, Shamsaei E, Kandil S, Cherblanc FL, Payne L, Bell E, Ganesh T, Srimongkolpithak N, Caron J, Li F, Uren AG, Snyder JP, Vedadi M, Fuchter MJ, Brown R (2015) Dual EZH2 and EHMT2 histone methyltransferase inhibition increases biological efficacy in breast cancer cells. Clin Epigenetics 7(1):84. doi:10.1186/s13148-015-0118-9

Dawson MA, Kouzarides T (2012) Cancer epigenetics: from mechanism to therapy. Cell 150(1):12–27. doi:10.1016/j.cell.2012.06.013

Dedeurwaerder S, Fuks F (2012) DNA methylation markers for breast cancer prognosis: unmasking the immune component. Oncoimmunology 1(6):962–964. doi:10.4161/onci.19996

Fan J, Yin WJ, Lu JS, Wang L, Wu J, Wu FY, Di GH, Shen ZZ, Shao ZM (2008) ER alpha negative breast cancer cells restore response to endocrine therapy by combination treatment with both HDAC inhibitor and DNMT inhibitor. J Cancer Res Clin Oncol 134 (8):883–890. doi:10.1007/s00432-008-0354-x

Feng W, Lu Z, Luo RZ, Zhang X, Seto E, Liao WS, Yu Y (2007) Multiple histone deacetylases repress tumor suppressor gene ARHI in breast cancer. Int J Cancer 120(8):1664–1668. doi:10.1002/ijc.22474

Gallenkamp D, Gelato KA, Haendler B, Weinmann H (2014) Bromodomains and their pharmacological inhibitors. ChemMedChem 9(3):438–464. doi:10.1002/cmdc.201300434

Gheibi A, Kazemi M, Baradaran A, Akbari M, Salehi M (2012) Study of promoter methylation pattern of 14-3-3 sigma gene in normal and cancerous tissue of breast: a potential biomarker for detection of breast cancer in patients. Adv Biomed Res 1:80. doi:10.4103/2277-9175.102990

Girault I, Tozlu S, Lidereau R, Bieche I (2003) Expression analysis of DNA methyltransferases 1, 3A, and 3B in sporadic breast carcinomas. Clin Cancer Res 9 (12):4415–4422

Glaros S, Cirrincione GM, Muchardt C, Kleer CG, Michael CW, Reisman D (2007) The reversible epigenetic silencing of BRM: implications for clinical targeted therapy. Oncogene 26(49):7058–7066. doi:10.1038/sj.onc.1210514

Goll MG, Kirpekar F, Maggert KA, Yoder JA, Hsieh CL, Zhang X, Golic KG, Jacobsen SE, Bestor TH (2006) Methylation of tRNAAsp by the DNA methyltransferase homolog Dnmt2. Science 311(5759):395–398. doi:10.1126/science.1120976

Gupta S, Jaworska-Bieniek K, Narod SA, Lubinski J, Wojdacz TK, Jakubowska A (2014) Methylation of the BRCA1 promoter in peripheral blood DNA is associated with triple-negative and medullary breast cancer. Breast Cancer Res Treat 148(3):615–622. doi:10.1007/s10549-014-3179-0

Hagrass HA, Pasha HF, Ali AM (2014) Estrogen receptor alpha (ERalpha) promoter methylation status in tumor and serum DNA in Egyptian breast cancer patients. Gene 552(1):81–86. doi:10.1016/j.gene.2014.09.016

Hodges-Gallagher L, Valentine CD, Bader SE, Kushner PJ (2007) Inhibition of histone deacetylase enhances the anti-proliferative action of antiestrogens on breast cancer cells and blocks tamoxifen-induced proliferation of uterine cells. Breast Cancer Res Treat 105 (3):297–309. doi:10.1007/s10549-006-9459-6

Houseman EA, Ince TA (2014) Normal cell-type epigenetics and breast cancer classification: a case study of cell mixture-adjusted analysis of DNA methylation data from tumors. Cancer Inform 13(Suppl 4):53–64. doi:10.4137/CIN.S13980

Huang X, Wang S, Lee CK, Yang X, Liu B (2011) HDAC inhibitor SNDX-275 enhances efficacy of trastuzumab in erbB2-overexpressing breast cancer cells and exhibits potential to overcome trastuzumab resistance. Cancer Lett 307(1):72–79. doi:10.1016/j.canlet.2011.03.019

Huang Y, Vasilatos SN, Boric L, Shaw PG, Davidson NE (2012) Inhibitors of histone demethylation and histone deacetylation cooperate in regulating gene expression and inhibiting growth in human breast cancer cells. Breast Cancer Res Treat 131(3):777–789. doi:10.1007/s10549-011-1480-8

Iannone C, Pohl A, Papasaikas P, Soronellas D, Vicent GP, Beato M, ValcaRcel J (2015) Relationship between nucleosome positioning and progesterone-induced alternative splicing in breast cancer cells. RNA 21(3):360–374. doi:10.1261/rna.048843.114

Jang ER, Lim SJ, Lee ES, Jeong G, Kim TY, Bang YJ, Lee JS (2004) The histone deacetylase inhibitor trichostatin A sensitizes estrogen receptor alpha-negative breast cancer cells to tamoxifen. Oncogene 23(9):1724–1736. doi:10.1038/sj.onc.1207315

Jang KS, Paik SS, Chung H, Oh YH, Kong G (2006) MTA1 overexpression correlates significantly with tumor grade and angiogenesis in human breast cancers. Cancer Sci 97(5):374–379. doi:10.1111/j.1349-7006.2006.00186.x

Jin Q, Mao X, Li B, Guan S, Yao F, Jin F (2015) Overexpression of SMARCA5 correlates with cell proliferation and migration in breast cancer. Tumour Biol 36(3):1895–1902. doi:10.1007/s13277-014-2791-2

Jones S, Li M, Parsons DW, Zhang X, Wesseling J, Kristel P, Schmidt MK, Markowitz S, Yan H, Bigner D, Hruban RH, Eshleman JR, Iacobuzio-Donahue CA, Goggins M, Maitra A, Malek SN, Powell S, Vogelstein B, Kinzler KW, Velculescu VE, Papadopoulos N (2012) Somatic mutations in the chromatin remodeling gene ARID1A occur in several tumor types. Hum Mutat 33(1):100–103. doi:10.1002/humu.21633

Kadoch C, Hargreaves DC, Hodges C, Elias L, Ho L, Ranish J, Crabtree GR (2013) Proteomic and bioinformatic analysis of mammalian SWI/SNF complexes identifies extensive roles in human malignancy. Nat Genet 45(6):592–601. doi:10.1038/ng.2628

Kastl L, Brown I, Schofield AC (2010) Altered DNA methylation is associated with docetaxel resistance in human breast cancer cells. Int J Oncol 36(5):1235–1241

Kastl L, Brown I, Schofield AC (2012) miRNA-34a is associated with docetaxel resistance in human breast cancer cells. Breast Cancer Res Treat 131(2):445–454. doi:10.1007/s10549-011-1424-3

Kim SH, Kang HJ, Na H, Lee MO (2010) Trichostatin A enhances acetylation as well as protein stability of ERalpha through induction of p300 protein. Breast Cancer Res 12(2):R22. doi:10.1186/bcr2562

Kogan SB, Kato M, Kiyama R, Trifonov EN (2006) Sequence structure of human nucleosome DNA. J Biomol Struct Dyn 24(1):43–48. doi:10.1080/07391102.2006.10507097

Komatsu S, Moriya S, Che XF, Yokoyama T, Kohno N, Miyazawa K (2013) Combined treatment with SAHA, bortezomib, and clarithromycin for concomitant targeting of aggresome formation and intracellular proteolytic pathways enhances ER stress-mediated cell death in breast cancer cells. Biochem Biophys Res Commun 437(1):41–47. doi:10.1016/j.bbrc.2013.06.032

Krawczyk B, Fabianowska-Majewska K (2006) Alteration of DNA methylation status in K562 and MCF-7 cancer cell lines by nucleoside analogues. Nucleosides, Nucleotides Nucleic Acids 25(9–11):1029–1032. doi:10.1080/15257770600890764

Krawczyk B, Rudnicka K, Fabianowska-Majewska K (2007) The effects of nucleoside analogues on promoter methylation of selected tumor suppressor genes in MCF-7 and MDA-MB-231 breast cancer cell lines. Nucleosides, Nucleotides Nucleic Acids 26(8–9):1043–1046. doi:10.1080/15257770701509594

Kullmann K, Deryal M, Ong MF, Schmidt W, Mahlknecht U (2013) DNMT1 genetic polymorphisms affect breast cancer risk in the central European Caucasian population. Clin Epigenetics 5(1):7. doi:10.1186/1868-7083-5-7

Kumar R, Li DQ, Muller S, Knapp S (2016) Epigenomic regulation of oncogenesis by chromatin remodeling. Oncogene. doi:10.1038/onc.2015.513

Lai AY, Wade PA (2011) Cancer biology and NuRD: a multifaceted chromatin remodelling complex. Nat Rev Cancer 11(8):588–596. doi:10.1038/nrc3091

Langst G, Manelyte L (2015) Chromatin remodelers: from function to dysfunction. Genes (Basel) 6(2):299–324. doi:10.3390/genes6020299

Lee YM, Lee JY, Ho CC, Hong QS, Yu SL, Tzeng CR, Yang PC, Chen HW (2011) miRNA-34b as a tumor suppressor in estrogen-dependent growth of breast cancer cells. Breast Cancer Res 13(6):R116. doi:10.1186/bcr3059

Lehmann BD, Pietenpol JA (2014) Identification and use of biomarkers in treatment strategies for triple-negative breast cancer subtypes. J Pathol 232 (2):142–150. doi:10.1002/path.4280

Li ZH, Zhang XB, Han XQ, Feng CR, Wang FS, Wang PG, Shen J, Shi YK (2013) Antitumor effects of a novel histone deacetylase inhibitor NK-HDAC-1 on breast cancer. Oncol Rep 30(1):499–505. doi:10.3892/or.2013.2434

Liu Y, Mayo MW, Nagji AS, Smith PW, Ramsey CS, Li D, Jones DR (2012) Phosphorylation of RelA/p65 promotes DNMT-1 recruitment to chromatin and represses transcription of the tumor metastasis suppressor gene BRMS1. Oncogene 31(9):1143–1154. doi:10.1038/onc.2011.308

Liu L, Kimball S, Liu H, Holowatyj A, Yang ZQ (2015) Genetic alterations of histone lysine methyltransferases and their significance in breast cancer. Oncotarget 6(4):2466–2482

Marcotte R, Sayad A, Brown KR, Sanchez-Garcia F, Reimand J, Haider M, Virtanen C, Bradner JE, Bader GD, Mills GB, Pe'er D, Moffat J, Neel BG (2016) Functional genomic landscape of human breast cancer drivers, vulnerabilities, and resistance. Cell 164 (1–2):293–309. doi:10.1016/j.cell.2015.11.062

Martinez-Galan J, Torres-Torres B, Nunez MI, Lopez-Penalver J, Del Moral R, Ruiz De Almodovar JM, Menjon S, Concha A, Chamorro C, Rios S, Delgado JR (2014) ESR1 gene promoter region methylation in free circulating DNA and its correlation with estrogen receptor protein expression in tumor tissue in breast cancer patients. BMC Cancer 14:59. doi:10.1186/1471-2407-14-59

Maruyama R, Suzuki H (2012) Long noncoding RNA involvement in cancer. BMB Rep 45(11):604–611

Mikkelsen TS, Ku M, Jaffe DB, Issac B, Lieberman E, Giannoukos G, Alvarez P, Brockman W, Kim TK, Koche RP, Lee W, Mendenhall E, O'Donovan A, Presser A, Russ C, Xie X, Meissner A, Wernig M, Jaenisch R, Nusbaum C, Lander ES, Bernstein BE (2007) Genome-wide maps of chromatin state in pluripotent and lineage-committed cells. Nature 448 (7153):553–560. doi:10.1038/nature06008

Min A, Im SA, Kim DK, Song SH, Kim HJ, Lee KH, Kim TY, Han SW, Oh DY, Kim TY, O'Connor MJ, Bang YJ (2015) Histone deacetylase inhibitor, suberoylanilide hydroxamic acid (SAHA), enhances anti-tumor effects of the poly (ADP-ribose) polymerase (PARP) inhibitor olaparib in triple-negative breast cancer cells. Breast Cancer Res 17:33. doi:10.1186/s13058-015-0534-y

Ning X, Shi Z, Liu X, Zhang A, Han L, Jiang K, Kang C, Zhang Q (2015) DNMT1 and EZH2 mediated methylation silences the microRNA-200b/a/429 gene and promotes tumor progression. Cancer Lett 359 (2):198–205. doi:10.1016/j.canlet.2015.01.005

Okano M, Bell DW, Haber DA, Li E (1999) DNA methyltransferases Dnmt3a and Dnmt3b are essential for de novo methylation and mammalian development. Cell 99(3):247–257

Pathania R, Ramachandran S, Elangovan S, Padia R, Yang P, Cinghu S, Veeranan-Karmegam R, Arjunan P, Gnana-Prakasam JP, Sadanand F, Pei L, Chang CS, Choi JH, Shi H, Manicassamy S, Prasad PD, Sharma S, Ganapathy V, Jothi R, Thangaraju M (2015) DNMT1 is essential for mammary and cancer stem cell maintenance and tumorigenesis. Nat Commun 6:6910. doi:10.1038/ncomms7910

Pathiraja TN, Stearns V, Oesterreich S (2010) Epigenetic regulation in estrogen receptor positive breast cancer–role in treatment response. J Mammary Gland Biol Neoplasia 15(1):35–47. doi:10.1007/s10911-010-9166-0

Rafique S, Thomas JS, Sproul D, Bickmore WA (2015) Estrogen-induced chromatin decondensation and nuclear re-organization linked to regional epigenetic regulation in breast cancer. Genome Biol 16:145. doi:10.1186/s13059-015-0719-9

Reid G, Metivier R, Lin CY, Denger S, Ibberson D, Ivacevic T, Brand H, Benes V, Liu ET, Gannon F (2005) Multiple mechanisms induce transcriptional silencing of a subset of genes, including oestrogen receptor alpha, in response to deacetylase inhibition by valproic acid and trichostatin A. Oncogene 24 (31):4894–4907. doi:10.1038/sj.onc.1208662

Rothbart SB, Strahl BD (2014) Interpreting the language of histone and DNA modifications. Biochim Biophys Acta 1839(8):627–643. doi:10.1016/j.bbagrm.2014.03.001

Severi G, Southey MC, English DR, Jung CH, Lonie A, McLean C, Tsimiklis H, Hopper JL, Giles GG, Baglietto L (2014) Epigenome-wide methylation in DNA from peripheral blood as a marker of risk for breast cancer. Breast Cancer Res Treat 148(3):665–673. doi:10.1007/s10549-014-3209-y

Song SJ, Poliseno L, Song MS, Ala U, Webster K, Ng C, Beringer G, Brikbak NJ, Yuan X, Cantley LC, Richardson AL, Pandolfi PP (2013) MicroRNA-antagonism regulates breast cancer stemness and metastasis via

TET-family-dependent chromatin remodeling. Cell 154 (2):311–324. doi:10.1016/j.cell.2013.06.026

Srivastava RK, Kurzrock R, Shankar S (2010) MS-275 sensitizes TRAIL-resistant breast cancer cells, inhibits angiogenesis and metastasis, and reverses epithelial-mesenchymal transition in vivo. Mol Cancer Ther 9(12):3254–3266. doi:10.1158/1535-7163.MCT-10-0582

Subramaniam D, Thombre R, Dhar A, Anant S (2014) DNA methyltransferases: a novel target for prevention and therapy. Front Oncol 4:80. doi:10.3389/fonc.2014.00080

Sun MY, Yang XX, Xu WW, Yao GY, Pan HZ, Li M (2012) Association of DNMT1 and DNMT3B polymorphisms with breast cancer risk in Han Chinese women from South China. Genet Mol Res 11 (4):4330–4341. doi:10.4238/2012.September.26.1

Szyf M (2009) Epigenetics, DNA methylation, and chromatin modifying drugs. Annu Rev Pharmacol Toxicol 49:243–263. doi:10.1146/annurev-pharmtox-061008-103102

Tessarz P, Kouzarides T (2014) Histone core modifications regulating nucleosome structure and dynamics. Nat Rev Mol Cell Biol 15(11):703–708. doi:10.1038/nrm3890

Thakur S, Feng X, Qiao Shi Z, Ganapathy A, Kumar Mishra M, Atadja P, Morris D, Riabowol K (2012) ING1 and 5-azacytidine act synergistically to block breast cancer cell growth. PLoS ONE 7(8):e43671. doi:10.1371/journal.pone.0043671

Travers AA, Vaillant C, Arneodo A, Muskhelishvili G (2012) DNA structure, nucleosome placement and chromatin remodelling: a perspective. Biochem Soc Trans 40(2):335–340. doi:10.1042/BST20110757

Tsai HC, Li H, Van Neste L, Cai Y, Robert C, Rassool FV, Shin JJ, Harbom KM, Beaty R, Pappou E, Harris J, Yen RW, Ahuja N, Brock MV, Stearns V, Feller-Kopman D, Yarmus LB, Lin YC, Welm AL, Issa JP, Minn I, Matsui W, Jang YY, Sharkis SJ, Baylin SB, Zahnow CA (2012) Transient low doses of DNA-demethylating agents exert durable antitumor effects on hematological and epithelial tumor cells. Cancer Cell 21(3):430–446. doi:10.1016/j.ccr.2011.12.029

Tu Z, Li H, Ma Y, Tang B, Tian J, Akers W, Achilefu S, Gu Y (2012) The enhanced antiproliferative response to combined treatment of trichostatin A with raloxifene in MCF-7 breast cancer cells and its relevance to estrogen receptor beta expression. Mol Cell Biochem 366(1–2):111–122. doi:10.1007/s11010-012-1288-9

Vad-Nielsen J, Nielsen AL (2015) Beyond the histone tale: HP1alpha deregulation in breast cancer epigenetics. Cancer Biol Ther 16(2):189–200. doi:10.1080/15384047.2014.1001277

Vasilatos SN, Katz TA, Oesterreich S, Wan Y, Davidson NE, Huang Y (2013) Crosstalk between lysine-specific demethylase 1 (LSD1) and histone deacetylases mediates antineoplastic efficacy of HDAC inhibitors in human breast cancer cells. Carcinogenesis 34(6):1196–1207. doi:10.1093/carcin/bgt033

Veeck J, Esteller M (2010) Breast cancer epigenetics: from DNA methylation to microRNAs. J Mammary Gland Biol Neoplasia 15(1):5–17. doi:10.1007/s10911-010-9165-1

Wee EJ, Peters K, Nair SS, Hulf T, Stein S, Wagner S, Bailey P, Lee SY, Qu WJ, Brewster B, French JD, Dobrovic A, Francis GD, Clark SJ, Brown MA (2012) Mapping the regulatory sequences controlling 93 breast cancer-associated miRNA genes leads to the identification of two functional promoters of the Hsa-mir-200b cluster, methylation of which is associated with metastasis or hormone receptor status in advanced breast cancer. Oncogene 31(38):4182–4195. doi:10.1038/onc.2011.584

Wei J, Han B, Mao XY, Wei MJ, Yao F, Jin F (2012) Promoter methylation status and expression of estrogen receptor alpha in familial breast cancer patients. Tumour Biol 33(2):413–420. doi:10.1007/s13277-011-0234-x

Weng M, Song F, Chen J, Wu J, Qin J, Jin T, Xu J (2015) The high-mobility group nucleosome-binding domain 5 is highly expressed in breast cancer and promotes the proliferation and invasion of breast cancer cells. Tumour Biol 36(2):959–966. doi:10.1007/s13277-014-2715-1

Wong AK, Shanahan F, Chen Y, Lian L, Ha P, Hendricks K, Ghaffari S, Iliev D, Penn B, Woodland AM, Smith R, Salada G, Carillo A, Laity K, Gupte J, Swedlund B, Tavtigian SV, Teng DH, Lees E (2000) BRG1, a component of the SWI-SNF complex, is mutated in multiple human tumor cell lines. Cancer Res 60(21):6171–6177

Wozniak RJ, Klimecki WT, Lau SS, Feinstein Y, Futscher BW (2007) 5-Aza-2'-deoxycytidine-mediated reductions in G9A histone methyltransferase and histone H3 K9 di-methylation levels are linked to tumor suppressor gene reactivation. Oncogene 26(1):77–90. doi:10.1038/sj.onc.1209763

Xhemalce B (2013) From histones to RNA: role of methylation in cancer. Brief Funct Genomics 12 (3):244–253. doi:10.1093/bfgp/els064

Xiao K, Li YP, Wang C, Ahmad S, Vu M, Kuma K, Cheng YQ, Lam KS (2015) Disulfide cross-linked micelles of novel HDAC inhibitor thailandepsin A for the treatment of breast cancer. Biomaterials 67:183–193. doi:10.1016/j.biomaterials.2015.07.033

Xu C, Corces VG (2015) Towards a predictive model of chromatin 3D organization. Semin Cell Dev Biol. doi:10.1016/j.semcdb.2015.11.013

Xu J, Zhou JY, Tainsky MA, Wu GS (2007) Evidence that tumor necrosis factor-related apoptosis-inducing ligand induction by 5-Aza-2'-deoxycytidine sensitizes human breast cancer cells to adriamycin. Cancer Res 67(3):1203–1211. doi:10.1158/0008-5472.CAN-06-2310

Yamamoto N, Nakayama T, Kajita M, Miyake T, Iwamoto T, Kim SJ, Sakai A, Ishihara H, Tamaki Y, Noguchi S (2012) Detection of aberrant promoter methylation of GSTP1, RASSF1A, and RARbeta2 in serum DNA of patients with breast cancer by a newly established one-step methylation-specific PCR assay. Breast Cancer Res Treat 132(1):165–173. doi:10.1007/s10549-011-1575-2

Yang XJ, Seto E (2007) HATs and HDACs: from structure, function and regulation to novel strategies for therapy and prevention. Oncogene 26(37):5310–5318. doi:10.1038/sj.onc.1210599

Yarosh W, Barrientos T, Esmailpour T, Lin L, Carpenter PM, Osann K, Anton-Culver H, Huang T (2008) TBX3 is overexpressed in breast cancer and represses p14 ARF by interacting with histone deacetylases. Cancer Res 68(3):693–699. doi:10.1158/0008-5472.CAN-07-5012

Yazici H, Terry MB, Cho YH, Senie RT, Liao Y, Andrulis I, Santella RM (2009) Aberrant methylation of RASSF1A in plasma DNA before breast cancer diagnosis in the Breast Cancer Family Registry. Cancer Epidemiol Biomarkers Prev 18(10):2723–2725. doi:10.1158/1055-9965.EPI-08-1237

Ye C, Beeghly-Fadiel A, Lu W, Long J, Shu XO, Gao YT, Zheng W, Cai Q (2010) Two-stage case-control study of DNMT-1 and DNMT-3B gene variants and breast cancer risk. Breast Cancer Res Treat 121(3):765–769. doi:10.1007/s10549-009-0569-9

Yokoyama Y, Matsumoto A, Hieda M, Shinchi Y, Ogihara E, Hamada M, Nishioka Y, Kimura H, Yoshidome K, Tsujimoto M, Matsuura N (2014) Loss of histone H4K20 trimethylation predicts poor prognosis in breast cancer and is associated with invasive activity. Breast Cancer Res 16(3):R66. doi:10.1186/bcr3681

Yu Z, Xiao Q, Zhao L, Ren J, Bai X, Sun M, Wu H, Liu X, Song Z, Yan Y, Mi X, Wang E, Jin F, Wei M (2015) DNA methyltransferase 1/3a overexpression in sporadic breast cancer is associated with reduced expression of estrogen receptor-alpha/breast cancer susceptibility gene 1 and poor prognosis. Mol Carcinog 54(9):707–719. doi:10.1002/mc.22133

Zhang L, Deng L, Chen F, Yao Y, Wu B, Wei L, Mo Q, Song Y (2014) Inhibition of histone H3K79 methylation selectively inhibits proliferation, self-renewal and metastatic potential of breast cancer. Oncotarget 5(21):10665–10677

Zhong R, Roeder RG, Heintz N (1983) The primary structure and expression of four cloned human histone genes. Nucleic Acids Res 11(21):7409–7425

Zhu X, Shan L, Wang F, Wang J, Wang F, Shen G, Liu X, Wang B, Yuan Y, Ying J, Yang H (2015) Hypermethylation of BRCA1 gene: implication for prognostic biomarker and therapeutic target in sporadic primary triple-negative breast cancer. Breast Cancer Res Treat 150(3):479–486. doi:10.1007/s10549-015-3338-y

Noncoding RNAs in Breast Cancer

22

Yesim Gökmen-Polar and Sunil Badve

Abstract

Recent advances in RNA sequencing technologies have unveiled the complexity of RNA world outdating the traditional view that many noncoding RNA (ncRNA) transcripts are transcriptional noise, while the protein coding genes are important players in cancer signaling. Accumulating evidence suggests that they are not only key regulators of gene expression, but also direct targets of cancer pathways. These are mainly classified according to their size: microRNAs (miRNAs) and long noncoding RNAs (lncRNAs) being the most studied. The field has rapidly expanded and it is impossible to cover all the nuances in a single chapter. Noncoding RNAs, including miRNAs ($\sim$22 nucleotides long RNAs) and lncRNAs (>200 nucleotides), regulate gene expression at the transcriptional levels or post-transcriptionally by modulating the function of transcription factors, directing chromatin reorganization and modification, or by inhibiting the translation or stability of messenger RNA (mRNA). Here, we provide an overview of the role of ncRNAs in breast cancer and their prognostic and predictive potential in the clinical practice.

Keywords

Gene regulation · RNA-sequencing · Human genome and whole transcriptome · Noncoding RNA · Transcriptional noise · Long-noncoding RNA · Small RNA · Breast cancer

Y. Gökmen-Polar (✉)
Department of Pathology and Laboratory Medicine, Indiana University School of Medicine, 635 Barnhill Dr. MS A128, Indianapolis, IN 46202, USA
e-mail: ypolar@iu.edu

S. Badve (✉)
Department of Pathology and Laboratory Medicine, Indiana University School of Medicine, 350 West 11th Street, IUHPL 4050, Indianapolis, IN 46202, USA
e-mail: sbadve@iupui.edu

S. Badve and Y. Gökmen-Polar (eds.), *Molecular Pathology of Breast Cancer*, DOI 10.1007/978-3-319-41761-5_22

Abbreviations

lncRNA	Noncoding RNA
lncRNA	Long noncoding RNA
miRNA	MicroRNA

22.1 Introduction

High-throughput RNA sequencing technologies have identified that the majority of human genome is transcribed as short and long non-protein–coding RNAs (ncRNAs), whereas only 1–2 % of the genome encodes mRNAs which are translated to proteins (Carninci et al. 2005; Djebali et al. 2012; Birney 2007; Jia et al. 2010; Derrien et al. 2012; Banfai et al. 2012). Discovery of these ncRNAs has increased the overall complexity in understanding their role in the developmental processes and diseases such as cancer. (Mattick 2001, 2007; Clark et al. 2013; Prensner and Chinnaiyan 2011). NcRNAs are conventionally divided into two major groups based on their size as small or short noncoding RNAs (<200 bp) or long noncoding RNAs (lncRNAs) (200 bp) (Fig. 22.1). Small ncRNAs are further categorized into microRNAs (miRNAs), small interfering RNAs (siRNAs), PIWI-interacting RNAs (piRNAs), small nuclear RNAs (snRNAs) and small nucleolar RNAs (snoRNAs) (Taft et al. 2010). Other ncRNAs include rRNAs and tRNAs representing intracytoplasmic ncRNAs and are highly abundant, functionally important, and constitutively expressed and required for normal functions. Regulatory RNAs are expressed low in abundancy and altered in response to a condition or stimuli. They can affect the expression of other

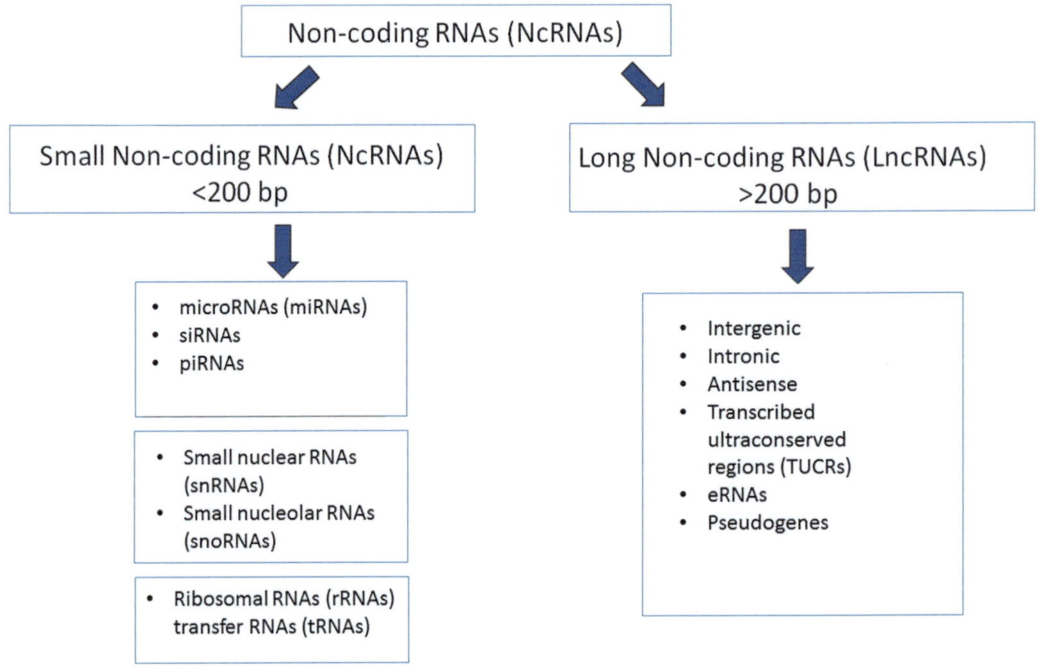

Fig. 22.1 Classification of ncRNAs based on their size and structure

genes at the level of transcription and translation. However, emerging data also suggests that intracytoplasmic or nuclear ncRNAs may be aberrant in diseases including cancer. Long non-coding RNAs (lncRNAs; >200 bp) can be categorized into different classes, such as intronic, intergenic, antisense lncRNAs, transcribed ultra-conserved regions (TUCRs), enhancer RNAs (eRNAs) and pseudogenes. (Prensner and Chinnaiyan 2011) (Fig. 22.1). Accumulating evidence suggests that the majority of ncRNAs play a role in regulating gene expression at multiple levels such as transcriptional and translational regulators. Among the ncRNAs, most of the data pertaining to breast cancer deals with miRNAs, siRNAs and lncRNAs, which will be discussed in detail.

22.2 Classes of Noncoding RNAs

22.2.1 Small Noncoding RNAs

22.2.1.1 miRNAs, siRNAs and piRNAs

miRNAs, siRNAs and piRNAs are small noncoding RNAs that are involved in RNA silencing (Ghildiyal and Zamore 2009; Ha and Kim 2014; Kim et al. 2009; Mattick and Makunin 2006). miRNAs (~22 nucleotides long RNAs) are derived from either short hairpin RNAs or double-stranded RNA precursors by two RNase III proteins (Drosha and Dicer). siRNAs (~21 nucleotides long) are derived from long double-stranded RNAs or long stem–loop structures through Dicer processing. The biogenesis of miRNAs is regulated at multiple levels including its transcription, nuclear processing, export and cytoplasmic processing (Fig. 22.2a). Its deregulation can impact the development of cancer. Briefly, miRNAs are transcribed from miRNA genes by RNA polymerase II (Pol II) in the nucleus as pri-miRNA (primary miRNA) of ~1000 nt. They are m7G capped and polyadenylated, and the long primary transcript has a local hairpin structure, where miRNA sequences are embedded. In the nucleus, the RNase III–type enzyme Drosha processes the long primary transcripts (pri-miRNA), yielding the hairpin precursors (pre-miRNA). The pre-miRNA hairpins (approximately 70 nt) are exported to the cytoplasm, where they are further processed into unstable, 19–25 nt miRNA duplex structures by

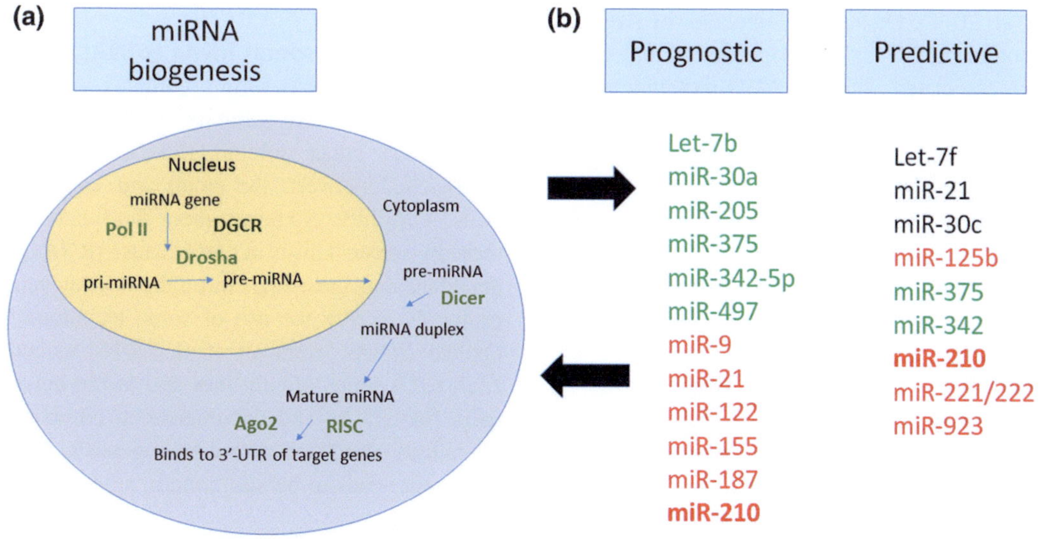

Fig. 22.2 miRNAs in breast cancer (**a**) genes involved in miRNA biogenesis, (**b**) prognostic and predictive miRNAs in breast cancer. *Green* (downregulation) and *red* (upregulation)

the RNase III protein Dicer (Sontheimer 2005). The less stable strand in the duplex is incorporated into a multiple-protein nuclease complex, the RNA-induced silencing complex (RISC), which regulates protein expression. miRNAs silence translation via non-perfect pairing with target mRNAs (mostly six to eight nucleotides in length) (Lewis et al. 2005). It has been implied that miRNAs control approximately one-third of human protein-coding genes (Du and Zamore 2005).

siRNAs ($\sim$21 nucleotides long) are derived from long double-stranded RNAs or long stem–loop structures through Dicer processing (Ghildiyal and Zamore 2009). siRNAs mainly contribute to the RNA interference (RNAi) pathway, and silence the expression of specific genes with complementary nucleotide sequences. siRNAs also mediate the post-transcriptional suppression of transcripts and transposons, and contribute to antiviral defense. piRNAs, on the other hand, differ from miRNAs and siRNAs in size (24–30 nucleotides rather than 22 and 21 nucleotides, respectively), in association with different Argonaute family of proteins and lack of sequence conservation (Ishizu et al. 2012; Siomi et al. 2011). The main function of piRNAs is to silence transposable elements in germline cells, although the roles of some piRNAs are still unclear (Siomi et al. 2011). Of the two subclades of Argonaute proteins (AGO and PIWI), miRNAs and siRNAs are associated with the AGO proteins, whereas piRNAs bind to PIWI proteins. Detailed reviews of miRNA and siRNA biogenesis can be read in the following recent reviews (Mattick and Makunin 2005; Berezikov and Plasterk 2005; Bartel 2005; Zamore and Haley 2005). piRNAs are the least studied among the small noncoding RNAs in humans.

22.2.1.2 Small Nuclear RNAs (snRNAs)

A number of small RNAs are found within the nucleus that are shorter than 200 nucleotides (nt); these can function as miRNAs, piRNAs and siRNAs. Additional classes of RNAs such as small nucleolar RNAs (snoRNAs), Y-RNAs, and small Cajal body specific RNAs (scaRNAs) are present in the nucleus. snoRNAs are a class of small RNA molecules that guide chemical modifications of other RNAs, mainly rRNAs, tRNAs and other small nuclear RNAs. The central function of snoRNAs is to modify, mature and stabilize rRNAs; abnormal ribosomal biosynthesis could result in chromosomal instability that is typically noted in cancers. snoRNAs could also be precursors to miRNAs (Scott and Ono 2011). snoRNAs are frequently overexpressed in both murine and human breast cancer as well as in prostate cancers, and its overexpression is essential for tumorigenicity in vitro and in vivo (Su et al. 2014). Some snoRNAs have been shown to have oncogenic potential. *U50* snoRNA gene is subject to frequent copy number loss and transcriptional down regulation in breast cancer. Re-expression of *U50* snoRNA in breast cancer cell lines (MDA-MB-231 and Hs 578T) resulted in dramatically decreased colony formation (Dong et al. 2009). snoRNAs have also been used as biomarkers in plasma and serum. Our group has documented that the ratio of *U6*: *SNORD44* was persistently elevated in patients with active or inactive breast cancer (Appaiah et al. 2011). Low expressions of *RNU43*, *RNU44*, and *RNU48* in the tumors including breast cancer were significantly associated with poor prognosis of cancer patients (Hall et al. 2006).

22.2.1.3 Ribosomal RNAs (rRNAs)

The ribosomal RNAs form a complex with proteins to generate two subunits, the large subunit (LSU) and small subunit (SSU). mRNA is sandwiched between the small and large subunits. Very little is known about the function of these in cancer. This is in part because rRNAs are abundant and most high throughput sequencing protocols require the use of some technique to deplete rRNAs. Karahan et al. (2015) recently analyzed a series of cell lines and tumor-normal pairs for rRNAs and documented a number of alterations associated with carcinogenesis. It is a topic that needs to be additionally studied.

22.2.1.4 Transfer RNAs (tRNAs)

tRNAs are adaptor molecules that are typically 76–90 nucleotides in length. They serve as the physical link between the mRNA and the amino acid sequence of proteins. Enzyme- catalyzed modifications of tRNAs affect the codon-anticodon interactions (Murphy et al. 2004; Yarian et al. 2002) and have been at least indirectly implicated in cancer. Begley et al. (2013) have documented that tRNA methyltransferase 9-like, hTRM9L/KIAA1456, is downregulated in several cancers including breast cancer. Pavon-Eternod et al. (2009) showed that there was global overexpression of tRNA species in breast cancer. Specifically, the expression levels of nuclear-encoded tRNAs increase by up to threefold, and mitochondrial-encoded tRNAs increase by up to fivefold in breast cancer. Polymorphisms in mitochondrial tRNA have been studied for their association with development of breast cancer (Meng et al. 2015; Grzybowska-Szatkowska and Slaska 2012). This topic is also less explored in cancers including breast cancer.

22.2.2 Functional Relevance of Small Noncoding RNAs in Breast Cancer: miRNAs as Prognostic and Predictive Markers

Deregulation of miRNAs can affect multiple hallmarks of cancer (Goh et al. 2015) and can serve as prognostic and predictive markers in multiple cancers including breast cancer (Van Schooneveld et al. 2015). miRNAs can play a role in oncogenesis, metastasis, and resistance to various therapies. They can be categorized as oncogenes (oncomiRs) or tumor-suppressor genes (Ahmad et al. 2011; Chen and Bourguignon 2014; Tang et al. 2012). Additionally, they can affect metastasis ('metastamiRs') and metastasis suppression. (O'Day and Lal 2010; Baffa et al. 2009). OncomiRs usually target tumor-suppressor genes and activate oncogenic transcription factors (Corcoran et al. 2011; Tang et al. 2012). microRNAs have also been categorized based on the molecular subtypes of breast cancer (Blenkiron et al. 2007). A miRNA profile has been established to classify basal versus luminal tumor subtypes. Subsequently, additional miRNA signatures have been reported to distinguish these molecular subtypes (Dvinge et al. 2013; de Rinaldis et al. 2013). Furthermore, miRNAs can be differentially expressed between histological subtypes such as ductal carcinoma in situ (DCIS) versus invasive ductal carcinoma (IDC) (Volinia et al. 2012), lobular carcinoma in situ versus invasive lobular carcinoma (Giricz et al. 2012), and inflammatory breast cancer (IBC) versus non-IBC (Lerebours et al. 2013; Van der Auwera et al. 2010).

Altered expression of enzymes in miRNA biogenesis has also been reported in aggressive breast cancers (Blenkiron et al. 2007). Higher levels of *AGO2* and *Drosha* and lower levels of *Dicer1* were associated with most aggressive ER-breast cancers. These alterations can be prognostic and predictive as shown in a number studies in breast cancer (Grelier et al. 2009; Sung et al. 2012; Leaderer et al. 2011; Khoshnaw et al. 2013). They can also affect the prognostic and predictive ability of miRNAs.

Some of the miRNAs have been well established as prognostic and/or predictive markers in breast cancer (Fig. 22.2b). High expression of let-7b and miR-205 have been associated with good prognosis in breast cancer, in particular in luminal subtype (Quesne et al. 2012). Downregulation of let-7b occurs early in breast cancer. In a cohort of 80 breast cancer and 22 benign breast disease (BBD) cases, low let-7b expression was associated with poor prognosis (Ma et al. 2014). Downregulation of miR-205 is associated with reduced disease-free interval (DFI) and overall survival (OS) in another study of 84 patients diagnosed with early breast cancer compared to 13 cancer-free breast tissue. These results were verified by both univariate and multivariate analysis (Markou et al. 2014). Other good prognostic miRNAs include miR30a, miR-375, miR-342-5p, and miR-497 (Wang et al. 2013; Shen et al. 2012; Leivonen et al. 2014; Zhang et al. 2014a; Cheng et al. 2012; Wu et al. 2012), whereas miR-9, miR-21, miR-122, miR-155, miR-187, and miR-210 were identified as poor prognostic miRNAs (Kong et al. 2014; Song et al. 2012; Wang et al. 2014; Mulrane et al. 2012; Zhou et al. 2012; Li et al. 2014; Lee et al. 2011; Si et al. 2007) (Fig. 22.2b). For detailed information, please see the reviews (Van Schooneveld et al. 2015; Bertoli et al. 2015).

Some of the above prognostic miRNAs are also predictive of response rate and treatment benefit. Some of them are only predictive. In particular, a set of miRNAs (miR-128a, miR-342, miR-221/222 and let-7f) have been useful in predicting response to hormone therapies (Shibahara et al. 2012; Rao et al. 2011; Gan et al. 2014; Wei et al. 2014; Zhao et al. 2008; Ward et al. 2013; He et al. 2013; Masri et al. 2010). Further information can be obtained by the reviews for endocrine resistance (Egeland et al. 2015; Muluhngwi and Klinge 2015). Besides endocrine therapy, microRNAs, such as miR-210, are also associated with response to targeted therapies. High miR-210 plasma baseline expression was associated with resistance to trastuzumab-included chemotherapy (Jung et al. 2012). Other microRNAs such as miR-21, miR-30c, miR-125b, miR-221/222, and miR-923, have been associated with altered response to chemotherapeutic agents. (Zhou et al. 2010; Chen and Bourguignon 2014; Climent et al. 2007; Bockhorn et al. 2013; Mei et al. 2010). A few miRNAs such as miR-205 and miR-34a, are associated with response or resistance to radiotherapy (Kato et al. 2009; Zhang et al. 2014b). miR-205 can radiosensitize the tumors, whereas low miR34a levels are associated with resistance to radiotherapy.

MicroRNAs identified as being highly expressed in breast cancer tumors can also be detected in the circulation. Detection of circulating miRNA is an emerging field that provides non-invasive method to rapidly (and cheaply) monitor cancer (refer to Chap. 16 for a detailed review).

miRNAs can exhibit additional potential in the clinical field as tools for miRNA-based therapeutics, mainly as miRNA antagonists or miRNA mimics (Bader et al. 2011). miRNA antagonists inhibit endogenous miRNAs that show a gain-of-function in cancer as an alternative to small molecule inhibitors or short interfering RNAs (siRNAs). In general, a highly chemically-modified miRNA passenger strand (anti-miR or antagomiR) binds with high affinity to the active miRNA strand. However, the binding is irreversible and can generate unwanted side effects.

miRNA mimics, on the other hand, are designed to restore loss of function, an approach also known as 'miRNA replacement therapy'. MicroRNA-34 (miR-34) is a master regulator of tumor suppression. It is required to inhibit malignant growth and repress multiple genes in oncogenic signaling pathways (Bader 2012). For example, MRX34 is a double-stranded RNA mimic of the tumor suppressor microRNA developed by Mirna Therapeutics. miR-34 is encapsulated in a liposomal nanoparticle formulation called Smarticles®. MRX34 is a first-in-class cancer therapy and the first microRNA mimic to enter clinical trials. A Multicenter Phase I Study of MRX34 is currently recruiting patients with primary liver cancer or other selected solid tumors or hematologic malignancies. It is aimed to be completed by the end of 2016. The primary objectives of this clinical trial are to establish the maximum tolerated dose and the recommended Phase 2 dose for future clinical trials. The secondary objectives are to assess the safety, tolerability and pharmacokinetic profile of MRX34, as well as to assess any biological and clinical activity. For clinical study information, please see clinicaltrials.gov.

22.2.3 Long Noncoding RNAs

Long noncoding RNAs (lncRNAs) are mostly transcribed via RNA polymerase II and have characteristics similar to mRNAs. Common features of lncRNAs include polyadenylation, alternative splicing of multiple exons via canonical genomic splice site motifs, regulation by transcription factors and expression in a tissue-specific manner (Derrien et al. 2012; Mattick and Rinn 2015). However, they do not have a recognizable trait, like the seed region as in the case of miRNA. Many small RNAs, such as microRNAs or snoRNAs, exhibit strong conservation across diverse species (Birney 2007).

LncRNAs may lack strong conservation (Johnsson et al. 2014).

LncRNAs are mainly categorized by their genomic location and orientation with respect to protein coding genes, such as intronic, intergenic, or antisense (Cabili et al. 2011; Derrien et al. 2012; Wright 2014; Kung et al. 2013). They can present as stand-alone transcription units, or may be transcribed from enhancers, promoters, or antisense to other genes with some degree of overlap. They may also contain small RNAs. Another major categorization scheme of lncRNAs is based on their regulatory function on the protein coding genes (Cabili et al. 2011; Kung et al. 2013) such as the following: (1) they can play a role in regulating transcription in "cis" or "trans" by targeting genomically close or distant genes, respectively (Osato et al. 2007; Wang and Chang 2011; Bak and Mikkelsen 2014). (2) they can act as decoys or as coregulators for transcription factors (Wang and Chang 2011), (3) they can regulate posttranscriptional processing of mRNAs such as splicing, editing, and translation; or (4) they can induce chromatin remodeling and histone modifications (Rinn and Chang 2012), and (5) inversely, they can be regulated by protein coding genes or transcription factors exhibiting a complex regulatory network (Guttman and Rinn 2012).

Several lncRNAs have been associated with developmental processes and diseases (Kung et al. 2013). Accumulating evidence suggests that lncRNAs may play a role in the development of cancer and metastasis and may serve as new potential targets for improving cancer prognosis or treatment (Du et al. 2013; Cabili et al. 2011; Kung et al. 2013; Iyer et al. 2015; Serviss et al. 2014; Murphy et al. 2004). In particular, recent advances in RNA sequencing (RNA-seq) and computational methods accelerated the identification of lncRNAs in various tissues and cell types. Among them, large intergenic noncoding RNAs (lincRNAs) are the most annotated group in the human genome (Cabili et al. 2011). Furthermore, Iyer et al. (2015) applied RNA-seq technology to identify more than 58,000 lncRNA genes across normal tissue and a range of common cancer types. 7942 of these genes have been linked directly or indirectly to cancer. Some long noncoding RNAs tend to be exquisitely specific for cancer (Gutschner and Diederichs 2012b). Another study characterized alterations in lncRNAs in 5037 tumor specimens comprising 13 cancer types from The Cancer Genome Atlas (TCGA). They looked at differential changes to lncRNAs at the transcriptional, genomic, and epigenomic level to identify cancer-driving lncRNAs and predict their function (Yan et al. 2015). Several lncRNAs have also been linked to hallmarks of cancer (Gutschner and Diederichs 2012a). The emerging evidence of lncRNAs can be read in further detailed reviews (Prensner and Chinnaiyan 2011). The current review will focus on lncRNAs that have been identified in breast cancer.

22.2.4 Functional Relevance of Long Noncoding RNAs in Breast Cancer: lncRNAs as Prognostic and Predictive Markers

LncRNAs have now been documented to be involved in a diverse set of specific functional roles with multiple mechanisms as detailed below. Sets of lncRNAs have been identified in breast cancer that can be grouped based on their regulatory function, and expression (Hansji et al. 2014). LncRNAs have been shown to act as protein–DNA or protein–protein scaffolds, miRNA sponges, and protein decoys, as well as regulators of translation (Hu et al. 2012). Examples for each regulatory function are shown in Table 22.1.

22.2.4.1 Chromatin Modifying LncRNAs

LncRNAs are critical for chromosomal organization and are likely to be responsible for guiding chromosomal factors to critical genomic loci that are important for the maintenance of pluripotency. Several studies have shown that lncRNAs can interact with chromatin modification complexes and modify the transcription of target genes in *cis* or *trans* leading to gene silencing (Wang and

Table 22.1 Summary of selected lncRNAs that play a role in breast cancer

Functional role	lncRNA name	References
Chromatin modification	*HOTAIR*	Gupta et al. (2010), Chisholm et al. (2012), Gokmen-Polar et al. (2015)
	XIST	Yang et al. (2014), Ganesan et al. (2002, 2004), Richardson et al. (2006), Vincent-Salomon et al. (2007)
	PINC	Ginger et al. (2001, 2006), Shore et al. (2012)
Nuclear Organization	*MALAT1*	Jin et al. (2015), Gutschner et al. (2013), Guffanti et al. (2009), Ellis et al. (2012)
	LSINCT5	Silva et al. (2011)
Protein or miRNA decoys	*GAS5*	Mourtada-Maarabouni et al. (2009)
	BC200	Chen et al. (1997), Iacoangeli et al. (2004)
	SRA1	Lanz et al. (1999), Kurisu et al. (2006)
snoRNA hosts	*RNU44*	Gee et al. (2011)
	ZFAS1	Askarian-Amiri et al. (2011)
Ribosome-associated	*treRNA*	Gumireddy et al. (2013)
	UCA1	Huang et al. (2014)
Signaling	*H19*	Hayes and Lewis-Wambi (2015), Lottin et al. (2002), Adriaenssens et al. (1998)
	BCAR4	Godinho et al. (2010, 2012), Meijer et al (Meijer et al. 2006)

Chang 2011; Rinn and Chang 2012). Human HOX antisense intergenic RNA (*HOTAIR*), one of the most studied lincRNAs in various cancers and responsible for metastasis in breast and epithelial cancers, (Gupta et al. 2010; Yang et al. 2011; Kogo et al. 2011; Niinuma et al. 2012) belongs to this group. *HOTAIR* directly associates with the polycomb repressive complex 2 (PRC2), a histone modifying complex, and modulates the PRC2 and H3K27me3 localization throughout the genome (Rinn et al. 2007; Tsai et al. 2010). *HOTAIR* is transcribed in an antisense orientation from the *HOXC* locus. It acts in *trans* as a repressor of the *HOXD* locus by recruiting PRC2, leading to trimethylation of H3K27 and subsequent transcriptional silencing such as tumor suppressors. Overexpression of *HOTAIR* has been shown to be a poor prognostic factor in breast tumors (Gupta et al. 2010; Chisholm et al. 2012). We have also shown that *HOTAIR* is a poor prognostic indicator in node-positive ER-negative patients (Gokmen-Polar et al. 2015).

XIST, X inactive specific transcript, is another lncRNA regulating the chromatin-modifying complexes. *XIST* expression is lost in breast cancer as well as other female cancers such as ovarian cancer (Yang et al. 2014). However, its role in breast cancer is controversial. Some studies reported that *XIST* interacts with tumor suppressor *BRCA* and its loss associated with *BRCA1* (Ganesan et al. 2002, 2004), whereas other studies imply that they are not co-localized. Similar controversial results was also observed in other breast cancer studies (Richardson et al. 2006; Vincent-Salomon et al. 2007).

Pregnancy induced noncoding RNA (*PINC*) is another lncRNA that was originally identified in the mammary glands of estrogen and progesterone-treated rats (Ginger et al. 2001). *PINC* is expressed in the developing embryo and in the mammary glands of adult mice, but it is conserved in other mammalian genomes including human. Its expression in the mammary gland is induced by pregnancy and drops during lactation. Loss of functions studies have indicated a role in cell survival and in the regulation of cell cycle progression (Ginger et al. 2006). *PINC* interacts with retinoblastoma binding protein 46

(RbAp46) which belongs to *PRC2*. This further indicates its role in chromatin modification and repression of gene expression (Shore et al. 2012). However, its role in breast tumors needs to be investigated.

22.2.4.2 LncRNAs Organizing Nuclear Structure

The mammalian cell nucleus is compartmentalized into nonmembranous subnuclear domains including nucleoli, nuclear speckles, paraspeckles, and Cajal bodies that contain specific subsets of proteins and RNAs (Spector 2006; Matera et al. 2009). Nuclear speckles are highly dynamic subnuclear domains enriched with pre-mRNA splicing/processing factors (Hall et al. 2006; Lamond and Spector 2003). It has been suggested that splicing factors are recruited to active sites of transcription from nuclear speckles (Lamond and Spector 2003; Misteli 2000).

Alterations in proteins and RNAs that regulate the cycling of splicing factors between nuclear speckles and sites of transcription may contribute to cancer development. Few lncRNAs have been identified in nuclear organization that is also important in breast cancer. Metastasis associated lung adenocarcinoma transcript 1 (*MALAT1*), also known as *NEAT2* (noncoding nuclear-enriched abundant transcript 2), is highly conserved among mammals and predominantly localizes to nuclear speckles (Tripathi et al. 2010). *MALAT1* is originally identified based upon its overexpression in numerous cancers including lung and breast cancer (Ji et al. 2003; Jin et al. 2015; Gutschner et al. 2013; Guffanti et al. 2009). In preclinical models, *MALAT1* has been shown to interact with SR splicing factors and modulates their distribution to nuclear speckles. *MALAT1* also regulates alternative splicing of pre-mRNAs by controlling the functional levels of SR splicing factors (Tripathi et al. 2010). Mutations and deletions in the human *MALAT1* gene have also been identified in luminal breast cancer (Ellis et al. 2012). These alterations are localized in the region that could mediate *SRSF1* interaction of *MALAT1* (Tripathi et al. 2010).

Long stress induced noncoding transcript 5 (*LSINCT5*), localized in the nucleus, serves as an oncogenic lncRNA in breast, ovarian, and gastrointestinal cancers and involved in many cellular processes, including proliferation and tumorigenesis (Xu et al. 2014; Silva et al. 2011). *LSINCT5* is overexpressed in both breast and ovarian cancer cell lines and tumor tissues, compared to their normal counterparts. Furthermore, knockdown of *LSINCT5* expression decreased cellular proliferation in cancer cell lines (Silva et al. 2011). Knockdown of *LSINCT5* altered genes that are involved in breast cancer metastasis including CXCR4, and lncRNA *NEAT1* and *PSPC1*. Its role needs to be further explored.

22.2.4.3 Protein or miRNA Decoys

LncRNAs can act as molecular decoys and can either bind to regulatory molecules like miRNAs, transcription factors (TF) and splicing factors or to the enhancer and promoter regions and prevent the action of regulatory molecules. LncRNAs can act as molecular decoys by binding to and titrating away proteins. These lncRNAs can "sponge" proteins such as transcription factors and chromatin modifiers, which inhibit protein functions. Growth arrest-specific 5 (*GAS5*) is such a lncRNA that functions as a protein decoy by binding to the glucocorticoid receptor (GR) and preventing it from interacting with the glucocorticoid response element (GRE) (Kino et al. 2010). This interaction modifies the transcriptional activity of the GR and affects cell survival and metabolic activities of GR during starvation. Therefore, *GAS5* functions as a starvation-linked or growth arrest–linked riborepressor of the GR and suppresses the transcription of GR target genes, such as *cIAP2*, *PEPCK*, and *G6Pase*. *GAS5* acts as a tumor suppressor gene in breast cancer and its expression is significantly reduced in breast tumors compared to normal breast epithelium (Mourtada-Maarabouni et al. 2009).

BC200, brain-associated lncRNA, is expressed in normal brain tissue, but it is deregulated in many human tumors including breast (Chen et al. 1997). *BC200* expression is highly elevated in invasive tumors but not in benign tumors. In addition, its high expression is associated with high nuclear grade in invasive breast carcinomas. In ductal carcinomas in situ (DCIS), *BC200* expression levels were nuclear grade dependent; high grade (HG) DCIS expressed BC200 levels similar to invasive carcinoma. In contrast, its expression in non-high grade DCIS did not reach statistical significance when compared with normal breast tissue (Iacoangeli et al. 2004). *BC200* also functions as a decoy for proteins such as poly(A)-binding protein 1 (PABP), a translation initiation regulator, repress translation (Kondrashov et al. 2005).

Steroid receptor RNA activator 1 (*SRA1*) is another decoy lncRNA that can bind steroid receptors, non-steroid receptors and transcription factors, and modify their expression (reviewed in (Colley and Leedman 2011). *SRA1* functions as a nuclear coactivator for steroid hormone receptors, such as the estrogen, progesterone and androgen receptors (Lanz et al. 1999; Kurisu et al. 2006).

22.2.4.4 LncRNAs as SnoRNA Hosts

Small nucleolar RNAs can be located within the introns of protein coding and lncRNA genes. SnoRNA *RNU44* is an intronic gene in a cluster of highly conserved snoRNAs in the growth arrest specific 5 (*GAS5*) transcript, which is normally upregulated to arrest cell growth under stress. Low levels of *RNU44* were associated with a poor prognosis in breast cancer and head and neck squamous cell carcinoma (Gee et al. 2011). *GAS5* also acts as protein decoy for GRE as mentioned above.

ZNFX1 antisense RNA 1 (*ZFAS1*) overlaps the promoter region of the gene *ZNFX1*, which encodes a zinc finger protein with unknown function. *ZFAS1* hosts three snoRNAs in three consecutive introns. *ZFAS1* is highly expressed in the mammary gland and is downregulated in breast tumors compared to normal tissue, being a putative tumor suppressor (Askarian-Amiri et al. 2011).

22.2.4.5 Ribosome Associated LncRNAs

Genome wide ribosome profiling revealed that all lncRNAs including the intergenic lncRNAs can be bound to ribosomes (Ingolia et al. 2011; van Heesch et al. 2014). Interestingly, these lncRNAs are not actively translated (Guttman et al. 2013). Their role is under investigation. Ribosome associated lncRNAs have also been identified in breast cancer and might regulate ribosome function in breast cancer. Translational regulatory lncRNA (TreRNA) is an example for these lncRNAs. Upregulation of treRNA stimulates tumor invasion in vitro and metastasis in vivo (Gumireddy et al. 2013). Overexpression of treRNA in breast cancer preclinical models significantly promoted invasion and lung metastases, respectively, whereas knockdown suppressed cellular migration, invasion, and metastasis in mouse (Gumireddy et al. 2013). TreRNA also suppressed epithelial markers, which is associated with epithelial to a mesenchymal transition (EMT) and metastasis. TreRNA play roles in both nucleus and cytoplasm and have different roles based on their localization. TreRNA acts as an enhancer for neighboring genes such as Snail in the nucleus (Orom et al. 2010). Cytoplasmic treRNA, on the other hand, acts to regulate E-cadherin by modulating its translation. Other than primary breast tumors, treRNA has been upregulated in lymph-node metastatic human breast cancer samples compared their primary matched tumors (Gumireddy et al. 2013).

Urothelial carcinoma-associated 1 (*UCA1*), originally identified in bladder cancer, is also upregulated in breast cancer (Wang et al. 2008; Huang et al. 2014). Its expression is mostly in the nucleus, but a small amount is also expressed in the cytoplasm. *UCA1* promotes breast cancer cell growth both in vitro and in vivo. This is achieved by suppressing the tumor suppressor p27 through interaction with heterogeneous nuclear ribonucleoprotein 1 (*hnRNP-1*). There is a negative correlation between *UCA1* and p27 in breast cancer suggesting an important role in growth regulation (Huang et al. 2014). In the cytoplasm, *UCA1* inhibits the interaction between the p27 mRNA and *hnRNP-1*, preventing the translation of p27.

22.2.4.6 LncRNAs Playing a Role in Estrogen Receptor Signaling and Endocrine Resistance

Estrogen receptor plays the central role in the development of ER+ breast cancer as well as in response to endocrine therapy. Upon binding to its ligand estrogen (17β-estradiol), ER is activated and functions as a transcription factor. ER is involved in regulation of multiple genes, many of which are associated with increased growth and survival (Ali and Coombes 2002; Osborne and Schiff 2011). Targeted therapy for endocrine responsive tumors is directed to inhibit activation of ER. LncRNAs have been also implicated in aberrant ER signaling and endocrine resistance (Hayes and Lewis-Wambi 2015). Using lncRNA Disease Database (Chen et al. 2013), 16 lncRNAs have been identified that may play a role in endocrine resistance including *H19*, *GAS5*, *HOTAIR*, and breast cancer antiestrogen resistance 4 (*BCAR4*) (Lottin et al. 2002; Mourtada-Maarabouni et al. 2009; Gupta et al. 2010; Godinho et al. 2010). *HOTAIR* and *GAS5* have been described earlier in the chapter. LncRNA *H19* expression, which is differentially regulated during mammary gland development, can be induced by estradiol (Adriaenssens et al. 1998). It has been reported to have an oncogenic role in breast cancer cells as well tumor suppressive roles in breast cancer in vivo (Lottin et al. 2002; Yoshimizu et al. 2008). H19 is upregulated in breast cancer, in over 70 % of breast adenomas and in the stroma of ER+ and PR+breast tumors (Adriaenssens et al. 1998). H19 is also shown to be induced by the transcription factor *E2F1*, which promotes cell cycle progression and c-Myc, a well-known oncogene. Further studies are necessary to understand the role of *H19* in breast tumors.

The lncRNA *BCAR4* was discovered in a functional screen of ZR-75-1 derived tamoxifen resistant colonies (Meijer et al. 2006). Furthermore, overexpression of *BCAR4* in tamoxifen-sensitive ZR-75-1 cells blocked the anti-proliferative effects of tamoxifen. In primary breast tumors, high *BCAR4* has been associated with poor distant metastasis-free survival and overall survival after tamoxifen therapy, suggesting its role in invasiveness and tamoxifen resistance (Godinho et al. 2010; Meijer et al. 2006). Mechanistic studies also showed that the role of *BCAR4* in tamoxifen resistance is dependent on the presence of HER2 expression, but not ERα (Godinho et al. 2010, 2012).

SOX2OT (SOX2 overlapping transcript) is a lncRNA that contains the *SOX2* gene within its intron. Ectopic expression of SOX2OT induced *SOX2* expression, suggesting a positive regulatory role (Askarian-Amiri et al. 2014). Together, SOX2OT plays a key role in the induction and/or maintenance of *SOX2* expression in breast cancer. *SOX2* is essential for maintaining pluripotency and might be important in ER+ tumors.

Newer techniques such as single-molecule sequencing revealed that other lncRNAs (i.e., *LINC00160*) are regulated by ER-alpha. There is a need to further investigate as potential biomarkers in breast cancer.

22.3 Challenges and Future Directions: The Clinical Relevance of Noncoding RNAs?

RNA sequencing has revealed the existence of large noncoding transcriptome data and identification of novel regulatory ncRNA classes. Emerging preclinical and clinical data suggest the potential clinical relevance for several ncRNAs as prognostic and predictive markers. In particular, miRNAs are the closest to clinical application for a number of reasons. First, miRNAs are stable in the cell-free body fluids such as plasma, serum, and urine which has been also considered as circulating miRNAs. Second, they do not only serve as prognostic and predictive markers, but they can be used as therapeutic tools such as specific knockdown of miRNAs using anti-miRNA oligonucleotides (antagomiRs) or miRNA mimetics. These approaches have been shown successful in mouse models (Galasso et al. 2010). In particular, *MRX34* is the first microRNA mimic to enter clinical trials. However, there are still challenges to improve assay standardization technology as well as the delivery of small RNAs into human tissues.

Experimental studies have also identified several functional lncRNAs, their mechanisms and target genes. However, the diversity of regulatory roles, and lack of functional assays hamper the transition of the lncRNAs into the clinical setting. They also exhibit tissue specificity and lower expression when compared with protein coding genes. To overcome the current limitations, it is important to develop novel computational methods to elucidate functional role of lncRNAs. Few methods have been developed for the functional annotation of lncRNAs (Guo et al. 2016; Liao et al. 2011). These methods predict functions of lncRNAs based on functional annotations of their associated mRNAs. The transcripts (lncRNAs and mRNAs) that are co-expressed have a high chance of being involved in the same functions. Integrating more biologically relevant information to coexpression data can greatly improve the quality of the functional roles of predictions. Combination of computational and experimental data will improve the understanding and translational relevance of lncRNAs.

22.4 Conclusions and Future Directions

Recent studies have shown that the eukaryotic transcriptome consists of large numbers of non-protein coding transcripts with unknown functions. Increasing evidence suggests that their diverse set of functions increase the complexity of post-transcriptional regulation (Guttman and Rinn 2012; Sumazin et al. 2011). Although the field of ncRNAs has come a long way with the advent of genomics, our understanding of the dynamic nature of their transcription is still evolving. However, the developments in high resolution sequencing technologies, have lead to a rapid increase in the number of high-quality genome-wide transcriptome maps in both healthy and disease states (Derrien et al. 2012; Djebali et al. 2012; Brunner et al. 2012). These maps, together with consortium projects (such as the NIH Roadmap Epigenomics consortium), are not only going to revolutionize our current understanding of lncRNAs, but genomic organization. In addition, this is going to result in improvements in the annotation of their functions by using integrated computational approaches, identification of novel lncRNA genes, elucidation of condition-specific expression patterns, and potential regulatory elements which contribute to their behavior. These new technologies and approaches will prove to be invaluable means for furthering our understanding of the principles governing RNA-based regulatory mechanisms in a genome-wide manner. Given the decreasing cost and unprecedented detail at which these high-throughput technologies can reveal the regulatory elements and expression levels specific to conditions, it is possible to use these approaches in the coming years to interrogate the prevalence of these phenomena in different states and thereby study their relevance to regulation, physiology and disease in order to link the genotype of lncRNAs with their phenotypes.

References

Adriaenssens E, Dumont L, Lottin S, Bolle D, Lepretre A, Delobelle A, Bouali F, Dugimont T, Coll J, Curgy JJ (1998) H19 overexpression in breast adenocarcinoma stromal cells is associated with tumor values and steroid receptor status but independent of p53 and Ki-67 expression. Am J Pathol 153(5):1597–1607. doi:10.1016/S0002-9440(10)65748-3

Ahmad A, Aboukameel A, Kong D, Wang Z, Sethi S, Chen W, Sarkar FH, Raz A (2011) Phosphoglucose isomerase/autocrine motility factor mediates epithelial-mesenchymal transition regulated by miR-200 in breast cancer cells. Cancer Res 71 (9):3400–3409. doi:10.1158/0008-5472.CAN-10-0965

Ali S, Coombes RC (2002) Endocrine-responsive breast cancer and strategies for combating resistance. Nat Rev Cancer 2(2):101–112. doi:10.1038/nrc721

Appaiah HN, Goswami CP, Mina LA, Badve S, Sledge GW Jr, Liu Y, Nakshatri H (2011) Persistent upregulation of U6:SNORD44 small RNA ratio in the serum of breast cancer patients. Breast Cancer Res 13(5):R86. doi:10.1186/bcr2943

Askarian-Amiri ME, Crawford J, French JD, Smart CE, Smith MA, Clark MB, Ru K, Mercer TR, Thompson ER, Lakhani SR, Vargas AC, Campbell IG, Brown MA, Dinger ME, Mattick JS (2011) SNORD-host RNA Zfas1 is a regulator of mammary development and a potential marker for breast cancer. RNA 17(5):878–891. doi:10.1261/rna.2528811

Askarian-Amiri ME, Seyfoddin V, Smart CE, Wang J, Kim JE, Hansji H, Baguley BC, Finlay GJ, Leung EY (2014) Emerging role of long non-coding RNA SOX2OT in SOX2 regulation in breast cancer. PLoS ONE 9(7):e102140. doi:10.1371/journal.pone.0102140

Bader AG, Brown D, Stoudemire J, Lammers P (2011) Developing therapeutic microRNAs for cancer. Gene Ther 18(12):1121–1126. doi:10.1038/gt.2011.79

Bader AG (2012) miR-34-a microRNA replacement therapy is headed to the clinic. Front Genet 3:120. doi:10.3389/fgene.2012.00120. eCollection

Baffa R, Fassan M, Volinia S, O'Hara B, Liu CG, Palazzo JP, Gardiman M, Rugge M, Gomella LG, Croce CM, Rosenberg A (2009) MicroRNA expression profiling of human metastatic cancers identifies cancer gene targets. J Pathol 219(2):214–221. doi:10.1002/path.2586

Bak RO, Mikkelsen JG (2014) miRNA sponges: soaking up miRNAs for regulation of gene expression. Wiley Interdiscip Rev RNA 5(3):317–333. doi:10.1002/wrna.1213

Banfai B, Jia H, Khatun J, Wood E, Risk B, Gundling WE Jr, Kundaje A, Gunawardena HP, Yu Y, Xie L, Krajewski K, Strahl BD, Chen X, Bickel P, Giddings MC, Brown JB, Lipovich L (2012) Long noncoding RNAs are rarely translated in two human cell lines. Genome Res 22(9):1646–1657. doi:10.1101/gr.134767.111

Bartel B (2005) MicroRNas directing siRNA biogenesis. Nat Struct Mol Biol 12(7):569–571. doi:10.1038/nsmb0705-569

Begley U, Sosa MS, Avivar-Valderas A, Patil A, Endres L, Estrada Y, Chan CT, Su D, Dedon PC, Aguirre-Ghiso JA, Begley T (2013) A human tRNA methyltransferase 9-like protein prevents tumour growth by regulating LIN9 and HIF1-alpha. EMBO Mol Med 5(3):366–383. doi:10.1002/emmm.201201161

Berezikov E, Plasterk RH (2005) Camels and zebrafish, viruses and cancer: a microRNA update. Hum Mol Genet 14(Spec No 2):R183–190. doi:10.1093/hmg/ddi271

Bertoli G, Cava C, Castiglioni I (2015) MicroRNAs: new biomarkers for diagnosis, prognosis, therapy prediction and therapeutic tools for breast cancer. Theranostics 5(10):1122–1143. doi:10.7150/thno.11543

Birney E (2007) Evolutionary genomics: come fly with us. Nature 450(7167):184–185. doi:10.1038/450184a

Blenkiron C, Goldstein LD, Thorne NP, Spiteri I, Chin SF, Dunning MJ, Barbosa-Morais NL, Teschendorff AE, Green AR, Ellis IO, Tavare S, Caldas C, Miska EA (2007) MicroRNA expression profiling of human breast cancer identifies new markers of tumor subtype. Genome Biol 8(10):R214. doi:10.1186/gb-2007-8-10-r214

Bockhorn J, Dalton R, Nwachukwu C, Huang S, Prat A, Yee K, Chang YF, Huo D, Wen Y, Swanson KE, Qiu T, Lu J, Park SY, Dolan ME, Perou CM, Olopade OI, Clarke MF, Greene GL, Liu H (2013) MicroRNA-30c inhibits human breast tumour chemotherapy resistance by regulating TWF1 and IL-11. Nat Commun 4:1393. doi:10.1038/ncomms2393

Brunner AL, Beck AH, Edris B, Sweeney RT, Zhu SX, Li R, Montgomery K, Varma S, Gilks T, Guo X, Foley JW, Witten DM, Giacomini CP, Flynn RA, Pollack JR, Tibshirani R, Chang HY, van de Rijn M, West RB (2012) Transcriptional profiling of lncRNAs and novel transcribed regions across a diverse panel of archived human cancers. Genome Biol 13(8):R75. doi:10.1186/gb-2012-13-8-r75

Cabili MN, Trapnell C, Goff L, Koziol M, Tazon-Vega B, Regev A, Rinn JL (2011) Integrative annotation of human large intergenic noncoding RNAs reveals global properties and specific subclasses. Genes Dev 25(18):1915–1927. doi:10.1101/gad.17446611

Carninci P, Kasukawa T, Katayama S, Gough J, Frith MC, Maeda N, Oyama R, Ravasi T, Lenhard B, Wells C, Kodzius R, Shimokawa K, Bajic VB, Brenner SE, Batalov S, Forrest AR, Zavolan M, Davis MJ, Wilming LG, Aidinis V, Allen JE, Ambesi-Impiombato A, Apweiler R, Aturaliya RN, Bailey TL, Bansal M, Baxter L, Beisel KW, Bersano T, Bono H, Chalk AM, Chiu KP, Choudhary V, Christoffels A, Clutterbuck DR, Crowe ML, Dalla E, Dalrymple BP, de Bono B, Della Gatta G, di Bernardo D, Down T, Engstrom P, Fagiolini M, Faulkner G, Fletcher CF, Fukushima T, Furuno M, Futaki S, Gariboldi M, Georgii-Hemming P, Gingeras TR, Gojobori T, Green RE, Gustincich S, Harbers M, Hayashi Y, Hensch TK, Hirokawa N, Hill D, Huminiecki L, Iacono M, Ikeo K, Iwama A, Ishikawa T, Jakt M, Kanapin A, Katoh M, Kawasawa Y, Kelso J, Kitamura H, Kitano H, Kollias G, Krishnan SP, Kruger A, Kummerfeld SK, Kurochkin IV, Lareau LF, Lazarevic D, Lipovich L, Liu J, Liuni S, McWilliam S, Madan Babu M, Madera M, Marchionni L, Matsuda H, Matsuzawa S, Miki H, Mignone F, Miyake S, Morris K, Mottagui-Tabar S, Mulder N, Nakano N, Nakauchi H, Ng P, Nilsson R, Nishiguchi S, Nishikawa S, Nori F, Ohara O, Okazaki Y, Orlando V, Pang KC, Pavan WJ, Pavesi G, Pesole G, Petrovsky N, Piazza S, Reed J, Reid JF, Ring BZ, Ringwald M, Rost B, Ruan Y, Salzberg SL,

Sandelin A, Schneider C, Schonbach C, Sekiguchi K, Semple CA, Seno S, Sessa L, Sheng Y, Shibata Y, Shimada H, Shimada K, Silva D, Sinclair B, Sperling S, Stupka E, Sugiura K, Sultana R, Takenaka Y, Taki K, Tammoja K, Tan SL, Tang S, Taylor MS, Tegner J, Teichmann SA, Ueda HR, van Nimwegen E, Verardo R, Wei CL, Yagi K, Yamanishi H, Zabarovsky E, Zhu S, Zimmer A, Hide W, Bult C, Grimmond SM, Teasdale RD, Liu ET, Brusic V, Quackenbush J, Wahlestedt C, Mattick JS, Hume DA, Kai C, Sasaki D, Tomaru Y, Fukuda S, Kanamori-Katayama M, Suzuki M, Aoki J, Arakawa T, Iida J, Imamura K, Itoh M, Kato T, Kawaji H, Kawagashira N, Kawashima T, Kojima M, Kondo S, Konno H, Nakano K, Ninomiya N, Nishio T, Okada M, Plessy C, Shibata K, Shiraki T, Suzuki S, Tagami M, Waki K, Watahiki A, Okamura-Oho Y, Suzuki H, Kawai J, Hayashizaki Y (2005) The transcriptional landscape of the mammalian genome. Science 309(5740):1559–1563. doi:10.1126/science.1112014

Chen G, Wang Z, Wang D, Qiu C, Liu M, Chen X, Zhang Q, Yan G, Cui Q (2013) LncRNADisease: a database for long-non-coding RNA-associated diseases. Nucleic Acids Res 41(Database issue):D983–986. doi:10.1093/nar/gks1099

Chen L, Bourguignon LY (2014) Hyaluronan-CD44 interaction promotes c-Jun signaling and miRNA21 expression leading to Bcl-2 expression and chemoresistance in breast cancer cells. Mol Cancer 13:52. doi:10.1186/1476-4598-13-52

Chen W, Bocker W, Brosius J, Tiedge H (1997) Expression of neural BC200 RNA in human tumours. J Pathol 183(3):345–351. doi:10.1002/(SICI)1096-9896(199711)183:3<345::AID-PATH930>3.0.CO;2-8 [pii]

Cheng CW, Wang HW, Chang CW, Chu HW, Chen CY, Yu JC, Chao JI, Liu HF, Ding SL, Shen CY (2012) MicroRNA-30a inhibits cell migration and invasion by downregulating vimentin expression and is a potential prognostic marker in breast cancer. Breast Cancer Res Treat 134(3):1081–1093. doi:10.1007/s10549-012-2034-4

Chisholm KM, Wan Y, Li R, Montgomery KD, Chang HY, West RB (2012) Detection of long non-coding RNA in archival tissue: correlation with polycomb protein expression in primary and metastatic breast carcinoma. PLoS ONE 7(10):e47998. doi:10.1371/journal.pone.0047998

Clark MB, Choudhary A, Smith MA, Taft RJ, Mattick JS (2013) The dark matter rises: the expanding world of regulatory RNAs. Essays Biochem 54:1–16. doi:10.1042/bse0540001

Climent J, Dimitrow P, Fridlyand J, Palacios J, Siebert R, Albertson DG, Gray JW, Pinkel D, Lluch A, Martinez-Climent JA (2007) Deletion of chromosome 11q predicts response to anthracycline-based chemotherapy in early breast cancer. Cancer Res 67 (2):818–826. doi:10.1158/0008-5472.CAN-06-3307

Colley SM, Leedman PJ (2011) Steroid Receptor RNA activator—a nuclear receptor coregulator with multiple partners: insights and challenges. Biochimie 93 (11):1966–1972. doi:10.1016/j.biochi.2011.07.004

Corcoran C, Friel AM, Duffy MJ, Crown J, O'Driscoll L (2011) Intracellular and extracellular microRNAs in breast cancer. Clin Chem 57(1):18–32. doi:10.1373/clinchem.2010.150730

de Rinaldis E, Gazinska P, Mera A, Modrusan Z, Fedorowicz GM, Burford B, Gillett C, Marra P, Grigoriadis A, Dornan D, Holmberg L, Pinder S, Tutt A (2013) Integrated genomic analysis of triple-negative breast cancers reveals novel microRNAs associated with clinical and molecular phenotypes and sheds light on the pathways they control. BMC Genom 14:643. doi:10.1186/1471-2164-14-643

Derrien T, Johnson R, Bussotti G, Tanzer A, Djebali S, Tilgner H, Guernec G, Martin D, Merkel A, Knowles DG, Lagarde J, Veeravalli L, Ruan X, Ruan Y, Lassmann T, Carninci P, Brown JB, Lipovich L, Gonzalez JM, Thomas M, Davis CA, Shiekhattar R, Gingeras TR, Hubbard TJ, Notredame C, Harrow J, Guigo R (2012) The GENCODE v7 catalog of human long noncoding RNAs: Analysis of their gene structure, evolution, and expression. Genome Res 22(9):1775–1789. doi:10.1101/gr.132159.111

Djebali S, Davis CA, Merkel A, Dobin A, Lassmann T, Mortazavi A, Tanzer A, Lagarde J, Lin W, Schlesinger F, Xue C, Marinov GK, Khatun J, Williams BA, Zaleski C, Rozowsky J, Roder M, Kokocinski F, Abdelhamid RF, Alioto T, Antoshechkin I, Baer MT, Bar NS, Batut P, Bell K, Bell I, Chakrabortty S, Chen X, Chrast J, Curado J, Derrien T, Drenkow J, Dumais E, Dumais J, Duttagupta R, Falconnet E, Fastuca M, Fejes-Toth K, Ferreira P, Foissac S, Fullwood MJ, Gao H, Gonzalez D, Gordon A, Gunawardena H, Howald C, Jha S, Johnson R, Kapranov P, King B, Kingswood C, Luo OJ, Park E, Persaud K, Preall JB, Ribeca P, Risk B, Robyr D, Sammeth M, Schaffer L, See LH, Shahab A, Skancke J, Suzuki AM, Takahashi H, Tilgner H, Trout D, Walters N, Wang H, Wrobel J, Yu Y, Ruan X, Hayashizaki Y, Harrow J, Gerstein M, Hubbard T, Reymond A, Antonarakis SE, Hannon G, Giddings MC, Ruan Y, Wold B, Carninci P, Guigo R, Gingeras TR (2012) Landscape of transcription in human cells. Nature 489(7414):101–108. doi:10.1038/nature11233

Dong XY, Guo P, Boyd J, Sun X, Li Q, Zhou W, Dong JT (2009) Implication of snoRNA U50 in human breast cancer. J Genet Genomics 36(8):447–454. doi:10.1016/S1673-8527(08)60134-4

Du T, Zamore PD (2005) microPrimer: the biogenesis and function of microRNA. Development 132(21):4645–4652. doi:10.1242/dev.02070

Du Z, Fei T, Verhaak RG, Su Z, Zhang Y, Brown M, Chen Y, Liu XS (2013) Integrative genomic analyses reveal clinically relevant long noncoding RNAs in

human cancer. Nat Struct Mol Biol 20(7):908–913. doi:10.1038/nsmb.2591
Dvinge H, Git A, Graf S, Salmon-Divon M, Curtis C, Sottoriva A, Zhao Y, Hirst M, Armisen J, Miska EA, Chin SF, Provenzano E, Turashvili G, Green A, Ellis I, Aparicio S, Caldas C (2013) The shaping and functional consequences of the microRNA landscape in breast cancer. Nature 497(7449):378–382. doi:10.1038/nature12108
Egeland NG, Lunde S, Jonsdottir K, Lende TH, Cronin-Fenton D, Gilje B, Janssen EA, Soiland H (2015) The role of MicroRNAs as predictors of response to tamoxifen treatment in breast cancer patients. Int J Mol Sci 16(10):24243–24275. doi:10.3390/ijms161024243
Ellis MJ, Ding L, Shen D, Luo J, Suman VJ, Wallis JW, Van Tine BA, Hoog J, Goiffon RJ, Goldstein TC, Ng S, Lin L, Crowder R, Snider J, Ballman K, Weber J, Chen K, Koboldt DC, Kandoth C, Schierding WS, McMichael JF, Miller CA, Lu C, Harris CC, McLellan MD, Wendl MC, DeSchryver K, Allred DC, Esserman L, Unzeitig G, Margenthaler J, Babiera GV, Marcom PK, Guenther JM, Leitch M, Hunt K, Olson J, Tao Y, Maher CA, Fulton LL, Fulton RS, Harrison M, Oberkfell B, Du F, Demeter R, Vickery TL, Elhammali A, Piwnica-Worms H, McDonald S, Watson M, Dooling DJ, Ota D, Chang LW, Bose R, Ley TJ, Piwnica-Worms D, Stuart JM, Wilson RK, Mardis ER (2012) Whole-genome analysis informs breast cancer response to aromatase inhibition. Nature 486(7403):353–360. doi:10.1038/nature11143
Galasso M, Sana ME, Volinia S (2010) Non-coding RNAs: a key to future personalized molecular therapy? Genome Med 2(2):12. doi:10.1186/gm133
Gan R, Yang Y, Yang X, Zhao L, Lu J, Meng QH (2014) Downregulation of miR-221/222 enhances sensitivity of breast cancer cells to tamoxifen through upregulation of TIMP3. Cancer Gene Ther 21(7):290–296. doi:10.1038/cgt.2014.29
Ganesan S, Silver DP, Drapkin R, Greenberg R, Feunteun J, Livingston DM (2004) Association of BRCA1 with the inactive X chromosome and XIST RNA. Philos Trans R Soc Lond B Biol Sci 359(1441):123–128. doi:10.1098/rstb.2003.1371
Ganesan S, Silver DP, Greenberg RA, Avni D, Drapkin R, Miron A, Mok SC, Randrianarison V, Brodie S, Salstrom J, Rasmussen TP, Klimke A, Marrese C, Marahrens Y, Deng CX, Feunteun J, Livingston DM (2002) BRCA1 supports XIST RNA concentration on the inactive X chromosome. Cell 111(3):393–405
Gee HE, Buffa FM, Camps C, Ramachandran A, Leek R, Taylor M, Patil M, Sheldon H, Betts G, Homer J, West C, Ragoussis J, Harris AL (2011) The small-nucleolar RNAs commonly used for microRNA normalisation correlate with tumour pathology and prognosis. Br J Cancer 104(7):1168–1177. doi:10.1038/sj.bjc.6606076
Ghildiyal M, Zamore PD (2009) Small silencing RNAs: an expanding universe. Nat Rev Genet 10(2):94–108. doi:10.1038/nrg2504
Ginger MR, Gonzalez-Rimbau MF, Gay JP, Rosen JM (2001) Persistent changes in gene expression induced by estrogen and progesterone in the rat mammary gland. Mol Endocrinol 15(11):1993–2009. doi:10.1210/mend.15.11.0724
Ginger MR, Shore AN, Contreras A, Rijnkels M, Miller J, Gonzalez-Rimbau MF, Rosen JM (2006) A noncoding RNA is a potential marker of cell fate during mammary gland development. Proc Natl Acad Sci U S A 103(15):5781–5786. doi:10.1073/pnas.0600745103
Giricz O, Reynolds PA, Ramnauth A, Liu C, Wang T, Stead L, Childs G, Rohan T, Shapiro N, Fineberg S, Kenny PA, Loudig O (2012) Hsa-miR-375 is differentially expressed during breast lobular neoplasia and promotes loss of mammary acinar polarity. J Pathol 226(1):108–119. doi:10.1002/path.2978
Godinho MF, Sieuwerts AM, Look MP, Meijer D, Foekens JA, Dorssers LC, van Agthoven T (2010) Relevance of BCAR4 in tamoxifen resistance and tumour aggressiveness of human breast cancer. Br J Cancer 103(8):1284–1291. doi:10.1038/sj.bjc.6605884
Godinho MF, Wulfkuhle JD, Look MP, Sieuwerts AM, Sleijfer S, Foekens JA, Petricoin EF 3rd, Dorssers LC, van Agthoven T (2012) BCAR4 induces antioestrogen resistance but sensitises breast cancer to lapatinib. Br J Cancer 107(6):947–955. doi:10.1038/bjc.2012.351
Goh JN, Loo SY, Datta A, Siveen KS, Yap WN, Cai W, Shin EM, Wang C, Kim JE, Chan M, Dharmarajan AM, Lee AS, Lobie PE, Yap CT, Kumar AP (2015) microRNAs in breast cancer: regulatory roles governing the hallmarks of cancer. Biol Rev Camb Philos Soc. doi:10.1111/brv.12176
Gokmen-Polar Y, Vladislav IT, Neelamraju Y, Janga SC, Badve S (2015) Prognostic impact of HOTAIR expression is restricted to ER-negative breast cancers. Sci Rep 5:8765. doi:10.1038/srep08765
Grelier G, Voirin N, Ay AS, Cox DG, Chabaud S, Treilleux I, Leon-Goddard S, Rimokh R, Mikaelian I, Venoux C, Puisieux A, Lasset C, Moyret-Lalle C (2009) Prognostic value of Dicer expression in human breast cancers and association with the mesenchymal phenotype. Br J Cancer 101(4):673–683. doi:10.1038/sj.bjc.6605193
Grzybowska-Szatkowska L, Slaska B (2012) Polymorphisms in genes encoding mt-tRNA in female breast cancer in Poland. Mitochondrial DNA 23(2):106–111. doi:10.3109/19401736.2012.660925
Guffanti A, Iacono M, Pelucchi P, Kim N, Solda G, Croft LJ, Taft RJ, Rizzi E, Askarian-Amiri M, Bonnal RJ, Callari M, Mignone F, Pesole G, Bertalot G, Bernardi LR, Albertini A, Lee C, Mattick JS, Zucchi I, De Bellis G (2009) A transcriptional sketch of a primary human breast cancer by 454 deep sequencing. BMC Genom 10:163. doi:10.1186/1471-2164-10-163

Gumireddy K, Li A, Yan J, Setoyama T, Johannes GJ, Orom UA, Tchou J, Liu Q, Zhang L, Speicher DW, Calin GA, Huang Q (2013) Identification of a long non-coding RNA-associated RNP complex regulating metastasis at the translational step. EMBO J 32 (20):2672–2684. doi:10.1038/emboj.2013.188

Guo X, Gao L, Wang Y, Chiu DK, Wang T, Deng Y (2016) Advances in long noncoding RNAs: identification, structure prediction and function annotation. Brief Funct Genomics 15(1):38–46. doi:10.1093/bfgp/elv022

Gupta RA, Shah N, Wang KC, Kim J, Horlings HM, Wong DJ, Tsai MC, Hung T, Argani P, Rinn JL, Wang Y, Brzoska P, Kong B, Li R, West RB, van de Vijver MJ, Sukumar S, Chang HY (2010) Long non-coding RNA HOTAIR reprograms chromatin state to promote cancer metastasis. Nature 464 (7291):1071–1076. doi:10.1038/nature08975

Gutschner T, Diederichs S (2012a) The hallmarks of cancer: a long non-coding RNA point of view. RNA Biol 9(6)

Gutschner T, Diederichs S (2012b) The hallmarks of cancer: a long non-coding RNA point of view. RNA Biol 9(6):703–719. doi:10.4161/rna.20481

Gutschner T, Hammerle M, Diederichs S (2013) MALAT1—a paradigm for long noncoding RNA function in cancer. J Mol Med (Berl) 91(7):791–801. doi:10.1007/s00109-013-1028-y

Guttman M, Rinn JL (2012) Modular regulatory principles of large non-coding RNAs. Nature 482 (7385):339–346. doi:10.1038/nature10887

Guttman M, Russell P, Ingolia NT, Weissman JS, Lander ES (2013) Ribosome profiling provides evidence that large noncoding RNAs do not encode proteins. Cell 154(1):240–251. doi:10.1016/j.cell.2013.06.009

Ha M, Kim VN (2014) Regulation of microRNA biogenesis. Nat Rev Mol Cell Biol 15(8):509–524. doi:10.1038/nrm3838

Hall LL, Smith KP, Byron M, Lawrence JB (2006) Molecular anatomy of a speckle. Anat Rec A Discov Mol Cell Evol Biol 288(7):664–675. doi:10.1002/ar.a.20336

Hansji H, Leung EY, Baguley BC, Finlay GJ, Askarian-Amiri ME (2014) Keeping abreast with long non-coding RNAs in mammary gland development and breast cancer. Front Genet 5:379. doi:10.3389/fgene.2014.00379

Hayes EL, Lewis-Wambi JS (2015) Mechanisms of endocrine resistance in breast cancer: an overview of the proposed roles of noncoding RNA. Breast Cancer Res 17:40. doi:10.1186/s13058-015-0542-y

He YJ, Wu JZ, Ji MH, Ma T, Qiao EQ, Ma R, Tang JH (2013) miR-342 is associated with estrogen receptor-alpha expression and response to tamoxifen in breast cancer. Exp Ther Med 5(3):813–818. doi:10.3892/etm.2013.915

Hu W, Alvarez-Dominguez JR, Lodish HF (2012) Regulation of mammalian cell differentiation by long non-coding RNAs. EMBO Rep 13(11):971–983. doi:10.1038/embor.2012.145

Huang J, Zhou N, Watabe K, Lu Z, Wu F, Xu M, Mo YY (2014) Long non-coding RNA UCA1 promotes breast tumor growth by suppression of p27 (Kip1). Cell Death Dis 5:e1008. doi:10.1038/cddis.2013.541

Iacoangeli A, Lin Y, Morley EJ, Muslimov IA, Bianchi R, Reilly J, Weedon J, Diallo R, Bocker W, Tiedge H (2004) BC200 RNA in invasive and preinvasive breast cancer. Carcinogenesis 25(11):2125–2133. doi:10.1093/carcin/bgh228

Ingolia NT, Lareau LF, Weissman JS (2011) Ribosome profiling of mouse embryonic stem cells reveals the complexity and dynamics of mammalian proteomes. Cell 147(4):789–802. doi:10.1016/j.cell.2011.10.002

Ishizu H, Siomi H, Siomi MC (2012) Biology of PIWI-interacting RNAs: new insights into biogenesis and function inside and outside of germlines. Genes Dev 26(21):2361–2373. doi:10.1101/gad.203786.112

Iyer MK, Niknafs YS, Malik R, Singhal U, Sahu A, Hosono Y, Barrette TR, Prensner JR, Evans JR, Zhao S, Poliakov A, Cao X, Dhanasekaran SM, Wu YM, Robinson DR, Beer DG, Feng FY, Iyer HK, Chinnaiyan AM (2015) The landscape of long noncoding RNAs in the human transcriptome. Nat Genet 47(3):199–208. doi:10.1038/ng.3192

Ji P, Diederichs S, Wang W, Boing S, Metzger R, Schneider PM, Tidow N, Brandt B, Buerger H, Bulk E, Thomas M, Berdel WE, Serve H, Muller-Tidow C (2003) MALAT-1, a novel noncoding RNA, and thymosin beta4 predict metastasis and survival in early-stage non-small cell lung cancer. Oncogene 22(39):8031–8041. doi:10.1038/sj.onc.1206928

Jia H, Osak M, Bogu GK, Stanton LW, Johnson R, Lipovich L (2010) Genome-wide computational identification and manual annotation of human long noncoding RNA genes. RNA 16(8):1478–1487. doi:10.1261/rna.1951310 [pii]

Jin C, Yan B, Lu Q, Lin Y, Ma L (2015) Reciprocal regulation of Hsa-miR-1 and long noncoding RNA MALAT1 promotes triple-negative breast cancer development. Tumour Biol. doi:10.1007/s13277-015-4605-6

Johnsson P, Lipovich L, Grander D, Morris KV (2014) Evolutionary conservation of long non-coding RNAs; sequence, structure, function. Biochim Biophys Acta 1840(3):1063–71. doi:10.1016/j.bbagen.2013.10.035

Jung EJ, Santarpia L, Kim J, Esteva FJ, Moretti E, Buzdar AU, Di Leo A, Le XF, Bast RC Jr, Park ST, Pusztai L, Calin GA (2012) Plasma microRNA 210 levels correlate with sensitivity to trastuzumab and tumor presence in breast cancer patients. Cancer 118 (10):2603–2614. doi:10.1002/cncr.26565

Karahan G, Sayar N, Gozum G, Bozkurt B, Konu O, Yulug IG (2015) Relative expression of rRNA transcripts and 45S rDNA promoter methylation status are dysregulated in tumors in comparison with matched-normal tissues in breast cancer. Oncol Rep 33(6):3131–3145. doi:10.3892/or.2015.3940

Kato M, Paranjape T, Muller RU, Nallur S, Gillespie E, Keane K, Esquela-Kerscher A, Weidhaas JB, Slack FJ

(2009) The mir-34 microRNA is required for the DNA damage response in vivo in C. elegans and in vitro in human breast cancer cells. Oncogene 28(25):2419–2424. doi:10.1038/onc.2009.106

Khoshnaw SM, Rakha EA, Abdel-Fatah T, Nolan CC, Hodi Z, Macmillan RD, Ellis IO, Green AR (2013) The microRNA maturation regulator Drosha is an independent predictor of outcome in breast cancer patients. Breast Cancer Res Treat 137(1):139–153. doi:10.1007/s10549-012-2358-0

Kim VN, Han J, Siomi MC (2009) Biogenesis of small RNAs in animals. Nat Rev Mol Cell Biol 10(2):126–139. doi:10.1038/nrm2632

Kino T, Hurt DE, Ichijo T, Nader N, Chrousos GP (2010) Noncoding RNA gas5 is a growth arrest- and starvation-associated repressor of the glucocorticoid receptor. Sci Signal 3(107):ra8. doi:10.1126/scisignal.2000568. 3/107/ra8 [pii]

Kogo R, Shimamura T, Mimori K, Kawahara K, Imoto S, Sudo T, Tanaka F, Shibata K, Suzuki A, Komune S, Miyano S, Mori M (2011) Long noncoding RNA HOTAIR regulates polycomb-dependent chromatin modification and is associated with poor prognosis in colorectal cancers. Cancer Res 71(20):6320–6326. doi:10.1158/0008-5472.CAN-11-1021

Kondrashov AV, Kiefmann M, Ebnet K, Khanam T, Muddashetty RS, Brosius J (2005) Inhibitory effect of naked neural BC1 RNA or BC200 RNA on eukaryotic in vitro translation systems is reversed by poly(A)-binding protein (PABP). J Mol Biol 353(1):88–103. doi:10.1016/j.jmb.2005.07.049

Kong W, He L, Richards EJ, Challa S, Xu CX, Permuth-Wey J, Lancaster JM, Coppola D, Sellers TA, Djeu JY, Cheng JQ (2014) Upregulation of miRNA-155 promotes tumour angiogenesis by targeting VHL and is associated with poor prognosis and triple-negative breast cancer. Oncogene 33 (6):679–689. doi:10.1038/onc.2012.636

Kung JT, Colognori D, Lee JT (2013) Long noncoding RNAs: past, present, and future. Genetics 193(3):651–669. doi:10.1534/genetics.112.146704

Kurisu T, Tanaka T, Ishii J, Matsumura K, Sugimura K, Nakatani T, Kawashima H (2006) Expression and function of human steroid receptor RNA activator in prostate cancer cells: role of endogenous hSRA protein in androgen receptor-mediated transcription. Prostate Cancer Prostatic Dis 9(2):173–178. doi:10.1038/sj.pcan.4500867

Lamond AI, Spector DL (2003) Nuclear speckles: a model for nuclear organelles. Nat Rev Mol Cell Biol 4 (8):605–612. doi:10.1038/nrm1172

Lanz RB, McKenna NJ, Onate SA, Albrecht U, Wong J, Tsai SY, Tsai MJ, O'Malley BW (1999) A steroid receptor coactivator, SRA, functions as an RNA and is present in an SRC-1 complex. Cell 97(1):17–27

Leaderer D, Hoffman AE, Zheng T, Fu A, Weidhaas J, Paranjape T, Zhu Y (2011) Genetic and epigenetic association studies suggest a role of microRNA biogenesis gene exportin-5 (XPO5) in breast tumorigenesis. Int J Mol Epidemiol Genet 2(1):9–18

Lee JA, Lee HY, Lee ES, Kim I, Bae JW (2011) Prognostic Implications of MicroRNA-21 Overexpression in Invasive Ductal Carcinomas of the Breast. J Breast Cancer 14(4):269–275. doi:10.4048/jbc.2011.14.4.269

Leivonen SK, Sahlberg KK, Makela R, Due EU, Kallioniemi O, Borresen-Dale AL, Perala M (2014) High-throughput screens identify microRNAs essential for HER2 positive breast cancer cell growth. Mol Oncol 8(1):93–104. doi:10.1016/j.molonc.2013.10.001

Lerebours F, Cizeron-Clairac G, Susini A, Vacher S, Mouret-Fourme E, Belichard C, Brain E, Alberini JL, Spyratos F, Lidereau R, Bieche I (2013) miRNA expression profiling of inflammatory breast cancer identifies a 5-miRNA signature predictive of breast tumor aggressiveness. Int J Cancer 133(7):1614–1623. doi:10.1002/ijc.28171

Lewis BP, Burge CB, Bartel DP (2005) Conserved seed pairing, often flanked by adenosines, indicates that thousands of human genes are microRNA targets. Cell 120(1):15–20. doi:10.1016/j.cell.2004.12.035

Li M, Ma X, Li M, Zhang B, Huang J, Liu L, Wei Y (2014) Prognostic role of microRNA-210 in various carcinomas: a systematic review and meta-analysis. Dis Markers 2014:106197. doi:10.1155/2014/106197

Liao Q, Liu C, Yuan X, Kang S, Miao R, Xiao H, Zhao G, Luo H, Bu D, Zhao H, Skogerbo G, Wu Z, Zhao Y (2011) Large-scale prediction of long non-coding RNA functions in a coding-non-coding gene co-expression network. Nucleic Acids Res 39 (9):3864–3878. doi:10.1093/nar/gkq1348

Lottin S, Adriaenssens E, Dupressoir T, Berteaux N, Montpellier C, Coll J, Dugimont T, Curgy JJ (2002) Overexpression of an ectopic H19 gene enhances the tumorigenic properties of breast cancer cells. Carcinogenesis 23(11):1885–1895

Ma L, Li GZ, Wu ZS, Meng G (2014) Prognostic significance of let-7b expression in breast cancer and correlation to its target gene of BSG expression. Med Oncol 31(1):773. doi:10.1007/s12032-013-0773-7

Markou A, Yousef GM, Stathopoulos E, Georgoulias V, Lianidou E (2014) Prognostic significance of metastasis-related microRNAs in early breast cancer patients with a long follow-up. Clin Chem 60(1):197–205. doi:10.1373/clinchem.2013.210542

Masri S, Liu Z, Phung S, Wang E, Yuan YC, Chen S (2010) The role of microRNA-128a in regulating TGFbeta signaling in letrozole-resistant breast cancer cells. Breast Cancer Res Treat 124(1):89–99. doi:10.1007/s10549-009-0716-3

Matera AG, Izaguire-Sierra M, Praveen K, Rajendra TK (2009) Nuclear bodies: random aggregates of sticky proteins or crucibles of macromolecular assembly? Dev Cell 17(5):639–647. doi:10.1016/j.devcel.2009.10.017

Mattick JS (2001) Non-coding RNAs: the architects of eukaryotic complexity. EMBO Rep 2(11):986–991. doi:10.1093/embo-reports/kve230

Mattick JS (2007) A new paradigm for developmental biology. J Exp Biol 210(Pt 9):1526–1547. doi:10.1242/jeb.005017

Mattick JS, Makunin IV (2005) Small regulatory RNAs in mammals. Hum Mol Genet 14(Spec No 1):R121–132. doi:10.1093/hmg/ddi101
Mattick JS, Makunin IV (2006) Non-coding RNA. Hum Mol Genet 15(Spec No 1):R17–29. doi:10.1093/hmg/ddl046
Mattick JS, Rinn JL (2015) Discovery and annotation of long noncoding RNAs. Nat Struct Mol Biol 22(1):5–7. doi:10.1038/nsmb.2942
Mei M, Ren Y, Zhou X, Yuan XB, Han L, Wang GX, Jia Z, Pu PY, Kang CS, Yao Z (2010) Downregulation of miR-21 enhances chemotherapeutic effect of taxol in breast carcinoma cells. Technol Cancer Res Treat 9 (1):77–86
Meijer D, van Agthoven T, Bosma PT, Nooter K, Dorssers LC (2006) Functional screen for genes responsible for tamoxifen resistance in human breast cancer cells. Mol Cancer Res 4(6):379–386. doi:10.1158/1541-7786.MCR-05-0156
Meng XL, Meng H, Zhang W, Qin YH, Zhao NM (2015) The role of mitochondrial tRNA variants in female breast cancer. Mitochondrial DNA 1–3. doi:10.3109/19401736.2015.1007332
Misteli T (2000) Cell biology of transcription and pre-mRNA splicing: nuclear architecture meets nuclear function. J Cell Sci 113(Pt 11):1841–1849
Mourtada-Maarabouni M, Pickard MR, Hedge VL, Farzaneh F, Williams GT (2009) GAS5, a non-protein-coding RNA, controls apoptosis and is downregulated in breast cancer. Oncogene 28(2):195–208. doi:10.1038/onc.2008.373
Mulrane L, Madden SF, Brennan DJ, Gremel G, McGee SF, McNally S, Martin F, Crown JP, Jirstrom K, Higgins DG, Gallagher WM, O'Connor DP (2012) miR-187 is an independent prognostic factor in breast cancer and confers increased invasive potential in vitro. Clin Cancer Res 18(24):6702–6713. doi:10.1158/1078-0432.CCR-12-1420
Muluhngwi P, Klinge CM (2015) Roles for miRNAs in endocrine resistance in breast cancer. Endocr Relat Cancer 22(5):R279–300. doi:10.1530/ERC-15-0355
Murphy FV, Ramakrishnan V, Malkiewicz A, Agris PF (2004) The role of modifications in codon discrimination by tRNA(Lys)UUU. Nat Struct Mol Biol 11 (12):1186–1191. doi:10.1038/nsmb861
Niinuma T, Suzuki H, Nojima M, Nosho K, Yamamoto H, Takamaru H, Yamamoto E, Maruyama R, Nobuoka T, Miyazaki Y, Nishida T, Bamba T, Kanda T, Ajioka Y, Taguchi T, Okahara S, Takahashi H, Nishida Y, Hosokawa M, Hasegawa T, Tokino T, Hirata K, Imai K, Toyota M, Shinomura Y (2012) Upregulation of miR-196a and HOTAIR drive malignant character in gastrointestinal stromal tumors. Cancer Res 72(5):1126–1136. doi:10.1158/0008-5472.CAN-11-1803
O'Day E, Lal A (2010) MicroRNAs and their target gene networks in breast cancer. Breast Cancer Res 12 (2):201. doi:10.1186/bcr2484
Orom UA, Derrien T, Beringer M, Gumireddy K, Gardini A, Bussotti G, Lai F, Zytnicki M, Notredame C, Huang Q, Guigo R, Shiekhattar R (2010) Long noncoding RNAs with enhancer-like function in human cells. Cell 143(1):46–58. doi:10.1016/j.cell.2010.09.001
Osato N, Suzuki Y, Ikeo K, Gojobori T (2007) Transcriptional interferences in cis natural antisense transcripts of humans and mice. Genetics 176(2):1299–1306. doi:10.1534/genetics.106.069484
Osborne CK, Schiff R (2011) Mechanisms of endocrine resistance in breast cancer. Annu Rev Med 62:233–247. doi:10.1146/annurev-med-070909-182917
Pavon-Eternod M, Gomes S, Geslain R, Dai Q, Rosner MR, Pan T (2009) tRNA over-expression in breast cancer and functional consequences. Nucleic Acids Res 37(21):7268–7280. doi:10.1093/nar/gkp787
Prensner JR, Chinnaiyan AM (2011) The emergence of lncRNAs in cancer biology. Cancer Discov 1(5):391–407. doi:10.1158/2159-8290.CD-11-0209
Quesne JL, Jones J, Warren J, Dawson SJ, Ali HR, Bardwell H, Blows F, Pharoah P, Caldas C (2012) Biological and prognostic associations of miR-205 and let-7b in breast cancer revealed by in situ hybridization analysis of micro-RNA expression in arrays of archival tumour tissue. J Pathol 227(3):306–314. doi:10.1002/path.3983
Rao X, Di Leva G, Li M, Fang F, Devlin C, Hartman-Frey C, Burow ME, Ivan M, Croce CM, Nephew KP (2011) MicroRNA-221/222 confers breast cancer fulvestrant resistance by regulating multiple signaling pathways. Oncogene 30(9):1082–1097. doi:10.1038/onc.2010.487
Richardson AL, Wang ZC, De Nicolo A, Lu X, Brown M, Miron A, Liao X, Iglehart JD, Livingston DM, Ganesan S (2006) X chromosomal abnormalities in basal-like human breast cancer. Cancer Cell 9(2):121–132. doi:10.1016/j.ccr.2006.01.013
Rinn JL, Chang HY (2012) Genome regulation by long noncoding RNAs. Annu Rev Biochem 81:145–166. doi:10.1146/annurev-biochem-051410-092902
Rinn JL, Kertesz M, Wang JK, Squazzo SL, Xu X, Brugmann SA, Goodnough LH, Helms JA, Farnham PJ, Segal E, Chang HY (2007) Functional demarcation of active and silent chromatin domains in human HOX loci by noncoding RNAs. Cell 129 (7):1311–1323. doi:10.1016/j.cell.2007.05.022
Scott MS, Ono M (2011) From snoRNA to miRNA: Dual function regulatory non-coding RNAs. Biochimie 93 (11):1987–1992. doi:10.1016/j.biochi.2011.05.026
Serviss JT, Johnsson P, Grander D (2014) An emerging role for long non-coding RNAs in cancer metastasis. Front Genet 5:234. doi:10.3389/fgene.2014.00234
Shen L, Li J, Xu L, Ma J, Li H, Xiao X, Zhao J, Fang L (2012) miR-497 induces apoptosis of breast cancer cells by targeting Bcl-w. Exp Ther Med 3(3):475–480. doi:10.3892/etm.2011.428
Shibahara Y, Miki Y, Onodera Y, Hata S, Chan MS, Yiu CC, Loo TY, Nakamura Y, Akahira J, Ishida T, Abe K, Hirakawa H, Chow LW, Suzuki T, Ouchi N, Sasano H (2012) Aromatase inhibitor treatment of breast cancer cells increases the expression of let-7f, a microRNA targeting CYP19A1. J Pathol 227(3):357–366. doi:10.1002/path.4019

Shore AN, Kabotyanski EB, Roarty K, Smith MA, Zhang Y, Creighton CJ, Dinger ME, Rosen JM (2012) Pregnancy-induced noncoding RNA (PINC) associates with polycomb repressive complex 2 and regulates mammary epithelial differentiation. PLoS Genet 8(7): e1002840. doi:10.1371/journal.pgen.1002840

Si ML, Zhu S, Wu H, Lu Z, Wu F, Mo YY (2007) miR-21-mediated tumor growth. Oncogene 26 (19):2799–2803. doi:10.1038/sj.onc.1210083

Silva JM, Boczek NJ, Berres MW, Ma X, Smith DI (2011) LSINCT5 is over expressed in breast and ovarian cancer and affects cellular proliferation. RNA Biol 8(3):496–505

Siomi MC, Sato K, Pezic D, Aravin AA (2011) PIWI-interacting small RNAs: the vanguard of genome defence. Nat Rev Mol Cell Biol 12(4):246–258. doi:10.1038/nrm3089

Song CG, Wu XY, Fu FM, Han ZH, Wang C, Shao ZM (2012) Correlation of miR-155 on formalin-fixed paraffin embedded tissues with invasiveness and prognosis of breast cancer. Zhonghua Wai Ke Za Zhi 50(11):1011–1014

Sontheimer EJ (2005) Assembly and function of RNA silencing complexes. Nat Rev Mol Cell Biol 6(2):127–138. doi:10.1038/nrm1568

Spector DL (2006) SnapShot: cellular bodies. Cell 127 (5):1071. doi:10.1016/j.cell.2006.11.026

Su H, Xu T, Ganapathy S, Shadfan M, Long M, Huang TH, Thompson I, Yuan ZM (2014) Elevated snoRNA biogenesis is essential in breast cancer. Oncogene 33 (11):1348–1358. doi:10.1038/onc.2013.89

Sumazin P, Yang X, Chiu HS, Chung WJ, Iyer A, Llobet-Navas D, Rajbhandari P, Bansal M, Guarnieri P, Silva J, Califano A (2011) An extensive microRNA-mediated network of RNA-RNA interactions regulates established oncogenic pathways in glioblastoma. Cell 147(2):370–381. doi:10.1016/j.cell.2011.09.041

Sung H, Jeon S, Lee KM, Han S, Song M, Choi JY, Park SK, Yoo KY, Noh DY, Ahn SH, Kang D (2012) Common genetic polymorphisms of microRNA biogenesis pathway genes and breast cancer survival. BMC Cancer 12:195. doi:10.1186/1471-2407-12-195

Taft RJ, Pang KC, Mercer TR, Dinger M, Mattick JS (2010) Non-coding RNAs: regulators of disease. J Pathol 220(2):126–139. doi:10.1002/path.2638

Tang J, Ahmad A, Sarkar FH (2012) The role of microRNAs in breast cancer migration, invasion and metastasis. Int J Mol Sci 13(10):13414–13437. doi:10.3390/ijms131013414

Tripathi V, Ellis JD, Shen Z, Song DY, Pan Q, Watt AT, Freier SM, Bennett CF, Sharma A, Bubulya PA, Blencowe BJ, Prasanth SG, Prasanth KV (2010) The nuclear-retained noncoding RNA MALAT1 regulates alternative splicing by modulating SR splicing factor phosphorylation. Mol Cell 39(6):925–938. doi:10.1016/j.molcel.2010.08.011

Tsai MC, Manor O, Wan Y, Mosammaparast N, Wang JK, Lan F, Shi Y, Segal E, Chang HY (2010) Long noncoding RNA as modular scaffold of histone modification complexes. Science 329(5992):689–693. doi:10.1126/science.1192002 [pii]

Van der Auwera I, Limame R, van Dam P, Vermeulen PB, Dirix LY, Van Laere SJ (2010) Integrated miRNA and mRNA expression profiling of the inflammatory breast cancer subtype. Br J Cancer 103(4):532–541. doi:10.1038/sj.bjc.6605787

van Heesch S, van Iterson M, Jacobi J, Boymans S, Essers PB, de Bruijn E, Hao W, MacInnes AW, Cuppen E, Simonis M (2014) Extensive localization of long noncoding RNAs to the cytosol and mono- and polyribosomal complexes. Genome Biol 15(1): R6. doi:10.1186/gb-2014-15-1-r6

van Schooneveld E, Wildiers H, Vergote I, Vermeulen PB, Dirix LY, Van Laere SJ (2015) Dysregulation of microRNAs in breast cancer and their potential role as prognostic and predictive biomarkers in patient management. Breast Cancer Res 17:21. doi:10.1186/s13058-015-0526-y

Vincent-Salomon A, Ganem-Elbaz C, Manie E, Raynal V, Sastre-Garau X, Stoppa-Lyonnet D, Stern MH, Heard E (2007) X inactive-specific transcript RNA coating and genetic instability of the X chromosome in BRCA1 breast tumors. Cancer Res 67(11):5134–5140. doi:10.1158/0008-5472.CAN-07-0465

Volinia S, Galasso M, Sana ME, Wise TF, Palatini J, Huebner K, Croce CM (2012) Breast cancer signatures for invasiveness and prognosis defined by deep sequencing of microRNA. Proc Natl Acad Sci U S A 109(8):3024–3029. doi:10.1073/pnas.1200010109

Wang F, Li X, Xie X, Zhao L, Chen W (2008) UCA1, a non-protein-coding RNA up-regulated in bladder carcinoma and embryo, influencing cell growth and promoting invasion. FEBS Lett 582(13):1919–1927. doi:10.1016/j.febslet.2008.05.012

Wang J, Zhao J, Shi M, Ding Y, Sun H, Yuan F, Zou Z (2014) Elevated expression of miR-210 predicts poor survival of cancer patients: a systematic review and meta-analysis. PLoS ONE 9(2):e89223. doi:10.1371/journal.pone.0089223

Wang KC, Chang HY (2011) Molecular mechanisms of long noncoding RNAs. Mol Cell 43(6):904–914. doi:10.1016/j.molcel.2011.08.018

Wang S, Li H, Wang J, Wang D (2013) Expression of microRNA-497 and its prognostic significance in human breast cancer. Diagn Pathol 8:172. doi:10.1186/1746-1596-8-172

Ward A, Balwierz A, Zhang JD, Kublbeck M, Pawitan Y, Hielscher T, Wiemann S, Sahin O (2013) Re-expression of microRNA-375 reverses both tamoxifen resistance and accompanying EMT-like properties in breast cancer. Oncogene 32(9):1173–1182. doi:10.1038/onc.2012.128

Wei Y, Lai X, Yu S, Chen S, Ma Y, Zhang Y, Li H, Zhu X, Yao L, Zhang J (2014) Exosomal miR-221/222 enhances tamoxifen resistance in recipient ER-positive breast cancer cells. Breast Cancer Res Treat 147(2):423–431. doi:10.1007/s10549-014-3037-0

Wright MW (2014) A short guide to long non-coding RNA gene nomenclature. Hum Genomics 8:7. doi:10.1186/1479-7364-8-7

Wu X, Somlo G, Yu Y, Palomares MR, Li AX, Zhou W, Chow A, Yen Y, Rossi JJ, Gao H, Wang J, Yuan YC, Frankel P, Li S, Ashing-Giwa KT, Sun G, Wang Y, Smith R, Robinson K, Ren X, Wang SE (2012) De novo sequencing of circulating miRNAs identifies novel markers predicting clinical outcome of locally advanced breast cancer. J Transl Med 10:42. doi:10.1186/1479-5876-10-42

Xu MD, Qi P, Weng WW, Shen XH, Ni SJ, Dong L, Huang D, Tan C, Sheng WQ, Zhou XY, Du X (2014) Long non-coding RNA LSINCT5 predicts negative prognosis and exhibits oncogenic activity in gastric cancer. Medicine (Baltimore) 93(28):e303. doi:10.1097/MD.0000000000000303

Yan X, Hu Z, Feng Y, Hu X, Yuan J, Zhao SD, Zhang Y, Yang L, Shan W, He Q, Fan L, Kandalaft LE, Tanyi JL, Li C, Yuan CX, Zhang D, Yuan H, Hua K, Lu Y, Katsaros D, Huang Q, Montone K, Fan Y, Coukos G, Boyd J, Sood AK, Rebbeck T, Mills GB, Dang CV, Zhang L (2015) Comprehensive Genomic Characterization of Long Non-coding RNAs across Human Cancers. Cancer Cell 28(4):529–540. doi:10.1016/j.ccell.2015.09.006

Yang L, Froberg JE, Lee JT (2014) Long noncoding RNAs: fresh perspectives into the RNA world. Trends Biochem Sci 39(1):35–43. doi:10.1016/j.tibs.2013.10.002

Yang Z, Zhou L, Wu LM, Lai MC, Xie HY, Zhang F, Zheng SS (2011) Overexpression of long non-coding RNA HOTAIR predicts tumor recurrence in hepatocellular carcinoma patients following liver transplantation. Ann Surg Oncol 18(5):1243–1250. doi:10.1245/s10434-011-1581-y

Yarian C, Townsend H, Czestkowski W, Sochacka E, Malkiewicz AJ, Guenther R, Miskiewicz A, Agris PF (2002) Accurate translation of the genetic code depends on tRNA modified nucleosides. J Biol Chem 277(19):16391–16395. doi:10.1074/jbc.M200253200

Yoshimizu T, Miroglio A, Ripoche MA, Gabory A, Vernucci M, Riccio A, Colnot S, Godard C, Terris B, Jammes H, Dandolo L (2008) The H19 locus acts in vivo as a tumor suppressor. Proc Natl Acad Sci U S A 105(34):12417–12422. doi:10.1073/pnas.0801540105

Zamore PD, Haley B (2005) Ribo-gnome: the big world of small RNAs. Science 309(5740):1519–1524. doi:10.1126/science.1111444

Zhang N, Wang X, Huo Q, Sun M, Cai C, Liu Z, Hu G, Yang Q (2014a) MicroRNA-30a suppresses breast tumor growth and metastasis by targeting metadherin. Oncogene 33(24):3119–3128. doi:10.1038/onc.2013.286

Zhang P, Wang L, Rodriguez-Aguayo C, Yuan Y, Debeb BG, Chen D, Sun Y, You MJ, Liu Y, Dean DC, Woodward WA, Liang H, Yang X, Lopez-Berestein G, Sood AK, Hu Y, Ang KK, Chen J, Ma L (2014b) miR-205 acts as a tumour radiosensitizer by targeting ZEB1 and Ubc13. Nat Commun 5:5671. doi:10.1038/ncomms6671

Zhao JJ, Lin J, Yang H, Kong W, He L, Ma X, Coppola D, Cheng JQ (2008) MicroRNA-221/222 negatively regulates estrogen receptor alpha and is associated with tamoxifen resistance in breast cancer. J Biol Chem 283(45):31079–31086. doi:10.1074/jbc.M806041200

Zhou M, Liu Z, Zhao Y, Ding Y, Liu H, Xi Y, Xiong W, Li G, Lu J, Fodstad O, Riker AI, Tan M (2010) MicroRNA-125b confers the resistance of breast cancer cells to paclitaxel through suppression of pro-apoptotic Bcl-2 antagonist killer 1 (Bak1) expression. J Biol Chem 285(28):21496–21507. doi:10.1074/jbc.M109.083337

Zhou X, Marian C, Makambi KH, Kosti O, Kallakury BV, Loffredo CA, Zheng YL (2012) MicroRNA-9 as potential biomarker for breast cancer local recurrence and tumor estrogen receptor status. PLoS ONE 7(6):e39011. doi:10.1371/journal.pone.0039011

Alternative Splicing in Breast Cancer 23

Yesim Gökmen-Polar

Abstract

Alternative splicing of pre-mRNA is an essential event that leads to protein diversity and regulation of the cellular processes in mammals. With the advent of the next generation sequencing technologies, the role of alternative splicing is gaining a momentum. Regulation of alternative splicing is a complex process involving the core spliceosome machinery and multiple regulatory factors that enable the tightly controlled splicing of introns/exons. Any aberrant alteration in this process can result in diseases such as cancer. Indeed, accumulating evidence suggests that alternative splicing plays an important role in all hallmarks of cancer including proliferative signaling, resisting cell death, inducing angiogenesis, and activating invasion and metastasis. These changes may occur due to mutations or altered expression levels of key regulatory genes of spliceosome machinery or splicing factors. In this review, we summarize recent findings that have implicated the critical role of alternative splicing in breast cancer and discuss current understandings and its potential utility in breast cancer.

Keywords

Alternative splicing · Breast cancer · Alternative splicing events · Spliceosome machinery · Splicing factors

23.1 Introduction

The splicing mechanism is the process in which introns are separated from the exons; the latter go on to form mature mRNAs. Alternative splicing (AS) is a mechanism by which selective inclusion/ exclusion of exons and introns during splicing of the pre-mRNAs leads to the production of more than one isoform. It plays an

Y. Gökmen-Polar (✉)
Department of Pathology and Laboratory Medicine, Indiana University School of Medicine, 635 Barnhill Drive, MS 0038, Indianapolis, IN 46202, USA
e-mail: ypolar@iu.edu

S. Badve and Y. Gökmen-Polar (eds.), *Molecular Pathology of Breast Cancer*, DOI 10.1007/978-3-319-41761-5_23

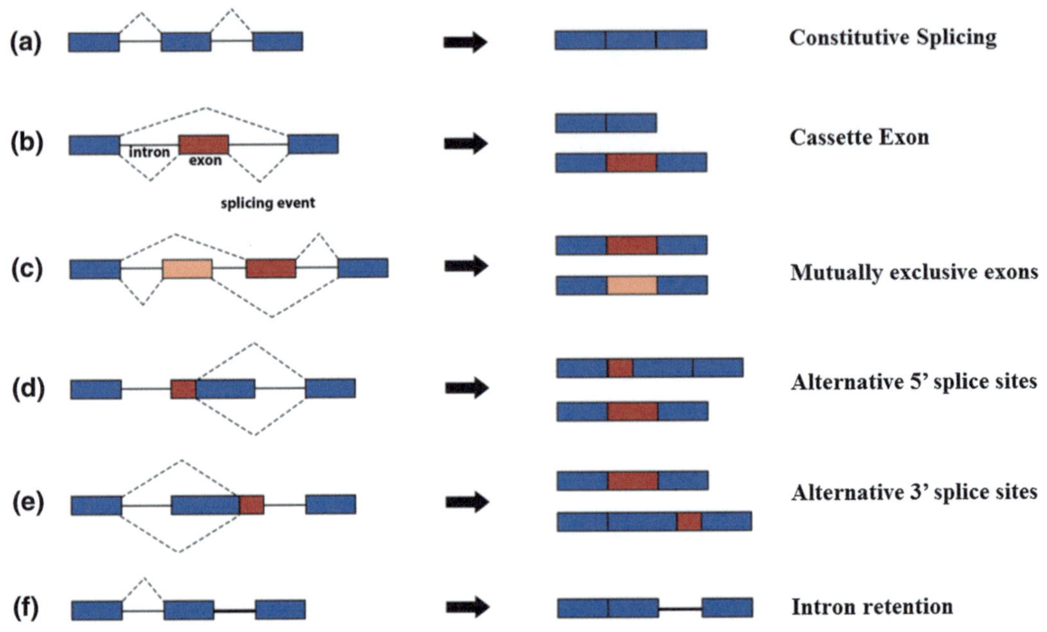

Fig. 23.1 Main alternative splicing events **a** Constitutive splicing; **b** cassette alternative exon; **c** mutually exclusive exons; **d** alternative 5′ splice site; **e** alternative 3′ splice site and **f** intron retention

important role in regulating cellular processes in a tissue-specific manner (Black 2003; Pan et al. 2008). In particular, recent high-throughput sequencing technologies revealed that about 92–94 % of human genes are alternatively spliced (Blencowe 2006; Pan et al. 2008; Wang et al. 2011; Irimia and Blencowe 2012). In this process, inclusion or exclusion of exons or portions of exons or introns within a pre-mRNA transcript can result in multiple protein isoforms being encoded by a single gene. This process is tightly regulated in normal cells. Most exons are constitutive, being always spliced or included in the mature mRNA (Fig. 23.1a). However, aberrant regulation of AS may result in several diseases including cancer. The major alternative splicing patterns or events (Fig. 23.1b–f) are grouped into five types. If an exon is sometimes excluded or included, this indicates that the exon expression is regulated and also termed as cassette exon (Fig. 23.1b). In some cases, cassette exons are mutually exclusive (Fig. 23.1c); this might hold true for more than one exons. Exons can be longer or shorter affecting their splice sites. Alterations in 5′-terminal exons result in alternative promoter sites (Fig. 23.1d). On the other hand, alternative splicing of the 3′-terminal exons can lead to alternative polyadenylation sites (Fig. 23.1e). In addition, some regulatory events result in inclusion of an intron, a splicing pattern called intron retention (Fig. 23.1f).

Aberrant alternative splicing events in cancer may impact the alteration of genes and proteins both at the expression and functional level. These events are regulated by a complex process involving the core spliceosome machinery and multiple regulatory factors (Irimia and Blencowe 2012). A schematic was depicted in Fig. 23.2 to summarize the key regulatory players at the exon level.

The core spliceosome machinery is a large dynamic macromolecular RNA-protein complex composed of five small nuclear RNAs (snRNAs) and over 100 associated proteins. The association of these small RNAs with the protein factors comprise the RNA-protein-complex called small nuclear ribonucleic proteins (snRNPs). Splice sites of a gene are the binding sites for the spliceosome machinery. Splicing factors (SFs), a subset of RNA binding proteins (RBPs), control

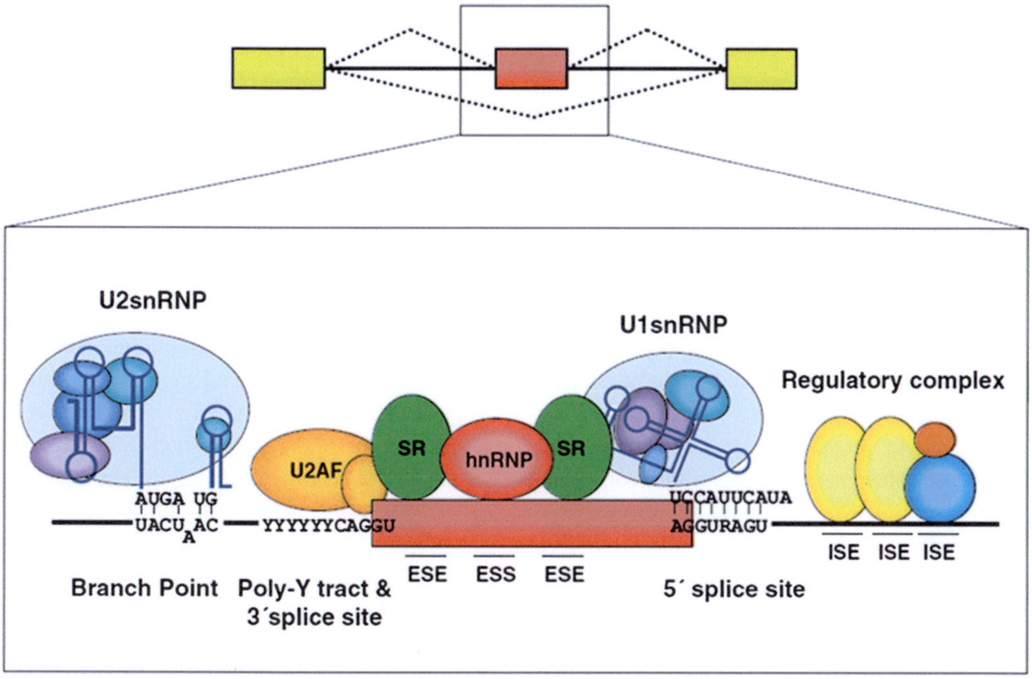

Fig. 23.2 Schematic representation of core spliceosomal components and its binding proteins. Splicing factors can either promote or repress splice site selection depending on the location of their binding sites with respect to splicing signals. *ISE* Intronic splicing\enhancer; *ISS* Intronic splicing silencer; *ESE* Exonic splicing enhancer; *ESS* Exonic splicing silencer; SR, Ser/Arg-repeat containing protein; *hnRNP* Heterogeneous ribonucleoprotein (hnRNP); and U2AF, U2 snRNP auxiliary factor. Adapted from Irimia and Blencowe Current Opinion in Cell Biology

the choice of splice sites and impact the recruitment of the spliceosome to splice sites (Chen and Weiss 2015; Liu and Cheng 2013; Zhang and Manley 2013; Cartegni et al. 2002; Irimia and Blencowe 2012). SFs exert their effect by binding specific RNA sequences, or motifs, known as exonic splicing enhancers (ESEs), exonic splicing silencers (ESS), intronic splicing enhancers (ISEs) and intronic splicing silencers (ISSs) (Cartegni et al. 2002; Irimia and Blencowe 2012). Bound SFs can either activate or inhibit the interaction between spliceosome and pre-mRNAs (McManus and Graveley 2011). Some of them can have dual function based on the location of the motifs they bind. Several splicing factors have been well established in humans (Venables et al. 2008; Twyffels et al. 2011), and categorized into two major families: serine-arginine protein (SR) and heterogeneous ribonucleoprotein (hnRNP). SRs usually promotes splicing, while hnRNPs usually inhibit the splicing process by binding to silencer sequences (Cartegni et al. 2002; David and Manley 2010; Irimia and Blencowe 2012). The decision of alternative splicing also requires cis-acting RNA splicing regulatory elements (SREs) which influence the splicing of exons/introns in the mRNA (Cho et al. 2014). Cis-acting regulatory elements are located on 200–300 nucleotides adjacent to observed splice sites. They also can alter splicing by binding to different *trans*-acting proteins which are remotely located and act as splicing enhancers or silencers. The ultimate decision for splicing regulation is combinatorial and context-dependent based on the cooperation and competition of splicing factors. All these factors increase the diversity and functional capacity of a gene during post-transcriptional processing and exert tight gene regulation.

Mutations of SF genes or alterations in expression levels of the proteins may contribute to aberrant AS. These proteins are guided by additional factors that can also interact with mRNAs at specific motifs to regulate the inclusion or exclusion of exons in the final transcript. Alterations in the levels and activity of these SFs thus provide another means of AS deregulation. Changes in splice sites or motifs of SFs in a given gene may also affect the alternative splicing. Besides binding to SFs, other characteristics of the protein may be altered including ligand binding, enzymatic activity, subcellular localization, and/or protein-protein interactions. This further may alter many processes that can switch cells from normal to malignant phenotype.

Deregulation of alternative splicing due to these factors may result in cancers including breast cancer. Several studies have revealed splice variants specific to tumors in several cancers including breast cancer which impact hallmarks of cancer such as proliferation, apoptosis, cell-cycle-control, metabolism, angiogenesis, and invasion (Chen and Weiss 2015; Dutertre et al. 2010; Germann et al. 2012; Swami et al. 2009; Liu and Cheng 2013; Oltean and Bates 2014; Venables et al. 2008; Zhang and Manley 2013). In this chapter, we will review the regulatory factors and alternative splicing events in breast cancer, its promises and limitations in the clinical practice.

23.2 Alternative Splicing in Breast Cancer

23.2.1 Mutations in RNA Splicing Factors

Recent next-generation sequencing technologies have revealed the presence of somatic mutations in the components of spliceosome machinery and splicing factors (Malcovati et al. 2011; Papaemmanuil et al. 2011; Yoshida and Ogawa 2014; Yoshida et al. 2011). These mutations mostly involve components that are involved in the initial steps of pre-mRNA splicing, such as 3' splice-site recognition and occur in a mutually exclusive manner. Among the mutated splicing factors, *U2AF1, SRSF2, SF3B1, and ZRSR2* genes were common mutational hotspots in myeloid neoplasms such as myelodysplastic syndrome (MDS). Although these mutations were frequent (45–85 %) in myeloid neoplasms, they exist in other hematologic malignancies and solid tumors, albeit at different frequencies (Quesada et al. 2012; Ramsay et al. 2013; Scott and Rebel 2013; Wang et al. 2011; Yoshida and Ogawa 2014). Mutations in splicing factor 3b, subunit 1 (*SF3B1*) occurred in 15 % of chronic lymphocytic leukemias (CLLs) (Quesada et al. 2012), and in solid cancers such as uveal melanomas (9.7 %) (Furney et al. 2013; Harbour et al. 2013), pancreatic cancers (4 %) (Biankin et al. 2012), and breast cancers (2 %) (Cancer Genome Atlas 2012; Stephens et al. 2012). Mutations in other splicing genes, such as the U2 small nuclear RNA auxiliary factor 1 gene (*U2AF1*), the serine/arginine-rich splicing factor 2 gene (*SRSF2*), and the U2 small nuclear ribonucleoprotein auxiliary factor 35 kDa subunit-related protein 2 gene (*ZRSR2*), have also been identified in a lower frequency than *SF3B1* mutations (Yoshida and Ogawa 2014; Yoshida et al. 2011).

SF3B1 is the only splicing factor that has been reported to be among the top 35 mutated genes using next-generation sequencing on 510 breast tumors (Cancer Genome Atlas 2012). However, the frequency was low (2 % of all tumors). Of the 15 non-silent mutations, the majority were missense mutations. Patients with estrogen receptor ER+ and HER-2+ subtypes harbored the majority of these mutations. The *SF3B1* was also among the 18 significantly mutated genes in untreated ER+ breast tumors from 77 patients accrued from two neo-adjuvant aromatase inhibitor clinical trials (Ellis et al. 2012). A recent study re-analyzed the mutations in spliceosomal components using public exome and whole genome sequencing data (Maguire et al. 2015). Their data also confirmed that *SF3B1* was the most commonly mutated gene in the spliceosomal complex in breast cancer, in particular in ER + breast tumors. Furthermore, *SF3B1* mutations were associated with differential splicing of genes in ER+ breast tumors including

TMEM14C, *RPL31*, *DYNLL1*, *UQCC*, *ABCC5* and *CRNDE*. Some of these splice variants have also been observed in other cancers with *SF3B1* mutations (Furney et al. 2013).

23.2.2 Altered Gene Expression Levels in RNA Splicing Factors

Accumulating evidence implicates that aberrant expression of genes regulating alternative splicing is another factor that impacts the alternative splicing events in breast cancer. In our study, the splicing factor *SF3B1* was upregulated in acquired endocrine resistant models as well as in cases with Onco*type* DX high-recurrence scores (Gokmen-Polar et al. 2015). However, we did not observe any prognostic correlation of *SF3B1* expression in our analyses using breast tumors from TCGA and Affymetrix microarray datasets. Interestingly, splicing factor 3b, subunit 3 (*SF3B3*), a SF3B subunit interacting with SF3B1, was also upregulated in these models. As in the case of *SF3B1*, high expression of *SF3B3* correlated with the Onco*type* DX high-recurrence cases. In contrast to *SF3B1*, high expression of *SF3B3* correlated with poor prognosis in patients with ER+ breast cancer.

Other alterations in expression of splicing factors or components of spliceosome machinery, have also been reported in breast cancer (Grosso et al. 2008). These alterations are assumed to affect the splicing pattern of other genes that are involved in tumor development and progression. Alternatively, they might act as oncogenes. For example, splicing factor SF2/ASF is upregulated in various human tumors, and impacts alternative splicing of the tumor suppressor *BIN1* and the kinases *MNK2* and *S6K1*. While *BIN1* isoforms lost their tumor-suppressor activity, the *MNK2* isoform promotes MAPK-independent eIF4E phosphorylation and the *S6K1* isoform has demonstrated oncogenic properties (Karni et al. 2007).

Heterogeneous ribonucleoproteins (hnRNPs) are another major group of splicing factors that are involved in different steps of pre-mRNA processing and cellular functions (Carpenter et al. 2006; Grosso et al. 2008). The hnRNP proteins are also involved in various biological processes required for tumor progression. Splicing factor *SRSF1* is upregulated in human breast tumors, and its overexpression promotes transformation of mammary cells (Anczukow et al. 2015). A recent study reported the expression profile of ten splicing factors (both SRs and hnRNPs) and eight RNA-binding proteins in breast cancer cells (Silipo 2015). Taken together, these studies emphasize that alterations (mutations or altered expression) in core spliceosomal complex genes and its associated genes may contribute to aberrant alternative splicing in breast cancer progression.

23.3 Alternative Splicing Events in Breast Cancer

Aberrant alternative splicing events have been associated with the initiation and progression in breast cancer (Dutertre et al. 2010). We will enumerate some examples for each type of alternative splicing events and emphasize their contribution in breast cancer development and progression (Table 23.1).

23.3.1 Cassette Exons

23.3.1.1 Exon Skipping

The breast cancer susceptibility genes, *BRCA1* and *BRCA2*, are good illustrative examples for exon skipping. *BRCA1* RNAs from most tumors show splicing alterations (Bonnet et al. 2008; Easton et al. 2007; Lovelock et al. 2006; Tommasi et al. 2008; Caux-Moncoutier et al. 2009; Anczukow et al. 2008). For example, the full-length *BRCA1* gene encodes 24 exons. Exon 18 skipping in *BRCA1* can enhance (SF2/ASF) or inhibit (hnRNPA1 and hnRNPH/F) binding of splicing factors to the mRNA (Liu et al. 2001; Millevoi et al. 2010). In addition, skipping of exon 11 has been associated with cell death and proliferation. Besides exon 11 and 18 skipping, other splice variants of *BRCA1* have been

Table 23.1 Aberrant alternative splicing events in breast cancer

Gene name	Alternative splicing event	References
BRCA1	**Cassette exon** Skipping of exon 18 and exon 11 IRIS isoform- skipping of multiple exons	Liu et al (2001), Millevoi et al. (2010), Tammaro et al. (2012), Ahlborn et al. (2015), Romero et al. (2015)
CD44	**Cassette exon** Inclusion of variable exons 9 (exon 6–14) in humans	Inoue and Fry (2015), Olsson et al. (2011), Screaton et al. (1993)
FGFR2	**Mutually exclusive exons** FGFR2 IIIb or IIIc	Fletcher et al (2013)
HER-2	**Intron retention** Herstatin-retention of intron 18, p100-retention of intron 15	Jackson et al. (2013), Doherty et al. (1999), Aigner et al. (2001)
Bcl- 2-like Bcl-xL versus Bcl-xS	**Alternative 5′ splice sites** 5′ splice sites in exon 2	Boise et al. (1993), Adams and Cory (2007), Akgul et al. (2004)
VEGF	**Alternative 3′ splice sites** Proximal/distal 3′ splice site	Biselli-Chicote et al. (2012), Harper and Bates (2008), Nowak et al. (2008)

identified including *BRCA1* full length (inclusion of all exons), partial skipping of exon 11, skipping of exons 9, 10, and partial skipping of exon 11 and IRIS isoforms (skipping of exons 12–24, but retaining a short segment from intron 11) (Tammaro et al. 2012). Additional studies are emerging regarding novel *BRCA1* variants inducing splicing defects (Ahlborn et al. 2015; Romero et al. 2015; Tammaro et al. 2012). However, the clinical significance of these variants and the relevance of these mutations are unknown. With the exception of IRIS, the importance of other *BRCA1* splicing events in cancer development needs to be further determined.

23.3.1.2 Exon Inclusion and Complex Splicing Patterns

CD44, a cell surface receptor, has been gained attention as a breast cancer stem cell marker and chemo-resistance and is under extensive study as a therapeutic target. CD44 has been used as biomarkers to identify and characterize the breast cancer stem cell (CSC) phenotype (Al-Hajj et al. 2003; Shipitsin et al. 2007). Breast cancer cells with *CD44+/CD24-* subpopulation express higher levels of pro-invasive genes and have highly invasive properties specific to ER− cell lines (Sheridan et al. 2006). However, overexpression of *CD44* has been implicated in both tumor suppression and progression (Horak et al. 2008). Relevance of *CD44* in breast carcinomas is still unclear in part due to the complex splice pattern observed in breast cancer.

CD44 pre-mRNA contains 19 exons, 9 of which are alternatively spliced (Loh et al. 2015). Based on the inclusion of variable exons, a number of isoforms are generated. The standard isoform of *CD44 (CD44s)* contains 10 constant exons (exons 1–5 and 15–20), whereas the variant *CD44v* isoforms includes exons 5a and 14 (exon v1–v10). Exon 5a (v1) is not expressed in humans (Screaton et al. 1993; Inoue and Fry 2015). Several groups have assessed the role of *CD44* in breast cancer progression in vivo using mouse models (Brown et al. 2011; Warzecha et al. 2009). Different splice variants of *CD44* have also been associated with different subtypes of breast cancer (Olsson et al. 2011). High expression of standard (CD44s) isoform was present in tumors with strong HER-2 staining and in a subgroup of basal-like tumors. Expression was associated with ALDH1 expression. In contrast, other *CD44* variants are associated with luminal A subtype and with tumors with high CD44+/CD24- subpopulation. In breast cancer cell lines, the untransformed (MCF10A) and non-metastatic (MCF-7) cell lines harbor different isoform pattern (*CD44v6* isoform, which includes all of the v6-containing mRNA isoforms- c5v6v7v8v9v10c6) compared to metastatic MDA-MB-231 cell lines. The splicing factor epithelial splicing regulatory protein 1 (*ESRP1*) and *hnRNPA1* are important in controlling the *CD44* isoform switch and critical for regulating the EMT phenotype in cell line models (Warzecha et al. 2009). The switch of *CD44v* to *CD44s* variants has been reported to induce EMT phenotype (Brown et al. 2011). In contrast, other studies reported that *CD44v* isoforms can mediate metastasis (Zhang et al. 2014, 2015; Tjhay et al. 2015). Orthotropic transplantation of a *CD44v*(+) subpopulation of 4T1 breast cancer cells, but not that of a *CD44v*(−) subpopulation, in mice results in efficient lung metastasis accompanied by expansion of stem-like cancer cells proving the role of the variant isoform in cancer metastasis (Yae et al. 2012). In summary, *CD44* splicing is very complex and further analysis is necessary to understand the role of *CD44* splice variants in breast cancer.

23.3.2 Mutually Exclusive Exons

Fibroblast Growth Factor Receptor 2 (*FGFR2*), a member of the fibroblast growth factor receptors, has been shown to be altered in breast cancer (Fletcher et al. 2013). *FGFR2* is one of the examples in breast cancer where the alternative splicing of two mutually exclusive exons (FGFR2 IIIb or IIIc) alters its ligand binding ability and its biological function. Switching of FGFR2 IIIb to IIIc plays a role in EMT process and results in mammary tumor development (Cha et al. 2008; Moffa et al. 2004; Wei et al. 2012).

23.3.3 Intron Retention

Intron retention is common in most of the tumors except in breast tumors (Dvinge and Bradley 2015). Breast tumors were associated with decreased intron retention relative to normal controls. For example, Herstatin is a naturally occurring truncated HER-2 protein generated from alternative *HER-2* mRNA transcripts that retain intron 8 (Jackson et al. 2013; Doherty et al. 1999). Herstatin can act as an inhibitor of full-length HER-2 by interfering with dimerization, and tyrosine phosphorylation (Guidi et al. 1997). In particular, Herstatin levels are significantly higher in noncancerous breast cells compared to carcinoma cells (Koletsa et al. 2008), p100, another truncated HER2 mRNA splice variant, exhibits the retention of intron 15 and inhibits the tumor cell proliferation and oncogenic signaling (Aigner et al. 2001). Further studies are necessary to understand its prognostic and predictive value in breast cancer.

23.3.4 Alternative 5′ Splice Sites

The apoptosis regulator gene Bcl-2-like 1 or Bcl-x, which belongs to the Bcl-2 family of proteins, can act as an anti-apoptotic (Bcl-xL) or pro-apoptotic (Bcl-xS) protein by regulating caspase activation. These two isoforms are generated based on the alternative splicing pattern of Bcl-x in the 5′ splice sites in exon 2. Overexpression of the longer isoform Bcl-xL has been reported in several cancers including breast cancer, whereas the shorter isoform Bcl-xS is downregulated in cancer (Boise et al. 1993; Adams and Cory 2007; Akgul et al. 2004; Cloutier et al. 2008; Ma et al. 2010). The alternative splicing of Bcl-x has been well documented in affecting survival or evading apoptosis, one of the key hallmarks of cancer (Hanahan and Weinberg 2000, 2011).

23.3.5 Alternative 3′ Splice Sites

Vascular endothelial growth factor (VEGF) is a well-known stimulator of tumor angiogenesis, tumor growth and metastasis in cancer, all of which are hallmarks of cancer. Overexpression of VEGF is an early event in breast cancer progression and a prerequisite step to tumor invasion (Guidi et al. 1997). Elevated expression of VEGF can be associated with shorter relapse-free survival and overall survival times in breast cancer patients with both positive and negative lymph nodes (Gasparini et al. 1997; Konecny et al. 2004; Relf et al. 1997). *VEGF* pre-mRNA is regulated by alternative splicing (Biselli-Chicote et al. 2012; Harper and Bates 2008). The *VEGF* gene contains eight exons having two competing 3′ splice sites (proximal and distal) in exon 8 (Houck et al. 1991). The proximal 3′ splice site of exon 8 generates the *VEGF* isoforms that are pro-angiogenic, whereas the distal 3′ splice site produces the *VEGF*β isoforms that are anti-angiogenic. Splicing factors *SRSF1* and *SRSF5* (SRp40) have been shown to control the splicing of *VEGF* exon 8 proximal 3′ splice site and promote the production of *VEGF* (Nowak et al. 2008). *VEGF* splicing is complex and alternative splicing of other exons (exon 6 and 7) increases its functional diversity.

23.4 Future Directions; Promises and Limitations

High throughput technologies such as massively parallel RNA-sequencing have emphasized the importance of alternative splicing in biological models and human disease by providing an extensive information of small RNAs and associated proteins that are involved in RNA splicing process. Alterations of these proteins by mutations or gene expression level affect the alternative splicing events leading to altered function and protein-protein interactions of several proteins. In particular, mutations in spliceosome components have opened new therapeutic opportunities in cancer. Much work needs to be done to understand the clinical utility of key splice variants in tumor development, progression and metastasis. In particular, major challenges need to be overcome to remove significant bottlenecks for the clinical utility of cancer-specific splice variants. First, computational biology methods need to be refined and standardized among the different databases and platforms. Second, identification of gene expression alterations at the exon level need to be coupled with biological endpoints such as proliferation, apoptosis or recurrence/metastasis. For example, in breast cancer, a decrease in the proliferation rate following neoadjuvant endocrine therapies can be associated with alterations at the exon level. Exon markers can unravel the dual roles of some of the prognostic and predictive markers in breast cancer initiation, progression and metastasis. Third, experimental models need to be developed that can determine and validate the biological significance of these exon markers. However, the complexity arises when multiple exons are skipped or included. This might suggest that it is important to not only identify clinical significance at the exon level as well as at the transcript level. Fourth, databases at the transcript level need to be developed from tumors of retrospective and prospective clinical trials with the outcome follow-up. These databases are critical to understand their ultimate clinical utility both at the discovery and validation stage.

In conclusion, overcoming of all of these challenges requires the extensive collaboration of computational scientists, mathematicians, cancer biologists, pathologists and clinicians.

References

Adams JM, Cory S (2007) The Bcl-2 apoptotic switch in cancer development and therapy. Oncogene 26 (9):1324–1337. doi:10.1038/sj.onc.1210220

Ahlborn LB, Dandanell M, Steffensen AY, Jonson L, Nielsen FC, Hansen TV (2015) Splicing analysis of 14

BRCA1 missense variants classifies nine variants as pathogenic. Breast Cancer Res Treat 150(2):289–298. doi:10.1007/s10549-015-3313-7
Aigner A, Juhl H, Malerczyk C, Tkybusch A, Benz CC, Czubayko F (2001) Expression of a truncated 100 kDa HER2 splice variant acts as an endogenous inhibitor of tumour cell proliferation. Oncogene 20 (17):2101–2111. doi:10.1038/sj.onc.1204305
Akgul C, Moulding DA, Edwards SW (2004) Alternative splicing of Bcl-2-related genes: functional consequences and potential therapeutic applications. Cell Mol Life Sci 61(17):2189–2199. doi:10.1007/s00018-004-4001-7
Al-Hajj M, Wicha MS, Benito-Hernandez A, Morrison SJ, Clarke MF (2003) Prospective identification of tumorigenic breast cancer cells. Proc Natl Acad Sci U S A 100(7):3983–3988. doi:10.1073/pnas.0530291100
Anczukow O, Akerman M, Clery A, Wu J, Shen C, Shirole NH, Raimer A, Sun S, Jensen MA, Hua Y, Allain FH, Krainer AR (2015) SRSF1-regulated alternative splicing in breast cancer. Mol Cell 60 (1):105–117. doi:10.1016/j.molcel.2015.09.005
Anczukow O, Buisson M, Salles MJ, Triboulet S, Longy M, Lidereau R, Sinilnikova OM, Mazoyer S (2008) Unclassified variants identified in BRCA1 exon 11: consequences on splicing. Genes Chromosomes Cancer 47(5):418–426. doi:10.1002/gcc.20546
Biankin AV, Waddell N, Kassahn KS, Gingras MC, Muthuswamy LB, Johns AL, Miller DK, Wilson PJ, Patch AM, Wu J, Chang DK, Cowley MJ, Gardiner BB, Song S, Harliwong I, Idrisoglu S, Nourse C, Nourbakhsh E, Manning S, Wani S, Gongora M, Pajic M, Scarlett CJ, Gill AJ, Pinho AV, Rooman I, Anderson M, Holmes O, Leonard C, Taylor D, Wood S, Xu Q, Nones K, Fink JL, Christ A, Bruxner T, Cloonan N, Kolle G, Newell F, Pinese M, Mead RS, Humphris JL, Kaplan W, Jones MD, Colvin EK, Nagrial AM, Humphrey ES, Chou A, Chin VT, Chantrill LA, Mawson A, Samra JS, Kench JG, Lovell JA, Daly RJ, Merrett ND, Toon C, Epari K, Nguyen NQ, Barbour A, Zeps N, Australian Pancreatic Cancer Genome I, Kakkar N, Zhao F, Wu YQ, Wang M, Muzny DM, Fisher WE, Brunicardi FC, Hodges SE, Reid JG, Drummond J, Chang K, Han Y, Lewis LR, Dinh H, Buhay CJ, Beck T, Timms L, Sam M, Begley K, Brown A, Pai D, Panchal A, Buchner N, De Borja R, Denroche RE, Yung CK, Serra S, Onetto N, Mukhopadhyay D, Tsao MS, Shaw PA, Petersen GM, Gallinger S, Hruban RH, Maitra A, Iacobuzio-Donahue CA, Schulick RD, Wolfgang CL, Morgan RA, Lawlor RT, Capelli P, Corbo V, Scardoni M, Tortora G, Tempero MA, Mann KM, Jenkins NA, Perez-Mancera PA, Adams DJ, Largaespada DA, Wessels LF, Rust AG, Stein LD, Tuveson DA, Copeland NG, Musgrove EA, Scarpa A, Eshleman JR, Hudson TJ, Sutherland RL, Wheeler DA, Pearson JV, McPherson JD, Gibbs RA, Grimmond SM (2012) Pancreatic cancer genomes reveal aberrations in axon guidance pathway genes. Nature 491(7424):399–405. doi:10.1038/nature11547
Biselli-Chicote PM, Oliveira AR, Pavarino EC, Goloni-Bertollo EM (2012) VEGF gene alternative splicing: pro- and anti-angiogenic isoforms in cancer. J Cancer Res Clin Oncol 138(3):363–370. doi:10.1007/s00432-011-1073-2
Black DL (2003) Mechanisms of alternative pre-messenger RNA splicing. Annu Rev Biochem 72:291–336. doi:10.1146/annurev.biochem.72.121801.161720
Blencowe BJ (2006) Alternative splicing: new insights from global analyses. Cell 126(1):37–47. doi:10.1016/j.cell.2006.06.023
Boise LH, Gonzalez-Garcia M, Postema CE, Ding L, Lindsten T, Turka LA, Mao X, Nunez G, Thompson CB (1993) bcl-x, a bcl-2-related gene that functions as a dominant regulator of apoptotic cell death. Cell 74(4):597–608
Bonnet C, Krieger S, Vezain M, Rousselin A, Tournier I, Martins A, Berthet P, Chevrier A, Dugast C, Layet V, Rossi A, Lidereau R, Frebourg T, Hardouin A, Tosi M (2008) Screening BRCA1 and BRCA2 unclassified variants for splicing mutations using reverse transcription PCR on patient RNA and an ex vivo assay based on a splicing reporter minigene. J Med Genet 45 (7):438–446. doi:10.1136/jmg.2007.056895
Brown RL, Reinke LM, Damerow MS, Perez D, Chodosh LA, Yang J, Cheng C (2011) CD44 splice isoform switching in human and mouse epithelium is essential for epithelial-mesenchymal transition and breast cancer progression. J Clin Invest 121(3):1064–1074. doi:10.1172/JCI44540
Cancer Genome Atlas N (2012) Comprehensive molecular portraits of human breast tumours. Nature 490 (7418):61–70. doi:10.1038/nature11412
Carpenter B, MacKay C, Alnabulsi A, MacKay M, Telfer C, Melvin WT, Murray GI (2006) The roles of heterogeneous nuclear ribonucleoproteins in tumour development and progression. Biochim Biophys Acta 1765(2):85–100. doi:10.1016/j.bbcan.2005.10.002
Cartegni L, Chew SL, Krainer AR (2002) Listening to silence and understanding nonsense: exonic mutations that affect splicing. Nat Rev Genet 3(4):285–298. doi:10.1038/nrg775
Caux-Moncoutier V, Pages-Berhouet S, Michaux D, Asselain B, Castera L, De Pauw A, Buecher B, Gauthier-Villars M, Stoppa-Lyonnet D, Houdayer C (2009) Impact of BRCA1 and BRCA2 variants on splicing: clues from an allelic imbalance study. Eur J Hum Genet 17(11):1471–1480. doi:10.1038/ejhg.2009.89
Cha JY, Lambert QT, Reuther GW, Der CJ (2008) Involvement of fibroblast growth factor receptor 2 isoform switching in mammary oncogenesis. Mol Cancer Res 6(3):435–445. doi:10.1158/1541-7786.MCR-07-0187
Chen J, Weiss WA (2015) Alternative splicing in cancer: implications for biology and therapy. Oncogene 34 (1):1–14. doi:10.1038/onc.2013.570

Cho H, Davis J, Li X, Smith KS, Battle A, Montgomery SB (2014) High-resolution transcriptome analysis with long-read RNA sequencing. PLoS ONE 9(9):e108095. doi:10.1371/journal.pone.0108095

Cloutier P, Toutant J, Shkreta L, Goekjian S, Revil T, Chabot B (2008) Antagonistic effects of the SRp30c protein and cryptic 5′ splice sites on the alternative splicing of the apoptotic regulator Bcl-x. J Biol Chem 283(31):21315–21324. doi:10.1074/jbc.M800353200

David CJ, Manley JL (2010) Alternative pre-mRNA splicing regulation in cancer: pathways and programs unhinged. Genes Dev 24(21):2343–2364. doi:10.1101/gad.1973010

Doherty JK, Bond C, Jardim A, Adelman JP, Clinton GM (1999) The HER-2/neu receptor tyrosine kinase gene encodes a secreted autoinhibitor. Proc Natl Acad Sci U S A 96(19):10869–10874

Dutertre M, Vagner S, Auboeuf D (2010) Alternative splicing and breast cancer. RNA Biol 7(4):403–411

Dvinge H, Bradley RK (2015) Widespread intron retention diversifies most cancer transcriptomes. Genome Med 7(1):45. doi:10.1186/s13073-015-0168-9

Easton DF, Deffenbaugh AM, Pruss D, Frye C, Wenstrup RJ, Allen-Brady K, Tavtigian SV, Monteiro AN, Iversen ES, Couch FJ, Goldgar DE (2007) A systematic genetic assessment of 1,433 sequence variants of unknown clinical significance in the BRCA1 and BRCA2 breast cancer-predisposition genes. Am J Hum Genet 81(5):873–883. doi:10.1086/521032

Ellis MJ, Ding L, Shen D, Luo J, Suman VJ, Wallis JW, Van Tine BA, Hoog J, Goiffon RJ, Goldstein TC, Ng S, Lin L, Crowder R, Snider J, Ballman K, Weber J, Chen K, Koboldt DC, Kandoth C, Schierding WS, McMichael JF, Miller CA, Lu C, Harris CC, McLellan MD, Wendl MC, DeSchryver K, Allred DC, Esserman L, Unzeitig G, Margenthaler J, Babiera GV, Marcom PK, Guenther JM, Leitch M, Hunt K, Olson J, Tao Y, Maher CA, Fulton LL, Fulton RS, Harrison M, Oberkfell B, Du F, Demeter R, Vickery TL, Elhammali A, Piwnica-Worms H, McDonald S, Watson M, Dooling DJ, Ota D, Chang LW, Bose R, Ley TJ, Piwnica-Worms D, Stuart JM, Wilson RK, Mardis ER (2012) Whole-genome analysis informs breast cancer response to aromatase inhibition. Nature 486(7403):353–360. doi:10.1038/nature11143

Fletcher MN, Castro MA, Wang X, de Santiago I, O'Reilly M, Chin SF, Rueda OM, Caldas C, Ponder BA, Markowetz F, Meyer KB (2013) Master regulators of FGFR2 signalling and breast cancer risk. Nat Commun 4:2464. doi:10.1038/ncomms3464

Furney SJ, Pedersen M, Gentien D, Dumont AG, Rapinat A, Desjardins L, Turajlic S, Piperno-Neumann S, de la Grange P, Roman-Roman S, Stern MH, Marais R (2013) SF3B1 mutations are associated with alternative splicing in uveal melanoma. Cancer Discov 3 (10):1122–1129. doi:10.1158/2159-8290.CD-13-0330

Gasparini G, Toi M, Gion M, Verderio P, Dittadi R, Hanatani M, Matsubara I, Vinante O, Bonoldi E, Boracchi P, Gatti C, Suzuki H, Tominaga T (1997) Prognostic significance of vascular endothelial growth factor protein in node-negative breast carcinoma. J Natl Cancer Inst 89(2):139–147

Germann S, Gratadou L, Dutertre M, Auboeuf D (2012) Splicing programs and cancer. J Nucleic Acids 2012:269570. doi:10.1155/2012/269570

Gokmen-Polar Y, Neelamraju Y, Goswami CP, Gu X, Nallamothu G, Janga SC, Badve S (2015) Expression levels of SF3B3 correlate with prognosis and endocrine resistance in estrogen receptor-positive breast cancer. Mod Pathol 28(5):677–685. doi:10.1038/modpathol.2014.146

Grosso AR, Martins S, Carmo-Fonseca M (2008) The emerging role of splicing factors in cancer. EMBO Rep 9(11):1087–1093. doi:10.1038/embor.2008.189

Guidi AJ, Schnitt SJ, Fischer L, Tognazzi K, Harris JR, Dvorak HF, Brown LF (1997) Vascular permeability factor (vascular endothelial growth factor) expression and angiogenesis in patients with ductal carcinoma in situ of the breast. Cancer 80(10):1945–1953

Hanahan D, Weinberg RA (2000) The hallmarks of cancer. Cell 100(1):57–70

Hanahan D, Weinberg RA (2011) Hallmarks of cancer: the next generation. Cell 144(5):646–674. doi:10.1016/j.cell.2011.02.013

Harbour JW, Roberson ED, Anbunathan H, Onken MD, Worley LA, Bowcock AM (2013) Recurrent mutations at codon 625 of the splicing factor SF3B1 in uveal melanoma. Nat Genet 45(2):133–135. doi:10.1038/ng.2523

Harper SJ, Bates DO (2008) VEGF-A splicing: the key to anti-angiogenic therapeutics? Nat Rev Cancer 8 (11):880–887. doi:10.1038/nrc2505

Horak CE, Lee JH, Marshall JC, Shreeve SM, Steeg PS (2008) The role of metastasis suppressor genes in metastatic dormancy. APMIS 116(7–8):586–601. doi:10.1111/j.1600-0463.2008.01213.x

Houck KA, Ferrara N, Winer J, Cachianes G, Li B, Leung DW (1991) The vascular endothelial growth factor family: identification of a fourth molecular species and characterization of alternative splicing of RNA. Mol Endocrinol 5(12):1806–1814. doi:10.1210/mend-5-12-1806

Inoue K (2015) Fry EA (2015) Aberrant splicing of estrogen receptor, HER2, and CD44 genes in breast cancer. Genet Epigenet. 2(7):19–32. doi:10.4137/GEG.S35500

Irimia M, Blencowe BJ (2012) Alternative splicing: decoding an expansive regulatory layer. Curr Opin Cell Biol 24(3):323–332. doi:10.1016/j.ceb.2012.03.005

Jackson C, Browell D, Gautrey H, Tyson-Capper A (2013) Clinical significance of HER-2 splice variants in breast cancer progression and drug resistance. Int J Cell Biol 2013:973584. doi:10.1155/2013/973584

Karni R, de Stanchina E, Lowe SW, Sinha R, Mu D, Krainer AR (2007) The gene encoding the splicing factor SF2/ASF is a proto-oncogene. Nat Struct Mol Biol 14(3):185–193. doi:10.1038/nsmb1209

Koletsa T, Kostopoulos I, Charalambous E, Christoforidou B, Nenopoulou E, Kotoula V (2008) A splice variant of HER2 corresponding to Herstatin is expressed in the noncancerous breast and in breast carcinomas. Neoplasia 10(7):687–696

Konecny GE, Meng YG, Untch M, Wang HJ, Bauerfeind I, Epstein M, Stieber P, Vernes JM, Gutierrez J, Hong K, Beryt M, Hepp H, Slamon DJ, Pegram MD (2004) Association between HER-2/neu and vascular endothelial growth factor expression predicts clinical outcome in primary breast cancer patients. Clin Cancer Res 10(5):1706–1716

Liu HX, Cartegni L, Zhang MQ, Krainer AR (2001) A mechanism for exon skipping caused by nonsense or missense mutations in BRCA1 and other genes. Nat Genet 27(1):55–58. doi:10.1038/83762

Liu S, Cheng C (2013) Alternative RNA splicing and cancer. Wiley Interdiscip Rev RNA 4(5):547–566. doi:10.1002/wrna.1178

Loh TJ, Moon H, Cho S, Jang H, Liu YC, Tai H, Jung DW, Williams DR, Kim HR, Shin MG, Liao DJ, Zhou J, Shi W, Zheng X, Shen H (2015) CD44 alternative splicing and hnRNP A1 expression are associated with the metastasis of breast cancer. Oncol Rep 34(3):1231–1238. doi:10.3892/or.2015.4110

Lovelock PK, Healey S, Au W, Sum EY, Tesoriero A, Wong EM, Hinson S, Brinkworth R, Bekessy A, Diez O, Izatt L, Solomon E, Jenkins M, Renard H, Hopper J, Waring P, Tavtigian SV, Goldgar D, Lindeman GJ, Visvader JE, Couch FJ, Henderson BR, Southey M, Chenevix-Trench G, Spurdle AB, Brown MA, kConFab I (2006) Genetic, functional, and histopathological evaluation of two C-terminal BRCA1 missense variants. J Med Genet 43(1):74–83. doi:10.1136/jmg.2005.033258

Ma X, Zhao Y, Li Y, Lu H, He Y (2010) Relevance of Bcl-x expression in different types of endometrial tissues. J Exp Clin Cancer Res 29:14. doi:10.1186/1756-9966-29-14

Maguire SL, Leonidou A, Wai P, Marchio C, Ng CK, Sapino A, Salomon AV, Reis-Filho JS, Weigelt B, Natrajan RC (2015) SF3B1 mutations constitute a novel therapeutic target in breast cancer. J Pathol 235(4):571–580. doi:10.1002/path.4483

Malcovati L, Papaemmanuil E, Bowen DT, Boultwood J, Della Porta MG, Pascutto C, Travaglino E, Groves MJ, Godfrey AL, Ambaglio I, Galli A, Da Via MC, Conte S, Tauro S, Keenan N, Hyslop A, Hinton J, Mudie LJ, Wainscoat JS, Futreal PA, Stratton MR, Campbell PJ, Hellstrom-Lindberg E, Cazzola M, Chronic Myeloid Disorders Working Group of the International Cancer Genome C, of the Associazione Italiana per la Ricerca sul Cancro Gruppo Italiano Malattie M (2011) Clinical significance of SF3B1 mutations in myelodysplastic syndromes and myelodysplastic/myeloproliferative neoplasms. Blood 118(24):6239–6246. doi:10.1182/blood-2011-09-377275

McManus CJ, Graveley BR (2011) RNA structure and the mechanisms of alternative splicing. Curr Opin Genet Dev 21(4):373–379. doi:10.1016/j.gde.2011.04.001

Millevoi S, Bernat S, Telly D, Fouque F, Gladieff L, Favre G, Vagner S, Toulas C (2010) The c.5242C> A BRCA1 missense variant induces exon skipping by increasing splicing repressors binding. Breast Cancer Res Treat 120(2):391–399. doi:10.1007/s10549-009-0392-3

Moffa AB, Tannheimer SL, Ethier SP (2004) Transforming potential of alternatively spliced variants of fibroblast growth factor receptor 2 in human mammary epithelial cells. Mol Cancer Res 2(11):643–652

Nowak DG, Woolard J, Amin EM, Konopatskaya O, Saleem MA, Churchill AJ, Ladomery MR, Harper SJ, Bates DO (2008) Expression of pro- and anti-angiogenic isoforms of VEGF is differentially regulated by splicing and growth factors. J Cell Sci 121(Pt 20):3487–3495. doi:10.1242/jcs.016410

Olsson E, Honeth G, Bendahl PO, Saal LH, Gruvberger-Saal S, Ringner M, Vallon-Christersson J, Jonsson G, Holm K, Lovgren K, Ferno M, Grabau D, Borg A, Hegardt C (2011) CD44 isoforms are heterogeneously expressed in breast cancer and correlate with tumor subtypes and cancer stem cell markers. BMC Cancer 11:418. doi:10.1186/1471-2407-11-418

Oltean S, Bates DO (2014) Hallmarks of alternative splicing in cancer. Oncogene 33(46):5311–5318. doi:10.1038/onc.2013.533

Pan Q, Shai O, Lee LJ, Frey BJ, Blencowe BJ (2008) Deep surveying of alternative splicing complexity in the human transcriptome by high-throughput sequencing. Nat Genet 40(12):1413–1415. doi:10.1038/ng.259

Papaemmanuil E, Cazzola M, Boultwood J, Malcovati L, Vyas P, Bowen D, Pellagatti A, Wainscoat JS, Hellstrom-Lindberg E, Gambacorti-Passerini C, Godfrey AL, Rapado I, Cvejic A, Rance R, McGee C, Ellis P, Mudie LJ, Stephens PJ, McLaren S, Massie CE, Tarpey PS, Varela I, Nik-Zainal S, Davies HR, Shlien A, Jones D, Raine K, Hinton J, Butler AP, Teague JW, Baxter EJ, Score J, Galli A, Della Porta MG, Travaglino E, Groves M, Tauro S, Munshi NC, Anderson KC, El-Naggar A, Fischer A, Mustonen V, Warren AJ, Cross NC, Green AR, Futreal PA, Stratton MR, Campbell PJ, Chronic Myeloid Disorders Working Group of the International Cancer Genome C (2011) Somatic SF3B1 mutation in myelodysplasia with ring sideroblasts. N Engl J Med 365(15):1384–1395. doi:10.1056/NEJMoa1103283

Quesada V, Conde L, Villamor N, Ordonez GR, Jares P, Bassaganyas L, Ramsay AJ, Bea S, Pinyol M, Martinez-Trillos A, Lopez-Guerra M, Colomer D, Navarro A, Baumann T, Aymerich M, Rozman M, Delgado J, Gine E, Hernandez JM, Gonzalez-Diaz M, Puente DA, Velasco G, Freije JM, Tubio JM, Royo R,

Gelpi JL, Orozco M, Pisano DG, Zamora J, Vazquez M, Valencia A, Himmelbauer H, Bayes M, Heath S, Gut M, Gut I, Estivill X, Lopez-Guillermo A, Puente XS, Campo E, Lopez-Otin C (2012) Exome sequencing identifies recurrent mutations of the splicing factor SF3B1 gene in chronic lymphocytic leukemia. Nat Genet 44(1):47–52. doi:10.1038/ng.1032

Ramsay AJ, Rodriguez D, Villamor N, Kwarciak A, Tejedor JR, Valcarcel J, Lopez-Guillermo A, Martinez-Trillos A, Puente XS, Campo E, Lopez-Otin C, Quesada V (2013) Frequent somatic mutations in components of the RNA processing machinery in chronic lymphocytic leukemia. Leukemia 27(7):1600–1603. doi:10.1038/leu.2012.344

Relf M, LeJeune S, Scott PA, Fox S, Smith K, Leek R, Moghaddam A, Whitehouse R, Bicknell R, Harris AL (1997) Expression of the angiogenic factors vascular endothelial cell growth factor, acidic and basic fibroblast growth factor, tumor growth factor beta-1, platelet-derived endothelial cell growth factor, placenta growth factor, and pleiotrophin in human primary breast cancer and its relation to angiogenesis. Cancer Res 57(5):963–969

Romero A, Garcia-Garcia F, Lopez-Perolio I, Ruiz de Garibay G, Garcia-Saenz JA, Garre P, Ayllon P, Benito E, Dopazo J, Diaz-Rubio E, Caldes T, de la Hoya M (2015) BRCA1 Alternative splicing landscape in breast tissue samples. BMC Cancer 15:219. doi:10.1186/s12885-015-1145-9

Scott LM, Rebel VI (2013) Acquired mutations that affect pre-mRNA splicing in hematologic malignancies and solid tumors. J Natl Cancer Inst 105(20):1540–1549. doi:10.1093/jnci/djt257

Screaton GR, Bell MV, Bell JI, Jackson DG (1993) The identification of a new alternative exon with highly restricted tissue expression in transcripts encoding the mouse Pgp-1 (CD44) homing receptor. Comparison of all 10 variable exons between mouse, human, and rat. J Biol Chem 268(17):12235–12238

Sheridan C, Kishimoto H, Fuchs RK, Mehrotra S, Bhat-Nakshatri P, Turner CH, Goulet R Jr, Badve S, Nakshatri H (2006) CD44+/CD24- breast cancer cells exhibit enhanced invasive properties: an early step necessary for metastasis. Breast Cancer Res 8(5):R59. doi:10.1186/bcr1610

Shipitsin M, Campbell LL, Argani P, Weremowicz S, Bloushtain-Qimron N, Yao J, Nikolskaya T, Serebryiskaya T, Beroukhim R, Hu M, Halushka MK, Sukumar S, Parker LM, Anderson KS, Harris LN, Garber JE, Richardson AL, Schnitt SJ, Nikolsky Y, Gelman RS, Polyak K (2007) Molecular definition of breast tumor heterogeneity. Cancer Cell 11(3):259–273. doi:10.1016/j.ccr.2007.01.013

Silipo M, Gautrey H, Tyson-Capper A (2015) Deregulation of splicing factors and breast cancer development. J Mol Cell Biol 7(5): 388–401

Stephens PJ, Tarpey PS, Davies H, Van Loo P, Greenman C, Wedge DC, Nik-Zainal S, Martin S, Varela I, Bignell GR, Yates LR, Papaemmanuil E, Beare D, Butler A, Cheverton A, Gamble J, Hinton J, Jia M, Jayakumar A, Jones D, Latimer C, Lau KW, McLaren S, McBride DJ, Menzies A, Mudie L, Raine K, Rad R, Chapman MS, Teague J, Easton D, Langerod A, Oslo Breast Cancer C, Lee MT, Shen CY, Tee BT, Huimin BW, Broeks A, Vargas AC, Turashvili G, Martens J, Fatima A, Miron P, Chin SF, Thomas G, Boyault S, Mariani O, Lakhani SR, van de Vijver M, van 't Veer L, Foekens J, Desmedt C, Sotiriou C, Tutt A, Caldas C, Reis-Filho JS, Aparicio SA, Salomon AV, Borresen-Dale AL, Richardson AL, Campbell PJ, Futreal PA, Stratton MR (2012) The landscape of cancer genes and mutational processes in breast cancer. Nature 486(7403):400–404. doi:10.1038/nature11017

Swami V, Arteche A, Chamorro-Premuzic T, Maakip I, Stanistreet D, Furnham A (2009) Lay perceptions of current and future health, the causes of illness, and the nature of recovery: explaining health and illness in Malaysia. Br J Health Psychol 14(Pt 3):519–540. doi:10.1348/135910708X370781 308587 [pii]

Tammaro C, Raponi M, Wilson DI, Baralle D (2012) BRCA1 exon 11 alternative splicing, multiple functions and the association with cancer. Biochem Soc Trans 40(4):768–772. doi:10.1042/BST20120140

Tjhay F, Motohara T, Tayama S, Narantuya D, Fujimoto K, Guo J, Sakaguchi I, Honda R, Tashiro H, Katabuchi H (2015) CD44 variant 6 is correlated with peritoneal dissemination and poor prognosis in patients with advanced epithelial ovarian cancer. Cancer Sci 106(10):1421–1428. doi:10.1111/cas.12765

Tommasi S, Pilato B, Pinto R, Monaco A, Bruno M, Campana M, Digennaro M, Schittulli F, Lacalamita R, Paradiso A (2008) Molecular and in silico analysis of BRCA1 and BRCA2 variants. Mutat Res 644(1–2):64–70. doi:10.1016/j.mrfmmm.2008.07.005

Twyffels L, Gueydan C, Kruys V (2011) Shuttling SR proteins: more than splicing factors. FEBS J 278(18):3246–3255. doi:10.1111/j.1742-4658.2011.08274.x

Venables JP, Klinck R, Bramard A, Inkel L, Dufresne-Martin G, Koh C, Gervais-Bird J, Lapointe E, Froehlich U, Durand M, Gendron D, Brosseau JP, Thibault P, Lucier JF, Tremblay K, Prinos P, Wellinger RJ, Chabot B, Rancourt C, Elela SA (2008) Identification of alternative splicing markers for breast cancer. Cancer Res 68(22):9525–9531. doi:10.1158/0008-5472.CAN-08-1769

Wang L, Lawrence MS, Wan Y, Stojanov P, Sougnez C, Stevenson K, Werner L, Sivachenko A, DeLuca DS, Zhang L, Zhang W, Vartanov AR, Fernandes SM, Goldstein NR, Folco EG, Cibulskis K, Tesar B, Sievers QL, Shefler E, Gabriel S, Hacohen N, Reed R, Meyerson M, Golub TR, Lander ES, Neuberg D, Brown JR, Getz G, Wu CJ (2011) SF3B1 and other novel cancer genes in chronic lymphocytic leukemia. N Engl J Med 365(26):2497–2506. doi:10.1056/NEJMoa1109016

Warzecha CC, Sato TK, Nabet B, Hogenesch JB, Carstens RP (2009) ESRP1 and ESRP2 are epithelial cell-type-specific regulators of FGFR2 splicing. Mol Cell 33(5):591–601. doi:10.1016/j.molcel.2009.01.025

Wei W, Liu W, Cassol CA, Zheng W, Asa SL, Ezzat S (2012) The breast cancer susceptibility gene product fibroblast growth factor receptor 2 serves as a scaffold for regulation of NF-kappaB signaling. Mol Cell Biol 32(22):4662–4673. doi:10.1128/MCB.00935-12

Yae T, Tsuchihashi K, Ishimoto T, Motohara T, Yoshikawa M, Yoshida GJ, Wada T, Masuko T, Mogushi K, Tanaka H, Osawa T, Kanki Y, Minami T, Aburatani H, Ohmura M, Kubo A, Suematsu M, Takahashi K, Saya H, Nagano O (2012) Alternative splicing of CD44 mRNA by ESRP1 enhances lung colonization of metastatic cancer cell. Nat Commun 3:883. doi:10.1038/ncomms1892

Yoshida K, Ogawa S (2014) Splicing factor mutations and cancer. Wiley Interdiscip Rev RNA 5(4):445–459. doi:10.1002/wrna.1222

Yoshida K, Sanada M, Shiraishi Y, Nowak D, Nagata Y, Yamamoto R, Sato Y, Sato-Otsubo A, Kon A, Nagasaki M, Chalkidis G, Suzuki Y, Shiosaka M, Kawahata R, Yamaguchi T, Otsu M, Obara N, Sakata-Yanagimoto M, Ishiyama K, Mori H, Nolte F, Hofmann WK, Miyawaki S, Sugano S, Haferlach C, Koeffler HP, Shih LY, Haferlach T, Chiba S, Nakauchi H, Miyano S, Ogawa S (2011) Frequent pathway mutations of splicing machinery in myelodysplasia. Nature 478(7367):64–69. doi:10.1038/nature10496

Zhang J, Manley JL (2013) Misregulation of pre-mRNA alternative splicing in cancer. Cancer Discov 3 (11):1228–1237. doi:10.1158/2159-8290.CD-13-0253

Zhang P, Fu C, Bai H, Song E, Dong C, Song Y (2014) CD44 variant, but not standard CD44 isoforms, mediate disassembly of endothelial VE-cadherin junction on metastatic melanoma cells. FEBS Lett 588 (24):4573–4582. doi:10.1016/j.febslet.2014.10.027

Zhang P, Fu C, Bai H, Song E, Dong C, Song Y (2015) Corrigendum to "CD44 variant, but not standard CD44 isoforms, mediate disassembly of endothelial VE-cadherin junction on metastatic melanoma cells" [FEBS Lett 588(24) (2014) 4573–4582]. FEBS Lett 589(4):553. doi:10.1016/j.febslet.2015.01.016

24 Pharmacogenomics of Breast Cancer

Mark Abramovitz, Casey Williams and Brian Leyland-Jones

Abstract

Pharmacogenomic markers may be able to identify subgroups of patients who will optimally benefit from a particular therapy, other patients who might derive little or no benefit, and/or individuals who are at elevated risk for serious adverse events. It is expected that these studies will enable optimization of risk-benefit ratios for therapeutic agents. In order to fully realize the potential of these markers, it is important to understand the biology underlying drug response. Full realization of the potential of this approach will require the integration of basic discoveries in drug development and pharmacogenomic variability, genomic and outcome data from phase I–III randomized clinical trials, and data on the effects of drugs and their interactions with genomic variants in large populations. In this Chapter, polymorphic genes that have been implicated in both ER-positive and ER-negative cancers will be discussed, as well as other genes that have been implicated through genome-wide association studies (GWAS) in breast cancer.

Keywords

Taxanes CYP2D6 · CYP19A1 · SULTA1 · Aromatases · Tamoxifen · Estrogen receptors

24.1 Introduction

Pharmacogenomics is having an important impact on the clinical management of cancer patients. In breast cancer, these pharmacogenomic markers may be able to identify subgroups of patients who will optimally benefit from a particular therapy, other patients who might derive little or no benefit, and/or individuals who are at elevated risk for serious adverse events. It

M. Abramovitz
VM Institute of Research, Montreal, QC, Canada
e-mail: mark.abramovitz@gmail.com

C. Williams
Avera Cancer Institute, Sioux Falls, SD, USA
e-mail: Casey.Williams@avera.org

B. Leyland-Jones (✉)
Molecular and Experimental Medicine, Avera Cancer Institute, 1000 E 23rd Street, Sioux Falls, SD 57105, USA
e-mail: bleylandj@aol.com

S. Badve and Y. Gökmen-Polar (eds.), *Molecular Pathology of Breast Cancer*, DOI 10.1007/978-3-319-41761-5_24

is expected that discoveries from cancer pharmacogenomics and pharmacoepidemiology research will help optimize the benefit to risk ratio of treatment strategies in clinical practice. The ability to translate these discoveries may more efficiently target therapies to patients who will benefit and avoid or anticipate potentially serious adverse events, among high-risk patients and thus may reduce breast cancer morbidity and mortality as well as reduce the cost of cancer care. Of equal import, these novel discoveries may provide insights into the underlying biology of drug response phenotypes. Full realization of the potential of pharmacogenomics research and the validation of potential pharmacogenomic markers in breast cancer will require the integration of basic discoveries in drug development and pharmacogenomic variability, genomic and outcome data from phase I–III randomized clinical trials, and data on the effects of drugs and their interactions with genomic variants in large populations. In this Chapter, polymorphic genes that have been implicated in tamoxifen, estrogen and taxane activity and metabolism that include CYP2D6, CYP19A1, SULTA1, aromatases and estrogen receptors will be discussed, as well as other genes that have been implicated through genome-wide association studies (GWAS) in breast cancer. Although a great deal of progress has been made, the clinical utility for the most promising pharmacogenomic breast cancer markers is still being investigated and the jury is still out on if and when they will be integrated into clinical practice.

24.2 Tamoxifen Metabolism—The CYP2D6 Story

Tamoxifen, the groundbreaking antiestrogenic medicine targeted to the tumor estrogen receptor (ER), is widely used to prevent recurrence in patients with ER or progesterone receptor (PGR)-positive breast cancer due to its ER blocking effect (Fisher et al. 1996) and has been used as the standard adjuvant endocrine therapy for postmenopausal women with ER and/or PGR-positive breast cancer. Women treated for five years with tamoxifen showed improved disease-free survival (DFS), and tamoxifen reduced the annual breast cancer death rate by 31 % (Early Breast Cancer Trialists' Collaborative et al. 2011; Jordan 2003).

It has also been shown in a number of recent reports from the Breast International Group (BIG) 1-98 trial that adjuvant therapy with the third generation aromatase inhibitor letrozole given as a single agent for five years improves DFS and overall survival (OS) compared with five years of tamoxifen in this population (Breast International Group 1-98 Collaborative et al. 2005; Coates et al. 2007; Colleoni et al. 2011; Group et al. 2009). It has also been determined that there may be groups of patients, for example, those at lower risk for recurrence, for whom tamoxifen or a sequence of the two agents represents a reasonable choice (Group et al. 2009; Viale et al. 2011), and others for whom the availability and/or side effects of aromatase inhibitor therapy make tamoxifen the preferable treatment. Thus, there is considerable interest in defining the population of patients who have the greatest chance of benefiting from tamoxifen. The ability to improve survivorship in ER-positive patients treated with tamoxifen, in an era of personalized medicine, is justification for conducting rigorous investigations.

Tamoxifen is described as a prodrug, given that two of its metabolites, 4-hydroxy-tamoxifen (4-OHT) and 4-hydroxy-N-desmethyltamoxifen (endoxifen) (Fig. 24.1), are formed as a result of hepatic cytochrome P450 2D6 (CYP2D6) metabolism, the rate-limiting enzymatic step in the formation of endoxifen (Fig. 24.2). Both metabolites have an affinity for ER that markedly exceeds that of tamoxifen itself (Johnson et al. 2004). Comprehensive analysis of tamoxifen and 22 of its metabolites confirms that endoxifen is the most abundant and clinically active metabolite of tamoxifen (Jordan et al. 1977; Murdter et al. 2011; Jin et al. 2005; Lim et al. 2005; Wu et al. 2009) with an estrogen receptor affinity that is 100-fold that of tamoxifen (Johnson et al. 2004; Jordan 1982) and serum levels that are 10-fold those of 4-OHT (Gjerde et al. 2005).

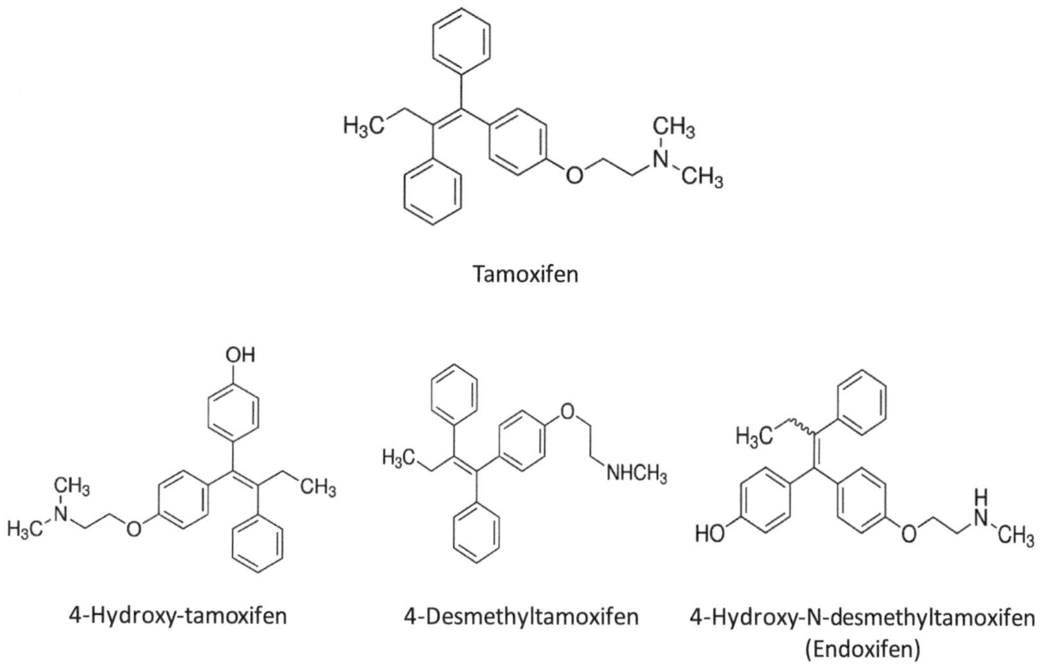

Fig. 24.1 Chemical structures of tamoxifen and three of its metabolites, 4-hydroxy-tamoxifen, 4-desmethyl-tamoxifen and 4-hydroxy-N-desmethyltamoxifen (endoxifen), the most potent and clinically active of the more than 20 metabolites formed through the action of various cytochrome P450s including CYP2D6

Genetic variability of CYP-regulated drug metabolism is common, and this can result in different levels of activity of a given enzyme from normal, to low or null. CYP2D6 (Desta et al. 2004), the main enzyme responsible for 4OH-tamoxifen and endoxifen formation, is encoded by a highly polymorphic gene (Brauch et al. 2009; Desta et al. 2004) with greater than 80 different alleles resulting in reduced or impaired CYP2D6 activity being reported (Sim and Ingelman-Sundberg 2010). CYP2D6 isozymes range in activity from splice variants without metabolic capability to gene duplications that possess 10–30-fold greater activity than that of the wild-type enzyme (Ingelman-Sundberg et al. 2007). Knowledge of the *CYP2D6* genotype facilitates classification of patients as a poor metabolizer (PM), intermediate metabolizer (IM), extensive metabolizer (EM), or ultrarapid metabolizer (UM), specifying the extent of drug metabolism (Zanger et al. 2004).

Early clinical investigation of the pharmacogenetics of tamoxifen metabolism showed promise, and pharmacogenetic testing of the *CYP2D6* phenotype to identify patients with reduced tamoxifen metabolism could predict poorer responsiveness to tamoxifen in terms of disease recurrence (Goetz et al. 2005). A modeling study further suggested that patients with a phenotype of extensive tamoxifen metabolism might receive equal benefit from tamoxifen as from an aromatase inhibitor (Punglia et al. 2008).

With the availability of CYP2D6 pharmacogenetic clinical testing, there is uncertainty among patients, health-care providers, health authorities and insurers about its utility for patient care. The underlying hypothesis is that *CYP2D6* polymorphisms leading to reduced CYP2D6 enzyme activity result in lower plasma concentrations of endoxifen, which adversely affects tamoxifen efficacy and reduces onset of tamoxifen-induced hot flushes. Patients' plasma concentrations of tamoxifen, endoxifen and

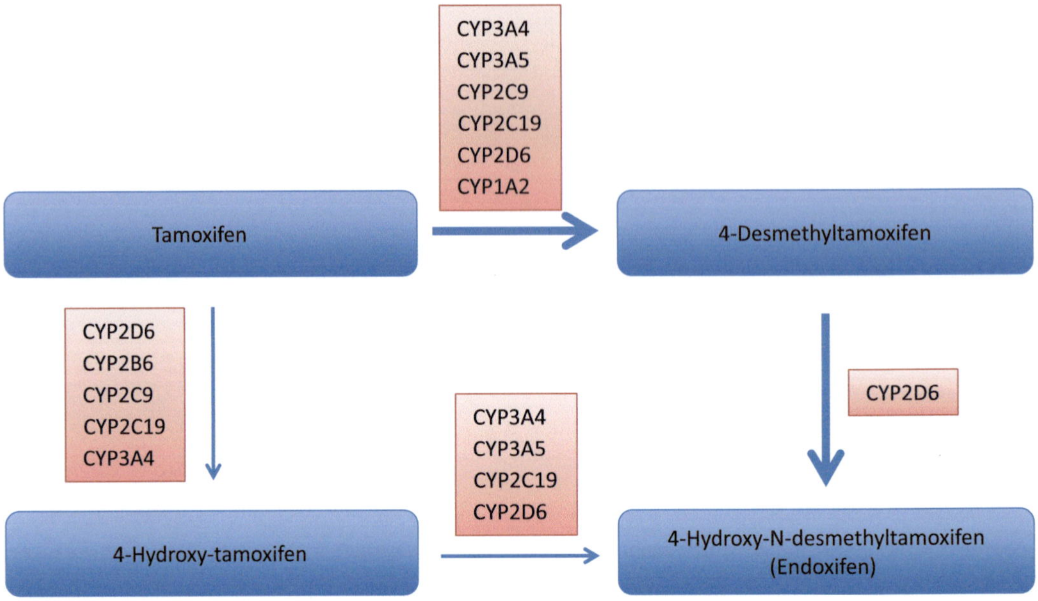

Fig. 24.2 CYP2D6 plays a major role in the metabolism of tamoxifen. It is solely responsible for the metabolism of 4-desmethyltamoxifen to endoxifen, the major active tamoxifen metabolite. Tamoxifen undergoes oxidative metabolism to either *N*-desmethyltamoxifen or 4-hydroxytamoxifen. *N*-desmethyltamoxifen is then activated to endoxifen via metabolism by CYP2D6. Endoxifen undergoes sulfation and glucuronidation before elimination. Abbreviations: *CYP2C9* cytochrome P450 2C9; *CYP2D6* cytochrome P450 2D6; *CYP3A4* cytochrome P450 3A4 enzyme; *CYP3A5* cytochrome P450, family 3, subfamily A, polypeptide 5. Major metabolic pathways are highlighted with *bold arrows*

4-hydroxytamoxifen have been found to vary widely, but studies have indicated that lower endoxifen levels are associated with CYP2D6 reduced metabolism phenotypes (Borges et al. 2006; Jin et al. 2005; Stearns et al. 2003). Lower endoxifen levels are also hypothesized to result in fewer or less severe tamoxifen-induced hot flushes (Bonanni et al. 2006; Goetz et al. 2005; Henry et al. 2009).

However, in more than one dozen subsequent clinical investigations, the results have been conflicting (Ferraldeschi and Newman 2010; Higgins and Stearns 2011) and the evidence base inconclusive. Thus, there has been great inconsistency among studies that have reported the association of known genetic and drug factors influencing CYP2D6 enzyme activity with tamoxifen efficacy (Hertz et al. 2012a).

In a more recent large BIG 1-98 trial, the clinical relevance of the CYP2D6 metabolism phenotype was evaluated (Regan et al. 2012). In this study, unlike previous ones that mostly focused on patients who received tamoxifen without prior chemotherapy, patients were separated according to previous chemotherapy use. Interestingly, no association of CYP2D6 metabolism phenotypes with breast cancer-free interval (BCFI) among postmenopausal patients treated with tamoxifen, with or without prior chemotherapy, was found in the BIG 1-98 trial. Patients who received five years of tamoxifen and were classified as having a PM or IM phenotype did not have poorer disease control than those classified as having an EM phenotype.

Furthermore, a treatment-by-phenotype interaction in the study was not observed; therefore, the magnitude of benefit of letrozole over tamoxifen was the same among EMs as in the study as a whole. This result contradicts the modeling supposition put forth by Punglia et al. (Punglia et al. 2008) that EMs might receive similar or perhaps greater benefit from adjuvant tamoxifen than an aromatase inhibitor. However, in the Austrian Breast and Colorectal Study 8 (ABCSG trial 8), a prospective, multicenter, randomized, open-label trial, postmenopausal women with ER-positive breast cancer with the *CYP2D6* PM/PM phenotype only had significantly higher odds (OR, 2.45; 95 % CI, 1.05–5.73; $P = 0.04$) of having a disease event relative to those with the *CYP2D6* EM/EM phenotype (Goetz et al. 2013). The authors suggested that prospective studies were required to validate the use of the CYP2D6 genotype in the selection of dose, duration or choice of adjuvant hormonal therapy in postmenopausal women with ER-positive, early-stage breast cancer.

A greater incidence of tamoxifen-induced hot flushes was observed in patients with PM and IM *CYP2D6* phenotypes, which is in contrast to the hypothesis that lower endoxifen levels would result in fewer or less severe tamoxifen-induced hot flushes, as observed in 13 patients with *CYP2D6**4/*4 genotype (PM phenotype), none of whom had moderate or severe hot flushes (Goetz et al. 2005). In two additional studies, results have been mixed (Bonanni et al. 2006; Henry et al. 2009), with one of the studies also reporting hot flushes in the IM group (Henry et al. 2009). If there is an association of hot flushes to breast cancer outcome (Cuzick et al. 2008; Mortimer et al. 2008), the mechanism is more likely related to other causes rather than just tamoxifen metabolism.

The role of endoxifen in tamoxifen efficacy is controversial. Several groups have shown that endoxifen has greater affinity for ER than does tamoxifen (Johnson et al. 2004; Jordan 1982), and endoxifen could be the most important tamoxifen metabolite, with higher plasma concentrations than 4-OHT (Borges et al. 2006; Jin et al. 2005; Lim et al. 2005; Stearns et al. 2003) is similar ER affinity (Johnson et al. 2004; Jordan 1982). Furthermore, endoxifen appears to have a different mechanism of action from 4-OHT through targeting ERα for degradation, as opposed to stabilizing ERα, and inhibiting estradiol-mediated upregulation of amphiregulin, an epidermal growth factor receptor ligand (Wu et al. 2009). In fact, endoxifen in the forms of endoxifen citrate (Ahmad et al. 2010) and z-endoxifen hydrochloride (Stearns et al. 2003) is being developed as therapeutics and being evaluated in ongoing clinical trials (clintrials.gov NCT01273168). However, plasma concentrations of endoxifen and 4-hydroxytamoxifen are lower than those of tamoxifen and the primary metabolite N-desmethyltamoxifen (Borges et al. 2006; Jin et al. 2005; Lim et al. 2005; Stearns et al. 2003). Furthermore, tamoxifen and metabolites N-desmethyltamoxifen, didesmethyltamoxifen, and 4-OHT have been estimated to nearly saturate ER with 99.94 % occupancy (Dowsett and Haynes 2003). In addition, ER degradation has not been examined in neoadjuvant tamoxifen trials (Smith et al. 2005). Thus, further elucidation of tamoxifen metabolism and efficacy are needed.

There have been more than 20 published studies that have investigated the potential association between *CYP2D6* polymorphisms and tamoxifen treatment outcomes, with highly variable results. Hertz et al. examined which factors contributed most to these discrepancies and they identified several factors including tamoxifen combination therapy, insufficient genotyping, lack of tamoxifen adherence and CYP2D6 inhibitor coadministration (Ferraldeschi and Newman 2010) that may have accounted for some of the inconsistent results of past pharmacogenomic studies (Hertz et al. 2012a).

One of the issues raised is the concomitant administration of tamoxifen and CYP2D6 inhibitors and whether patients should avoid these inhibitors when possible (Brauch et al. 2009; Ferraldeschi and Newman 2010; Higgins and Stearns 2011), for example, selective serotonin reuptake inhibitors like paroxetine (Stearns et al. 2003). This is based not only on studies showing variation in plasma endoxifen levels according to a CYP2D6 metabolism phenotype that includes CYP2D6 inhibitor drugs but also on the purported association of phenotype with outcome. Although this suggestion is controversial (Lash et al. 2011; Rae et al. 2012), use of CYP2D6 inhibitors will more likely than not complicate the analysis. In a recent study, the Arimidex, Tamoxifen, Alone or in Combination (ATAC) trial, that controlled for the use of potent

CYP2D6 inhibitors, although it did not employ the AmpliChip or incorporate tamoxifen adherence into its analysis, no association between *CYP2D6* genotype and tamoxifen efficacy was found (Rae et al. 2012).

The role of CYP2D6 in premenopausal women is relatively unknown; however, in an analysis of just the premenopausal patients in 17 CYPD26 pharmacogenomic studies (of mostly postmenopausal patients) evaluated by Hertz et al. (2012a), an association between CYP2D6 genotype and tamoxifen efficacy did not appear to be substantial. In a recently published study, however, that investigated a purely premenopausal breast cancer population (306 tamoxifen compliant patients; median age 39 years) and looked at tamoxifen metabolism and germline variations in a number of CYPs, an association was found between endoxifen formation and CYP2D6, irrespective of ethnicity. They also showed that a low endoxifen concentration and decreased CYP2D6 activity predicted shorter distant relapse-free survival (DRFS) (Saladores et al. 2015). Thus, their data support the idea that tamoxifen efficacy in premenopausal breast cancer patients is influenced by CYP2D6-mediated metabolism. Whether this result will be reproducible is currently being tested in an ongoing investigation using pharmacogenetic testing that is targeting premenopausal patients, the Tamoxifen and Exemestane Trial (TEXT; identifier NCT00066703 at clinicaltrials.gov) and Suppression of Ovarian Function Trial (SOFT; identifier NCT00066690 at clinicaltrials.gov).

A major bone of contention regarding the BIG 1-98 and ATAC trials, both of which failed to detect an association between *CYP2D6* genotype and tamoxifen response, raised by Brauch et al. (Brauch et al. 2013), was the fact that in both studies certain CYP2D6 alleles deviated from Hardy-Weinberg equilibrium (HWE) and that the basis for this may have resulted from the genotyping of the tumor (somatic) genome and not the host genome (germline DNA) (Nakamura et al. 2012).

In fact, this is contrary to what has been demonstrated over the past decade by different groups in that *CYP2D6* genotypes derived from tumor versus blood consistently resulted in 100 % concordance (Ahern et al. 2010; Goetz et al. 2005; Rae et al. 2003; Thompson et al. 2011). More recently, Rae et al. showed that CYP2D6 genotyping using DNA prepared from FFPE breast tumor, lymph node sections or blood gave comparable results with high concordance (>94 %) as were the predicted CYP2D6 metabolic phenotypes (>98 %) (Rae et al. 2015), thus establishing convincingly that tumor DNA is appropriate for germline *CYP2D6* genotype determinations.

This would strongly suggest that other factors were at play that could account for the deviations from HWE, which can also occur in large datasets that involve population admixture and germline copy number variants, as happened for example in the study by Schroth et al. (2009). Thus, it has been shown that in other studies, HWE deviations for *CYP2D6*4* were not uniformly or exclusively found in studies using tumor DNA, but occurred as a statistical consequence of combining genotypes from heterogeneous populations (Schroth et al. 2009), as was observed in the multi-institution BIG 1-98 and ATAC studies. In an interesting meta-analysis study that evaluated the association between CYP2D6 inhibition and tamoxifen effectiveness, Cronin-Fenton et al. (2014) found minimal effect of either drug-induced and/or gene-induced inhibition of CYP2D6 activity. They suggested that given the numerous enzymes involved in the complex tamoxifen metabolic pathway, it would be difficult to ascribe the effectiveness of tamoxifen to only one allelic variant in a gene encoding a single enzyme. Taken together, these findings reaffirm the validity of the BIG 1-98 and ATAC analyses and support inclusion of these studies to rigorously assess the association between *CYP2D6* genotypes and tamoxifen efficacy.

Based upon the results from the above studies, there is no compelling data to suggest that the CYP2D6 metabolism phenotype is the correct surrogate for predicting symptoms and outcome of tamoxifen-treated postmenopausal women, and therefore, it is reasonable to conclude that the complex relationship of tamoxifen metabolism with symptoms and disease control is not adequately understood. Based on these collective results, CYP2D6 pharmacogenetic testing has not been recommended to determine whether adjuvant tamoxifen should be given to postmenopausal women with endocrine-responsive breast cancer. The jury is still out with regard to premenopausal women.

Prospective clinical trials are needed to better understand the relationship between CYP2D6 metabolism phenotypes, active metabolite concentrations, and outcomes. An ongoing prospective trial in the United States is the Eastern Cooperative Oncology Group (ECOG) Trial 3108 (clinicaltrials.gov NCT01124695). This phase 2 trial plans to enroll 240 patients with metastatic breast cancer treated with single-agent tamoxifen and the relationship of CYP2D6 activity with progression-free survival (PFS) and response, and of endoxifen concentration with response will be assessed. Dr. Stearns noted that the study has been on hold for over a year after it enrolled 124 patients, but should have metabolite data soon.

Any future studies, though, should ensure that they take into account combination therapy and CYP2D6 inhibition as well as interrogate as many CY2D6 polymorphisms as possible using, for example, the AmpliChip in assessing a more comprehensive set of CYP2D6 alleles.

24.3 SULT1A1

Phase II sulfotransferase enzymes (SULTs) are involved in the breakdown and clearance of tamoxifen, another key component of its metabolism in addition to CYP2D6. Active tamoxifen metabolites are converted to inactive and soluble metabolites by UDP-glucuronosyl-transferase (UGT) and sulfotransferase 1A1 (SULT1A1).

The human phenol *SULT* gene, *SULT1A1*, has a functional SNP that confers decreased enzymatic activity and thermostability of the expressed protein when measured in liver or in blood platelets (Ozawa et al. 1998; Raftogianis et al. 1997). This common genetic variant results in the change of arginine to histidine at residue 213 of the translated protein, and the common allele has been designated as *SULT1A1*1* and the variant as *SULT1A1*2*, representing either Arg213 or His213, respectively. There are additional SNPs that have since been identified in *SULT1A1*, as well as other SULT isoforms. A number of *SULT1A1* SNPs have also been identified in both the distal and proximal promoter region that imparts differential promoter activity and platelet enzymatic activity levels (Lin et al. 2012; Ning et al. 2005).

Most pharmacogenomic studies have been conducted on *SULT1A1*, though some of these other SNPs have been investigated in regard to disease etiology, and in the pharmacogenomics of tamoxifen response. With regard to breast cancer risk, a large study was conducted in a mixed population of African-American and Caucasian women (1644 cases/1451 controls), but no association between *SULT1A1* and breast cancer risk was found (Reding et al. 2012). When a large meta-analysis was performed on 14 case–control studies with a total of 8454 cases and 11,800 controls, again no significant overall correlation was uncovered; however, interestingly there was some suggestion that *SULT1A1*2* was a breast cancer risk factor for Asian women (Wang et al. 2010). Similarly, in another larger meta-analysis of 10,362 cases and 14,250 controls there was no association between *SULT1A1* and breast cancer risk (odds ratio (OR) = 1.07, 95 % confidence interval (CI): 0.97–1.17, $p = 0.164$) (Jiang et al. 2010). In this same study though, analysis of just postmenopausal women suggested that there was an increased breast cancer risk associated with *SULT1A1*2* (OR = 1.28, 95 % CI: 1.04–1.58, $p = 0.019$), but not among premenopausal breast cancer women (OR = 1.06, 95 % CI: 0.88–1.27, $p = 0.537$). Jiang et al. (2010) performed a subgroup analysis by race and also found a significant increase in breast cancer risk among Asian women (OR = 2.03, 95 % CI: 1.00–4.14, $p = 0.051$) in the recessive model.

In a third large meta-analysis (9881 cases/13,564 controls), and consistent with the above two meta-analysis studies, there was no significant association of *SULT1A1* with breast cancer risk (Sun et al. 2011). A number of factors may have contributed to the lack of association given that studies that were included in these meta-analyses used different selection methods and analysis criteria and did not consider potential confounding gene–environment interactions that could profoundly alter the *SULT1A1* phenotype. What will be needed going forward are large-scale studies among different ethnic groups with the necessary environmental data, otherwise it will be almost impossible to truly determine the role that *SULT1A1* genetic variability plays in relation to breast cancer risk.

Few studies, however, have examined the pharmacogenomic role in breast cancer patients that genes encoding for these enzymes play in terms of response to tamoxifen, even though it has been established that tamoxifen and its metabolites undergo phase II conjugation reactions including glucuronidation and sulfation. SULT1A1, for which 4-OH-tamoxifen and endoxifen are known substrates (Hildebrandt et al. 2009; Nowell et al. 2005), has the potential to markedly influence the efficacy of tamoxifen (Hildebrandt et al. 2009).

An early report in 2002, in which an association between the SULT1A1*2 allele and OS in a cohort of 337 women with breast cancer who received tamoxifen (n = 160) or who did not (n = 177) was assessed, indicated that *SULT1A1*1* was significantly associated with improved OS in breast cancer patients receiving adjuvant tamoxifen therapy (Nowell et al. 2002). In a subsequent study, 677 tamoxifen-treated postmenopausal patients with breast cancer, of whom 238 were randomized to either two or five years of tamoxifen, were genotyped. No association was found between the *SULT1A1* genotype with recurrence-free survival (RFS) at five years (Wegman et al. 2007). In another study, researchers reported an increased risk of recurrence and death in tamoxifen-treated patients with variation in SULT1A1 and UGT2B15 alleles (Nowell et al. 2005). However, in the Italian Tamoxifen Prevention Trial, an association of variants of SULT1A1 with tamoxifen efficacy could not be shown (Serrano et al. 2011). This null association between SULT1A1 copy number and DFS was also reported in another small study (Moyer et al. 2011).

The mechanistic basis for any potential improved outcomes associated with the high activity *SULT1A1*2* allele could be attributed to the observation that the sulfated tamoxifen metabolite, 4-OHT, has been shown to induce apoptosis in breast cancer cell lines (Mercer et al. 2010). Mercer et al. showed that within 24 h of treatment with 4-OHT, an 80 % increase in apoptosis occurred in SULT1A1-expressing cells, but not in cells similarly treated that did not express SULT1A1. In this case, rapid sulfation of an active metabolite of tamoxifen in breast tumor cells could result in an increase in apoptosis and hence, could potentially improve survival in individuals with the high activity *SULT1A1* genotype. Later studies, however, have not supported the involvement of *SULT1A1* genotype or copy number in tamoxifen response. One study did report improved OS with the *SULT1A1*2* allele (Tengstrom et al. 2012) in patients also receiving chemotherapy. All of these studies were done with small cohorts of patients and exhibited heterogeneity in terms of disease stage and patient ethnicity. Larger studies will be necessary to truly define the role that the *SULT1A1* genotype plays, if any, in the tamoxifen response.

24.4 CYP19A1 and Estrogen Metabolism

The *CYP19A1* gene encodes the enzyme aromatase, which is responsible for the final step in the biosynthesis of estrogens (Fig. 24.3). This complex gene has many polymorphic and splice variants. Several of these polymorphisms have been associated with abnormal activity of aromatase (Ma et al. 2005), breast cancer risk (Tempfer et al. 2006), aromatase inhibitor-associated arthralgia (Mao et al. 2011) and bone mineral density (Enjuanes et al. 2006; Napoli et al. 2005; Zarrabeitia et al. 2004). Relationships between genetic variants of ERs and their ligand, the hormone estrogen, and the enzymes that synthesize it, are not well understood. There are a number of genetically determined variants in sex steroid hormone pathways

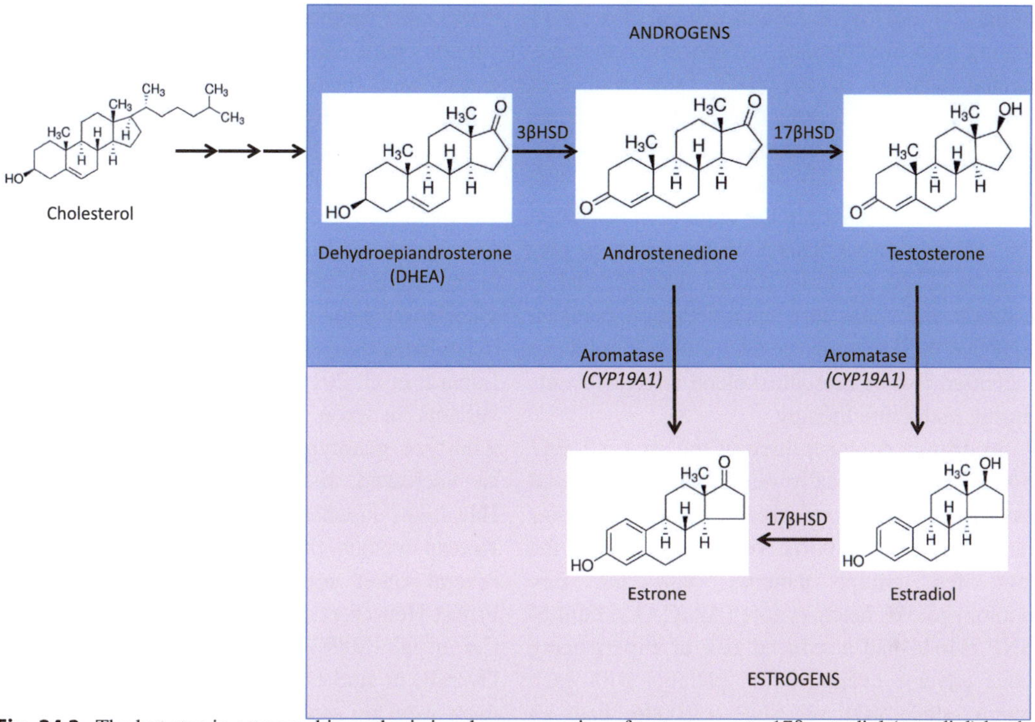

Fig. 24.3 The last step in estrogen biosynthesis involves conversion of testosterone to 17ß-estradiol (estradiol) by the aromatase enzyme encoded by the *CYP19A1* gene. Abbreviations: *CYP19A1* cytochrome P450 19A1; *17βHSD* 17β-hydroxysteroid dehydrogenase; *3βHSD* 3β-hydroxysteroid dehydrogenase

that have recently been connected to several measures of health status (e.g. circulating hormone concentrations, menstrual cycle profiles, lipids, diabetes mellitus, depressive symptoms, measures of cognition, bone mineral density and vasomotor symptoms) in a community-based population of premenopausal women (Sowers et al. 2006b).

There is also evidence that genetic variation may explain the difference in the degree of side effects among women receiving aromatase inhibitors for early breast cancer. For example, Ingle et al. found that four SNPs (rs7158782, rs7159713, rs2369049 and rs6637820), that were closest to the T-cell leukemia 1A (TCL1A) gene, were associated with a certain degree of musculoskeletal symptoms using a genome-wide association case-control study (Ingle et al. 2010). In a second study, a *CYP19A1* SNP was associated with a decrease in bone mineral density in postmenopausal women with ER-positive breast cancer treated with aromatase inhibitors (Napoli et al. 2013), while in a third study, an association was found between a *CYP19A1* polymorphism and aromatase inhibitor-associated arthralgia in postmenopausal women with ER-positive breast cancer (Mao et al. 2011).

The clinical relevance of *CYP19A1* SNPs in the BIG 1–98 trial comparing adjuvant treatment with letrozole and tamoxifen, alone or in sequence, was investigated in postmenopausal women (Leyland-Jones et al. 2015). In this study, it was hypothesized that *CYP19A1* genotypes that affect enzyme activity would be associated with worse disease outcomes among postmenopausal hormone receptor-positive breast cancer patients, and that the association may vary by type of endocrine therapy. Potential associations between *CYP19A1* SNPs and musculoskeletal adverse events (arthralgia and myalgia) during treatment, and bone adverse events (osteoporosis and bone fractures) during and subsequent to treatment were also investigated. No statistically significant association between any of the *CYP19A1* SNP variants and BCFI or DRFI among postmenopausal, endocrine therapy-treated patients in the BIG 1–98 trial was found. However, it was observed that patients with SNP rs700518 variants CC and TC, compared with those with the wild type TT, had better BCFI and DRFI in the tamoxifen but not in the letrozole group. This SNP has not been previously linked to breast cancer outcome. Interestingly, there was also an association between SNP rs700518 variants CC and TC and an increased risk of musculoskeletal adverse events during endocrine therapy.

In distinct contrast, three of the six *CYP19A1* SNPs had statistically significant differential associations with bone adverse events in patients randomized to tamoxifen versus letrozole. In the tamoxifen group, patients with the rare homozygote or heterozygote (AA/CA) variant of SNP rs4646 had a reduced risk of experiencing bone adverse events, while patients with each minor allele (C) of SNP rs10046 had an increased risk of reporting a bone adverse event. On the other hand, patients with the rare homozygote or heterozygote (GG/GC) variant of SNP rs936308 had a reduced risk of bone adverse events in the letrozole group, in contrast to an increased risk in the tamoxifen group.

Of note, no association between the three most studied SNPs, rs4646, rs10046 and rs700519, and BCFI or DRFI outcomes was detected. In a number of analyses in which these three SNPs have been investigated, conflicting results have been reported, raising the question of whether these SNPs are prognostic or predictive factors in endocrine therapy-treated breast cancer patients (Chen et al. 2008; Fasching et al. 2008; Garcia-Casado et al. 2010; Lunardi et al. 2013; Colomer et al. 2008; Ferraldeschi et al. 2012; Liu et al. 2013a). In one study, (Colomer et al. 2008) only rs4646 was found to be associated with greater efficacy in 67 letrozole-treated advanced hormone receptor-positive breast cancer patients. Patients with the rs4646 SNP variant had median time to progression that was three times that of patients with the wild-type aromatase gene; but whether rs4646 was a prognostic or predictive factor could not be assessed (Colomer et al. 2008). In another study, 95 postmenopausal women with stage II–III ER-positive breast cancer were treated with neoadjuvant letrozole, and only rs4646 was associated with a poor response ($P = 0.03$) (Garcia-Casado et al. 2010); PFS was reduced in patients carrying (CA/AA) variants compared with those with the reference CC variant (Garcia-Casado et al. 2010). In other recent studies, rs4646 was shown to have no association with breast cancer outcome or risk (Clendenen et al. 2013; Ferraldeschi et al. 2012; Lunardi et al. 2013). In addition, rs700519 SNP variants in exon 7, when compared with the wild-type genotype, have been associated with an increased risk of breast cancer among Hawaiian, Japanese (Haiman et al. 2003) and Korean women (Lee et al. 2003). However, in several other reports (Miyoshi et al. 2000; Probst-Hensch et al. 1999; Watanabe et al. 1997; Cai et al. 2008), no association was found. Overall, in studies that were not underpowered, there were no associations found between these three SNPs and disease outcomes.

Very few studies have evaluated the role that *CYP19A1* SNPs play with respect to either musculoskeletal or bone adverse events in postmenopausal women with endocrine-responsive breast cancer. In one study, 390 Caucasian postmenopausal women were genotyped for several SNPs and one 7 and one 8-repeat allele (Mao et al. 2011); 50.8 % reported having an adverse event-associated arthralgia and women carrying at least one 8-repeat allele had a significantly lower risk of having an adverse event-associated arthralgia. They also confirmed previous results (Mao et al. 2009) that women who went into menopause more recently (within five years) were significantly more likely to report having an adverse event-associated arthralgia than those greater than ten years post menopause. Napoli et al. (2013) investigated 97 postmenopausal women with ER-positive breast cancer who were treated with aromatase inhibitors and observed that women with the AA genotype for the *CYP19A1* SNP rs700518 (G/A at Val80) developed significant bone loss at both the lumbar spine and total hip at 12 months relative to patients with the GA/GG variants. On the other hand, no associations between bone AEs and *CYP19A1* SNP rs700518 genotype variants were observed in the study by Leyland-Jones et al. (2015). The reason for the discrepancy between these two studies may be related to the small sample size used in the Napoli et al. study and the subsequently few bone adverse events recorded over the study period. Fontein et al. found that the CYP19A1 SNP rs934635 was associated with increased musculoskeletal adverse events and vasomotor symptoms in patients treated with exemestane (Fontein et al. 2014).

The *CYP19A1* pharmacogenomic studies discussed provide increasing evidence that genes involved in estrogen synthesis may modify outcomes and the risk of adverse events, and enhance both quality of life and survival in women with breast cancer. Furthermore, other genetic factors may influence estradiol concentrations. For example, the gene TSPYL5 has been recently identified through a GWAS to be associated with elevated plasma estradiol in postmenopausal breast cancer patients. SNP rs2583506 was identified and shown to create a functional estrogen response element (ERE). The authors suggested that estradiol-induced expression of TSPYL5 SNP rs2583506 might play a potential role, acting as a transcription factor, in modulating *CYP19A1* expression along with numerous other genes (Liu et al. 2013b). However, substantiation of any of these *CYP19A1* polymorphisms or genes linked to *CYP19A1* expression that will be clinically useful will require prospective investigations in larger and independent cohorts to confirm these associations between *CYP19A1* SNPs and breast cancer outcomes and adverse events in postmenopausal endocrine-responsive breast cancer patients.

24.5 Estrogen Receptors 1 and 2

The association between ERs and their ligand, the hormone estrogen (17β-estradiol) and the enzymes that synthesize it are poorly understood. The estrogen receptor genes, *ESR1* and *ESR2*, encode for the proteins ERα and ERβ, respectively, which mediate the effects of estrogens and are the therapeutic targets of selective estrogen receptor modulators (SERMs) including tamoxifen, the first targeted breast cancer agent. ER genes are complex with numerous polymorphic and splice variants. Genetically determined variants in sex steroid hormone pathways have recently been related to several measures of health status (i.e. circulating hormone concentrations, menstrual cycle profiles, lipids, diabetes mellitus, depressive symptoms, measures of cognition, BMD and vasomotor symptoms) in a community-based population of premenopausal women (Sowers et al. 2006b). Associations between polymorphisms in the *ESR1* and *ESR2* genes with multiple endocrine-mediated physiological mechanisms including lipid profile (Almeida and Hutz 2008; Hayes et al. 2010; Molvarec et al. 2007; Ntukidem et al. 2008; Sowers et al. 2006a), mammographic density (Crandall et al. 2009), venous thromboembolism (VTE) (Onitilo et al. 2009; Oger et al. 2007), cognition (Yaffe et al. 2009), and inconsistently associated with breast cancer risk and outcomes and bone mineral density (BMD) changes have been reported (Boyapati et al. 2005; Dunning et al. 2009; Gennari et al. 2005; Heilberg et al. 2005; Henry et al. 2010; Li et al. 2010; Rapuri et al. 2006).

No pharmacogenetic studies have been published so far on *ESR1* and *ESR2* polymorphisms and the differential effectiveness or side effect profile of SERMs or aromatase inhibitors in postmenopausal women with breast cancer. The role that *ESR1* and *ESR2* polymorphisms play in breast cancer outcomes and the effects that they exert on BMD in postmenopausal women requires further studies to confirm any effect they may have on other populations.

There are many published studies that have investigated the association of *ESR1* and *ESR2* polymorphisms with breast cancer risk and that have described varied and equivocal results in both Caucasian and Asian populations. Conversely, there has been only one study published on the association of *ERS1* polymorphisms and breast cancer survival (Boyapati et al. 2005), and although no overall association was observed between *ESR* gene polymorphisms and survival in this study, there were interactive effects of *ESR1* gene polymorphisms and ER status on breast cancer survival.

Two of the most extensively studied *ESR1* polymorphisms, rs2234693 and rs9340799 (PvuII and XbaI restriction fragment length polymorphisms (RFLPs), respectively), are found in intron 1, 50 bp apart, and have been investigated with regard to breast cancer risk with equivocal results overall being reported depending on patient ethnicity and age. In an early large-scale population-based case-control study, *ESR1* PvuII and XbaI RFLPs were investigated in 1069 Chinese breast cancer cases ($\sim$64 % ER-positive) and 1166 age-matched controls. The PvuII polymorphism was associated with an increased risk of breast cancer while the XbaI polymorphism was associated with a nonsignificantly elevated risk, which was mainly confined to postmenopausal women (Cai et al. 2003). However, this increase in breast cancer risk was not observed in another study in a similar Chinese population. Furthermore, no association was detected between *ESR1* PvuII and XbaI RFLPs and breast cancer risk among 614 women with breast cancer (Sakoda et al. 2011).

Genotyping of four *ESR1* SNPs, rs746432, rs2234693(PvuII), rs9340799(XbaI) and rs1801132, was performed on 1183 Caucasian postmenopausal women (393 breast cancer cases and 790 controls) from the Study of Osteoporotic Fractures (Wang et al. 2007). A protective effect of SNP rs9340799 (XbaI) was observed, while no statistically significant association was found for any of the other three SNPs and breast cancer risk in this population of postmenopausal women. In a case-control study conducted with a total of 846 pairs (388 Japanese, 79 Japanese Brazilians and 379 non-Japanese Brazilians) in pre and postmenopausal breast cancer women, none of the five *ESR1* SNPs (rs2234693, rs9340799, rs1801132, rs3798577 and rs2228480) or two *ESR2* SNPs (rs4986938 and rs1256049) genotyped were associated with breast cancer risk (Iwasaki et al. 2009). In a large meta-analysis of 1678 breast cancer cases and 1678 general population controls from Asian populations, the association between *ESR1* XbaI and PuvII SNPs and breast cancer risk was evaluated (Li and Xu 2012). The risk of breast cancer was not observed in pre-menopausal and postmenopausal individuals with the rs9340799 (XbaI) polymorphism; however, pre-menopausal breast cancer women with the rs2234693(PvuII) variant had a significantly elevated breast cancer risk, while postmenopausal women showed a non-significant increased risk.

There have also been several studies focused on *ESR2* SNPs and their association with breast cancer risk. In one study, three common *ESR2* polymorphisms, rs1256049 (G1082A), rs4986938 (G1730A) and rs928554 (Cx + 56 A $\rightarrow$ G), were not found to be significantly associated with breast cancer risk in 723 breast cancer cases (323 sporadic and 400 familial cases) (Maguire et al. 2005). In a meta-analysis of the two most commonly studied *ESR2* polymorphisms, rs4986938 and rs2987983 (nine studies of 10,837 cases and 16,021 controls for rs4986938; 8 studies of 11,652 cases and 15,726 controls for rs1256049), rs4986938 AA/AG versus GG was associated with a significant but small decreased breast cancer risk, while rs2987983 was not (Yu et al. 2011). In our study, the *ESR2* SNP rs4986938 was not prognostic or predictive of outcome in tamoxifen or letrozole-treated postmenopausal ER-positive women.

Taken together, the above studies suggest that the population of women involved may influence how *ESR1* and *ESR2* SNPs affect breast cancer risk and that no general conclusion can be drawn as to the role that they might play in breast cancer outcomes in either pre or postmenopausal women.

Musculoskeletal or bone adverse events (i.e., arthralgia, osteoporosis and bone fractures) have been shown to occur in postmenopausal women receiving adjuvant third-generation aromatase inhibitor therapy for hormone-sensitive breast cancer. However, there have been relatively few studies that have investigated the role of *ESR* SNPs as they relate to breast cancer adverse events. Aromatase inhibitors have been shown to profoundly reduce already low circulating estrogen levels in postmenopausal women by a further 80–90 % compared with tamoxifen, which is associated with a modest increase of deleterious effects on the musculoskeletal system, which has been shown to be an important reason for treatment discontinuation (Henry et al. 2008). In a recent study, the *ESR1* SNP rs2234693(PvuII) variants TT and TC were found to be associated with a lower risk of musculoskeletal adverse events, while SNP rs9340799(XbaI) variant TT was associated with a higher risk of musculoskeletal adverse events in 436 postmenopausal Chinese Han women receiving adjuvant AI therapy for early-stage hormone-sensitive breast cancer (Wang et al. 2013).

Both *ESR1* SNP rs2234693(PvuII) and *ESR2* SNP rs4986938 have been found to influence the prevalence of hot flushes in tamoxifen-treated postmenopausal women (Jin et al. 2008). In 297 participants at four months of tamoxifen treatment, postmenopausal women with *ESR1* rs4986938 CC and ESR2 rs4986938 GG genotypes had a 4.6-fold increase in the number of hot flush scores compared to other postmenopausal women. On the other hand, postmenopausal women with the *ESR2* AA genotype were significantly less likely to experience tamoxifen treatment-induced hot flushes than women who carried at least one *ESR2* G allele (Jin et al. 2008).

BMD has also been a concern for women on hormone replacement therapy. A few studies have been published that show that *ESR* SNPs can affect bone loss (Rapuri et al. 2006; Ryan et al. 2012; Salmen et al. 2000). Women with the *ESR1* PvuII genotypes PP and Pp were shown to have a greater risk of relatively fast bone loss after menopause and therefore, may derive more benefit from hormone replacement therapy (Salmen et al. 2000). A later study also found similar results and extended them to include the *ESR1* XX genotype as being associated with lower rates of bone loss and hence would benefit more from hormone replacement therapy (Rapuri et al. 2006). In a more recent study (Ryan et al. 2012), Ryan et al. found that women carrying the C allele of *ESR1* rs2234693(PvuII) had a decreased risk of all-cause mortality with hormone replacement therapy. They also showed in distinct contrast that women who were homozygous for the T allele had a significantly increased risk of cancer-related mortality. The findings were similar for *ESR1* rs9340799(XbaI) and ESR2 rs1271572.

Data from the above studies have implicated polymorphisms in ESR genes affecting outcomes and adverse events. These results provide increasing evidence that genes involved in estrogen signaling and synthesis may affect outcomes and adverse events, which if validated could then be incorporated into a therapeutic strategy that would increase both quality of life and survival in women with breast cancer. Future well-controlled large prospective pharmacogenomic studies will be needed to establish the clinical utility of ESR polymorphisms in breast cancer.

24.6 Pharmacogenetics and Taxane-Related Toxicities

Paclitaxel and docetaxel are taxanes that are highly effective, widely prescribed chemotherapeutic drugs for the treatment of breast cancer in the metastatic, adjuvant and neoadjuvant settings (Gines et al. 2011; Buzdar et al. 1999). A number of pharmacogenes are involved in the pharmacokinetics and pharmacodynamics of taxanes as depicted in Fig. 24.4. Taxanes block cell division by binding to α-tubulin, which along with β-tubulin, as heterodimers, form microtubules, and act as microtubule-stabilizing agents, which leads to cell death (Huizing et al. 1995; Jordan and Wilson 2004). Furthermore, in vitro studies have shown that taxanes can induce BCL2 phosphorylation and apoptosis, although docetaxel was effective at much lower concentrations than paclitaxel (Haldar et al. 1995, 1997).

Polymorphisms in genes in the taxane pathway have been studied; however, the impact of genetic variants on the taxane response is unclear. In a number of earlier studies, no

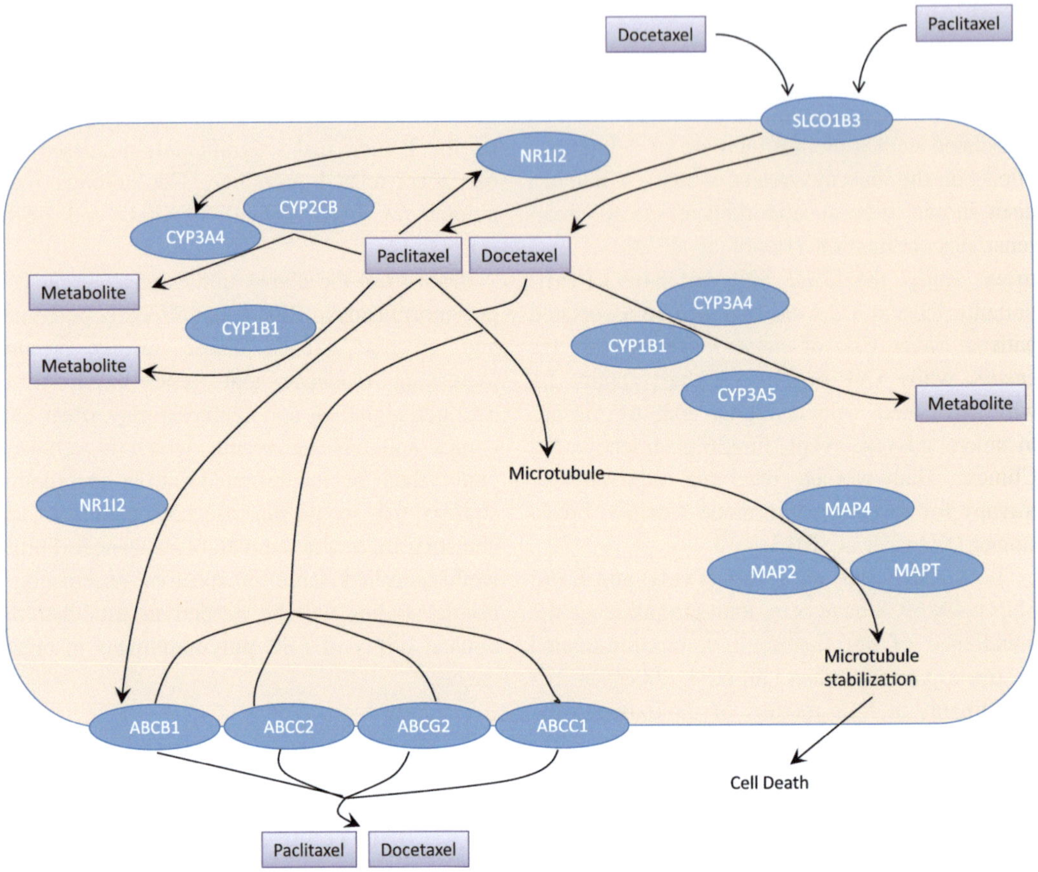

Fig. 24.4 Genes involved in the metabolism and transport of paclitaxel and docetaxel, and the downstream effects of the drugs. OATP1B3 (SLCO1B3) is an influx transporter for docetaxel. Taxanes are substrates for a number of ATP binding cassette multidrug transporters that include ABCB1 (multidrug resistance protein 1), ABCG2, ABCC1 and ABCC2. Cytochrome P450 3A4 enzyme (CYP3A4) is involved in the metabolism of both paclitaxel and docetaxel. Other cytochrome P450s (CYP2CB, CYP1B1, and CYP3A5) are also involved. Both taxanes appear to be substrates for the pregnane X receptor (PXR) that can result in the induction of CYP3A4 and ABCB1. The toxic activity of both paclitaxel and docetaxel involves the stabilization of microtubules that leads to cell death. Other abbreviations: *MAP2* microtubule-associated protein 2; *MAP4* microtubule-associated protein 4; *MAPT* microtubule-associated protein tau

definitive associations related to taxane response were found. For example, in a study of 93 patients with high-risk primary or stage IV breast cancer, who received dose-intense paclitaxel, doxorubicin and cyclophosphamide, no association between eight polymorphisms in six genes associated with metabolism and transport of paclitaxel and taxane response was found (Marsh et al. 2007). This study assessed polymorphisms in ABCB1, ABCG2, CYP1B1, CYP3A4, CYP3A5 and CYP2C8 genotypes and paclitaxel clearance.

In some studies, though, associations between polymorphisms of genes in the taxane pathway and either patient survival or drug response were observed. SNPs in CYP1B1 and ABCB1 were found to be correlated with survival of breast cancer patients. One study found rs1056836, CYP1B1*3 (4326 C > G; L432 V) allele, was significantly associated with PFS, independent of paclitaxel clearance (Marsh et al. 2007). In one study of patients with metastatic breast cancer, the synonymous variant rs1045642 (ABCB1: 3435 C > T) showed a significantly lower disease control rate and a lower overall survival rate than the CC genotype for the variant allele (Chang et al. 2009).

Taxane-induced peripheral neuropathy (TIPN) is a common AE associated with taxanes that often leads to therapeutic disruption and patient discomfort, which involves a tingling or burning sensation in the extremities that can lead to irreversible loss of function if treatment is continued (Postma et al. 1995). Many breast cancer patients are long-term survivors; therefore, ensuring that long-term TIPN does not develop, which could potentially compromise their quality of life, is an important therapeutic objective. Clinically, if a patient experiences grade 2 + neurotoxicity, paclitaxel therapy is usually stopped.

The main enzyme involved in the metabolism of paclitaxel is CYP2C8 (Rahman et al. 1994), which has been shown to correlate with exposure to paclitaxel in cancer patients (Hertz et al. 2012b). The CYP2C8*3 variant (rs11572080 R139 K and rs10509681 K399R) has been shown to display decreased paclitaxel metabolic activity that leads to increased drug exposure (Bergmann et al. 2011).

The notion that patients who were CYP2C8*3 carriers could have an increased risk of paclitaxel-induced neuropathy was first raised in an ovarian study by Green et al. (Green et al. 2009), which was subsequently shown in a breast cancer study carried out by Leskela et al. in a cohort of Spanish paclitaxel-treated cancer patients (n = 118), in which patients homozygous for the CYP2C8*3 allele were at a significantly increased neuropathy risk (Leskela et al. 2011). However, this was not confirmed in a study by Rizzo et al. (2010), in which 95 patients affected by breast cancer were treated with taxanes as adjuvant, metastatic or neo-adjuvant therapy. In their analysis, however, they combined patients on either paclitaxel (24 %) or docetaxel (76 %) and analyzed these groups together. Even though docetaxel has both structural and mechanistic similarities with paclitaxel, it does not have the higher incidence of neurotoxicity and in fact is not metabolized by CYP2C8. In the study by Hertz et al. (2013), they specifically tested the hypothesis that the CYP2C8*3 variant increases risk of paclitaxel-induced neuropathy in two cohorts (n = 411), one European-American (n = 209) and the other African-American (n = 107), that received neoadjuvant and/or adjuvant paclitaxel-containing regimens. The single SNP that was analyzed, the CYP2C8*3 K399R (rs10509681) variant, was found to increase the risk of grade 2+ paclitaxel-induced neuropathy in both cohorts and this approximate doubling was consistent across racial groups. This finding is clinically relevant in that patients, either heterozygous or homozygous for the CYP2C8*3 allele, would be at an increased risk of neuropathy and this may inform the use of an alternate to paclitaxel and/or the clinical management of this toxicity.

An alternative method for discovering polymorphisms that influence treatment outcome is the GWAS. This approach enables the simultaneous interrogation of a huge amount of the known genetic variation in humans. The benefit of a GWAS over the candidate gene approach is that it does not require previous knowledge of the genomic regions to be examined for alleles of interest.

Baldwin et al. published the first GWAS based on the largest prospective breast cancer pharmacogenetic study of paclitaxel treatment toxicities, reporting an association between an *FGD4* SNP and the onset of TIPN in a paclitaxel-treated discovery cohort (n = 855) from the CALGB 40101 phase 3 clinical trial randomized study comparing cyclophosphamide and doxorubicin versus single-agent paclitaxel as adjuvant therapy for patients with breast cancer at relatively low risk for relapse and two smaller independent replication cohorts, one European (n = 154) and African American (n = 117) (Baldwin et al. 2012). The *FGD4* rs10771973 SNP is located in the intronic region and is in tight linkage disequilibrium with a number of other SNPs. It was found to increase the risk of neuropathy by 57 % in the discovery cohort (hazard ratio [HR]: 1.57; 95 % CI: 1.30–1.91; $p = 2.6 \times 10^{-6}$) and an even larger increase in risk was detected in independent cohorts of European (HR: 1.72; 95 % CI: 1.06–2.80;

$p = 0.013$) and African–American (HR: 1.93; 95 % CI: 1.13–3.28; $p = 6.7 \times 10^{-3}$) patients. *FGD4* encodes for the protein FGD1-related F-actin binding protein (Frabin), a widely expressed guanine nucleotide exchange factor for Cdc42, a small rhoGTPase that regulates cellular morphogenesis, including myelination. *FGD4* has previously been linked with the congenital Charcot–Marie–Tooth disease, a condition that resembles TIPN, providing a plausible biological explanation for their finding. Other intriguing SNPs related to the onset or severity of neuropathy that were also identified in this study included *EPHA5* (rs7349683) and *FZD3* (rs10771973), although they did not meet genome-wide significance.

Perhaps surprisingly, no significant associations were observed for any SNPs residing in the candidate genes, including CYP2C8, known to influence paclitaxel metabolism that could alter paclitaxel pharmacokinetics and hence be involved in determining genetic susceptibility to this toxicity. The FGD4 variant, if validated, has potential to be used as a genetic predictor of paclitaxel-induced sensory peripheral neuropathy.

In another recent GWAS, Schneider et al. investigated genetic variants to predict TIPN using germline DNA samples from the ECOG-5103, a large phase 3 randomized adjuvant breast cancer trial (n = 4994 patients) and candidate SNPs were further validated using samples from the E1199 trial (Schneider et al. 2015). One SNP (rs3125923) was found to be associated with grade 3–4 TIPN ($p = 1.7 \times 10^{-3}$; OR = 1.8), although it did not meet genome-wide significance. Interestingly, being of African descent and obesity were also identified as independent predictors of this toxicity. The SNP, rs3125923, is a variant in a gene desert on chromosome 1 in a non-coding region of the genome. Functionality of the SNP was not established though a potential link to GPR177, a G-protein coupled receptor, and its expression has been identified through expression quantitative trait loci mapping (Fehrmann et al. 2011). Additional work, however, using other large data sets will be needed to confirm these findings. Dr. Schneider notes that he is planning a meta-analysis of all key reported taxane-related SNPs identified by several breast cancer groups, including SWOG, ECOG-ACRIN, Alliance and PGSNPS, after each of their primary work is published. This is expected to be published in early 2016.

24.7 Pharmacogenomics of Bevacizumab Treatment Breast Cancer

The ability to block angiogenesis has been found to be beneficial in the treatment of multiple malignancies, but to varying degrees depending on the type of cancer (Schneider and Sledge 2007). One of the most clinically tested antiangiogenesis agents is bevacizumab, a humanized monoclonal antibody against vascular endothelial growth factor (VEGF) (Keating 2014). With regard to breast cancer, the E2100, a North American breast intergroup phase 3 trial, examined bevacizumab in the treatment of patients receiving initial chemotherapy for metastatic, HER2-breast cancer (Miller et al. 2007). Patients were randomly assigned to receive weekly paclitaxel with or without bevacizumab as first-line therapy. The addition of bevacizumab was associated with an improved response rate from 21.2–36.9 % ($P = 0.001$) and PFS (the primary endpoint) time from 5.9–11.8 months ($P = 0.001$), but not with an improved mean OS. Grade 3 and 4 hypertension, the main AE associated with bevacizumab treatment, also increased.

An important issue is how to find biomarkers that are associated with efficacy and toxicity of bevacizumab. Hypertension is a common troubling toxicity induced by bevacizumab, which can cause drug discontinuation and requires treatment. The ability to screen patients would allow for closer monitoring with both early intervention and potentially prophylactic antihypertensive therapy as strategic treatment options.

In a study by Schneider et al. (2008), SNPs in the VEGFA gene and its receptor, VEGFR2, were evaluated in a retrospective analysis of samples from the E2100 clinical trial in order to identify such biomarkers. The five VEGFA SNPs were all in regulatory regions (no common non-synonymous polymorphisms have been found in VEGFA) and two non- synonymous exonic SNPs in VEGFR2, all with high minor allele frequencies.

VEGFA—2578 AA (HR = 0.58; 95 % CI, 0.36–0.93; $P = 0.023$) and—1154 AA (HR = 0.62; 95 % CI, 0.46–0.83; $P = 0.001$) genotypes were associated with better median OS in the combination arm when compared with the alternate genotypes combined. Similar effects were seen for PFS but were non-significant. Since no such effect was seen in the control groups, this would suggest that these SNPs had potential predictive value. However, the association between these SNPs in VEGFA and disease outcome in response to bevacizumab was not found in the AVADO study (Miles et al. 2013), despite the disease type (breast cancer) and setting being similar to those in E2100.

Another interesting finding was that two additional genotypes, VEGF-634 CC and VEGF-1498 TT, were associated with significantly less grade 3 or 4 hypertension, the most common non-hematological toxicity, in the combination arm when compared with the alternate genotypes combined (0 % vs. 19–22 %, $P = 0.005$; and 8 % vs. 22–23 %, $P = 0.022$, respectively) in the E2100, and were therefore protected from serious hypertension (Schneider et al. 2008). This association between SNPs in VEGFA and protection from grade 3/4 hypertension was examined using samples from the much larger E5103 phase 3 clinical trial (see below); however, no significant correlation could be found (Schneider et al. 2014) and thus, these prior results could not be validated.

A GWAS was undertaken using germline DNA samples from the ECOG-5103 (described above) that showed a convincing association between bevacizumab-induced hypertension and an intronic SNP in *SV2C* (rs6453204) and was further validated using DNA samples from the E2100 trial (Schneider et al. 2014). The *SV2C* gene encodes synaptic vesicle protein 2 (SV2C), one of three isoforms that make up a small gene family (Janz and Sudhof 1999). Although SNPs in this gene have been associated with some diseases (Hill-Burns et al. 2013; Ramsey et al. 2013) and suggests that SV2C has various biological and pharmacological activities, its role in hypertension is currently unknown. The identified SNP in SV2C, therefore, can be used to predict bevacizumab-induced hypertension and future studies will examine its use in early clinical intervention.

24.8 GWAS and Aromatase Inhibitor-Associated Adverse Effects

GWAS are also being applied to the investigation of pharmacogenetic relationships of AI-associated AEs. In a nested case-control assessment of patients enrolled in NCIC MA.27, a phase 3 trial comparing anastrozole with exemestane, cases with musculoskeletal toxicities or treatment discontinuation due to toxicity were genotyped and GWAS identified four SNPs closest to the TCL1A gene associated with musculoskeletal AEs in women treated with aromatase inhibitors (Ingle et al. 2010). One of the four SNPs (rs11849538) was only 926 bp from the 3' end of the gene and created an ERE (estrogen response element). The authors went on to show that in ERα-transfected cells, TCL1A expression was induced eight-fold at 24 h, with even higher levels of expression of TCL1A induced in lymphoblastoid cell lines containing the variant SNPs when compared with cells having the WT sequence after transient transfection with ERα. How these SNPs, through differential changes in TCL1A expression, might cause MS-AEs is still unknown; however, the relationship between TCL1A and IL17RA expression may be indicative of a role for cytokines and will require future studies to elucidate this intriguing data.

Several GWAS based on prospective cooperative group clinical trials are underway to search for genetic markers predictive of response and toxicity in breast cancer patients (Ingle 2013).

24.9 Conclusion

The ultimate goal of pharmacogenomics studies related to breast cancer is to use the information so that patients with particular germline genotype variants receive the optimal therapy, either selective ER modulators (SERMs) or aromatase inhibitors, for the optimal outcome with the fewest AEs. Clinicians who have at their disposal both genetic and hormonal information are in a better position to help maximize benefits, minimize AEs and determine which patients deserve close follow-up during long-term SERM or AI therapy. There is increasing evidence generated from numerous studies that suggests that estrogen synthesizing and metabolizing genes may modify outcomes and the risk of AEs, which can be applied in the clinical setting to enhance both quality of life and survival of women with breast cancer.

Thus, the promise of identifying which patients would be most likely to benefit from which therapies, and those who will experience significant AEs, remains an exciting prospect and allows us to foresee a time when cancer therapy is tailored not only to tumor characteristics, but also to individual patients' pharmacogenetics.

Though we have made substantial progress in understanding the role of pharmacogenomics in drug safety and efficacy, many questions remain unanswered and the lack of prospective, controlled trials designed to address pharmacogenomic questions that will translate into clinical benefits are still lacking. Several recent publications have called into question the significance of pharmacogenetic effects on outcomes; however, most studies reported to date were not designed to address pharmacogenetic questions, and have been based upon retrospective or monocentric studies with conflicting conclusions. In addition, the fact that most breast cancer patients are treated with several drugs given in combination, is a confounding factor likely to impede the comprehension of the actual impact of a given genetic polymorphism on the clinical outcome (toxicity, response and survival).

Therefore, truly assessing clinical utility will require validation of current hypotheses by prospective data collection. Some commercial tests are available to assess genetic polymorphisms that have been suggested to have pharmacogenetic significance; however, the current body of knowledge is still too limited to recommend testing in current practice. Thus, a great deal more needs to be done and ongoing prospective investigations in larger and independent cohorts will greatly contribute to our understanding of these associations between pharmacogenomics and breast cancer outcomes and AEs in breast cancer patients.

References

Ahern TP, Christensen M, Cronin-Fenton DP et al (2010) Concordance of metabolic enzyme genotypes assayed from paraffin-embedded, formalin-fixed breast tumors and normal lymphatic tissue. Clin Epidemiol 2:241–246

Ahmad A, Shahabuddin S, Sheikh S et al (2010) Endoxifen, a new cornerstone of breast cancer therapy: demonstration of safety, tolerability, and systemic bioavailability in healthy human subjects. Clin Pharmacol Ther 88(6):814–817

Almeida S, Hutz MH (2008) Estrogen receptor 1 gene polymorphisms in premenopausal women: interaction between genotype and smoking on lipid levels. Braz J Med Biol Res 41(10):872–876

Baldwin RM, Owzar K, Zembutsu H et al (2012) A genome-wide association study identifies novel loci for paclitaxel-induced sensory peripheral neuropathy in CALGB 40101. Clin Cancer Res 18(18):5099–5109

Bergmann TK, Brasch-Andersen C, Green H et al (2011) Impact of CYP2C8*3 on paclitaxel clearance: a population pharmacokinetic and pharmacogenomic study in 93 patients with ovarian cancer. Pharmacogenomics J 11(2):113–120

Bonanni B, Macis D, Maisonneuve P et al. (2006) Polymorphism in the CYP2D6 tamoxifen-metabolizing gene influences clinical effect but not hot flashes: data from the Italian Tamoxifen Trial. J Clin Oncol 24 (22):3708–3709; author reply 3709

Borges S, Desta Z, Li L et al (2006) Quantitative effect of CYP2D6 genotype and inhibitors on tamoxifen metabolism: implication for optimization of breast cancer treatment. Clin Pharmacol Ther 80(1):61–74

Boyapati SM, Shu XO, Ruan ZX et al (2005) Polymorphisms in ER-alpha gene interact with estrogen receptor status in breast cancer survival. Clin Cancer Res 11(3):1093–1098

Brauch H, Murdter TE, Eichelbaum M, Schwab M (2009) Pharmacogenomics of tamoxifen therapy. Clin Chem 55(10):1770–1782

Brauch H, Schroth W, Goetz MP et al (2013) Tamoxifen use in postmenopausal breast cancer: CYP2D6 matters. J Clin Oncol 31(2):176–180

Breast International Group 1-98 Collaborative G, Thurlimann B, Keshaviah A et al (2005) A comparison of letrozole and tamoxifen in postmenopausal women with early breast cancer. N Engl J Med 353(26): 2747–2757

Buzdar AU, Singletary SE, Theriault RL et al (1999) Prospective evaluation of paclitaxel versus combination chemotherapy with fluorouracil, doxorubicin, and cyclophosphamide as neoadjuvant therapy in patients with operable breast cancer. J Clin Oncol 17 (11):3412–3417

Cai Q, Shu XO, Jin F et al (2003) Genetic polymorphisms in the estrogen receptor alpha gene and risk of breast cancer: results from the Shanghai Breast Cancer Study. Cancer Epidemiol Biomarkers Prev 12 (9):853–859

Cai Q, Kataoka N, Li C et al (2008) Haplotype analyses of CYP19A1 gene variants and breast cancer risk: results from the Shanghai Breast Cancer Study. Cancer Epidemiol Biomarkers Prev 17(1):27–32

Chang H, Rha SY, Jeung HC et al (2009) Association of the ABCB1 gene polymorphisms 2677G > T/A and 3435C > T with clinical outcomes of paclitaxel monotherapy in metastatic breast cancer patients. Ann Oncol 20(2):272–277

Chen C, Sakoda LC, Doherty JA et al (2008) Genetic variation in CYP19A1 and risk of breast cancer and fibrocystic breast conditions among women in Shanghai. China. Cancer Epidemiol Biomarkers Prev 17 (12):3457–3466

Clendenen T, Zeleniuch-Jacquotte A, Wirgin I et al (2013) Genetic variants in hormone-related genes and risk of breast cancer. PLoS ONE 8(7):e69367

Coates AS, Keshaviah A, Thurlimann B et al (2007) Five years of letrozole compared with tamoxifen as initial adjuvant therapy for postmenopausal women with endocrine-responsive early breast cancer: update of study BIG 1-98. J Clin Oncol 25(5):486–492

Colleoni M, Giobbie-Hurder A, Regan MM et al (2011) Analyses adjusting for selective crossover show improved overall survival with adjuvant letrozole compared with tamoxifen in the BIG 1-98 study. J Clin Oncol 29(9):1117–1124

Colomer R, Monzo M, Tusquets I et al (2008) A single-nucleotide polymorphism in the aromatase gene is associated with the efficacy of the aromatase inhibitor letrozole in advanced breast carcinoma. Clin Cancer Res 14(3):811–816

Crandall CJ, Sehl ME, Crawford SL et al (2009) Sex steroid metabolism polymorphisms and mammographic density in pre- and early perimenopausal women. Breast Cancer Res 11(4):R51

Cronin-Fenton DP, Damkier P, Lash TL (2014) Metabolism and transport of tamoxifen in relation to its effectiveness: new perspectives on an ongoing controversy. Future Oncol 10(1):107–122

Cuzick J, Sestak I, Cella D, Fallowfield L, Group AT (2008) Treatment-emergent endocrine symptoms and the risk of breast cancer recurrence: a retrospective analysis of the ATAC trial. Lancet Oncol 9(12):1143–1148

Desta Z, Ward BA, Soukhova NV, Flockhart DA (2004) Comprehensive evaluation of tamoxifen sequential biotransformation by the human cytochrome P450 system in vitro: prominent roles for CYP3A and CYP2D6. J Pharmacol Exp Ther 310(3):1062–1075

Dowsett M, Haynes BP (2003) Hormonal effects of aromatase inhibitors: focus on premenopausal effects and interaction with tamoxifen. J Steroid Biochem Mol Biol 86(3–5):255–263

Dunning AM, Healey CS, Baynes C et al (2009) Association of ESR1 gene tagging SNPs with breast cancer risk. Hum Mol Genet 18(6):1131–1139

Early Breast Cancer Trialists' Collaborative G, Davies C, Godwin J et al (2011) Relevance of breast cancer hormone receptors and other factors to the efficacy of adjuvant tamoxifen: patient-level meta-analysis of randomised trials. Lancet 378(9793):771–784

Enjuanes A, Garcia-Giralt N, Supervia A et al (2006) A new SNP in a negative regulatory region of the CYP19A1 gene is associated with lumbar spine BMD in postmenopausal women. Bone 38(5):738–743

Fasching PA, Loehberg CR, Strissel PL et al (2008) Single nucleotide polymorphisms of the aromatase gene (CYP19A1), HER2/neu status, and prognosis in breast cancer patients. Breast Cancer Res Treat 112 (1):89–98

Fehrmann RS, Jansen RC, Veldink JH et al (2011) Trans-eQTLs reveal that independent genetic variants associated with a complex phenotype converge on intermediate genes, with a major role for the HLA. PLoS Genet 7(8):e1002197

Ferraldeschi R, Newman WG (2010) The impact of CYP2D6 genotyping on tamoxifen treatment. Pharmaceuticals 3(4):1122

Ferraldeschi R, Arnedos M, Hadfield KD et al (2012) Polymorphisms of CYP19A1 and response to aromatase inhibitors in metastatic breast cancer patients. Breast Cancer Res Treat 133(3):1191–1198

Fisher B, Dignam J, Bryant J et al (1996) Five versus more than five years of tamoxifen therapy for breast cancer patients with negative lymph nodes and estrogen receptor-positive tumors. J Natl Cancer Inst 88(21):1529–1542

Fontein DB, Houtsma D, Nortier JW et al (2014) Germline variants in the CYP19A1 gene are related to specific adverse events in aromatase inhibitor users: a substudy of Dutch patients in the TEAM trial. Breast Cancer Res Treat 144(3):599–606

Garcia-Casado Z, Guerrero-Zotano A, Llombart-Cussac A et al (2010) A polymorphism at the 3'-UTR region of the aromatase gene defines a subgroup of postmenopausal breast cancer patients with poor response to neoadjuvant letrozole. BMC Cancer 10:36

Gennari L, Merlotti D, De Paola V et al (2005) Estrogen receptor gene polymorphisms and the genetics of

osteoporosis: a HuGE review. Am J Epidemiol 161 (4):307–320
Gines J, Sabater E, Martorell C, Grau M, Monroy M, Casado MA (2011) Efficacy of taxanes as adjuvant treatment of breast cancer: a review and meta-analysis of randomised clinical trials. Clin Transl Oncol 13 (7):485–498
Gjerde J, Hauglid M, Breilid H, Lundgren S, Varhaug JE (2005) Relationship between CYP2D6 and SULT1A1 genotypes and serum concen- trations of tamoxifen and its metabolites during steady state treatment in breast cancer patients. In: 28th annual San Antonio breast cancer symposium, San Antonio, TX, 08–11 Dec 2005
Goetz MP, Rae JM, Suman VJ et al (2005) Pharmacogenetics of tamoxifen biotransformation is associated with clinical outcomes of efficacy and hot flashes. J Clin Oncol 23(36):9312–9318
Goetz MP, Suman VJ, Hoskin TL et al (2013) CYP2D6 metabolism and patient outcome in the Austrian Breast and Colorectal Cancer Study Group trial (ABCSG) 8. Clin Cancer Res 19(2):500–507
Green H, Soderkvist P, Rosenberg P et al (2009) Pharmacogenetic studies of paclitaxel in the treatment of ovarian cancer. Basic Clin Pharmacol Toxicol 104 (2):130–137
Group BIGC, Mouridsen H, Giobbie-Hurder A et al (2009) Letrozole therapy alone or in sequence with tamoxifen in women with breast cancer. N Engl J Med 361(8):766–776
Haiman CA, Stram DO, Pike MC et al (2003) A comprehensive haplotype analysis of CYP19 and breast cancer risk: the multiethnic cohort. Hum Mol Genet 12(20):2679–2692
Haldar S, Jena N, Croce CM (1995) Inactivation of Bcl-2 by phosphorylation. Proc Natl Acad Sci USA 92 (10):4507–4511
Haldar S, Basu A, Croce CM (1997) Bcl2 is the guardian of microtubule integrity. Cancer Res 57(2):229–233
Hayes DF, Skaar TC, Rae JM et al (2010) Estrogen receptor genotypes, menopausal status, and the effects of tamoxifen on lipid levels: revised and updated results. Clin Pharmacol Ther 88(5):626–629
Heilberg IP, Hernandez E, Alonzo E et al (2005) Estrogen receptor (ER) gene polymorphism may predict the bone mineral density response to raloxifene in postmenopausal women on chronic hemodialysis. Ren Fail 27(2):155–161
Henry NL, Giles JT, Ang D et al (2008) Prospective characterization of musculoskeletal symptoms in early stage breast cancer patients treated with aromatase inhibitors. Breast Cancer Res Treat 111(2):365–372
Henry NL, Rae JM, Li L et al (2009) Association between CYP2D6 genotype and tamoxifen-induced hot flashes in a prospective cohort. Breast Cancer Res Treat 117 (3):571–575
Henry NL, Nguyen A, Azzouz F et al (2010) Lack of association between oestrogen receptor polymorphisms and change in bone mineral density with tamoxifen therapy. Br J Cancer 102(2):294–300
Hertz DL, McLeod HL, Irvin WJ Jr (2012a) Tamoxifen and CYP2D6: a contradiction of data. Oncologist 17 (5):620–630
Hertz DL, Walko CM, Bridges AS et al (2012b) Pilot study of rosiglitazone as an in vivo probe of paclitaxel exposure. Br J Clin Pharmacol 74(1):197–200
Hertz DL, Roy S, Motsinger-Reif AA et al (2013) CYP2C8*3 increases risk of neuropathy in breast cancer patients treated with paclitaxel. Ann Oncol 24 (6):1472–1478
Higgins MJ, Stearns V (2011) Pharmacogenetics of endocrine therapy for breast cancer. Annu Rev Med 62:281–293
Hildebrandt M, Adjei A, Weinshilboum R et al (2009) Very important pharmacogene summary: sulfotransferase 1A1. Pharmacogenet Genomics 19(6):404–406
Hill-Burns EM, Singh N, Ganguly P et al (2013) A genetic basis for the variable effect of smoking/nicotine on Parkinson's disease. Pharmacogenomics J 13(6):530–537
Huizing MT, Misser VH, Pieters RC et al (1995) Taxanes: a new class of antitumor agents. Cancer Invest 13 (4):381–404
Ingelman-Sundberg M, Sim SC, Gomez A, Rodriguez-Antona C (2007) Influence of cytochrome P450 polymorphisms on drug therapies: pharmacogenetic, pharmacoepigenetic and clinical aspects. Pharmacol Ther 116(3):496–526
Ingle JN (2013) Pharmacogenomics of endocrine therapy in breast cancer. J Hum Genet 58(6):306–312
Ingle JN, Schaid DJ, Goss PE et al (2010) Genome-wide associations and functional genomic studies of musculoskeletal adverse events in women receiving aromatase inhibitors. J Clin Oncol 28(31):4674–4682
Iwasaki M, Hamada GS, Nishimoto IN et al (2009) Isoflavone, polymorphisms in estrogen receptor genes and breast cancer risk in case-control studies in Japanese, Japanese Brazilians and non-Japanese Brazilians. Cancer Sci 100(5):927–933
Janz R, Sudhof TC (1999) SV2C is a synaptic vesicle protein with an unusually restricted localization: anatomy of a synaptic vesicle protein family. Neuroscience 94(4):1279–1290
Jiang Y, Zhou L, Yan T, Shen Z, Shao Z, Lu J (2010) Association of sulfotransferase SULT1A1 with breast cancer risk: a meta-analysis of case-control studies with subgroups of ethnic and menopausal statue. J Exp Clin Cancer Res 29:101
Jin Y, Desta Z, Stearns V et al (2005) CYP2D6 genotype, antidepressant use, and tamoxifen metabolism during adjuvant breast cancer treatment. J Natl Cancer Inst 97 (1):30–39
Jin Y, Hayes DF, Li L et al (2008) Estrogen receptor genotypes influence hot flash prevalence and composite score before and after tamoxifen therapy. J Clin Oncol 26(36):5849–5854
Johnson MD, Zuo H, Lee KH et al (2004) Pharmacological characterization of 4-hydroxy-N-desmethyl tamoxifen, a novel active metabolite of tamoxifen. Breast Cancer Res Treat 85(2):151–159

Jordan VC (1982) Metabolites of tamoxifen in animals and man: identification, pharmacology, and significance. Breast Cancer Res Treat 2(2):123–138

Jordan VC (2003) Tamoxifen: a most unlikely pioneering medicine. Nat Rev Drug Discov 2(3):205–213

Jordan MA, Wilson L (2004) Microtubules as a target for anticancer drugs. Nat Rev Cancer 4(4):253–265

Jordan VC, Collins MM, Rowsby L, Prestwich G (1977) A monohydroxylated metabolite of tamoxifen with potent antioestrogenic activity. J Endocrinol 75 (2):305–316

Keating GM (2014) Bevacizumab: a review of its use in advanced cancer. Drugs 74(16):1891–1925

Lash TL, Cronin-Fenton D, Ahern TP et al (2011) CYP2D6 inhibition and breast cancer recurrence in a population-based study in Denmark. J Natl Cancer Inst 103(6):489–500

Lee KM, Abel J, Ko Y et al (2003) Genetic polymorphisms of cytochrome P450 19 and 1B1, alcohol use, and breast cancer risk in Korean women. Br J Cancer 88(5):675–678

Leskela S, Jara C, Leandro-Garcia LJ et al (2011) Polymorphisms in cytochromes P450 2C8 and 3A5 are associated with paclitaxel neurotoxicity. Pharmacogenomics J 11(2):121–129

Leyland-Jones B, Gray KP, Abramovitz M et al (2015) CYP19A1 polymorphisms and clinical outcomes in postmenopausal women with hormone receptor-positive breast cancer in the BIG 1-98 trial. Breast Cancer Res Treat 151(2):373–384

Li LW, Xu L (2012) Menopausal status modifies breast cancer risk associated with ESR1 PvuII and XbaI polymorphisms in Asian women: a HuGE review and meta-analysis. Asian Pac J Cancer Prev 13(10):5105–5111

Li N, Dong J, Hu Z, Shen H, Dai M (2010) Potentially functional polymorphisms in ESR1 and breast cancer risk: a meta-analysis. Breast Cancer Res Treat 121 (1):177–184

Lim YC, Desta Z, Flockhart DA, Skaar TC (2005) Endoxifen (4-hydroxy-N-desmethyl-tamoxifen) has anti-estrogenic effects in breast cancer cells with potency similar to 4-hydroxy-tamoxifen. Cancer Chemother Pharmacol 55(5):471–478

Lin ZN, Lin YC, Zhang X et al (2012) Differential promoter activities of functional haplotypes in the 5′-flanking region of human sulfotransferase 1A1. J Biochem Mol Toxicol 26(10):422–428

Liu L, Bai YX, Zhou JH et al (2013a) A Polymorphism at the 3′-UTR Region of the Aromatase Gene Is Associated with the Efficacy of the Aromatase Inhibitor, Anastrozole, in Metastatic Breast Carcinoma. Int J Mol Sci 14(9):18973–18988

Liu M, Ingle JN, Fridley BL et al (2013b) TSPYL5 SNPs: association with plasma estradiol concentrations and aromatase expression. Mol Endocrinol 27(4):657–670

Lunardi G, Piccioli P, Bruzzi P et al (2013) Plasma estrone sulfate concentrations and genetic variation at the CYP19A1 locus in postmenopausal women with early breast cancer treated with letrozole. Breast Cancer Res Treat 137(1):167–174

Ma CX, Adjei AA, Salavaggione OE et al (2005) Human aromatase: gene resequencing and functional genomics. Cancer Res 65(23):11071–11082

Maguire P, Margolin S, Skoglund J et al (2005) Estrogen receptor beta (ESR2) polymorphisms in familial and sporadic breast cancer. Breast Cancer Res Treat 94 (2):145–152

Mao JJ, Stricker C, Bruner D et al (2009) Patterns and risk factors associated with aromatase inhibitor-related arthralgia among breast cancer survivors. Cancer 115 (16):3631–3639

Mao JJ, Su HI, Feng R et al (2011) Association of functional polymorphisms in CYP19A1 with aromatase inhibitor associated arthralgia in breast cancer survivors. Breast Cancer Res 13(1):R8

Marsh S, Somlo G, Li X et al (2007) Pharmacogenetic analysis of paclitaxel transport and metabolism genes in breast cancer. Pharmacogenomics J 7(5):362–365

Mercer KE, Apostolov EO, da Costa GG et al (2010) Expression of sulfotransferase isoform 1A1 (SULT1A1) in breast cancer cells significantly increases 4-hydroxytamoxifen-induced apoptosis. Int J Mol Epidemiol Genet 1(2):92–103

Miles DW, de Haas SL, Dirix LY et al (2013) Biomarker results from the AVADO phase 3 trial of first-line bevacizumab plus docetaxel for HER2-negative metastatic breast cancer. Br J Cancer 108(5):1052–1060

Miller K, Wang M, Gralow J et al (2007) Paclitaxel plus bevacizumab versus paclitaxel alone for metastatic breast cancer. N Engl J Med 357(26):2666–2676

Miyoshi Y, Iwao K, Ikeda N, Egawa C, Noguchi S (2000) Breast cancer risk associated with polymorphism in CYP19 in Japanese women. Int J Cancer 89(4):325–328

Molvarec A, Nagy B, Kovacs M et al (2007) Lipid, haemostatic and inflammatory variables in relation to the estrogen receptor alpha (ESR1) PvuII and XbaI gene polymorphisms. Clin Chim Acta 380(1–2):157–164

Mortimer JE, Flatt SW, Parker BA et al (2008) Tamoxifen, hot flashes and recurrence in breast cancer. Breast Cancer Res Treat 108(3):421–426

Moyer AM, Suman VJ, Weinshilboum RM et al (2011) SULT1A1, CYP2C19 and disease-free survival in early breast cancer patients receiving tamoxifen. Pharmacogenomics 12(11):1535–1543

Murdter TE, Schroth W, Bacchus-Gerybadze L et al (2011) Activity levels of tamoxifen metabolites at the estrogen receptor and the impact of genetic polymorphisms of phase I and II enzymes on their concentration levels in plasma. Clin Pharmacol Ther 89(5):708–717

Nakamura Y, Ratain MJ, Cox NJ, McLeod HL, Kroetz DL, Flockhart DA (2012) Re: CYP2D6 genotype and tamoxifen response in postmenopausal women with endocrine-responsive breast cancer: the Breast International Group 1-98 trial. J Natl Cancer Inst 104(16):1264; author reply 1266–1268

Napoli N, Villareal DT, Mumm S et al (2005) Effect of CYP1A1 gene polymorphisms on estrogen metabolism and bone density. J Bone Miner Res 20(2):232–239

Napoli N, Rastelli A, Ma C et al (2013) Genetic polymorphism at Val80 (rs700518) of the CYP19A1 gene is associated with aromatase inhibitor associated bone loss in women with ER + breast cancer. Bone 55 (2):309–314

Ning B, Nowell S, Sweeney C et al (2005) Common genetic polymorphisms in the 5'-flanking region of the SULT1A1 gene: haplotypes and their association with platelet enzymatic activity. Pharmacogenet Genomics 15(7):465–473

Nowell S, Sweeney C, Winters M et al (2002) Association between sulfotransferase 1A1 genotype and survival of breast cancer patients receiving tamoxifen therapy. J Natl Cancer Inst 94(21):1635–1640

Nowell SA, Ahn J, Rae JM et al (2005) Association of genetic variation in tamoxifen-metabolizing enzymes with overall survival and recurrence of disease in breast cancer patients. Breast Cancer Res Treat 91 (3):249–258

Ntukidem NI, Nguyen AT, Stearns V et al (2008) Estrogen receptor genotypes, menopausal status, and the lipid effects of tamoxifen. Clin Pharmacol Ther 83 (5):702–710

Oger E, Lacut K, Mercier B et al (2007) Estrogen receptor alpha polymorphism and venous thromboembolism in male and female: data from the EDITH study. Thromb Res 119(4):433–439

Onitilo AA, McCarty CA, Wilke RA et al (2009) Estrogen receptor genotype is associated with risk of venous thromboembolism during tamoxifen therapy. Breast Cancer Res Treat 115(3):643–650

Ozawa S, Tang YM, Yamazoe Y, Kato R, Lang NP, Kadlubar FF (1998) Genetic polymorphisms in human liver phenol sulfotransferases involved in the bioactivation of N-hydroxy derivatives of carcinogenic arylamines and heterocyclic amines. Chem Biol Interact 109(1–3):237–248

Postma TJ, Vermorken JB, Liefting AJ, Pinedo HM, Heimans JJ (1995) Paclitaxel-induced neuropathy. Ann Oncol 6(5):489–494

Probst-Hensch NM, Ingles SA, Diep AT et al (1999) Aromatase and breast cancer susceptibility. Endocr Relat Cancer 6(2):165–173

Punglia RS, Burstein HJ, Winer EP, Weeks JC (2008) Pharmacogenomic variation of CYP2D6 and the choice of optimal adjuvant endocrine therapy for postmenopausal breast cancer: a modeling analysis. J Natl Cancer Inst 100(9):642–648

Rae JM, Cordero KE, Scheys JO, Lippman ME, Flockhart DA, Johnson MD (2003) Genotyping for polymorphic drug metabolizing enzymes from paraffin-embedded and immunohistochemically stained tumor samples. Pharmacogenetics 13(8):501–507

Rae JM, Drury S, Hayes DF et al (2012) CYP2D6 and UGT2B7 genotype and risk of recurrence in tamoxifen-treated breast cancer patients. J Natl Cancer Inst 104(6):452–460

Rae JM, Regan MM, Thibert JN et al (2015) CYP2D6 genotypes obtained from tumor-derived dna are highly concordant with germline DNA genotypes obtained from patient whole blood samples. CYP2D6 genotypes obtained from tumor-derived DNA are highly concordant with germline DNA genotypes obtained from patient whole blood samples. JNCI [Epub ahead of print]

Raftogianis RB, Wood TC, Otterness DM, Van Loon JA, Weinshilboum RM (1997) Phenol sulfotransferase pharmacogenetics in humans: association of common SULT1A1 alleles with TS PST phenotype. Biochem Biophys Res Commun 239(1):298–304

Rahman A, Korzekwa KR, Grogan J, Gonzalez FJ, Harris JW (1994) Selective biotransformation of taxol to 6 alpha-hydroxytaxol by human cytochrome P450 2C8. Cancer Res 54(21):5543–5546

Ramsey TL, Liu Q, Massey BW, Brennan MD (2013) Genotypic variation in the SV2C gene impacts response to atypical antipsychotics the CATIE study. Schizophr Res 149(1–3):21–25

Rapuri PB, Gallagher JC, Knezetic JA, Haynatzka V (2006) Estrogen receptor alpha gene polymorphisms are associated with changes in bone remodeling markers and treatment response to estrogen. Maturitas 53(4):371–379

Reding KW, Chen C, Lowe K et al (2012) Estrogen-related genes and their contribution to racial differences in breast cancer risk. Cancer Causes Control 23(5):671–681

Regan MM, Leyland-Jones B, Bouzyk M et al (2012) CYP2D6 genotype and tamoxifen response in postmenopausal women with endocrine-responsive breast cancer: the breast international group 1-98 trial. J Natl Cancer Inst 104(6):441–451

Rizzo R, Spaggiari F, Indelli M, Lelli G, Baricordi OR, Rimessi P, Ferlini A (2010) Association of CYP1B1 with hypersensitivity induced by taxane therapy in breast cancer patients. Breast Cancer Res Treat 124 (2):593–598

Ryan J, Canonico M, Carcaillon L et al (2012) Hormone treatment, estrogen receptor polymorphisms and mortality: a prospective cohort study. PLoS ONE 7(3): e34112

Sakoda LC, Blackston CR, Doherty JA et al (2011) Selected estrogen receptor 1 and androgen receptor gene polymorphisms in relation to risk of breast cancer and fibrocystic breast conditions among Chinese women. Cancer Epidemiol 35(1):48–55

Saladores P, Murdter T, Eccles D et al (2015) Tamoxifen metabolism predicts drug concentrations and outcome in premenopausal patients with early breast cancer. Pharmacogenomics J 15(1):84–94

Salmen T, Heikkinen AM, Mahonen A et al (2000) Early postmenopausal bone loss is associated with PvuII estrogen receptor gene polymorphism in Finnish women: effect of hormone replacement therapy. J Bone Miner Res 15(2):315–321

Schneider BP, Sledge GW Jr (2007) Drug insight: VEGF as a therapeutic target for breast cancer. Nat Clin Pract Oncol 4(3):181–189

Schneider BP, Wang M, Radovich M et al (2008) Association of vascular endothelial growth factor and vascular endothelial growth factor receptor-2 genetic polymorphisms with outcome in a trial of paclitaxel compared with paclitaxel plus bevacizumab in advanced breast cancer: ECOG 2100. J Clin Oncol 26(28):4672–4678

Schneider BP, Li L, Shen F et al (2014) Genetic variant predicts bevacizumab-induced hypertension in ECOG-5103 and ECOG-2100. Br J Cancer 111 (6):1241–1248

Schneider BP, Li L, Radovich M et al (2015) Genome-Wide Association Studies for Taxane-Induced Peripheral Neuropathy in ECOG-5103 and ECOG-1199. Clin Cancer Res 21(22):5082–5091

Schroth W, Goetz MP, Hamann U et al (2009) Association between CYP2D6 polymorphisms and outcomes among women with early stage breast cancer treated with tamoxifen. JAMA 302(13):1429–1436

Serrano D, Lazzeroni M, Zambon CF et al (2011) Efficacy of tamoxifen based on cytochrome P450 2D6, CYP2C19 and SULT1A1 genotype in the Italian tamoxifen prevention trial. Pharmacogenomics J 11 (2):100–107

Sim SC, Ingelman-Sundberg M (2010) The human cytochrome P450 (CYP) allele nomenclature website: a peer-reviewed database of CYP variants and their associated effects. Hum Genomics 4(4):278–281

Smith IE, Dowsett M, Ebbs SR et al (2005) Neoadjuvant treatment of postmenopausal breast cancer with anastrozole, tamoxifen, or both in combination: the immediate preoperative anastrozole, tamoxifen, or combined with tamoxifen (IMPACT) multicenter double-blind randomized trial. J Clin Oncol 23 (22):5108–5116

Sowers MR, Symons JP, Jannausch ML, Chu J, Kardia SR (2006a) Sex steroid hormone polymorphisms, high-density lipoprotein cholesterol, and apolipoprotein A-1 from the study of women's health across the nation (SWAN). Am J Med 119(9 Suppl 1):S61–S68

Sowers MR, Wilson AL, Karvonen-Gutierrez CA, Kardia SR (2006b) Sex steroid hormone pathway genes and health-related measures in women of 4 races/ ethnicities: the study of women's health across the nation (SWAN). Am J Med 119(9 Suppl 1):S103–S110

Stearns V, Johnson MD, Rae JM et al (2003) Active tamoxifen metabolite plasma concentrations after coadministration of tamoxifen and the selective serotonin reuptake inhibitor paroxetine. J Natl Cancer Inst 95(23):1758–1764

Sun Y, Zang Z, Xu X et al (2011) The association of SULT1A1 codon 213 polymorphism and breast cancer susceptibility: meta-analysis from 16 studies involving 23,445 subjects. Breast Cancer Res Treat 125(1):215–219

Tempfer CB, Hefler LA, Schneeberger C, Huber JC (2006) How valid is single nucleotide polymorphism (SNP) diagnosis for the individual risk assessment of breast cancer? Gynecol Endocrinol 22(3):155–159

Tengstrom M, Mannermaa A, Kosma VM, Hirvonen A, Kataja V (2012) SULT1A1 rs9282861 polymorphism-a potential modifier of efficacy of the systemic adjuvant therapy in breast cancer? BMC Cancer 12:257

Thompson AM, Johnson A, Quinlan P et al (2011) Comprehensive CYP2D6 genotype and adherence affect outcome in breast cancer patients treated with tamoxifen monotherapy. Breast Cancer Res Treat 125 (1):279–287

Viale G, Regan MM, Dell'Orto P et al (2011) Which patients benefit most from adjuvant aromatase inhibitors? Results using a composite measure of prognostic risk in the BIG 1-98 randomized trial. Ann Oncol 22 (10):2201–2207

Wang J, Higuchi R, Modugno F et al (2007) Estrogen receptor alpha haplotypes and breast cancer risk in older Caucasian women. Breast Cancer Res Treat 106 (2):273–280

Wang Z, Fu Y, Tang C, Lu S, Chu WM (2010) SULT1A1 R213H polymorphism and breast cancer risk: a meta-analysis based on 8,454 cases and 11,800 controls. Breast Cancer Res Treat 122(1):193–198

Wang J, Lu K, Song Y et al (2013) Indications of clinical and genetic predictors for aromatase inhibitors related musculoskeletal adverse events in Chinese Han women with breast cancer. PLoS ONE 8(7):e68798

Watanabe J, Harada N, Suemasu K, Higashi Y, Gotoh O, Kawajiri K (1997) Arginine-cysteine polymorphism at codon 264 of the human CYP19 gene does not affect aromatase activity. Pharmacogenetics 7(5):419–424

Wegman P, Elingarami S, Carstensen J, Stal O, Nordenskjold B, Wingren S (2007) Genetic variants of CYP3A5, CYP2D6, SULT1A1, UGT2B15 and tamoxifen response in postmenopausal patients with breast cancer. Breast Cancer Res 9(1):R7

Wu X, Hawse JR, Subramaniam M, Goetz MP, Ingle JN, Spelsberg TC (2009) The tamoxifen metabolite, endoxifen, is a potent antiestrogen that targets estrogen receptor alpha for degradation in breast cancer cells. Cancer Res 69(5):1722–1727

Yaffe K, Lindquist K, Sen S et al (2009) Estrogen receptor genotype and risk of cognitive impairment in elders: findings from the health ABC study. Neurobiol Aging 30(4):607–614

Yu KD, Rao NY, Chen AX, Fan L, Yang C, Shao ZM (2011) A systematic review of the relationship between polymorphic sites in the estrogen receptor-beta (ESR2) gene and breast cancer risk. Breast Cancer Res Treat 126(1):37–45

Zanger UM, Raimundo S, Eichelbaum M (2004) Cytochrome P450 2D6: overview and update on pharmacology, genetics, biochemistry. Naunyn Schmiedebergs Arch Pharmacol 369(1):23–37

Zarrabeitia MT, Hernandez JL, Valero C et al (2004) A common polymorphism in the 5'-untranslated region of the aromatase gene influences bone mass and fracture risk. Eur J Endocrinol 150(5):699–704

25 Applied Proteomics in Breast Cancer

Xianyin Lai and S. Badve

Abstract

Breast cancer is the most commonly diagnosed cancer and remains the second most common cause of cancer-related deaths in women. Proteomics has been used in biomedical research for 20 years. However, the application of proteomics in breast cancer remains a small fraction of breast cancer research. Comprehensive analysis of proteins is seldom used in clinical practice. Analysis of single proteins still remains the standard practice in clinical laboratories. Despite the use of multiplex methods for protein analysis in preclinical research, it is challenging to apply these techniques in the clinical setting. In this review, we summarize the commonly implemented array-based and mass spectrometry-based proteomic techniques, and the application of biomarkers for a specific purpose or mechanisms involved in breast cancer biology. The ultimate goal of this review is to help clinicians and scientists for choosing the right techniques and understanding their potential with respect to prognosis and prediction of the treatment outcome.

X. Lai (✉)
Department of Biochemistry and Molecular Biology, Indiana University School of Medicine, 635 Barnhill Drive, Room 0044, Indianapolis 46202, IN, USA
e-mail: xlai@iu.edu

X. Lai
Department of Cellular and Integrative Physiology, Indiana University School of Medicine, 635 Barnhill Drive, Room 0044, Indianapolis 46202, IN, USA

S. Badve
Department of Pathology and Laboratory Medicine, Indiana University School of Medicine, Indianapolis IN 46202, USA

S. Badve and Y. Gökmen-Polar (eds.), *Molecular Pathology of Breast Cancer*, DOI 10.1007/978-3-319-41761-5_25

Keywords
Breast · Cancer · Proteomics

Abbreviations

2-DE	Two-dimensional gel electrophoresis
MALDI-TOF	Matrix-assisted laser desorption ionization time-of-flight
MRM	Multiple reaction monitoring
MS	Mass spectrometry
MudPIT	Multidimensional protein identification technology
sCD14	Soluble CD14
SILAC	Stable isotope labeling with amino acids in cell culture
SRM	Selected reaction monitoring

25.1 Introduction

The most commonly diagnosed cancer in women is breast cancer and the second most common cause of cancer-related deaths in women. Recent studies have highlighted the clinical, histological and molecular heterogeneity in breast cancer. These differences can occur in different patients with the same tumor type, different geographical regions of a tumor within the same patient, or over time within the same tumor of the same patient (Zardavas et al. 2015). Thus, understanding the comprehensive molecular landscape of the tumor is critical.

Comprehensive evaluation of hundreds to thousands of proteins simultaneously, proteomics, is now possible using cutting edge, high-throughput technology. The original definition and goal of proteomics was to study "all proteins expressed by a genome, cell or tissue" (Wilkins et al. 1996). In practice, this is not always possible and the words large-scale and global have been used very often to substitute for comprehensive (Zhao et al. 2015; Guo et al. 2015).

Historically, the evaluation of proteins originated with the combination of two-dimensional gel electrophoresis (2-DE) and mass spectrometry (MS). Today, the field of proteomics is still driven by the development of new technologies and improvement of existing technologies for sample processing, protein identification, and quantification to improve accuracy, scale, or throughput capabilities. In the current review, we focus on the major aspects of proteomics as applicable to breast cancer. The goal is to provide researchers with the basic tools to understand proteomic techniques and enhance the understanding of the molecular processes that are altered in breast cancer. This will enable the translation of these findings into the clinical field.

25.2 Types of Platforms for Multiplex Protein Profiling

The expression levels of multiple proteins can be measured by using different approaches (Fig. 25.1).

25.2.1 Proteomic Technologies

According to the original or practical definition, any study that evaluates >10 proteins simultaneously should be considered as a proteomic study. The detection may include the protein identification and/or protein quantification. The analysis may include detection and quantification of the post-translational modifications of peptides/amino acids. Indeed, proteomics

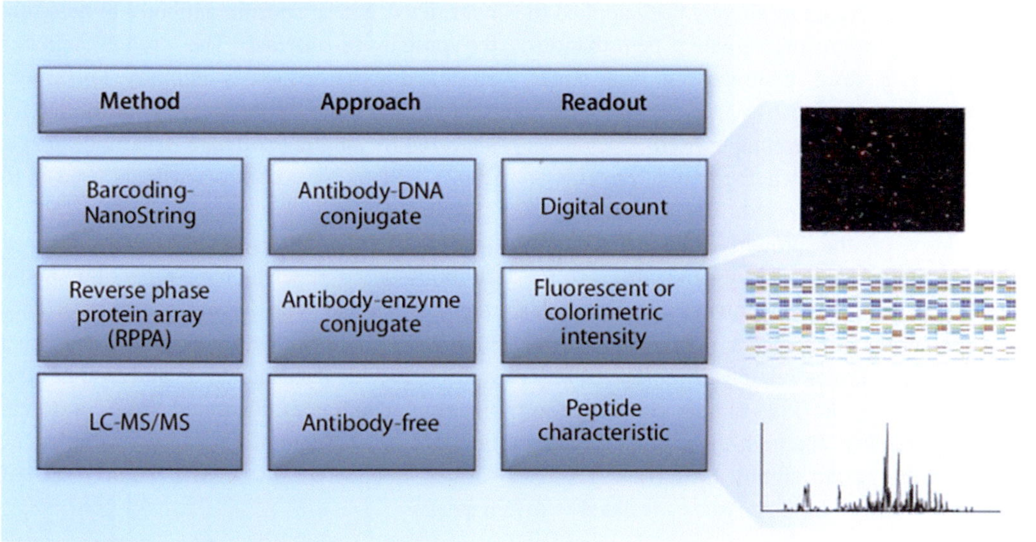

Fig. 25.1 Methods for multiplex protein profiling. The expression levels of multiple proteins can be measured by using different approaches. Barcoding-NanoString combines digital detection (NanoString's nCounter) with antibody-DNA conjugates. RPPA is a high-throughput antibody-based technique that uses colorimetric or fluorescent assay intensity. High-throughput antibody-free techniques consist of LC-MS/MS, which measures label-free peak peptide intensities, or stable-isotope labeling by tagging the mass of a protein or peptide. Recent modifications include SRM and MRM. Reprinted from Gokmen-Polar and Badve (2014)

fundamentally answers "who" and "what" questions of many proteins in one project. The "who" is the name of a protein or the post-translational modification of an amino acid. The "what" is the change in expression of a protein or posttranslational modification (Fig. 25.2).

Functional proteomics further improves the knowledge of conventional proteomics in that it incorporates the examination of protein activation, protein–protein interactions and activated pathway analysis. Functional proteomics can be further divided into distinct subtypes based on the types of protein analyzed such as exosomal proteins (exosome), secreted proteins (secretome), proteases (proteasome), kinases (kinome) and phosphorylated proteins (phosphoproteomics). Innovative MS approaches such as 5-plex stable isotope labeling with amino acids in

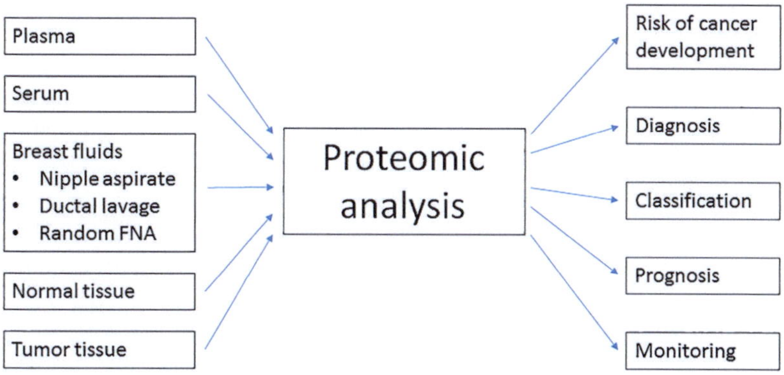

Fig. 25.2 Applications of proteomic technologies for breast cancer diagnosis, classification and assessment of risk of cancer as well as prediction of recurrence

cell culture (SILAC), has already been applied to monitor phosphotyrosine signaling perturbations induced by a drug treatment in one single experiment.

The choice of the technique used depends on the goals of study and whether whole proteins or peptides are being detected. The availability of the identity of the proteins and their corresponding antibodies may enable the use of array-based techniques. However, these techniques require bait molecules, which increase the cost and raises issues related to reproducibility. On the contrary, the low sample consumption, reduced variability, and high-throughput capacity of MS platforms are significant advantages for discovery, but have issues related to reproducibility.

25.2.2 Array-Based Technologies

Array analysis is based on binding between a bait molecule and an analyte, which are subsequently detected by a probe. The bait molecule can be an antibody, protein, peptide, drug, nucleic acid, cell, phage, etc. The analyte is a protein. The probe is a molecule with a signal-generating moiety, such as a labeled antibody. The intensity of the signal is proportional to the quantity of an analyte bound to the bait molecule. An image of the spot pattern is captured, analyzed, and interpreted (Liotta et al. 2003).

According to whether the analyte is captured from the solution phase or bound to the solid phase, protein microarrays include two major classes: forward-phase arrays and reverse-phase arrays. In forward-phase arrays, the analyte is captured from the solution phase, and the bait molecule, such as an antibody, is immobilized onto the solid support. Antibody microarray is a forward-phase array in which a number of antibodies are arrayed. The array is incubated with the test sample (containing the analyte) for analysis.

In the reverse-phase protein array (RPPA), the analyte is bound to the solid phase and detected by the probe (Liotta et al. 2003). After sample lysates are spotted onto an array, the array is then hybridized with a specific antibody to recognize the protein of interest. The protein signal is amplified with a secondary antibody. The array is scanned and the resulting image is quantified and analyzed by an array software (Charboneau et al. 2002). RPPAs have been extensively used in the TCGA analysis.

Tissue microarrays (TMA) are also an antibody-based reverse-phase array, but named after the sample type. Tissue microarrays allow high throughput molecular profiling of markers in cancer specimens and rapid validation of novel potential candidates identified from proteomic analyses in a large number of tumor samples. For further details on the TMA (Badve DAKO paper).

25.2.3 Mass Spectrometry (MS) Based Methods

MS is an analytical tool that generates spectra of the masses of proteins within a sample. It first ionizes compounds to generate charged molecules and then measures their mass to charge ratios. The apparatus acts as a high-accuracy ion scale that is mostly composed of an ionizing source, an analyzer [quadruplope or TOF (time of flight)], and one or more detectors, which records the mass-to-charge ratio of the ionized peptides (Domon and Aebersold 2006). The spectra are examined to determine the elemental composition of the sample and the masses of proteins and to depict the chemical structures of the proteins.

The commonly used separation methods for whole-protein (top-down) analysis include classic gel based methods or high-performance liquid chromatography (HPLC) and MudPIT (multidimensional protein identification technology). Ionization techniques include electrospray ionization, surface enhanced laser desorption, and matrix assisted laser desorption ionization (MALDI). This data can be automatically submitted to a database for peptide mass fingerprint. Alternatively, tandem MS or MS/MS may be performed to obtain peptide sequence. Electrospray methods are being adapted for rapid diagnostic purposes such as margin assessment during surgery (Ifa and Eberlin 2016) for details about methodologies.

The bottom-up (or shotgun) methods involve tryptic digestion. This provides more information per protein as peptides are easier to ionize than proteins. A peptide ion provides useful information, including its intensity at each time point in the MS/MS spectrum. Using this information, different label-free methods have been developed, including spectral counting, ion intensity, MS/MS fragment ion intensity, and a combination of spectral counting and ion intensity measurements. The principle of spectral counting is very simple: the number of mass spectra identified for a protein is used as a measure of the protein's abundance (Lundgren et al. 2010). It must be noted that the MS signal does not necessarily correlate with the abundance of the protein due to the variable ionization efficacy of proteins and peptides.

25.2.3.1 Label-Based and Label-Free MS Methods

Peptide centric proteomic approaches are broadly divided into isotope- and isobaric label based technologies (ICAT and iTRAQ, respectively) and label free MS-based proteomics. ICAT and iTRAQ methods have the potential for quantitative protein profiling of clinical samples, plasma and/or serum as well as tissues (Gromov et al. 2014). The ICAT platform has been used in conjunction with laser microdissection (LCM) in breast cancer (Zang et al. 2004). iTRAQ platform allows simultaneous assessment of differential abundance of proteins between several samples (up to 8) (Gromov et al. 2014). iTRAQ is still a discovery tool and the results need to be confirmed by other methods; SRM has been used for this purpose (Muraoka et al. 2012). Stable isotope labeling by amino acids in cell culture (SILAC) strategy is specifically tailored for detecting phosphoproteins. For example, this has been used by Tzouros et al. (2013) to identify 318 unique phosphopeptides belonging to 215 proteins from an erlotinib-treated breast cancer cell line model.

Label-free MS approaches allow for screening of proteomes on a global scale by quantitative measurement of peptide abundance by using peptide ion peak intensities or spectral counting without additional labeling of peptides. It is important to emphasize that the fold change of an individual peptide may be often different from the fold change for other peptides from the same protein. To detect and remove outlier peptides, multiple filters have been used to improve quantitation (Lai et al. 2011).

25.2.3.2 Selected and Multiple Reaction Monitoring (SRM and MRM)

Traditional label-free quantification methods quantify hundreds to thousands of proteins in a mixture. On the contrary, selected reaction monitoring (SRM) or multiple reaction monitoring (MRM), is a targeted protein quantification method. SRM/MRM is not a new mass spectrometry technique, but its application in proteomics is emerging as a complement to untargeted shotgun methods and is particularly useful in absolute quantification. When isotopically labeled peptides are used as internal standards, and SRM/MRM is able to absolutely quantify proteins (Chahrour et al. 2015). These methods have found commercial use and diagnostic and prognostic panels are available for clinical use. More specifically, tests for HER2 quantification as well as "comprehensive profiling" of tumors are offered by Nantomics.

25.3 Protein–Protein Interaction (PPI) Profiling

More than 80 % of proteins do not operate alone but in complexes (Berggard et al. 2007) so it is important to identify the interacting partners of proteins for deducing protein function (Phizicky et al. 2003). PPI can modify the kinetic properties of enzymes, act as mechanisms for substrate channeling, construct a new binding site for small effector molecules, inactivate or suppress protein, change the specificity of the protein for the substrate or serve as an upstream or downstream regulator of function (Phizicky et al. 2003). A number of in vitro, in vivo, and in silico methods are available to analyze PPIs (Rao et al. 2014). The in vitro methods include tandem affinity purification, affinity chromatography, co-immunoprecipitation, protein arrays, protein fragment complementation, phage display, X-ray crystallography, and NMR spectroscopy. In vivo methods include yeast-two-hybrid systems. A detailed discussion of these is beyond the scope of this chapter but a brief mention of fluorescence resonance energy transfer (FRET) will be made here.

FRET based methods have found their way in clinical practice because of the specificity of the reaction and the relative ease of analysis. The HERmark assay for HER2 is based on technology. Briefly, it is a proximity assay, which detects the binding of HER2 with its binding partners. Several studies have suggested that monitoring this interaction might be a better method for assessing HER2 activity (Duchnowska et al. 2012, 2014, 2015; Lipton et al. 2010).

25.3.1 Issues Related to Sample Preparation

Twenty-two most abundant blood-derived proteins constitute approximately 99 % of the total plasma protein mass. This makes it necessary to deplete these from clinical body fluid specimens in order to identify changes in less abundant proteins. Immunodepletion is a commonly employed technique (Prieto et al. 2014) to discover glycoproteins in breast cancer serum as biomarkers. This method has led to the identification of several biomarker candidates including thrombospondin-1 and 5, alpha-1B-glycoprotein, serum amyloid P-component, and tenascin-X (Zeng et al. 2011). These methods can be also applied to fresh frozen tissues.

In contrast to immunodepletion, pull-down technique selectively enriches a particular protein species and natural binding partners for the captured protein from a complex protein solution. It is particularly useful in determining protein–proteins interaction predicted by other research techniques or screening unknown protein–protein interactions.

Archival FFPE tissues require pretreatment to negate the effect of formalin fixation and processing. Detergent-based methods are commonly used to negate the effects of fixation; commercial kits such as Liquid Tissue® are also available for these purposes.

25.4 Applications

Excellent reviews summarizing the data from proteomics studies in relation to breast cancer have been published (Gromov et al. 2014; Lam et al. 2014; Zeidan et al. 2015). These reviews detail the methodology used for discovery, the type of samples and the technology used in the validation (if any) of the results. We shall highlight/summarize some of the critical studies below.

25.4.1 Biomarker for Breast Cancer Risk

The identification of biomarkers for the early detection of breast cancer has a major impact on reducing breast cancer mortality by removing the cancer early when it is most treatable. Because they can be monitored with minimal invasiveness, plasma biomarkers have additional value in early detection. Low abundance proteins in plasma collected from patients with stage I breast cancer or benign breast lesions have been enriched and analyzed using a proteomic approach, resulting in the identification of 397 proteins. Of these, 23 could be validated in an independent set of samples (Meng et al. 2011). Bohm et al. (2011) used an antibody microarray with 23 antibodies immobilized on nitrocellulose slides to determine the levels of acute phase proteins, interleukins and complement factors in the sera of 101 study participants (49 women with primary breast cancer and 52 healthy age-matched controls). Six proteins were found to be significantly different levels in breast cancer patients compared to healthy subjects. Garrisi et al. (2013) analyzed 292 serum samples (100 from healthy people, 100 from sporadic breast cancer patients, and 92 from familial breast cancer patients) to identify significant differentially expressed peptides.

In a tissue based approach, Chung et al. identified ubiquitin and S100P as differentially expressed in 82 breast cancer and 82 adjacent unaffected tissue samples (Chung et al. 2013). They confirmed the differential expression in an independent cohort of 89 patients. Proteomics of breast cancer-associated adipose tissue from freshly isolated tumors enabled the identification of paracrine secretion of oncostatin M by cancer-associated adipose tissue (Lapeire et al. 2014). Oncostatin M is known to phosphorylate STAT3 and induce transcription of several STAT3-dependent genes. Selective inhibition of oncostatin M by neutralizing antibody and Jak family kinases by tofacitinib inhibited STAT3 signaling, peritumoral angiogenesis, and cellular scattering (Lapeire et al. 2014).

Martinez-Lozano Sinues (2015) performed breath analysis in a cohort of 14 breast cancer patients and 11 healthy volunteers using secondary electrospray ionization-mass spectrometry (SESI-MS) to detect a cancer-related volatile profile. Supervised analysis of breath data identified a support vector machine (SVM) model including 8 features corresponding to m/z 106, 126, 147, 78, 148, 52, 128, 315 and able to discriminate exhaled breath from breast cancer patients from that of healthy individuals, with sensitivity and specificity above 0.9. Zhu et al. (2015) used electrospray ionization-linear ion trap quadrupole mass spectrometry (ESI-LTQ-MS) and liquid chromatography / electrospray ionization tandem mass spectrometry (LC/ESI-MS/MS) to determine the structure of a glycosphingolipids (α1,2 fucosidase and fucosyltransferases) in human breast cancer tissue. They identified the ion with m/z 1184 molecular ion as fucosyl-lactoceramide (Fuc-LacCer) was specific to breast cancer.

25.4.2 Biomarker for Classification

Brozkova et al. (2008) have used SELDI-TOF analysis of tumor tissue lysates to reproduce the DNA-based intrinsic classification of breast cancers. Tissue proteomic approaches have been used to determine prognosis in ER+, HER2+ and TNBC patients (Lam et al. 2014). In a number of these studies, validation has been performed using Western Blots or IHC. However, the end-points have been correlation with histology or IHC; the clinical significance of these classifiers has not always been analyzed. Similarly, RPPA data has been shown to be consistent with HER2 by IHC in a number of studies (Wulfkuhle et al. 2012). In the TCGA breast cancer cohort, RPPA analysis identified two novel protein expression-defined subgroups within the luminal tumors, possibly produced by stromal / microenvironmental factors. Seven clusters were identified in this TCGA analysis (HER2, Luminal A, Luminal A/B, X, reactive I and reactive II) (Cancer Genome Atlas 2012). Gujral et al. (2013) used RPPA to analyze 56 breast cancers and matched normal tissues using 71 signaling proteins. Using unsupervised hierarchical clustering, they were able to identify 12 clusters each composed of important signaling pathways that could be used for drug targeting.

A number of proteomics studies have correlated protein expression patterns with tumor stage (Villanueva et al. 2006; Li et al. 2002, 2005; Laronga et al. 2003). These studies have identified C-terminal truncated fragment of complement C3, FPA, fibrinogen, ITIH4, apoA-IV, bradykinin, factor XIIIa and transthyretin to be associated with stage (Gromov et al. 2014). Sonntag et al. (2014) have reported the use of proteomic signature composed of Caveolin-1, NDKA, RPS6, and Ki67 for prognostication and have resolved grade II patients into 2 subsets depending on their similarity to grade 1 or grade 3 tumors.

Recent years have seen the application of whole protein analysis in breast cancer including for margin assessment (Eberlin et al. 2011). Calligaris et al. (2014) used desorption electrospray ionization mass spectrometry imaging (DESI-MSI) for identifying and differentiating tumor from normal breast tissue. Several fatty acids, including oleic acid, were more abundant in the cancerous tissue than in normal tissues. Tumor margins were identified using the spatial distributions and varying intensities of different lipids were consistent with those margins obtained histology. They suggest the use of this method for the rapid intraoperative detection of residual cancer tissue during breast-conserving surgery.

25.4.3 Biomarker for Prognostics

UPA/PAI-1 is a well validated marker that has high levels of evidence for clinical use in breast cancer (Duffy et al. 1988a, b). It is also one of the few markers included in the ASCO biomarker guidelines based on the ELISA data confirmed using clinical trial materials (Harbeck et al. 2013).

Quiescin sulfhydryl oxidase 1 (QSOX1) has been documented to be useful in predicting relapse in Luminal B tumors (Katchman et al. 2013). Ferritin light chain levels have been correlated with node negative status (Descotes et al. 2012) and DCN and HSP90B1 levels with increased likelihood of metastases and poor overall survival (Cawthorn et al. 2012). He et al. (2013) used a 2D-LC coupled with HPLC-CHIP MS/MS approach to analysis of samples from $LN^{+}ER/PR^{-}HER2^{+}$ (n = 50) and $LN^{-}ER/PR^{+-}$ $HER2^{-}$ (n = 50) breast cancer patients. Of the 118 proteins differentially expressed, they were able to confirm the presence of an immune-related protein, serum soluble CD14 (sCD14) as a biomarker. High level of serum sCD14 at primary surgery was confirmed in an independent cohort of 183 breast cancer patients (90 $LN^{+}ER/PR^{-}$ $HER2^{+}$ and 93 patients with $LN^{-}ER/PR^{+}HER2^{-}$) to be associated with a significantly lower risk of relapse in 3 years. Naba et al. (2014) analyzed the extracellular matrix of human mammary carcinoma xenografts shows that primary tumors of differing metastatic potential differ in extracellular matrix composition. They confirmed that the mRNA levels of the identified targets (SNED1 and LTBP3) had prognostic relevance using an online Affymetrix microarray database.

Gonzalez-Angulo's group have profiled a large number of tumors with 146 antibodies (RPPA) to identify 6 clusters of breast tumors using a 10 protein panel (Hennessy et al. 2010; Gonzalez-Angulo et al. 2011, 2013; Sohn et al. 2013). These 10 proteins (ER, PR, BCL2, GATA3, CCNB1, CCNE1, EGFR, HER2, HERp1248 and EIG121) were shown to be useful in predicting the relapse free survival (RFS) in patients who underwent neoadjuvant chemotherapy.

25.4.4 Biomarker for Treatment Response Prediction

Majidzadeh and Gharechahi (2013) used plasma proteome signatures of 9 proteins to define a group of patients likely to have/develop tamoxifen resistance. The MD Anderson group has also reported that a panel of 3-proteins (CHK1pS345, Caveolin-1 and RAB25) could predict RFS after neoadjuvant system therapy. Yang et al. (2012) analyzed by mass spectrometry needle biopsies of tumor from patients prior to neoadjuvant (Doxorubicin-based) chemotherapy. Among 298 differentially expressed proteins (>1.5-fold) FKBP4 and S100A9 were validated by IHC as useful for predicting resistance to therapy.

25.5 Challenges to Proteomics

There are major advantages for the use of proteins as biomarkers for disease as they are the workhorses within the cellular environment. However, there are several limitations. Proteins, unlike DNA or RNA, cannot be amplified. Approximately 500,000 to 1,000,000 proteins are synthesized from the 35,000 genes in the human genome through processes of alternative splicing and posttranslational modifications. This makes identification of the structure critical. Most of the high-throughput techniques are based on peptide digestion and not intact proteins. Deciphering the identity of the protein can thus be challenging. Proteins/peptides having a mass between 4000 and 10,000 Da are difficult to identify. In addition, in most tissue/blood samples a small number of proteins account for the vast quantity of proteins detected. For example, approximately 20 proteins constitute more than 98 of the proteins identified in serum/plasma (Omenn et al. 2005; Anderson et al. 2004; Anderson and Anderson 2002). Detection of low abundance proteins is a major challenge that requires the use of depletion of major species or enrichment of rare proteins by variety of methods including fractionation. Protein expression can be transient in nature. This, in addition, to pre-analytical handling of the specimens can introduce significant reproducibility issues. The assays themselves are also not very reproducible and there can be significant variability between experiments resulting in descriptive studies.

The costs of proteomics studies is still fairly high resulting in studies that are composed of low number of samples. It is not always clear whether the differences noted in the studies are due to analytical system or low sample size, or due to tumor heterogeneity. The specimens used are often "samples of convenience" and lack detail annotations. Comparisons are often performed using surrogate variables such as histology or IHC rather than patient outcomes such as overall and disease free survival. In addition, in most studies the differences in the quantitative, the proteins/peptides are not exclusive to the disease state.

25.6 Conclusions

Proteomics has the capacity to help clinicians or scientists answer clinically and biologically relevant questions. These may involve the use of whole protein or peptide based analyses of cells, cell fractions or body fluids aided as necessary by fractionation and pull-down techniques. There is enormous scope for the use of these as biomarkers for early detection, diagnostics, classification, treatment response prediction, and prognostics, and for understanding mechanisms involved in cell proliferation, motility and survival. RPPA has been very successfully employed in multi-institutional studies such as the TCGA. Techniques that help elucidate protein–protein interactions are critical for defining molecular pathways; some of these have been also put towards clinical use. However, there is significant need for development of new technologies and improvement of existing technologies for sample processing, protein identification, and quantification to improve accuracy, scale, or throughput capabilities. These developments would lead to accurate identification of proteins and their isoforms as well as make the quantification more precise. Cost of analyses remain high and in many cases, prohibitive to large scale experimentation.

References

Anderson NL, Anderson NG (2002) The human plasma proteome: history, character, and diagnostic prospects. Mol Cell Proteomics 1(11):845–867

Anderson NL, Polanski M, Pieper R, Gatlin T, Tirumalai RS, Conrads TP, Veenstra TD, Adkins JN, Pounds JG, Fagan R, Lobley A (2004) The human plasma proteome: a nonredundant list developed by combination of four separate sources. Mol Cell Proteomics 3(4):311–326. doi:10.1074/mcp.M300127-MCP200

Berggard T, Linse S, James P (2007) Methods for the detection and analysis of protein–protein interactions. Proteomics 7(16):2833–2842. doi:10.1002/pmic.200700131

Bohm D, Keller K, Boehm N, Lebrecht A, Schmidt M, Kolbl H, Grus FH (2011) Antibody microarray analysis of the serum proteome in primary breast cancer patients. Cancer Biol Ther 12(9):772–779. doi:10.4161/cbt.12.9.17675

Brozkova K, Budinska E, Bouchal P, Hernychova L, Knoflickova D, Valik D, Vyzula R, Vojtesek B, Nenutil R (2008) Surface-enhanced laser desorption/ionization time-of-flight proteomic profiling of breast carcinomas identifies clinicopathologically relevant groups of patients similar to previously defined clusters from cDNA expression. Breast Cancer Res 10(3):R48. doi:10.1186/bcr2101

Calligaris D, Caragacianu D, Liu X, Norton I, Thompson CJ, Richardson AL, Golshan M, Easterling ML, Santagata S, Dillon DA, Jolesz FA, Agar NY (2014) Application of desorption electrospray ionization mass spectrometry imaging in breast cancer margin analysis. Proc Natl Acad Sci U S A 111(42):15184–15189. doi:10.1073/pnas.1408129111

Cancer Genome Atlas N (2012) Comprehensive molecular portraits of human breast tumours. Nature 490 (7418):61–70. doi:10.1038/nature11412

Cawthorn TR, Moreno JC, Dharsee M, Tran-Thanh D, Ackloo S, Zhu PH, Sardana G, Chen J, Kupchak P, Jacks LM, Miller NA, Youngson BJ, Iakovlev V,

Guidos CJ, Vallis KA, Evans KR, McCready D, Leong WL, Done SJ (2012) Proteomic analyses reveal high expression of decorin and endoplasmin (HSP90B1) are associated with breast cancer metastasis and decreased survival. PLoS ONE 7(2):e30992. doi:10.1371/journal.pone.0030992

Chahrour O, Cobice D, Malone J (2015) Stable isotope labelling methods in mass spectrometry-based quantitative proteomics. J Pharm Biomed Anal 113:2–20. doi:10.1016/j.jpba.2015.04.013

Charboneau L, Tory H, Chen T, Winters M, Petricoin EF 3rd, Liotta LA, Paweletz CP (2002) Utility of reverse phase protein arrays: applications to signalling pathways and human body arrays. Brief Funct Genomic Proteomic 1(3):305–315

Chung L, Shibli S, Moore K, Elder EE, Boyle FM, Marsh DJ, Baxter RC (2013) Tissue biomarkers of breast cancer and their association with conventional pathologic features. Br J Cancer 108(2):351–360. doi:10.1038/bjc.2012.552

Descotes F, Jezequel P, Spyratos F, Campion L, Grenot C, Lerebours F, Campone M, Guerin-Charbonnel C, Lanoe D, Adams M, Andre J, Carlioz A, Martin PM, Chassevent A, Jourdan ML, Guette C, Zanella-Cleon I, Ricolleau G (2012) Identification of potential prognostic biomarkers for node-negative breast tumours by proteomic analysis: a multicentric 2004 national PHRC study. Int J Oncol 41(1):92–104. doi:10.3892/ijo.2012.1456

Domon B, Aebersold R (2006) Mass spectrometry and protein analysis. Science 312(5771):212–217. doi:10.1126/science.1124619

Duchnowska R, Biernat W, Szostakiewicz B, Sperinde J, Piette F, Haddad M, Paquet A, Lie Y, Czartoryska-Arlukowicz B, Wysocki P, Jankowski T, Radecka B, Foszczynska-Kloda M, Litwiniuk M, Debska S, Weidler J, Huang W, Buyse M, Bates M, Jassem J (2012) Correlation between quantitative HER-2 protein expression and risk for brain metastases in HER-2+ advanced breast cancer patients receiving trastuzumab-containing therapy. Oncologist 17(1):26–35. doi:10.1634/theoncologist.2011-0212

Duchnowska R, Sperinde J, Chenna A, Haddad M, Paquet A, Lie Y, Weidler JM, Huang W, Winslow J, Jankowski T, Czartoryska-Arlukowicz B, Wysocki PJ, Foszczynska-Kloda M, Radecka B, Litwiniuk MM, Zok J, Wisniewski M, Zuziak D, Biernat W, Jassem J (2014) Quantitative measurements of tumoral p95HER2 protein expression in metastatic breast cancer patients treated with trastuzumab: independent validation of the p95HER2 clinical cutoff. Clin Cancer Res 20(10):2805–2813. doi:10.1158/1078-0432.CCR-13-2782

Duchnowska R, Sperinde J, Chenna A, Huang W, Weidler JM, Winslow J, Haddad M, Paquet A, Lie Y, Trojanowski T, Mandat T, Kowalczyk A, Czartoryska-Arlukowicz B, Radecka B, Jarosz B, Staszkiewicz R, Kalinka-Warzocha E, Chudzik M, Biernat W, Jassem J (2015) Quantitative HER2 and p95HER2 levels in primary breast cancers and matched brain metastases. Neuro Oncol 17(9):1241–1249. doi:10.1093/neuonc/nov012

Duffy MJ, O'Grady P, Devaney D, O'Siorain L, Fennelly JJ, Lijnen HJ (1988a) Urokinase-plasminogen activator, a marker for aggressive breast carcinomas. Preliminary report. Cancer 62(3):531–533

Duffy MJ, O'Grady P, Devaney D, O'Siorain L, Fennelly JJ, Lijnen HR (1988b) Tissue-type plasminogen activator, a new prognostic marker in breast cancer. Cancer Res 48(5):1348–1349

Eberlin LS, Ferreira CR, Dill AL, Ifa DR, Cooks RG (2011) Desorption electrospray ionization mass spectrometry for lipid characterization and biological tissue imaging. Biochim Biophys Acta 1811(11):946–960. doi:10.1016/j.bbalip.2011.05.006

Garrisi VM, Tommasi S, Facchiano A, Bongarzone I, De Bortoli M, Cremona M, Cafagna V, Abbate I, Tufaro A, Quaranta M, Paradiso A (2013) Proteomic profile in familial breast cancer patients. Clin Biochem 46(3):259–265. doi:10.1016/j.clinbiochem.2012.11.003

Gokmen-Polar Y, Badve S (2014) Multiplexed protein analysis. Sci Trans Med 6(219):219fs3. doi:10.1126/scitranslmed.3008407

Gonzalez-Angulo AM, Hennessy BT, Meric-Bernstam F, Sahin A, Liu W, Ju Z, Carey MS, Myhre S, Speers C, Deng L, Broaddus R, Lluch A, Aparicio S, Brown P, Pusztai L, Symmans WF, Alsner J, Overgaard J, Borresen-Dale AL, Hortobagyi GN, Coombes KR, Mills GB (2011) Functional proteomics can define prognosis and predict pathologic complete response in patients with breast cancer. Clin Proteomics 8(1):11. doi:10.1186/1559-0275-8-11

Gonzalez-Angulo AM, Liu S, Chen H, Chavez-Macgregor M, Sahin A, Hortobagyi GN, Mills GB, Do KA, Meric-Bernstam F (2013) Functional proteomics characterization of residual breast cancer after neoadjuvant systemic chemotherapy. Ann Oncol 24(4):909–916. doi:10.1093/annonc/mds530

Gromov P, Moreira JM, Gromova I (2014) Proteomic analysis of tissue samples in translational breast cancer research. Expert Rev Proteomics 11(3):285–302. doi:10.1586/14789450.2014.899469

Gujral TS, Karp RL, Finski A, Chan M, Schwartz PE, MacBeath G, Sorger P (2013) Profiling phospho-signaling networks in breast cancer using reverse-phase protein arrays. Oncogene 32(29):3470–3476. doi:10.1038/onc.2012.378

Guo L, Xiao Y, Fan M, Li JJ, Wang Y (2015) Profiling global kinome signatures of the radioresistant MCF-7/C6 breast cancer cells using MRM-based targeted proteomics. J Proteome Res 14(1):193–201. doi:10.1021/pr500919w

Harbeck N, Schmitt M, Meisner C, Friedel C, Untch M, Schmidt M, Sweep CG, Lisboa BW, Lux MP, Beck T, Hasmuller S, Kiechle M, Janicke F, Thomssen C, Chemo NSG (2013) Ten-year analysis of the prospective multicentre chemo-N0 trial validates American society of clinical oncology (ASCO)-recommended biomarkers uPA and PAI-1 for therapy decision making in node-negative breast cancer patients. Eur J Cancer 49(8):1825–1835. doi:10.1016/j.ejca.2013.01.007

He W, Tong Y, Wang Y, Liu J, Luo G, Wu J, Zhang J (2013) Serum soluble CD14 is a potential prognostic indicator of recurrence of human breast invasive ductal carcinoma with Her2-enriched subtype. PLoS ONE 8(9):e75366. doi:10.1371/journal.pone.0075366

Hennessy BT, Lu Y, Gonzalez-Angulo AM, Carey MS, Myhre S, Ju Z, Davies MA, Liu W, Coombes K, Meric-Bernstam F, Bedrosian I, McGahren M, Agarwal R, Zhang F, Overgaard J, Alsner J, Neve RM, Kuo WL, Gray JW, Borresen-Dale AL, Mills GB (2010) A technical assessment of the utility of reverse phase protein arrays for the study of the functional proteome in non-microdissected human breast cancers. Clin Proteomics 6(4):129–151. doi:10.1007/s12014-010-9055-y

Ifa DR, Eberlin LS (2016) Ambient ionization mass spectrometry for cancer diagnosis and surgical margin evaluation. Clin Chem 62(1):111–123. doi:10.1373/clinchem.2014.237172

Katchman BA, Ocal IT, Cunliffe HE, Chang YH, Hostetter G, Watanabe A, LoBello J, Lake DF (2013) Expression of quiescin sulfhydryl oxidase 1 is associated with a highly invasive phenotype and correlates with a poor prognosis in Luminal B breast cancer. Breast Cancer Res 15(2):R28. doi:10.1186/bcr3407

Lai X, Wang L, Tang H, Witzmann FA (2011) A novel alignment method and multiple filters for exclusion of unqualified peptides to enhance label-free quantification using peptide intensity in LC-MS/MS. J Proteome Res 10(10):4799–4812. doi:10.1021/pr2005633

Lam SW, Jimenez CR, Boven E (2014) Breast cancer classification by proteomic technologies: current state of knowledge. Cancer Treat Rev 40(1):129–138. doi:10.1016/j.ctrv.2013.06.006

Lapeire L, Hendrix A, Lambein K, Van Bockstal M, Braems G, Van Den Broecke R, Limame R, Mestdagh P, Vandesompele J, Vanhove C, Maynard D, Lehuede C, Muller C, Valet P, Gespach CP, Bracke M, Cocquyt V, Denys H, De Wever O (2014) Cancer-associated adipose tissue promotes breast cancer progression by paracrine oncostatin M and Jak/STAT3 signaling. Cancer Res 74(23):6806–6819. doi:10.1158/0008-5472.CAN-14-0160

Laronga C, Becker S, Watson P, Gregory B, Cazares L, Lynch H, Perry RR, Wright GL Jr, Drake RR, Semmes OJ (2003) SELDI-TOF serum profiling for prognostic and diagnostic classification of breast cancers. Dis Markers 19(4–5):229–238

Li J, Zhang Z, Rosenzweig J, Wang YY, Chan DW (2002) Proteomics and bioinformatics approaches for identification of serum biomarkers to detect breast cancer. Clin Chem 48(8):1296–1304

Li J, Orlandi R, White CN, Rosenzweig J, Zhao J, Seregni E, Morelli D, Yu Y, Meng XY, Zhang Z, Davidson NE, Fung ET, Chan DW (2005) Independent validation of candidate breast cancer serum biomarkers identified by mass spectrometry. Clin Chem 51(12):2229–2235. doi:10.1373/clinchem.2005.052878

Liotta LA, Espina V, Mehta AI, Calvert V, Rosenblatt K, Geho D, Munson PJ, Young L, Wulfkuhle J, Petricoin EF 3rd (2003) Protein microarrays: meeting analytical challenges for clinical applications. Cancer Cell 3(4):317–325

Lipton A, Kostler WJ, Leitzel K, Ali SM, Sperinde J, Weidler J, Paquet A, Sherwood T, Huang W, Bates M, Trastuzumab Response Biomarker G (2010) Quantitative HER2 protein levels predict outcome in fluorescence in situ hybridization-positive patients with metastatic breast cancer treated with trastuzumab. Cancer 116(22):5168–5178. doi:10.1002/cncr.25430

Lundgren DH, Hwang SI, Wu L, Han DK (2010) Role of spectral counting in quantitative proteomics. Expert Rev Proteomics 7(1):39–53. doi:10.1586/epr.09.69

Majidzadeh AK, Gharechahi J (2013) Plasma proteomics analysis of tamoxifen resistance in breast cancer. Med Oncol 30(4):753. doi:10.1007/s12032-013-0753-y

Martinez-Lozano Sinues P, Landoni E, Miceli R, Dibari VF, Dugo M, Agresti R, Tagliabue E, Cristoni S, Orlandi R (2015) Secondary electrospray ionization-mass spectrometry and a novel statistical bioinformatic approach identifies a cancer-related profile in exhaled breath of breast cancer patients: a pilot study. J Breath Res 9(3):031001. doi:10.1088/1752-7155/9/3/031001

Meng R, Gormley M, Bhat VB, Rosenberg A, Quong AA (2011) Low abundance protein enrichment for discovery of candidate plasma protein biomarkers for early detection of breast cancer. J Proteomics 75(2):366–374. doi:10.1016/j.jprot.2011.07.030

Muraoka S, Kume H, Watanabe S, Adachi J, Kuwano M, Sato M, Kawasaki N, Kodera Y, Ishitobi M, Inaji H, Miyamoto Y, Kato K, Tomonaga T (2012) Strategy for SRM-based verification of biomarker candidates discovered by iTRAQ method in limited breast cancer tissue samples. J Proteome Res 11(8):4201–4210. doi:10.1021/pr300322q

Naba A, Clauser KR, Lamar JM, Carr SA, Hynes RO (2014) Extracellular matrix signatures of human mammary carcinoma identify novel metastasis promoters. Elife 3:e01308. doi:10.7554/eLife.01308

Omenn GS, States DJ, Adamski M, Blackwell TW, Menon R, Hermjakob H, Apweiler R, Haab BB, Simpson RJ, Eddes JS, Kapp EA, Moritz RL, Chan DW, Rai AJ, Admon A, Aebersold R, Eng J, Hancock WS, Hefta SA, Meyer H, Paik YK, Yoo JS, Ping P, Pounds J, Adkins J, Qian X, Wang R, Wasinger V, Wu CY, Zhao X, Zeng R, Archakov A, Tsugita A, Beer I, Pandey A, Pisano M, Andrews P, Tammen H, Speicher DW, Hanash SM (2005) Overview of the HUPO plasma proteome project: results from the pilot phase with 35 collaborating laboratories and multiple analytical groups, generating a core dataset of 3020 proteins and a publicly-available database. Proteomics 5(13):3226–3245. doi:10.1002/pmic.200500358

Phizicky E, Bastiaens PI, Zhu H, Snyder M, Fields S (2003) Protein analysis on a proteomic scale. Nature 422(6928):208–215. doi:10.1038/nature01512

Prieto DA, Johann DJ Jr, Wei BR, Ye X, Chan KC, Nissley DV, Simpson RM, Citrin DE, Mackall CL, Linehan WM, Blonder J (2014) Mass spectrometry in cancer biomarker research: a case for immunodepletion of abundant blood-derived proteins from clinical tissue specimens. Biomark Med 8(2):269–286. doi:10.2217/bmm.13.101

Rao VS, Srinivas K, Sujini GN, Kumar GN (2014) Protein–protein interaction detection: methods and analysis. Int J Proteomics 2014:147648. doi:10.1155/2014/147648

Sohn J, Do KA, Liu S, Chen H, Mills GB, Hortobagyi GN, Meric-Bernstam F, Gonzalez-Angulo AM (2013) Functional proteomics characterization of residual triple-negative breast cancer after standard neoadjuvant chemotherapy. Ann Oncol 24(10):2522–2526. doi:10.1093/annonc/mdt248

Sonntag J, Bender C, Soons Z, von der Heyde S, König R, Wiemann S, Sinn H-P, Schneeweiss A, Beißbarth T, Korf U (2014) Reverse phase protein array based tumor profiling identifies a biomarker signature for risk classification of hormone receptor-positive breast cancer. Adv Integr Med 2:52–59

Tzouros M, Golling S, Avila D, Lamerz J, Berrera M, Ebeling M, Langen H, Augustin A (2013) Development of a 5-plex SILAC method tuned for the quantitation of tyrosine phosphorylation dynamics. Mol Cell Proteomics 12(11):3339–3349. doi:10.1074/mcp.O113.027342

Villanueva J, Shaffer DR, Philip J, Chaparro CA, Erdjument-Bromage H, Olshen AB, Fleisher M, Lilja H, Brogi E, Boyd J, Sanchez-Carbayo M, Holland EC, Cordon-Cardo C, Scher HI, Tempst P (2006) Differential exoprotease activities confer tumor-specific serum peptidome patterns. J Clin Invest 116(1):271–284. doi:10.1172/JCI26022

Wilkins MR, Pasquali C, Appel RD, Ou K, Golaz O, Sanchez JC, Yan JX, Gooley AA, Hughes G, Humphery-Smith I, Williams KL, Hochstrasser DF (1996) From proteins to proteomes: large scale protein identification by two-dimensional electrophoresis and amino acid analysis. Biotechnol (N Y) 14(1):61–65

Wulfkuhle JD, Berg D, Wolff C, Langer R, Tran K, Illi J, Espina V, Pierobon M, Deng J, DeMichele A, Walch A, Bronger H, Becker I, Waldhor C, Hofler H, Esserman L, Investigators IST, Liotta LA, Becker KF, Petricoin EF 3rd (2012) Molecular analysis of HER2 signaling in human breast cancer by functional protein pathway activation mapping. Clin Cancer Res 18(23):6426–6435. doi:10.1158/1078-0432.CCR-12-0452

Yang WS, Moon HG, Kim HS, Choi EJ, Yu MH, Noh DY, Lee C (2012) Proteomic approach reveals FKBP4 and S100A9 as potential prediction markers of therapeutic response to neoadjuvant chemotherapy in patients with breast cancer. J Proteome Res 11 (2):1078–1088. doi:10.1021/pr2008187

Zang L, Palmer Toy D, Hancock WS, Sgroi DC, Karger BL (2004) Proteomic analysis of ductal carcinoma of the breast using laser capture microdissection, LC-MS, and 16O/18O isotopic labeling. J Proteome Res 3(3):604–612

Zardavas D, Irrthum A, Swanton C, Piccart M (2015) Clinical management of breast cancer heterogeneity. Nat Rev Clin Oncol 12(7):381–394. doi:10.1038/nrclinonc.2015.73

Zeidan BA, Townsend PA, Garbis SD, Copson E, Cutress RI (2015) Clinical proteomics and breast cancer. Surgeon 13(5):271–278. doi:10.1016/j.surge.2014.12.003

Zeng Z, Hincapie M, Pitteri SJ, Hanash S, Schalkwijk J, Hogan JM, Wang H, Hancock WS (2011) A proteomics platform combining depletion, multi-lectin affinity chromatography (M-LAC), and isoelectric focusing to study the breast cancer proteome. Anal Chem 83(12):4845–4854. doi:10.1021/ac2002802

Zhao B, Xu B, Hu W, Song C, Wang F, Liu Z, Ye M, Zou H, Miao QR (2015) Comprehensive proteome quantification reveals NgBR as a new regulator for epithelial-mesenchymal transition of breast tumor cells. J Proteomics 112:38–52. doi:10.1016/j.jprot.2014.08.007

Zhu T, Xu L, Xu X, Wang Z, Zhu J, Xie Q, Zhang B, Wang Y, Ju L, He Y, Ye X, Zhou D, Li Y (2015) Analysis of breast cancer-associated glycosphingolipids using electrospray ionization-linear ion trap quadrupole mass spectrometry. Carbohydr Res 402:189–199. doi:10.1016/j.carres.2014.10.006

26 Biomarkers in the Clinic

Lida Mina and George W. Sledge

Abstract

The recent years has seen massive advances in technology that has helped better understand the biology of breast cancer. This understanding has resulted in the recognition that breast cancer is not a single disease but a group of diseases. The testing of biomarkers has become integral to therapeutics of breast cancer. These decisions are based not only on the extent of disease but on the specific the type of breast cancer. Terms unheard up a decade ago (luminal and TNBC) have become part of the language. However, only a few of the biomarkers have reached to the level of clinical practice. In this chapter we discuss the current status of biomarker usage and the limitations associated with the application of novel biomarkers to clinical practice.

Keywords

ER · PR · HER2 · Next gen sequencing · SHIVA

26.1 Introduction

An astonishing number of breast cancer biomarkers (certainly in the hundreds) have been evaluated since the discovery of the estrogen receptor in the late 1960s. Yet despite a half-century of work in this field, biomarkers that are both *validated* and *used* in the clinic remain few in number.

This chapter will review biomarker basics from a clinical standpoint, asking the question "what makes a biomarker both valid and useful."

26.2 Why Biomarkers?

Biomarkers represent not only the scientist's desire to understand the natural history or biology of a human cancer, but the clinician's desire to affect clinical outcome in some meaningful way. Breast cancer biomarkers fall into one of

L. Mina
Banner MD Anderson Cancer Center, Gilbert, AZ, USA

G.W. Sledge (✉)
Stanford University School of Medicine, 269 Campus Dr., CCSR-1115, Stanford, CA 94305, USA
e-mail: gsledge@stanford.edu

S. Badve and Y. Gökmen-Polar (eds.), *Molecular Pathology of Breast Cancer*, DOI 10.1007/978-3-319-41761-5_26

two main categories: prognostic and predictive (Table 26.1). *Prognostic* biomarkers define the natural history of a disease subset, either in the presence or absence of an intervening therapy. *Predictive* biomarkers, in contrast, define populations that benefit from (or lack benefit with) a specific therapeutic intervention.

Biomarkers may be both prognostic and predictive. For instance, the Oncotype Dx 21-gene assay defines prognosis (the natural history of estrogen-receptor positive breast cancer based on a recurrence score), but also predicts benefit (or lack thereof) to adjuvant chemotherapy in the same population.

There is no intrinsic reason why a biomarker need be both prognostic and predictive. Indeed, many prognostic biomarkers do not predict therapeutic benefit. This lack of predictive ability, however, diminishes clinician and patient interest in a biomarker. The reason is simple: physicians obtain biomarkers to affect clinical outcome, which typically involves making a specific therapeutic decision.

Even when a biomarker has biologic plausibility and predictive potential, that biomarker may not be readily embraced by either physicians or patients. Surveys of patients in both the adjuvant and metastatic settings suggest that many—perhaps the majority—of patients will accept significant therapeutic toxicity for even a small therapeutic benefit (Simes and Coates 2001; Smith et al. 2014). A biomarker that lacks "all-or-nothing" predictive ability may therefore be rejected despite scientific validity: at the end of the day clinical utility may not be easily defined or routinely accepted.

For instance, measures of circulating tumor cells (CTC) are well-validated determinants of patient outcome in the setting of metastatic disease, and indeed a rising circulating tumor cell count in the setting of a chemotherapy regimen demonstrates with fair certainty that that regimen will not benefit the patient. However, when the Southwest Oncology Group in its SWOG S0500 trial randomized patients with rising CTC levels to continue the same regimen or switch to a new regimen, no therapeutic benefit was seen for early biomarker-based therapeutic decision-making. While there are several potential reasons for this failure, the end result is that the biomarker, while prognostic, predictive, and highly validated, lacked sufficient utility to justify routine use (Smerage et al. 2014).

In the following narrative, we will study the most well established biomarkers shedding light on their prognostic, predictive as well as their clinical utility when applicable.

26.3 The Established Targets: ER, PR, and HER2

The estrogen receptor is the oldest established biomarker in breast cancer. The estrogen story began more than 100 years ago with a case report in the *Lancet* when the surgeon George Thomas Beatson described performing an oophorectomy on a young woman with inflammatory breast cancer, and that patient's clinical response. But it was not until the 1960s that the estrogen receptor (ER) was first characterized and measured by Jensen et al. (1971). In 1973, McGuire et al. described the DCC (dextran-coated charcoal) assay to quantify the estrogen receptor protein and suggested that quantifying ER was useful in guiding the therapeutic approach.

Table 26.1 Commonly used biomarkers in clinical practice and their functional utility

Markers	Prognostic	Predictive
Estrogen	Yes	Yes
Progesterone	Yes	No
HER2	Yes	Yes
BRCA1, BRCA2	No	Yes
CTC	Yes	No
Ki67	Yes	No
Androgen receptor	No	*Possibly*

Since then the ER story only got more interesting. We now know that more than 80 % of breast cancer is estrogen positive and potentially responsive to estrogen blockade. The Oxford Overview on adjuvant therapies for breast cancer did show that endocrine treatment is of benefit only in patients with tumors that are ER and/or progesterone receptor (PR) positive (Early Breast Cancer Trialists' Collaborative 2005). Testing of those markers has become a standard integral part of the initial assessment of a breast tumor in the cancer pathology laboratory. The old Dextran-Coated Charcoal (DCC) assay has now been replaced by the immunohistochemistry (IHC) test, which has proven to be more challenging than expected. The degree of estrogen sensitivity is currently quantified and may be expressed as the percentage of cells stained after incubation with anti-ER/PR antibodies. Despite all the hiccups of its testing, estrogen receptor positivity remains to date the best predictive marker of endocrine sensitivity in both the adjuvant and metastatic settings (Harvey et al. 1999).

The optimal algorithm for ER/PR testing has been recently summarized in the ASCO/CAP ER and PgR guideline recommendations (Table 26.2). The value of this marker for our patients goes beyond predicting endocrine therapy benefit; this marker defines the biology of this particular disease and helps avoid chemotherapy in innumerable patients. This is precious information because it has spared many women the harms of cytotoxic therapy that could be fatal or highly morbid.

Progesterone receptor status is, however, a more complicated story. Whereas the role of estrogen as a breast cancer mitogen is undisputed, the role of progesterone remains more controversial and less well understood (Hilton et al. 2012). Historically, the progesterone receptor was considered a marker for functional ER activity because PR is an ER target gene (Bal et al. 2015). Recent data however suggests that progesterone receptor function and target gene regulation may represent an independent driver of breast cancer cell proliferation as well as a predictor of mortality. These findings in humans are supported by numerous studies conducted in animal models of breast cancer (Chlebowski et al. 2003; Hilton et al. 2012; Carnevale et al. 2007; Labriola et al. 2003; Lanari et al. 1986a, b; Lydon et al. 1995; Michna et al. 1989; Molinolo et al. 1987; Poole et al. 2006).

26.4 Endocrine Resistance

Although the estrogen receptor status remains the strongest biomarker in breast cancer, its utility is limited by de novo as well as acquired resistance during endocrine therapy. About 30 % of front-line patients with metastatic disease have objective regression of tumor with initial endocrine treatment, while another 20 % have prolonged stable disease. Several different escape mechanisms account for the lack of sensitivity to hormonal therapy in the rest of those patients. Osborne and colleagues reviewed the different signaling pathways and suggested three principal mechanisms of estrogen resistance that should be considered when estrogen blockade fails (Giuliano et al. 2011; Osborne and Schiff 2011). These are: (1) Upregulation or downregulation of the cell cycle signaling molecules (such as overexpression of cyclins E1 and D1) can result in endocrine resistance either by activating cyclin-dependent kinases critical for G1 phase or by relieving the inhibitory effects of the negative cell cycle regulators p21 and p27 (Butt et al.

Table 26.2 Testing for ER/PR per ASCO/CAP guidelines

Positive for ER or PgR	If ≥1 % of tumor cell nuclei are immunoreactive
Negative for ER or PgR	If <1 % of tumor cell nuclei are immunoreactive in the presence of evidence that the sample can express ER or PgR (positive intrinsic controls are seen)
Uninterpretable for ER or PgR	If no tumor nuclei are immunoreactive and that internal epithelial elements present in the sample or separately submitted from the same sample lack any nuclear staining

2005; Span et al. 2003). (2) Loss of estrogen receptor expression through the upregulation or dysregulation of ER and PR coregulators; and finally (3) Growth factor receptor pathways such as the HER tyrosine kinase receptor family and receptors for insulin/IGF1, FGF, and VEGF, as well as cellular Src, AKT, and stress-related kinases have also been implicated (Arpino et al. 2008; Chakraborty et al. 2010; Kern et al. 1994; Morgan et al. 2009). More recently there has been growing evidence that ESR1 mutations are associated with resistance in patients progressing on adjuvant endocrine therapy (Fuqua et al. 2014).

Can we find new biomarkers based on those complex signaling pathways? Should we target both estrogen and other pathways at the same time? This is an important question. The answer will be in clinical trials built in around correlative studies requiring timely biopsies of breast or distant site tissue at multiple time points during therapy. Both physician and patients' selfless commitment is required to achieve that goal.

26.5 HER2

The human epidermal growth factor receptor type 2, or ERBB2 (and more frequently referred to as HER2), is an important prognostic as well as predictive tool in breast cancer. HER2 encodes a member of the epidermal growth factor receptor (EGFR) family of tyrosine kinases. Amplification of HER2 is the predominant mechanism of gene overexpression and abnormally high levels of this 185-kDa glycoprotein are seen in approximately 18–20 % of breast cancers (King et al. 1985; Yaziji et al. 2004; Slamon et al. 1987; Owens et al. 2004).

The HER2 story in breast cancer has been another great example on the successful transition of a targeted therapy from the laboratory to the clinic. HER2 was initially identified as a poor prognostic factor; its overexpression portends an overall dismal outcome for patients with breast cancer.

HER2 transitioned very quickly from being a prognostic biomarker to a valid predictive marker for response to anti-HER2 therapy. In September 1998, the FDA approved trastuzumab, an anti-HER2 monoclonal antibody, in combination with chemotherapy for women with metastatic breast cancers that overexpress HER2. This led to the rapid launching of four international trials (HERA, NCCTG 9831, NSABP-31, and BCIRG006) involving more than 10,000 women treated with trastuzumab-based therapy in the adjuvant setting. Those pivotal trials proved that 1 year of Trastuzumab plus standard adjuvant therapy significantly reduced the risk of disease recurrence and extended overall survival significantly (Puglisi and Piccart 2005; Romond et al. 2005; Piccart-Gebhart et al. 2005). Based on these trials, the FDA approval was expanded to include treatment of HER2 positive early stage breast cancer in the adjuvant setting.

Since then, there has been further significant progress in targeting the HER2 signaling pathway. Pertuzumab, another monoclonal antibody, prevents dimerization between HER2 and HER3, its preferential binding partner. Pertuzumab has already been approved in both the neoadjuvant as well as the first line metastatic setting based on results from the Neosphere as well as the Cleopatra study (Gianni et al. 2012; Swain et al. 2015; Baselga et al. 2012). Tyrosine kinase inhibitors are also being heavily investigated; lapatinib was approved in the metastatic setting, whereas neratinib has shown very promising results in the adjuvant setting (Geyer et al. 2006; Cameron et al. 2008, 2010). Finally, TDM1, a conjugate of trastuzumab with the cytotoxic agent, was approved in the second line metastatic setting (Verma et al. 2012; Krop et al. 2015, 2014).

The importance of identifying a population enriched with HER2 overexpressing breast cancer has led to more efforts to achieve an accurate and reproducible measurement of HER2 status. We are still far from mastering it however we have come a long way and we have finally a consensus on interpreting those tests based on recommendations from both the American Society of Clinical Oncology and the College of American Pathologists (Table 26.3).

Table 26.3 Testing for HER2 per ASCO/CAP guidelines

HER2 test result positive for HER2 if	– IHC 3+ based on circumferential membrane staining that is complete, intense Or – ISH positive based on • Single-probe average HER2 copy number ≥6.0 signals/cell • Dual-probe HER2/CEP17 ratio ≥2; with an average HER2 copy number ≥4.0 or <4 signals/cell • Dual-probe HER2/CEP17 ratio <2; with an average HER2 copy number >6 signals/cell
HER2 test result equivocal[a] for HER2 if	– IHC 2+ based on circumferential membrane staining that is incomplete and/or weak/moderate and within >10 % of the invasive tumor cells; or complete and circumferential membrane staining that is intense and within ≤10 % of the invasive tumor cells Or – ISH equivocal based on • Single-probe ISH average HER2 copy number ≥4.0 and <6 signals/cell • Dual-probe HER2/CEP17 ratio <2; with an average HER2 copy number ≥4.0 and <6 signals/cell
HER2 test result negative for HER2 if	– IHC 1+ as defined by incomplete membrane staining that is faint/barely perceptible and within >10 % of the invasive tumor cells Or – IHC 0 as defined by no staining observed or membrane staining that is incomplete and is faint/barely perceptible and within ≤10 % of the invasive tumor cells Or – ISH negative based on • Single-probe average HER2 copy number <4.0 signals/cell • Dual-probe HER2/CEP17 ratio <2.0 with an average HER2 copy number <4.0 signals/cell

[a]Must order reflex test (same specimen using the alternative test) or new test (new specimen, if available, using same or alternative test)

26.6 HER2 Resistance: When the Biomarker Fails Us

Although progress against HER2 is definitely palpable, several questions remain unanswered. Many women with HER2 positive disease either fail to respond to initial therapy or even progress following an initial response. Our knowledge of the mechanisms of resistance remains limited.

Molecular mechanisms that can play a role in trastuzumab resistance include but are not limited to the following: (1) Truncated HER2 receptor. When the HER2 receptor has aberrant epitopes, this will hinder trastuzumab binding and will interfere with its function (Arribas et al. 2011); (2) Genetic aberration in the downstream signaling pathway such as the PI3K/Akt pathway. Loss of function of PTEN or activating mutations of PI3K can possibly lead to trastuzumab resistance (Berns et al. 2007; Razis et al. 2011; Serra et al. 2008); (3) Compensatory activation of parallel signaling pathways (so-called "horizontal resistance") such as IGFR1 and HER3 pathways also can lead to loss of sensitivity to trastuzumab (Sergina et al. 2007; Lu et al. 2001).

At present there are no established biomarkers predicting resistance to therapy for any HER2-targeted agent. As such, the ASCO/ACP guidelines remain the standard approach to identifying HER2-sensitive tumors. We desperately need novel biomarkers that would reliably predict resistance. Increasingly there are suggestions that immune markers of response may ultimately prove beneficial in predicting adjuvant benefit (Perez et al. 2015).

26.7 Triple Negative Breast Cancer

Triple negative breast cancer is still defined clinically by its lack of a defined therapeutic target. Indeed, calling a tumor "triple negative" (i.e., negative for ER, PT and HER2 biomarkers) is virtually an admission of therapeutic futility, at least as regards targeted therapies such as estrogen blockade and HER2-targeted therapy. Finding predictive biomarkers to guide treatment in triple negative tumors remains a major challenge in breast cancer for both scientists and clinicians (Le Du et al. 2015).

Molecular studies of triple negative breast cancer have revealed the intrinsic heterogeneity of this disease. Gene expression profiling has identified over a decade ago that the majority of triple negative disease falls into the Basal-like subtype. Since then, Perou and colleagues have further dissected the molecular profiles of triple negative cancers, and other subtypes are emerging (Sorlie et al. 2001, 2003; Prat and Perou 2011). Recently, the Vanderbilt group defined 6 unique subsets through gene expression analysis of over 500 breast tumors from over 20 independent datasets (Lehmann et al. 2011). This analysis classified TNBC into the following clusters: two basal-like (BL1 and BL2), an immune-modulatory (IM), a mesenchymal (M), a mesenchymal stem-like (MSL), and a luminal androgen receptor (LAR) subtype. Each of those subgroups has a potential therapeutic targeted approach but none of them is clinically validated for standard practice at the present time.

Perhaps the most promising biomarkers at this juncture are genes involved in DNA damage repair, particularly BRCA mutations. An integrated molecular analysis of breast carcinomas in The Cancer Genome Atlas (TCGA) reported that ~20 % of Basal-like breast tumors harbored a BRCA1 or BRCA2 mutation, of which ~2/3 were germline and 1/3 somatic. BRCA carriers share a deficiency in Homologous recombination DNA pathway, a pathway uniquely involved in the repair of interstrand cross links. Using this pathway as a drug targetable biomarker is emerging as a new potential therapeutic approach (Schouten and Linn 2015).

Platinum agents are currently being investigated as a preferred treatment for BRCA-mutant triple negative disease because those agents can cause inter-strand crosslinks that would further damage cells that are vulnerable in that regard. Recently, the use of platinum in triple negative breast cancer was examined in two studies. The PrEcog 0105 trial treated patients with triple negative and/or BRCA, in the neoadjuvant setting with a regimen containing gemcitabine, carboplatin and Iniparib, a pCR of 36 % was achieved (Telli et al. 2015). In the TBCRC 009, a platinum was assessed for triple negative metastatic breast cancer and evaluation of p63/p73 as a biomarker for response. The overall response rate was around 25 %.

Many potential biomarkers for assessing HRD and specifically the HRD-LOH, and HRD-LST scores were investigated. Both markers unfortunately did not seem to be a reliable predictor of response as of yet (Isakoff et al. 2015). However, although no definitive data on their clinical utility is currently available, ongoing studies are still relentlessly looking into this question like the TBCRC 028.

In contrast, the BRCA mutation itself seems to be by far the most promising reproducible biomarker of the platinum effect in triple negative breast cancer. In the above studies the BRCA subpopulation seemed to derive the most benefit from platinum. This is also most illustrated in the TNT TRIAL (Tutt 2014). In that study, patients with locally advanced or metastatic TNBC were randomly assigned to therapy with Carboplatin AUC 6 or standard of care Docetaxel. A total of 376 patients were randomized, 43 had the BRCA1 or BRCA2 mutations. In the overall group there was no improvement in overall survival favoring platinum over the taxane. However, women with the BRCA mutation had a significantly higher response rate as well as a longer progression-free survival when treated with carboplatin (68 % vs. 30 %). At the same time, the composite score of the three tests for the HRD (LOH, LST and Telomeric allelic imbalance) was not predictive of benefit.

BRCA1 and BRCA2 mutations would seem to be appropriate biomarkers for sensitivity to

PARP inhibition. PARP (poly ADP ribose polymerase) is an enzyme intrinsically involved in base excision repair, a key pathway in DNA single strands breaks. Farmer and colleagues demonstrated that BRCA1 and BRCA2 deficient cells are particularly vulnerable to PARP depletion (Farmer et al. 2005). They proposed the following model: PARP inhibition can lead to inefficient base excision repair; this would cause persistent single-strand breaks in DNA. Those breaks could degenerate into double stranded breaks which repair is usually dependent on both BRCA1 and BRCA2. In the absence of BRCA, the repair of those breaks is compromised leading to death of the cells.

Based on the above "synthetic lethality" concept, several trials have been launched with different PARP inhibitors in the BRCA-mutant patient population. Olaparib was the first parp inhibitor with evidence of activity in BRCA1 and BRCA2 carriers with heavily pretreated breast cancer. In a phase 1 study of 27 patients, by Tutt et al. (2010), olaparib showed excellent results. Currently, there are more than 40 clinical trials with 4 different parp inhibitors actively recruiting, 3 of those PARP inhibitors are in phase III trials in metastatic breast cancer, talazoparib, olaparib, and niraparib.

Identifying non-BRCA associated TNBC tumors with similar phenotype and DNA damage repair defect with potential to benefit from PARP inhibition remains a subject of intense and ongoing research. HRD as mentioned above is one venue. Another possibility is identifying more specific mutations also involved in the DNA repair pathways like the PALB2. PALB2 has been recently identified as a partner of BRAC2 that encodes a BRCA2-interacting protein that helps in homologous recombination and double-strand breaks repair. A study by Rahman et al. demonstrated that PALB2 is a breast cancer susceptibility gene that is responsible for familial breast cancer. We argue that PALB2 could be a predictor of sensitivity to Parp inhibitors and should be potentially included in the trials with PARP inhibitors (Antoniou et al. 2014; Rahman et al. 2007).

Androgen receptor positivity is another biomarker being studied lately as a potential therapeutic target. Studies are promising; a recent study by Traina et al. showed that enzalutamide [a potent inhibitor of androgen receptor (AR)] is of potential benefit in women with advanced androgen receptor positive triple negative breast cancer (Proverbs-Singh et al. 2015).

The search for the targetable positives in the triple negative disease is still ongoing and an ideal biomarker is yet to be found. Triple negative breast cancer is not one disease, but instead a heterogeneous set of diseases. The answer will not lie in one biomarker but in multiple and possibly a combination of many before cure is achieved (Le Du and Ueno 2015).

26.8 The Multigene Assays

In recent years, biomarker discovery became more sophisticated as it moved slowly to the molecular level. Perou and colleagues analyzed breast cancer gene expression patterns derived from cDNA microarrays and identified 4 major intrinsic gene signatures: luminal (A and B), the basal-like, HER2-enriched and normal breast like. More recently other molecular subtypes have been described including the claudin low and the molecular apocrine tumors. Those subtypes have been shown to correlate not only with survival but also with therapeutic response.

Currently the field is becoming crowded with emerging novel gene expression prognostic tests for breast cancer however the power of prediction is still lacking in most of them. These include the Oncotype DX 21-gene array, followed closely by the MammaPrint, PAM 50, the Mapquant DX and the Theros Breast Cancer Index. Those gene assays add valuable prognostic information and can also provide an extra technical tool for testing of biomarkers that adds to the conventional IHC (although rarely used for that specific purpose and reasonably so).

The first FDA approved signature was the 70-gene MammaPrint, also called the Amsterdam 70-gene prognostic profile assay. It was developed using a supervised DNA microarray analysis of gene expression arrays on frozen tissue from 98 primary breast tumors.

A mathematical equation is then calculated to find a score which divides patients with breast cancer into the low risk group vs. the high risk group (van't Veer et al. 2002; van de Vijver et al. 2002). The clinical validity of this multi-gene biomarker has been proven in multiple studies where it was used in patients with early stage breast cancer, regardless of ER or HER2 status, to predict distant metastases at 10 years (Buyse et al. 2006; Mook et al. 2010). However, at this time it still lacks prospective data backing its clinical predictive utility. An ongoing international trial the MINDACT (Microarray in node negative disease may avoid chemotherapy) is currently being analyzed to answer that question (Cardoso et al. 2008).

The Oncotype DX is currently the most widely applied multigene assay in the adjuvant clinical setting. This 21-gene recurrence score has both prognostic but it and predictive value. The RS was developed by questioning the 250 most promising cancer tumors in 447 patient tumors using a reverse transcription polymerase chain reaction-based method. Investigators then identified 16 genes (with 5 reference genes) that could predict the risk of breast cancer recurrence in women with estrogen positive tumors receiving tamoxifen. Subsequent analyses demonstrated that the presence of a low recurrence score (approximately half of lymph-node negative, ER-positive breast cancers) predicted lack of benefit with adjuvant chemotherapy, results that significantly reduce the use of adjuvant chemotherapy in this group (Paik et al. 2004; Mamounas et al. 2010; Dowsett et al. 2010). While initial studies with this assay involved retrospective looks at prior clinical trials, the recent US Intergroup TAILORx trial prospectively validated the 21-gene recurrence score in lymph node-negative breast cancer for women with a low recurrence score (Sparano et al. 2015).

ASCO has suggested preference as far as using those tests in the clinic to guide treatment of early stage estrogen positive breast cancer (Burstein et al. 2010). While their use is still primarily limited to lymph node-negative disease, some studies have suggested that the predictive value of this multiplex biomarker might equally well be applied to lymph node-positive ER-positive disease in the adjuvant setting (Albain et al. 2010). This prospect is currently being examined in the Southwest Oncology Group's RxPONDER trial in patients with 1–3 positive lymph nodes. If this trial ultimately supports the use of multi-gene arrays in this population, the ultimate effect will be to reduce the use of adjuvant chemotherapy in ER-positive disease.

26.9 Proliferation as a Clinical Biomarker: Ki67

Ki67 remains at this time the most extensively studied marker of proliferation in early stage breast cancer. Data from 2 large meta-analyses have reported the prognostic implication of Ki67, with an elevated Ki67 being associated with an increased risk of recurrence (de Azambuja et al. 2007; Stuart-Harris et al. 2008).

A recurring issue with measures of Ki67 has been the lack of inter-observer reproducibility. Because of this, the American Society of Clinical Oncology (ASCO) tumor marker expert panel as well as the international IMPAKT working group recommend against the routine use of proliferation markers to assess prognosis (Harris et al. 2007; Guiu et al. 2012).

26.10 Biomarkers of the Future: The "Omics"

The Human Genome Project and its cancer-related offspring (such as The Cancer Genome Atlas, or TCGA) offer a novel and potentially exciting advance for the biomarker field. The ability to measure either the whole exome, or the whole genome, for the price of BRCA testing or of an Oncotype Dx offers exciting possibilities for biomarker analysis. Other "omics" (e.g., transcriptomics, proteomics and metabolomics) are following close behind.

The availability of (relatively) cheap genomic analyses has led to a proliferation of commercially available genomic testing focused on mutational analysis of so-called "driver mutations." Such panels (e.g., Paradigm, Foundation Medicine) provide information on specific cancer-related mutations that are—in the view of the providers—"actionable" in the clinic. "Actionable", however, is a slippery term. To the patient it means "this test will tell me which drug works for my cancer." In contrast, "actionable" currently means "we can identify a driver mutation or mutations, and there is a specific drug that inhibits the kinase or growth factor receptor coded for by that mutation and may have been used in some cancer with therapeutic benefit."

That such "actionable" mutations are tricky creatures is demonstrated by the recent SHIVA trial, which randomized patients with metastatic cancer to either a "doctor's best choice" regimen or to molecularly targeted therapy based on a genomic analysis performed as part of the trial. There was no statistically significant difference in progression-free survival between the two arms (Le Tourneau et al. 2015).

There are several reasons why such molecularly targeted therapy might fail patients. Much of cancer biology is contextual; i.e., organ-specific actions abound, and resistance patterns vary by organ. Resistance to EGFR-targeted therapy varies from colorectal to lung to head and neck cancer. Furthermore, targeting a single driver mutation may prove inadequate for breast cancers that have as many as six driver mutations (Stephens et al. 2012). Which mutation does one target, or which combination does one use? We are currently drowning in an "N of 1" sea of empiricism.

SHIVA was a nondefinitive randomized Phase II trial that tested agents across a broad array of cancers. The optimal drugs may not have been used (such trials tend to snatch what is available), and not enough mutations may have been targeted. Nevertheless, SHIVA suggests that genomic analyses should be used with caution. The clinical benefit (which, from a regulatory standpoint, is rarely just about objective tumor response) of random molecular testing/targeting remains unproven, though several active trials (e.g., the NCI MATCH trial) are ongoing.

Another exciting prospect involves the use of circulating tumor DNA to measure cancer in a dynamic fashion (Newman et al. 2014). While ctDNA is in its infancy, it is clear that we can measure cancer-related mutations in patients with advanced cancers, and can use such measures to predict early relapse (Garcia-Murillas et al. 2015). This opens the prospect of discovering emerging mutations at an early point in time, allowing for earlier and more appropriate therapeutic interventions.

The unparalleled explosion of data (so-called "big data") emerging from the "omics" revolutions are both exciting and challenging. Large quantities of potential biomarkers pose specific bioinformatics and clinical trials challenges. The endless profusion of "omics"-based biomarkers that the field is experiencing has not been an unmixed blessing. Small numbers of patients, lack of reproducibility, lack of appropriate quality assurance and quality control and lack of biologic plausibility have shadowed the biomarker field since its inception. These issues are magnified rather than reduced by the "big data" revolution. Yet their promise—the integrated, comprehensive look at the biology of the tumor—draws us forward.

What will the practice of oncology look like in a decade? The outlines of the future are already apparent. The rapid decline in the cost of genomic analysis will continue, rendering deep sequencing cheap and ubiquitous. The use of broad national databases (e.g., ASCO's CancerLinq) will support the rapid collection of "N of 1" outcomes into something like large (if unplanned) cohort studies identifying which targeted therapies benefit which patients with which specific mutation or mutations. The sequential use of genomic technologies (e.g., with circulating tumor DNA) will allow physicians to intervene at an early point in time with active agents, thwarting the cancer's Darwinian machinery. The demonstration that specific mutational patterns are associated with therapeutic failure will support the elimination of agents that are both expensive and toxic, reducing health care costs while promoting individual quality of life. While all this may seem incredible, the arc of medical history bends towards better health for all.

References

Albain KS, Barlow WE, Shak S et al (2010) Prognostic and predictive value of the 21-gene recurrence score assay in postmenopausal women with node-positive, oestrogen-receptor-positive breast cancer on chemotherapy: a retrospective analysis of a randomised trial. Lancet Oncol 11(1):55–65

Antoniou AC, Casadei S, Heikkinen T et al (2014) Breast-cancer risk in families with mutations in PALB2. N Engl J Med 371(6):497–506

Arpino G, Wiechmann L, Osborne CK, Schiff R (2008) Crosstalk between the estrogen receptor and the HER tyrosine kinase receptor family: molecular mechanism and clinical implications for endocrine therapy resistance. Endocr Rev 29(2):217–233

Arribas J, Baselga J, Pedersen K, Parra-Palau JL (2011) p95HER2 and breast cancer. Cancer Res 71(5):1515–1519

Bal O, Yalcintas Arslan U, Durnali A et al (2015) Progesterone receptor status in determining the prognosis of estrogen receptor positive/HER2 negative breast carcinoma patients. J BUON 20(1):28–34

Baselga J, Cortes J, Kim SB et al (2012) Pertuzumab plus trastuzumab plus docetaxel for metastatic breast cancer. N Engl J Med 366(2):109–119

Berns K, Horlings HM, Hennessy BT et al (2007) A functional genetic approach identifies the PI3K pathway as a major determinant of trastuzumab resistance in breast cancer. Cancer Cell 12(4):395–402

Burstein HJ, Prestrud AA, Seidenfeld J et al (2010) American Society of Clinical Oncology clinical practice guideline: update on adjuvant endocrine therapy for women with hormone receptor-positive breast cancer. J Clin Oncol 28(23):3784–3796

Butt AJ, McNeil CM, Musgrove EA, Sutherland RL (2005) Downstream targets of growth factor and oestrogen signalling and endocrine resistance: the potential roles of c-Myc, cyclin D1 and cyclin E. Endocr Relat Cancer 12(Suppl 1):S47–S59

Buyse M, Loi S, van't Veer L et al (2006) Validation and clinical utility of a 70-gene prognostic signature for women with node-negative breast cancer. J Natl Cancer Inst 98(17):1183–1192

Cameron D, Casey M, Press M et al (2008) A phase III randomized comparison of lapatinib plus capecitabine versus capecitabine alone in women with advanced breast cancer that has progressed on trastuzumab: updated efficacy and biomarker analyses. Breast Cancer Res Treat 112(3):533–543

Cameron D, Casey M, Oliva C, Newstat B, Imwalle B, Geyer CE (2010) Lapatinib plus capecitabine in women with HER-2-positive advanced breast cancer: final survival analysis of a phase III randomized trial. Oncologist 15(9):924–934

Cardoso F, Van't Veer L, Rutgers E, Loi S, Mook S, Piccart-Gebhart MJ (2008) Clinical application of the 70-gene profile: the MINDACT trial. J Clin Oncol 26 (5):729–735

Carnevale RP, Proietti CJ, Salatino M et al (2007) Progestin effects on breast cancer cell proliferation, proteases activation, and in vivo development of metastatic phenotype all depend on progesterone receptor capacity to activate cytoplasmic signaling pathways. Mol Endocrinol 21(6):1335–1358

Chakraborty A, Chatterjee S, Roy P (2010) Progesterone receptor agonists and antagonists as anticancer agents. Mini Rev Med Chem 10(6):506–517

Chlebowski RT, Hendrix SL, Langer RD et al (2003) Influence of estrogen plus progestin on breast cancer and mammography in healthy postmenopausal women: the women's health initiative randomized trial. JAMA 289(24):3243–3253

de Azambuja E, Cardoso F, de Castro G Jr et al (2007) Ki-67 as prognostic marker in early breast cancer: a meta-analysis of published studies involving 12,155 patients. Br J Cancer 96(10):1504–1513

Dowsett M, Cuzick J, Wale C et al (2010) Prediction of risk of distant recurrence using the 21-gene recurrence score in node-negative and node-positive postmenopausal patients with breast cancer treated with anastrozole or tamoxifen: a TransATAC study. J Clin Oncol 28(11):1829–1834

Early Breast Cancer Trialists' Collaborative G (2005) Effects of chemotherapy and hormonal therapy for early breast cancer on recurrence and 15-year survival: an overview of the randomised trials. Lancet 365 (9472):1687–1717

Farmer H, McCabe N, Lord CJ et al (2005) Targeting the DNA repair defect in BRCA mutant cells as a therapeutic strategy. Nature 434(7035):917–921

Fuqua SA, Gu G, Rechoum Y (2014) Estrogen receptor (ER) alpha mutations in breast cancer: hidden in plain sight. Breast Cancer Res Treat 144(1):11–19

Garcia-Murillas I, Schiavon G, Weigelt B et al (2015) Mutation tracking in circulating tumor DNA predicts relapse in early breast cancer. Sci Trans Med 7 (302):302ra133

Geyer CE, Forster J, Lindquist D et al (2006) Lapatinib plus capecitabine for HER2-positive advanced breast cancer. N Engl J Med 355(26):2733–2743

Gianni L, Pienkowski T, Im YH et al (2012) Efficacy and safety of neoadjuvant pertuzumab and trastuzumab in women with locally advanced, inflammatory, or early HER2-positive breast cancer (NeoSphere): a randomised multicentre, open-label, phase 2 trial. Lancet Oncol 13(1):25–32

Giuliano M, Schifp R, Osborne CK, Trivedi MV (2011) Biological mechanisms and clinical implications of endocrine resistance in breast cancer. Breast 20(Suppl 3):S42–S49

Guiu S, Michiels S, Andre F et al (2012) Molecular subclasses of breast cancer: how do we define them? The IMPAKT 2012 working group statement. Ann Oncol 23(12):2997–3006

Harris L, Fritsche H, Mennel R et al (2007) American Society of Clinical Oncology 2007 update of recommendations for the use of tumor markers in breast cancer. J Clin Oncol 25(33):5287–5312

Harvey JM, Clark GM, Osborne CK, Allred DC (1999) Estrogen receptor status by immunohistochemistry is superior to the ligand-binding assay for predicting response to adjuvant endocrine therapy in breast cancer. J Clin Oncol 17(5):1474–1481

Hilton HN, Graham JD, Kantimm S et al (2012) Progesterone and estrogen receptors segregate into different cell subpopulations in the normal human breast. Mol Cell Endocrinol 361(1–2):191–201

Isakoff SJ, Mayer EL, He L et al (2015) TBCRC009: a multicenter phase II clinical trial of platinum monotherapy with biomarker assessment in metastatic triple-negative breast cancer. J Clin Oncol 33 (17):1902–1909

Jensen EV, Block GE, Smith S, Kyser K, DeSombre ER (1971) Estrogen receptors and breast cancer response to adrenalectomy. Natl Cancer Inst Monogr 34:55–70

Kern FG, McLeskey SW, Zhang L et al (1994) Transfected MCF-7 cells as a model for breast-cancer progression. Breast Cancer Res Treat 31(2–3):153–165

King CR, Kraus MH, Aaronson SA (1985) Amplification of a novel v-erbB-related gene in a human mammary carcinoma. Science 229(4717):974–976

Krop IE, Kim SB, Gonzalez-Martin A et al (2014) Trastuzumab emtansine versus treatment of physician's choice for pretreated HER2-positive advanced breast cancer (TH3RESA): a randomised, open-label, phase 3 trial. Lancet Oncol 15(7):689–699

Krop IE, Lin NU, Blackwell K et al (2015) Trastuzumab emtansine (T-DM1) versus lapatinib plus capecitabine in patients with HER2-positive metastatic breast cancer and central nervous system metastases: a retrospective, exploratory analysis in EMILIA. Ann Oncol 26(1):113–119

Labriola L, Salatino M, Proietti CJ et al (2003) Heregulin induces transcriptional activation of the progesterone receptor by a mechanism that requires functional ErbB-2 and mitogen-activated protein kinase activation in breast cancer cells. Mol Cell Biol 23(3):1095–1111

Lanari C, Molinolo AA, Pasqualini CD (1986a) Induction of mammary adenocarcinomas by medroxyprogesterone acetate in BALB/c female mice. Cancer Lett 33 (2):215–223

Lanari C, Molinolo AA, Pasqualini CD (1986b) Inhibitory effect of medroxyprogesterone acetate on foreign body tumorigenesis in mice. J Natl Cancer Inst 77 (1):157–164

Le Du F, Ueno NT (2015) Targeted therapies in triple-negative breast cancer: failure and future. Womens Health (Lond Engl) 11(1):1–5

Le Du F, Eckhardt BL, Lim B et al (2015) Is the future of personalized therapy in triple-negative breast cancer based on molecular subtype? Oncotarget 6 (15):12890–12908

Le Tourneau C, Delord J-P, Gonçalves A, Gavoille C et al (2015) Molecularly targeted therapy based on tumour molecular profiling versus conventional therapy for advanced cancer (SHIVA): a multicentre, open-label, proof-of-concept, randomised, controlled phase 2 trial. Lancet Oncol 16:1324–1334 (Epub ahead of print)

Lehmann BD, Bauer JA, Chen X et al (2011) Identification of human triple-negative breast cancer subtypes and preclinical models for selection of targeted therapies. J Clin Invest 121(7):2750–2767

Lu Y, Condie A, Bennett JD, Fry MJ, Yuille MR, Shipley J (2001) Disruption of the ATM gene in breast cancer. Cancer Genet Cytogenet 126(2):97–101

Lydon JP, DeMayo FJ, Funk CR et al (1995) Mice lacking progesterone receptor exhibit pleiotropic reproductive abnormalities. Genes Dev 9(18):2266–2278

Mamounas EP, Tang G, Fisher B et al (2010) Association between the 21-gene recurrence score assay and risk of locoregional recurrence in node-negative, estrogen receptor-positive breast cancer: results from NSABP B-14 and NSABP B-20. J Clin Oncol 28(10):1677–1683

McGuire WL (1973) Estrogen receptors in human breast cancer. J Clin Invest 52(1):73–77

Michna H, Schneider MR, Nishino Y, El Etreby MF (1989) Antitumor activity of the antiprogestins ZK 98.299 and RU 38.486 in hormone dependent rat and mouse mammary tumors: mechanistic studies. Breast Cancer Res Treat 14(3):275–288

Molinolo AA, Lanari C, Charreau EH, Sanjuan N, Pasqualini CD (1987) Mouse mammary tumors induced by medroxyprogesterone acetate: immunohistochemistry and hormonal receptors. J Natl Cancer Inst 79(6):1341–1350

Mook S, Schmidt MK, Weigelt B et al (2010) The 70-gene prognosis signature predicts early metastasis in breast cancer patients between 55 and 70 years of age. Ann Oncol 21(4):717–722

Morgan L, Gee J, Pumford S et al (2009) Elevated Src kinase activity attenuates Tamoxifen response in vitro and is associated with poor prognosis clinically. Cancer Biol Ther 8(16):1550–1558

Newman AM, Bratman SV, To J et al (2014) An ultrasensitive method for quantitating circulating tumor DNA with broad patient coverage. Nat Med 20(5):548–554

Osborne CK, Schiff R (2011) Mechanisms of endocrine resistance in breast cancer. Annu Rev Med 62:233–247

Owens MA, Horten BC, Da Silva MM (2004) HER2 amplification ratios by fluorescence in situ hybridization and correlation with immunohistochemistry in a cohort of 6556 breast cancer tissues. Clin Breast Cancer 5(1):63–69

Paik S, Shak S, Tang G et al (2004) A multigene assay to predict recurrence of tamoxifen-treated, node-negative breast cancer. N Engl J Med 351(27):2817–2826

Perez EA, Thompson EA, Ballman KV et al (2015) Genomic analysis reveals that immune function genes are strongly linked to clinical outcome in the north central cancer treatment group n9831 adjuvant trastuzumab trial. J Clin Oncol 33(7):701–708

Piccart-Gebhart MJ, Procter M, Leyland-Jones B et al (2005) Trastuzumab after adjuvant chemotherapy in HER2-positive breast cancer. N Engl J Med 353 (16):1659–1672

Poole AJ, Li Y, Kim Y, Lin SC, Lee WH, Lee EY (2006) Prevention of BRCA1-mediated mammary tumorigenesis in mice by a progesterone antagonist. Science 314(5804):1467–1470

Prat A, Perou CM (2011) Deconstructing the molecular portraits of breast cancer. Mol Oncol 5(1):5–23

Proverbs-Singh T, Feldman JL, Morris MJ, Autio KA, Traina TA (2015) Targeting the androgen receptor in prostate and breast cancer: several new agents in development. Endocr Relat Cancer 22(3):R87–R106

Puglisi F, Piccart M (2005) Trastuzumab and breast cancer. Are we just beyond the prologue of a fascinating story? Onkologie 28(11):547–549

Rahman N, Seal S, Thompson D et al (2007) PALB2, which encodes a BRCA2-interacting protein, is a breast cancer susceptibility gene. Nat Genet 39 (2):165–167

Razis E, Bobos M, Kotoula V et al (2011) Evaluation of the association of PIK3CA mutations and PTEN loss with efficacy of trastuzumab therapy in metastatic breast cancer. Breast Cancer Res Treat 128(2):447–456

Romond EH, Perez EA, Bryant J et al (2005) Trastuzumab plus adjuvant chemotherapy for operable HER2-positive breast cancer. N Engl J Med 353 (16):1673–1684

Schouten PC, Linn SC (2015) Challenges in the use of DNA repair deficiency as a biomarker in breast cancer. J Clin Oncol 33(17):1867–1869

Sergina NV, Rausch M, Wang D et al (2007) Escape from HER-family tyrosine kinase inhibitor therapy by the kinase-inactive HER3. Nature 445(7126):437–441

Serra V, Markman B, Scaltriti M et al (2008) NVP-BEZ235, a dual PI3K/mTOR inhibitor, prevents PI3K signaling and inhibits the growth of cancer cells with activating PI3K mutations. Cancer Res 68 (19):8022–8030

Simes RJ, Coates AS (2001) Patient preferences for adjuvant chemotherapy of early breast cancer: how much benefit is needed? J Natl Cancer Inst Monogr 30:146–152

Slamon DJ, Clark GM, Wong SG, Levin WJ, Ullrich A, McGuire WL (1987) Human breast cancer: correlation of relapse and survival with amplification of the HER-2/neu oncogene. Science 235(4785):177–182

Smerage JB, Barlow WE, Hortobagyi GN et al (2014) Circulating tumor cells and response to chemotherapy in metastatic breast cancer: SWOG S0500. J Clin Oncol 32(31):3483–3489

Smith ML, White CB, Railey E, Sledge GW Jr (2014) Examining and predicting drug preferences of patients with metastatic breast cancer: using conjoint analysis to examine attributes of paclitaxel and capecitabine. Breast Cancer Res Treat 145(1):83–89

Sorlie T, Perou CM, Tibshirani R et al (2001) Gene expression patterns of breast carcinomas distinguish tumor subclasses with clinical implications. Proc Natl Acad Sci U S A 98(19):10869–10874

Sorlie T, Tibshirani R, Parker J et al (2003) Repeated observation of breast tumor subtypes in independent gene expression data sets. Proc Natl Acad Sci U S A 100(14):8418–8423

Span PN, Tjan-Heijnen VC, Manders P, Beex LV, Sweep CG (2003) Cyclin-E is a strong predictor of endocrine therapy failure in human breast cancer. Oncogene 22(31):4898–4904

Sparano JA, Gray RJ, Makower DF et al (2015) Prospective Validation of a 21-Gene Expression Assay in Breast Cancer. N Engl J Med 21:2005–2014

Stephens PJ, Tarpey PS, Davies H et al (2012) The landscape of cancer genes and mutational processes in breast cancer. Nature 486(7403):400–404

Stuart-Harris R, Caldas C, Pinder SE, Pharoah P (2008) Proliferation markers and survival in early breast cancer: a systematic review and meta-analysis of 85 studies in 32,825 patients. Breast 17(4):323–334

Swain SM, Baselga J, Kim SB et al (2015) Pertuzumab, trastuzumab, and docetaxel in HER2-positive metastatic breast cancer. N Engl J Med 372(8):724–734

Telli ML, Jensen KC, Vinayak S et al (2015) Phase II study of gemcitabine, carboplatin, and iniparib as neoadjuvant therapy for triple-negative and BRCA1/2 mutation-associated breast cancer with assessment of a tumor-based measure of genomic instability: PrECOG 0105. J Clin Oncol 33(17):1895–1901

Tutt A (2014) TNT: a randomized phase III trial of carboplatin compared with docetaxel for patients with metastatic or recurrent locally advanced triple negative breast cancer or BRCA1/2 breast cancer (Abstr S3-01). In: 37th annual San Antonio breast cancer symposium, 9–13 Dec, San Antonio, TX

Tutt A, Robson M, Garber JE et al (2010) Oral poly (ADP-ribose) polymerase inhibitor olaparib in patients with BRCA1 or BRCA2 mutations and advanced breast cancer: a proof-of-concept trial. Lancet 376 (9737):235–244

van de Vijver MJ, He YD, van't Veer LJ et al (2002) A gene-expression signature as a predictor of survival in breast cancer. N Engl J Med 347(25):1999–2009

van't Veer LJ, Dai H, van de Vijver MJ et al (2002) Gene expression profiling predicts clinical outcome of breast cancer. Nature 415(6871):530–536

Verma S, Miles D, Gianni L et al (2012) Trastuzumab emtansine for HER2-positive advanced breast cancer. N Engl J Med 367(19):1783–1791

Yaziji H, Goldstein LC, Barry TS et al (2004) HER-2 testing in breast cancer using parallel tissue-based methods. JAMA 291(16):1972–1977

Index

S. Badve and Y. Gökmen-Polar (eds.), *Molecular Pathology of Breast Cancer*, DOI 10.1007/978-3-319-41761-5

MIX
Papier aus verantwortungsvollen Quellen
Paper from responsible sources
FSC® C105338

If you have any concerns about our products,
you can contact us on
ProductSafety@springernature.com

In case Publisher is established outside the EU,
the EU authorized representative is:
Springer Nature Customer Service Center GmbH
Europaplatz 3, 69115 Heidelberg, Germany

Printed by Libri Plureos GmbH
in Hamburg, Germany